Multimodality Breast Imaging
A Correlative Atlas

Second Edition

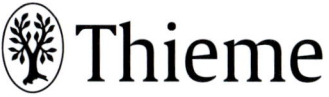

Multimodality Breast Imaging
A Correlative Atlas

Second Edition

Beverly E. Hashimoto, MD, FACR
Section Head, Ultrasound
Virginia Mason Medical Center
Seattle, Washington

Thieme
New York • Stuttgart

Thieme Medical Publishers, Inc.
333 Seventh Ave.
New York, NY 10001

Editorial Director: Michael Wachinger
Executive Editor: Timothy Y. Hiscock
Editorial Assistant: Jacquelyn DeSanti
International Production Director: Andreas Schabert
Production Editor: Kenneth L. Chumbley, Publication Services
Vice President, International Marketing and Sales: Cornelia Schulze
Chief Financial Officer: James W. Mitos
President: Brian D. Scanlan
Compositor: MPS Content Services
Printer: Everbest Printing Company, Ltd.

Library of Congress Cataloging-in-Publication Data

Hashimoto, Beverly.
  Multimodality breast imaging : a correlative atlas / Beverly Hashimoto. -- 2nd ed.
      p. ; cm.
  Rev. ed. of: Breast imaging / Beverly E. Hashimoto, Donald Bauermeister. c2003.
  Includes bibliographical references and index.
  ISBN 978-1-60406-171-0 (alk. paper)
  1. Breast—Imaging—Atlases. I. Hashimoto, Beverly. Breast imaging. II. Title.
  [DNLM: 1. Mammography—Atlases. 2. Mammography--Case Reports. 3. Breast Diseases—diagnosis—Atlases. 4. Breast Diseases—diagnosis—Case Reports. 5. Ultrasonography, Mammary—Atlases. 6. Ultrasonography, Mammary—Case Reports. WP 17 H3475m 2009]
  RG493.5.D52H37 2009
  618.1'90754—dc22
                      2009035372

Copyright © 2010 by Thieme Medical Publishers, Inc. This book, including all parts thereof, is legally protected by copyright. Any use, exploitation, or commercialization outside the narrow limits set by copyright legislation without the publisher's consent is illegal and liable to prosecution. This applies in particular to photostat reproduction, copying, mimeographing or duplication of any kind, translating, preparation of microfilms, and electronic data processing and storage.

Important note: Medical knowledge is ever-changing. As new research and clinical experience broaden our knowledge, changes in treatment and drug therapy may be required. The authors and editors of the material herein have consulted sources believed to be reliable in their efforts to provide information that is complete and in accord with the standards accepted at the time of publication. However, in view of the possibility of human error by the authors, editors, or publisher of the work herein or changes in medical knowledge, neither the authors, editors, nor publisher, nor any other party who has been involved in the preparation of this work, warrants that the information contained herein is in every respect accurate or complete, and they are not responsible for any errors or omissions or for the results obtained from use of such information. Readers are encouraged to confirm the information contained herein with other sources. For example, readers are advised to check the product information sheet included in the package of each drug they plan to administer to be certain that the information contained in this publication is accurate and that changes have not been made in the recommended dose or in the contraindications for administration. This recommendation is of particular importance in connection with new or infrequently used drugs.

Some of the product names, patents, and registered designs referred to in this book are in fact registered trademarks or proprietary names even though specific reference to this fact is not always made in the text. Therefore, the appearance of a name without designation as proprietary is not to be construed as a representation by the publisher that it is in the public domain.

Printed in China

5 4 3 2 1

ISBN 978-1-60406-171-0

To Doris and Claire Hashimoto for your positive spirit
and courage in facing breast cancer.

Contents

Pattern Approach to Breast Sonography Contents ix
Pattern Approach to MRI Contents xvii
Foreword xix
Preface xxi
Acknowledgments xxii
Contributors xxiii

1. Approach to Mammographic Analysis 1
2. Sonographic Technique and Cross-Correlation with Mammography 15
3. Approach to Magnetic Resonance Imaging 28
4. PET-CT in Breast Cancer Diagnosis 34

Circumscribed Masses

5. Circumscribed Masses: Fat-Containing Masses 42
6. Circumscribed Masses: Medium- or High-Density Masses 55

Irregular Masses

7. Irregular Masses: Benign Masses 132
8. Irregular Masses: Malignant Masses 155

Calcifications

9. Calcifications: Large Linear 190
10. Calcifications: Milk of Calcium 197
11. Calcifications: Large Round 201
12. Calcifications: Round Lucent Center 203
13. Calcifications: Eggshell/Rim 207
14. Calcifications: Coarse/Popcorn–Fibroadenoma 211
15. Calcifications: Dystrophic 216
16. Calcifications: Small Round/Punctate 224
17. Calcifications: Amorphous/Indistinct Microcalcifications 244

18. Calcifications: Heterogeneous/Pleomorphic Microcalcifications ... 260

19. Calcifications: Fine Linear/Branching Microcalcifications ... 290

Asymmetry

20. Global Asymmetry ... 306

21. Focal Asymmetry ... 324

Architectural Distortion

22. Peripheral Architectural Distortion ... 334

23. Central Architectural Distortion ... 348

Male Breast

24. Benign Male Breast ... 370

25. Malignant Male Breast ... 392

Postsurgical Findings

26. Augmentation Mammoplasty ... 402

27. Reduction Mammoplasty ... 450

28. After Diagnostic or Therapeutic Procedures for Neoplasm ... 458

Masses Poorly Identified Mammographically

29. Patient Unable to Tolerate Mammogram ... 494

30. Palpable Masses ... 496

31. Mammogram Underestimates Tumor Size ... 519

32. Mass in Unusual Locations ... 527

33. Ductal Abnormalities ... 531

34. Mammographically Occult MRI Lesions ... 541

Applications of PET-CT

35. Staging ... 570

36. Assessing Response to Therapy ... 592

37. Identifications of Recurrent Disease ... 602

38. Additional Malignancies ... 607

39. Unknown Primary ... 610

40. Pitfalls of PET ... 615

Index ... 629

Pattern Approach to Breast Sonography Contents

I. Fluid Collections

Simple Cysts
- Case 6.2 57
- Case 6.3 59

Complex Fluid Collection versus Solid Mass

Benign

Abscess
- Case 29.1... 494

Complex Cyst
- Case 6.4 61

Hematoma
- Case 6.9 72
- Case 7.6 143

Oil Cyst
- Case 5.6 51
- Case 5.7 53

Papilloma
- Case 6.13 81

Pseudoaneurysm
- Case 28.8... 473

Sebaceous Cyst
- Case 6.14 84

Malignant

Mucinous Carcinoma
- Case 6.31... 123

Papillary Carcinoma
- Case 6.25... 110

Ductal Carcinoma In Situ
- Case 39.1... 610

Dilated Duct

Ductal Carcinoma In Situ
- Case 19.2... 293
- Case 33.3... 535

Papilloma
    Case 33.1 531

II. Solid Masses

Ellipsoid/Round

Hyperechoic or Heterogeneous
Adenosis
    Case 7.1 132
Angiolipoma
    Case 6.1 55
Fibroadenoma
    Case 21.1 324
Fibrosis
    Case 6.8 70
Hamartoma
    Case 5.2 44
    Case 5.3 46
    Case 32.1 527
Lactating Adenoma
    Case 30.1 496
Lymph Node
    Case 6.11 76
Phyllodes Tumor
    Case 6.32 126

Isoechoic
Lypoma
    Case 5.4 48

Hypoechoic: Benign
Fibroadenoma
    Case 6.6 66
    Case 14.2 213
Hemangioma
    Case 6.18 92
Juvenile Fibroadenoma
    Case 30.2 498
Pseudoangiomatous Stroma
    Case 6.19 94

Hypoechoic: Malignant or Recurrent
Infiltrating Ductal Carcinoma
    Case 23.6 358
    Case 40.3 621
Lobular Carcinoma
    Case 6.26 112

Miscellaneous
Angiosarcoma
    Case 6.21 98

Granular Cell Tumor
　Case 6.33 129
Metaplastic Carcinoma
　Case 6.29 119

Lobulated

　Benign
　　Fibrocystic Change
　　　Case 6.7 68
　　Leiomyoma
　　　Case 6.10 74

　Malignant
　　Adenoid Cystic Carcinoma
　　　Case 6.20 96
　　Infiltrating Ductal Carcinoma
　　　Case 18.9 277
　　　Case 30.11 516
　　　Case 35.2 574
　　Metastases
　　　Case 6.30 121

Irregular

　Hyperechoic
　　Fat Necrosis
　　　Case 30.10 514
　　Fibroadenoma
　　　Case 7.4 138

　Hypoechoic/Heterogeneous: Benign
　　Adenosis
　　　Case 23.1 348
　　Diabetic Mastopathy
　　　Case 6.5 63
　　Fat Necrosis
　　　Case 7.2 134
　　　Case 20.5 316
　　Fibroadenoma
　　　Case 7.5 140
　　Myofibroadenoma
　　　Case 7.10 153
　　Radial Scar
　　　Case 23.2 351
　　Scar
　　　Case 15.3 220
　　　Case 18.5 268
　　　Case 27.3 453

　Hypoechoic/Heterogeneous: Malignant
　　Apocrine Carcinoma
　　　Case 18.11 284

After Augmentation Mammoplasty (Implants)
   Fat Necrosis
      Case 5.7 53
   Fluid
      Case 26.1 402
      Case 26.6 412
   Malignancy
      Case 26.19 442
      Case 26.20 445

VI. Implant Rupture
   Saline Implants
      Case 26.11 422
      Case 26.12 424
      Case 26.13 427
   Silicone Implants
      Case 26.17 436
      Case 26.18 439
   Scar
      Case 27.3 453

VII. Male Breast
   Abscess
      Case 24.1 370
   Fat Necrosis
      Case 24.3 373
   Gynecomastia
      Case 24.4 375
      Case 24.5 377
   Lipoma
      Case 24.8 384
   Metastases
      Case 25.3 396
   Myofibroblastoma
      Case 24.10 388
   Papillary Carcinoma
      Case 25.4 399
   Sabaceous Cyst
      Case 24.11 390

VIII. Masses Poorly Identified Sonographically
High Frequency Sonography Improves Image
   Infiltrating Ductal Carcinoma
      Case 6.24 107
      Case 16.7 237
   Infiltrating Ductal and Lobular Carcinoma
      Case 22.4 340
   Lobular Carcinoma
      Case 8.8 175

Lymph Node
    Case 6.11 76

Shadowing Interferes with Image
    Infiltrating Ductal
        Case 6.23 102
    Papilloma
        Case 7.7 145
    Scar
        Case 28.3 461
    Sclerosint Adenosis
        Case 23.1 348

IX. Masses Poorly Imaged Sonographically
    Ductal Carcinoma In Situ
        Case 30.6 506
    Fibroadenomatoid Hyperplasia
        Case 22.1 334
    Infiltrating Ductal Carcinoma
        Case 6.27 114
        Case 8.5 165
    Infiltrating Lobular Carcinoma
        Case 40.1 615

X. Second Look Sonographic Exam After MRI
Oval Mass
    Benign
        Case 18.10 280
    Malignant
        Case 22.5 343
        Case 34.2 543
        Case 34.3 546
        Case 34.4 550
        Case 34.7 561

Irregular Mass
    Case 6.23 102
    Case 36.2 596

Malignant Non-focal Sonographic Findings
    Ducts
        Case 34.6 556
        Case 39.1 610
    Increase Color Doppler
        Case 28.14 488
        Case 31.3 524

Pattern Approach to MRI Contents

I. Foci
    Case 6.23 102
    Case 22.5 343
    Case 34.5 553

II. Mass
  A. Oval
    1. Benign
      Case 18.10 280
    2. Malignant
      Case 6.23 102
      Case 34.4 550
      Case 34.2 543
      Case 34.3 546
  B. Irregular
    1. Benign
      Case 34.1 541
    2. Malignant
      Case 6.23 102
      Case 18.8 275
      Case 22.5 343
      Case 34.5 553
      Case 35.5 586
      Case 36.2 596

III. Non-Mass Enhancement
  A. Ductal
    Case 39.1 610
  B. Segmental
    1. Clumped
      Case 18.8 275
      Case 19.2 293
    2. Heterogeneous
      Case 31.3 524

C. Regional/Diffuse
1. Post Surgical
Case 28.14 488
2. Clumped
Case 18.7 273
3. Multiregional
Case 35.4 580

IV. Associated Findings
A. Nipple
Case 34.7 561

V. Technical Problems
A. Lack of Bolus
Case 8.6 168

Foreword

In the modern world of medical pedagogy, the practitioner must become a perpetual student. Through seminars, journals, meetings, day-to-day conversations with colleagues, and the wonderful new world of the Internet, today's radiologist is constantly challenged by an ever-expanding world of knowledge. The immense volume of complex information does not alter the need to quickly apply this information in daily casework. The textbook remains an integral part of this knowledge base. However, modern textbooks no longer can be simple repositories of information. Such texts are impractical considering the pace of modern medicine and the seemingly ever-increasing caseload. Current reality mandates that textbooks serve as a practical "desk reference," a tool that helps to rapidly answer questions as they arise in one's daily casework. This textbook, *Multimodality Breast Imaging, A Correlative Atlas,* in its second edition, meets this need brilliantly. It is timely, clearly written, excellently illustrated, and has the simplicity and brevity necessary to serve as a useful desk reference.

This textbook is well organized for the practicing radiologist who usually employs mammography primarily, and then uses sonography or other modalities to answer questions either raised or not addressed by the mammogram. Dr. Hashimoto organizes her textbook by mammographic findings and then effectively illustrates the pathologic entity. Each chapter carries the clinician radiologist through an analysis according to the specific mammographic abnormality.

This text documents the integral importance of sonography in breast imaging. Breast imaging now requires a multidisciplinary approach. The use of all modalities, as discussed in the text, must be brought to bear on the clinical problems encountered in the individual case. Increasing importance is being placed on the proposition that breast imagers not only attempt to find as many breast cancers as technically possible, but to find them without subjecting ten women to needless breast biopsies for every cancer detected. The surest means to this end is the appropriate application of alternative technologies to film mammography.

I first met Dr. Beverly Hashimoto as a resident in radiology at the University of California–San Francisco. I was very pleased when she accepted a fellowship in diagnostic sonography under my direction. She showed herself to be a student of extraordinary talent and to have an admirable dedication of purpose. I believed she was well suited to a typical academic post at a university. Instead, she opted to join the prestigious Virginia Mason Clinic. Beverly helped to teach me that an inquisitive mind could flourish anywhere. Many university academicians would envy her academic pursuits, publications, and national prominence. The responsibility to advance radiological imaging lies not only in academia but in private practices as well. I am most proud of my students who have achieved significant academic success in a non-university setting.

Although magnetic resonance imaging is likely to have an increasing impact on solving breast imaging problems as time goes on, currently sonography has the greatest ancillary benefit to film mammography. Breast sonography has a somewhat checkered past. In the early to mid-1980s, there was a strong push by several equipment developers to produce an automated, whole-breast, sonographic imaging device. Shortly after achieving success, claims of great ability in the detection of breast cancer began to appear. However, the data ultimately indicated the automated, whole-breast, sonographic imaging was not on a par with radiographic mammography. The experience left a bad taste in the mouths of many sonologists and mammographers. This episode undoubtedly retarded the growth and acceptance of sonographic breast imaging. However, to their credit, a small cadre of dedicated researchers took up the task of developing sonography in breast imaging for more than deciding whether a mass was cystic or not. Dr. Hashimoto figures prominently in this group of dedicated researchers. This book is the culmination of her years of excellent work in this medical arena.

Roy A. Filly, MD
Professor of Radiology, of Surgery, and of Obstetrics
Gynecology and Reproductive Sciences
Chief, Section of Diagnostic Sonography
University of California–San Francisco

Preface

One of the most important trends in breast imaging has been the expanding number of imaging technologies directed toward diagnosing breast cancer. This book is targeted for breast imagers who are interested in integrating these imaging techniques in breast cancer diagnosis. The initial didactic chapters are focused on teaching practical methods to analyze and integrate mammographic, sonographic, and magnetic resonance findings. These methods are based on developing familiarity with specific mammographic, sonographic, and magnetic resonance image patterns. After a radiologist is familiar with these patterns, the imager can approach mammographic, sonographic, and magnetic resonance lesions in a systematic manner and reach a logical assessment. To facilitate this process, imaging chapters 5–34 of this book are devoted to providing visual examples of these mammographic, sonographic, and magnetic resonance patterns.

Unlike mammography, sonography, and magnetic resonance imaging, positron emission tomography (PET) is currently utilized for patients with extensive disease, so this technique is treated independently. This book addresses the most common applications of PET in breast cancer (chapter 4) and illustrates these applications with clinical cases, which commonly also involve other modalities (chapters 35–40).

Because most breast problems initially present with a mammographic examination, the imaging chapters 5–34 are organized by specific mammographic findings according to the table of contents. Each mammographic pattern is illustrated by a variety of benign and malignant entities. Furthermore, the introduction of each chapter schematically illustrates the clinical approach to analyzing the mammographic abnormality. Since the clinical scenarios for PET are commonly different from those of mammography, imaging chapters 35–40 are devoted to illustrating applications of PET.

This book further promotes the goal of emphasizing the multidisciplinary nature of breast imaging by providing a framework of clinical indications for the modalities as illustrated by clinical cases. This multidisciplinary approach is emphasized by the Pattern Approach to Breast Sonography Contents and the Pattern Approach to MRI Contents that organize the individual cases into sonographic and MRI patterns. Furthermore, the cases in this book include multiple imaging modalities such as magnetic resonance and various nuclear medicine techniques. The utility of these modalities is discussed in the context of common clinical problems that are illustrated in the individual imaging cases.

The second purpose of this book is to demonstrate the importance of high-resolution sonography in breast imaging. Sonographic examination of the breast has become more important in breast imaging. As equipment improves, imagers are able to see lesions that previously were not visible sonographically. This improved detection not only enhances one's confidence in finding malignancies earlier, but also in identifying benign lesions. However, the potentially important contribution of sonography is greatly hindered by inadequate equipment, suboptimal imaging technique, and inconsistent operator training. Several cases show images of the same lesion with both high- and low-resolution equipment. These cases also demonstrate the importance of utilizing high-contrast, post-processing techniques in the detection of benign and malignant entities. Hopefully, this book will enhance the sonographic skills of breast imagers by encouraging the use of high-quality, high-resolution equipment and optimal technique. Furthermore, by reviewing the sonographic appearance of the numerous breast abnormalities presented in this book, one can broaden one's visual sonographic experience.

The final objective of this book is to provide an atlas of a wide variety of pathologic entities within the breast. This book includes both unusual mammographic and sonographic appearances of common pathologies, as well as examples of rare breast abnormalities. By grouping the pathologies within mammographic imaging patterns, one can use this book as a base for developing differential diagnoses.

In summary, I hope this book is used both as a quick reference guide to review the schematic work-up of a particular mammographic finding, as well as a more detailed reference to study methods to optimize sonographic technique and integrate alternative imaging modalities.

Acknowledgments

I could not have completed this book without the academic and emotional support of Shannon Boswell, ultrasound manager, Dr. Dawna Kramer, section head of breast imaging, and Dr. Marie Lee, section head of nuclear medicine. Motivated to improve patient care, they unselfishly give their time and energy to pursue new breast-imaging methods. I hope this book reflects their strong interest in integrating imaging technologies for breast diagnosis. I also have been dependent upon the help of my current research coordinator Erin Turpin, as well as my past coordinators Jennifer Sonntag and Lynn Wiitala and my research manager Anhaita Jamula. Their enthusiastic efforts allowed me to stay on schedule and their creative ideas solved many unanticipated logistical problems. Since I did much of my work from home, I am particularly indebted to Sharon Hemphill, manager of general imaging and office neighbor, who helped me maintain computer connections to the office. Dr. Donald Bauermeister contributed pathology expertise for this project. Our conversations cross-correlating specific cases have greatly improved my ability to understand the imaging appearance of benign and malignant lesions. The contributors, Drs. Kramer, Lee, Morgan, and Phinney, have not only written part of the material in this book, but also have helped choose images and edit text. I am also grateful for the radiologists at Virginia Mason Medical Center. They have unselfishly shared their clinical and technical expertise. I especially appreciate the administrative support from my department chiefs during this project: Drs. Michael Morishima and Lucy Glenn.

My sanity was saved by Morris Ferensen from Virginia Mason Medical Photography, who answered all my imaging questions and processed the sonographic images. Nancy Honssinger created all the schematic diagrams.

A special acknowledgment goes to the technical and support personnel of the John H. Walker Center for Diagnostic Imaging at Virginia Mason Medical Center. Although I am indebted to everyone in the section of imaging management, I want to express individual thanks to Alice Wirth, Jon Komatsu, Mary Ann Fernandez, Linda O'Connell, Rosalinda Argonza, Tino Ativalu, Agnes Celmar, Lucy Ferrer, Tracy Guster, Henock Kidane, Martin Medina, John Paul Morales, James Reyes, Valene Sanchez, and manager Najmah Messiah. Since digital imaging is so dependent upon computer systems, I highly appreciate the efforts of my information systems team: Michelle Ranous, Mitchell Murdock, Courtney Allen, Scott Hamilton, Peter Naglee, and manager Linda Seeley. I am also fortunate to be associated with wonderful imaging technologists including sonographers Irina Askerova, Stacy Buck, Chris Chapman, Tom Fasnacht, Lindsey Oram, Mary Gutkecht, Valerie Holland, Nancy Honssinger, Suzy Murray Dirks, Lynette Passey, Gisele Sodell, Ashley Little, Liesl Matthies, Debbie Noyes, Ann Polin, Emily Whiting, Elizabeth Ayers, Mary Frost, Jane Nova, Elizabeth Keating, Laurie McBryde, Cleo Llamas, and Ashleigh Joyce; mammography technologists, and Mary Anne Madsen, Diana Pearsall, Diane Sarver, Mary Ellen Bishop, Amy Chu, Patricia Dennis, Elena Ermolenko, Debra Krenzler, Kim Peery, Krystyna Wojtulewicz, and supervisor Dyan Blaiz; medical assistant Cheryl Childs; patient specialist Marsha Robb; radiology department administrative assistant Jean Nelson, radiology department adminstrative director Richard Lee.

At Thieme Publishers, I have been lucky to work with my editor Timothy Hiscock. He has been a great friend and colleague, providing guidance in developing and finalizing the project.

I also want to thank Drs. Roy Filly and Peter Callen. You have taught me the importance of approaching clinical questions in a creative yet systematic manner.

Finally, I am particularly grateful for the constant emotional support from my family: parents Doris and Ben, sister Claire, brothers Gary and Dean, husband Vincent, and children Ben, Dean, and Elissa. Without your cheerleading, I could never have attempted this project.

Contributors

Beverly E. Hashimoto, MD, FACR
Section Head, Ultrasound
Virginia Mason Medical Center
Seattle, Washington

Dawna J. Kramer, MD
Deputy Chief, Radiology
Virginia Mason Medical Center
Seattle, Washington

Marie E. Lee, MD, FACR
Section Head, Nuclear Medicine
Virginia Mason Medical Center
Seattle, Washington

Gail N. Morgan, MD
Section Head, Eastside Satellite Radiology Clinics
Virginia Mason Medical Center
Seattle, Washington

Alexi J. Phinney, MD
Radiologist
Virginia Mason Medical Center
Seattle, Washington

1 Approach to Mammographic Analysis

■ General Overview

There are three factors that lead to identifying mammographic abnormalities: production of high-quality images, perception of a lesion, and characterization of the finding. A team of professionals is needed to produce high-quality mammograms. The radiologist and the technologist should constantly be evaluating images for film contrast, exposure parameters, patient position, and image processing. Furthermore, a radiation physicist should work with the technologist to monitor equipment performance.

Perception of mammographic abnormality is the first step in identifying a breast malignancy. Perception is aided by a systematic review of the mammographic examination. Consistent systematic review of the mammogram is critical in avoiding perceptual errors. Tabar and Dean's *Teaching Atlas of Mammography*[1] has an excellent explanation of a horizontal and vertical masking technique that facilitates identification of abnormal mammographic asymmetries. Masking entails physically covering portions of the film so that only small corresponding regions of the two breasts are visible. In a busy practice or with digital mammography this technique is not practical, but one can develop the ability to visually mask by focusing on a small area of the breast and comparing it with the equivalent area on the contralateral side. My personal method involves this latter technique. I visually mask all breast views horizontally and then perform a second focused review of the axilla and the subareolar regions (**Fig. 1.1**).

During the review of the mammographic examination, one may identify asymmetries or calcifications. The breast imager should classify the asymmetry as a density or architectural distortion. The densities should be further analyzed and subdivided into either masses or asymmetric densities. Using the following methods, the breast imager then analyzes the lesion and assigns an assessment category according to the American College of Radiology (ACR) Breast Imaging Reporting and Data System (BI-RADS). These assessment categories are as follows:

- Category 0: Need additional imaging evaluation. This evaluation may include additional mammographic views (e.g., spot compression) or other imaging modalities (e.g., ultrasound).
- Category 1: Negative. The breasts are normal.
- Category 2: Benign finding. The mammogram is normal, but there is a finding that the interpreter wishes to describe.
- Category 3: Probably benign finding. Short-interval follow-up suggested. The finding has a high probability of being benign and is not expected to change in appearance. In this book, I generally assume that the patient will be reimaged approximately 6 months after this assessment is made.
- Category 4: Suspicious abnormality. Biopsy should be considered. The radiologist has enough concern about the lesion that biopsy is being recommended.
- Category 5: Highly suggestive of malignancy. Appropriate action should be taken.

■ Patterns of Mammographic Abnormality

After finding an asymmetry, the breast imager should classify the finding into one of four patterns: mass, focal asymmetry, calcifications, and architectural distortion.

Masses

If a density is identified, then the radiologist should first clarify if the density is a mass or a focal asymmetry. A mass is a density that has a consistent shape when imaged at different angles and with different patient positions. If the imager concludes that the lesion is a mass, then he or she should determine whether the shape of the mass is circumscribed or irregular. Circumscribed masses are round, oval, or lobulated (see Chapters 5 and 6). Circumscribed masses are commonly benign. Only 1.4% of well-defined circumscribed masses are malignant. As there are many benign lesions in this category, diagnostic evaluation should be directed toward excluding many of these benign lesions from being biopsied. The first step is to analyze the density of the mass. If the mass has a density equal to or greater than the parenchyma, then further examination is necessary. The next step is to examine the margins of the mass. If the margins are sharp or obscured by the surrounding parenchyma, then the mass should be examined sonographically. If the mass clearly has ill-defined or spiculated borders, then biopsy is indicated (category 4 or 5). This biopsy may be performed sonographically, as almost all of these lesions are sonographically visible, particularly if they are larger than 4 to 5 mm.

As noted earlier, circumscribed mammographic masses that have well-defined or obscured margins should be ex-

2 Approach to Mammographic Analysis

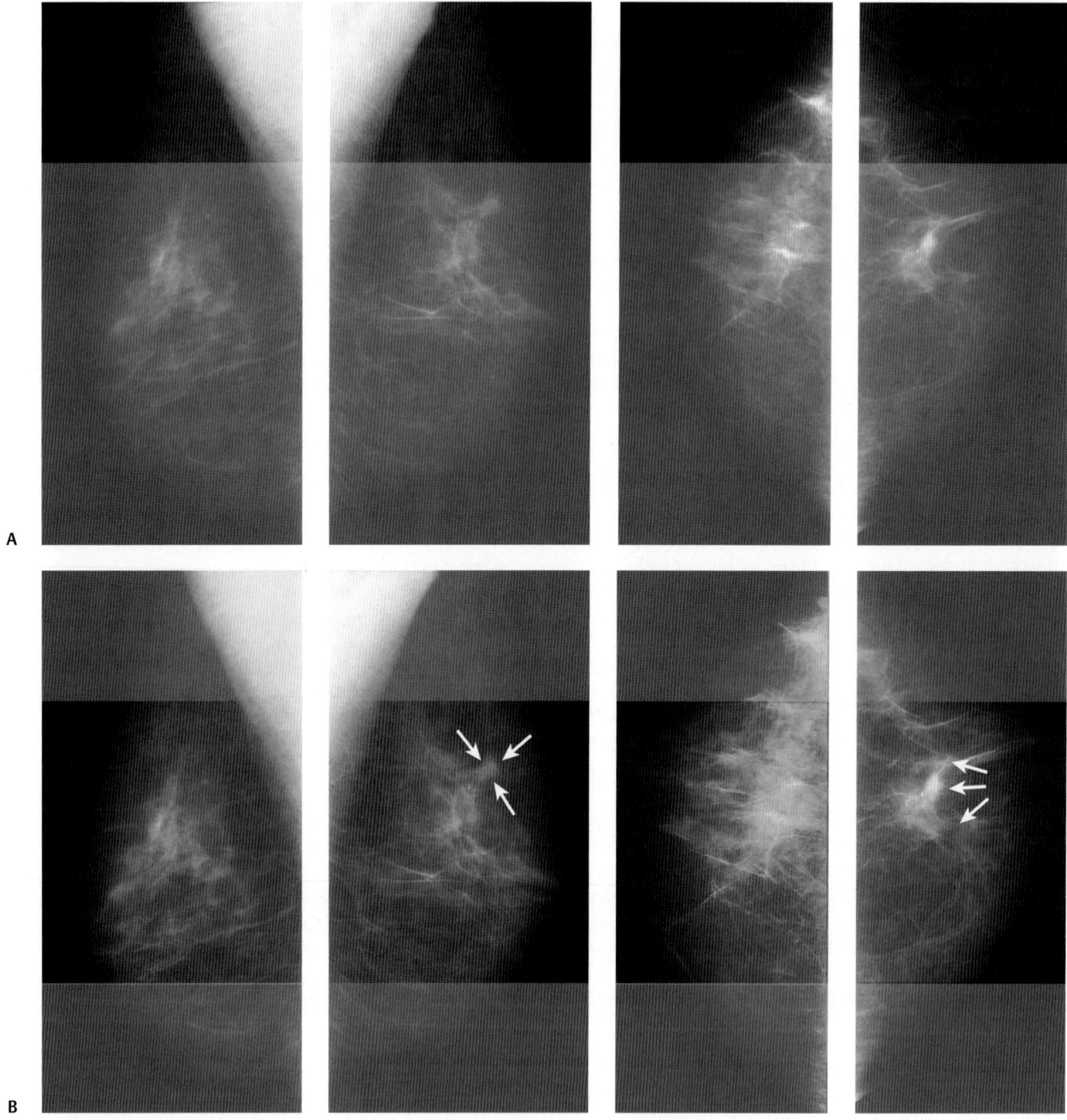

Fig. 1.1 **(A,B)** Systematic method to review mammograms. Horizontal examination: initially, you should focus on a small region in the superior section of the right film and then compare it with the comparable left side. You should then proceed inferiorly in the mammogram and continue the process. In this case, there is trabecular thickening and architectural distortion at the 12 o'clock position of the left breast (*arrows*). This lesion is an infiltrating ductal carcinoma.

amined sonographically. Of these masses, sonographically identified cysts are obviously benign (category 2). If the mass is well defined and uniformly hyperechoic to fat, it is probably benign (category 3). The mass is also probably benign (category 3) if it has all of the following characteristics: (1) shape: round, oval, or one or two lobulations; (2) margin: well defined with a hyperechoic thin capsule; (3) echogenicity: uniformly hypoechoic.

If the margin is extremely well defined but does not have a hyperechoic capsule, I also assess it as probably benign (category 3). To characterize whether a margin is well defined, you must have high-quality, high-resolution, and

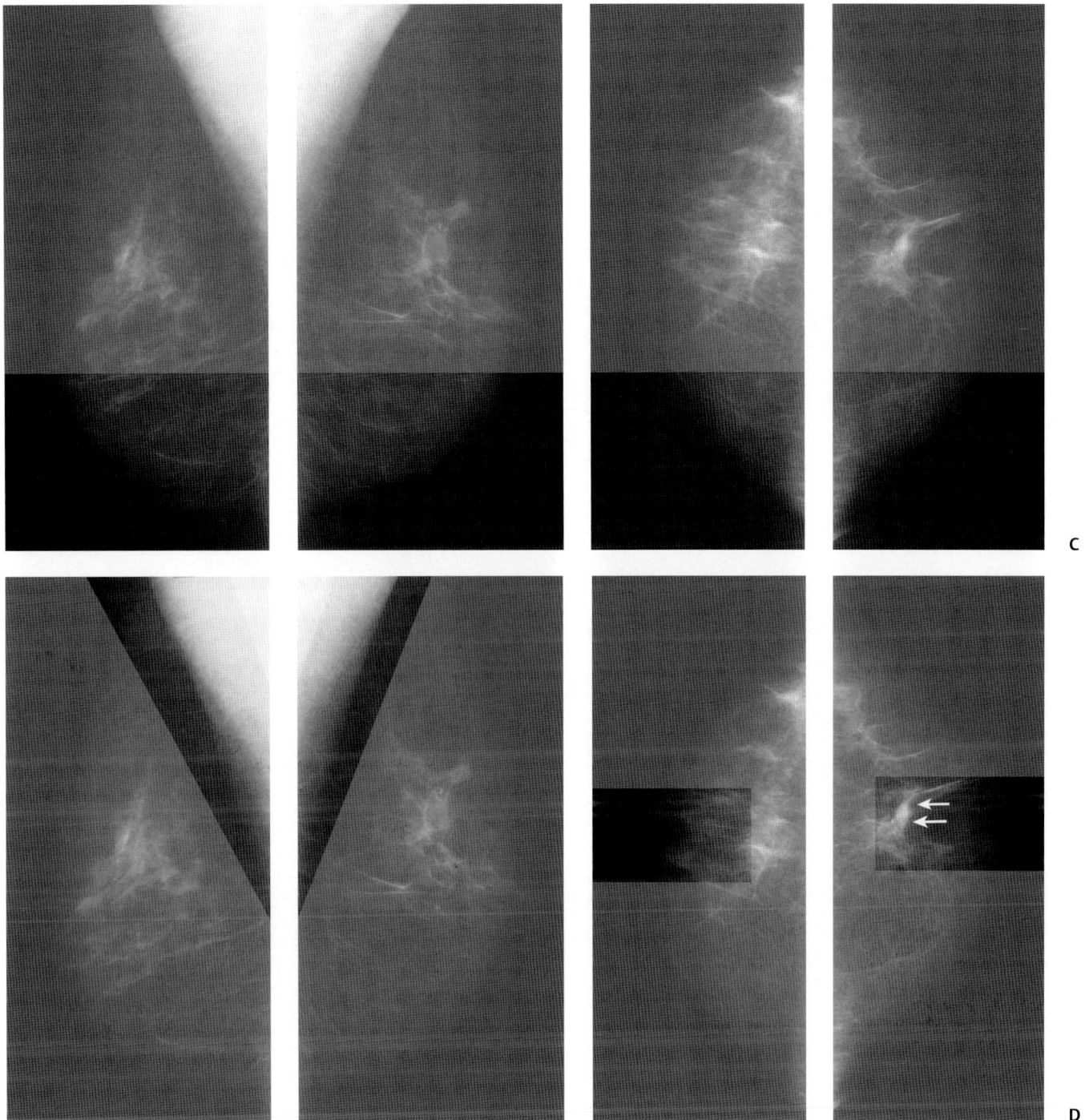

Fig. 1.1 (*Continued*) Systematic method to review mammograms. After the horizontal examination, (**C**) you should study the axillary and subareolar regions of each breast, (**D**) and compare each area with the contralateral side. The axillary region is important because the upper outer quadrant contains the highest percentage of breast cancers. Extra attention to the subareolar region is worthwhile, as this area exhibits a complex architecture consisting of numerous ductal lines. Subareolar architectural distortion is commonly difficult to identify. In this case, the malignancy produces left subareolar architectural distortion (*arrows*).

high-frequency (≥ 10 MHz) equipment. Furthermore, the entire margin must be well defined and clearly visible (**Fig. 1.2**). Finally, there should not be any other associated abnormality such as sonographic architectural distortion. In this situation, I am also assuming that I have seen the patient only once, and there is no evidence of growth. If the lesion has been identified on earlier imaging exams and has grown in size, then I will recommend biopsy (category 4).

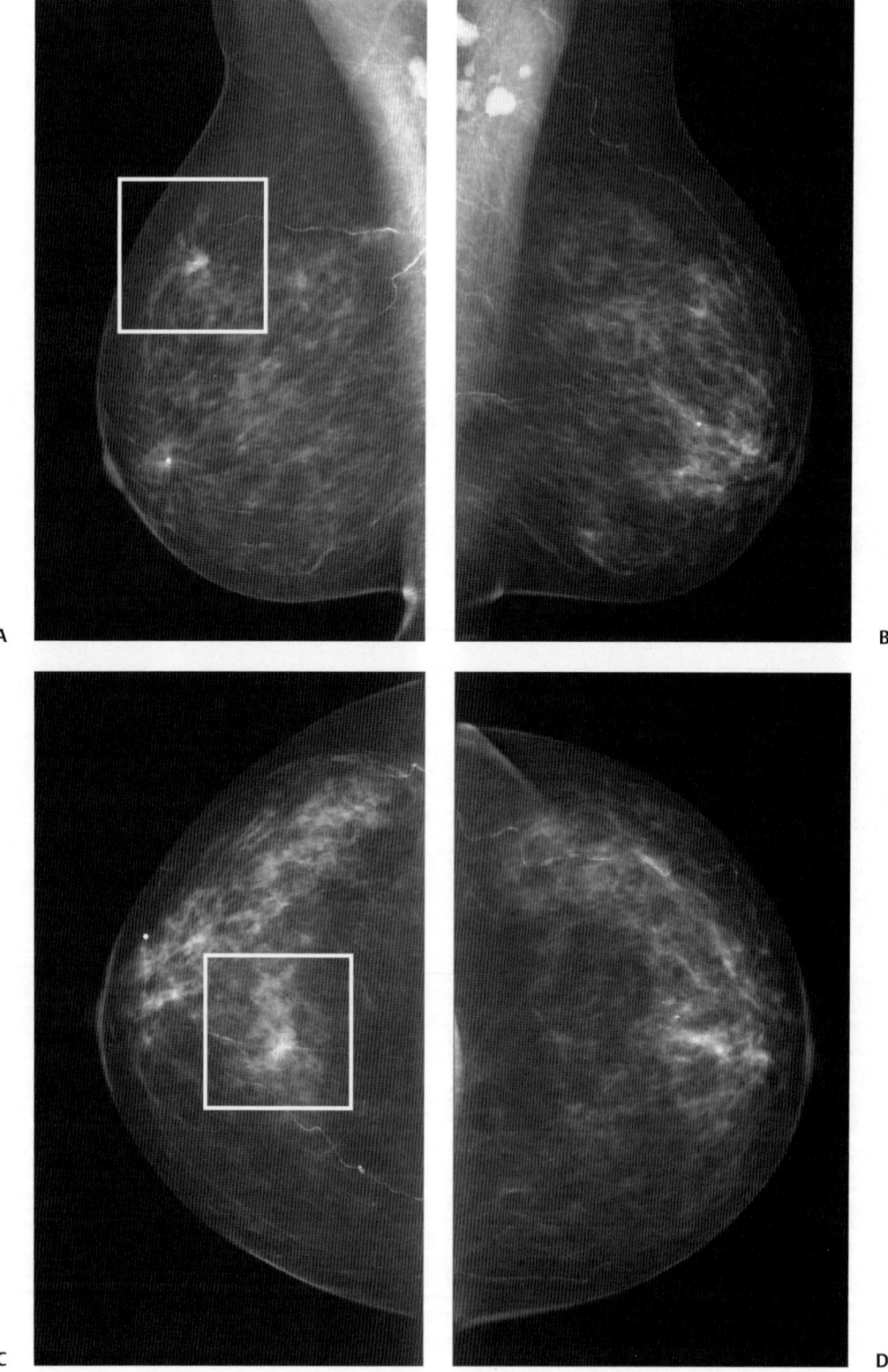

Fig. 1.2 Two breast cancers. (**A**) Right mediolateral oblique (MLO) digital mammogram. (**B**) Left MLO digital mammogram. (**C**) Right craniocaudal (CC) digital mammogram. (**D**) Left CC digital mammogram. There is a palpable right breast mass that is labeled with a radiopaque dot at the 3 o'clock position near the nipple. Independent of this palpable lump, there is an irregular mammographic mass (square).

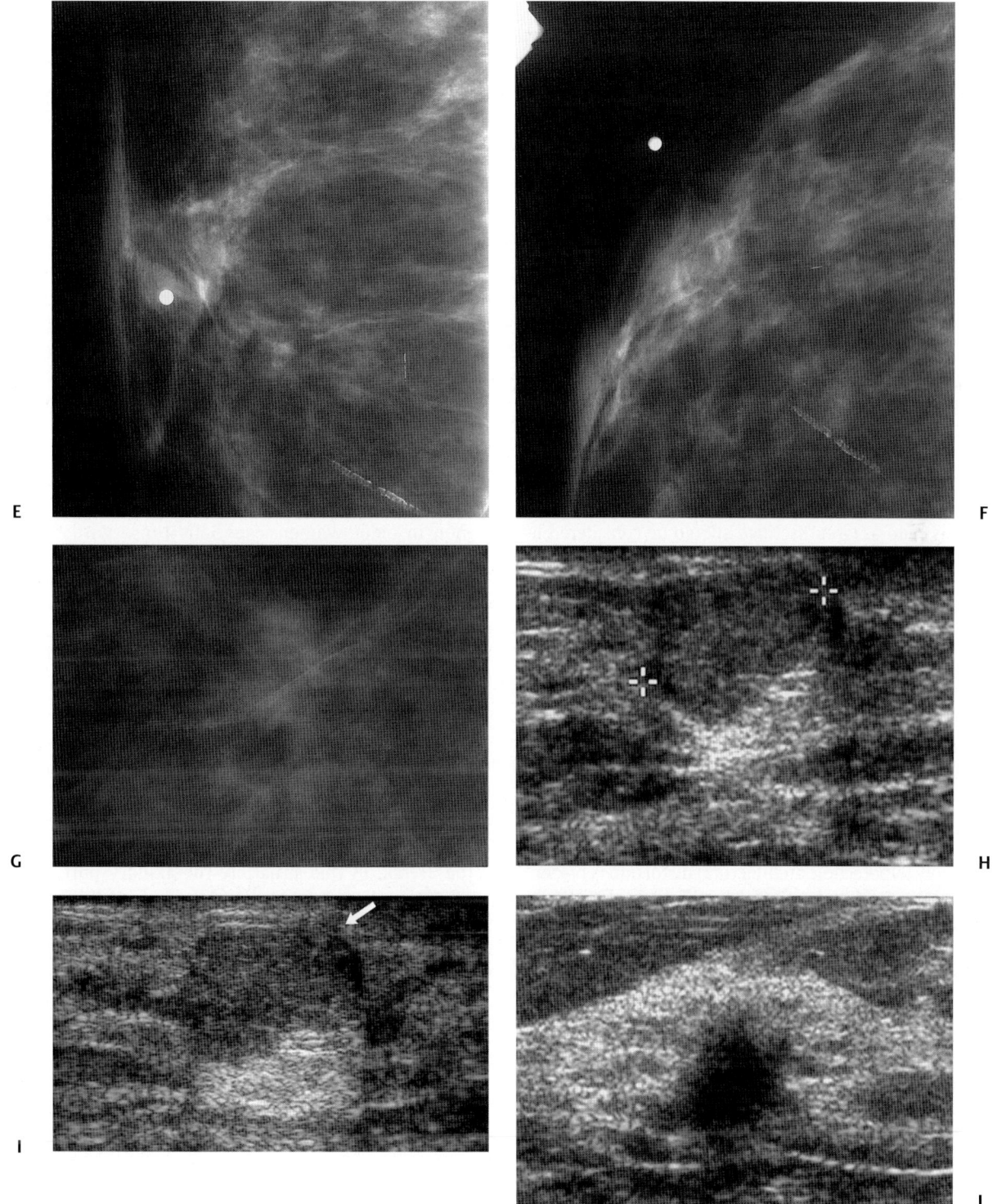

Fig. 1.2 (*Continued*) Two breast cancers. (**E**) Right MLO spot magnification mammogram of palpable lump. (**F**) Right CC spot magnification mammogram of mammographic mass. (**H**) Right antiradial breast sonogram of palpable lump. (**I**) Right antiradial breast sonogram of palpable lump. (**J**) Right antiradial breast sonogram of mammographic mass. (**E,F**) Although the palpable lump does not correspond to a mammographic mass, (**H**) sonography demonstrates that the lump is an oval mass. (**I**) Although most of the margins of the palpable sonographic mass are well defined, close inspection reveals subtle irregularity of the border (*arrow*). This palpable lump is infiltrating mucinous carcinoma. (**G**) The irregular mammographic mass corresponds to (**J**) an irregular sonographic mass that is infiltrating ductal carcinoma.

The reason for biopsying large or growing well-defined lesions is that some of the masses in this category will be malignant. As long as a malignancy is small, it has a good prognosis because the probability of metastasis is low. However, to have a good prognosis, it is best for the patient to be stage 1 (primary tumor < 2 cm) at the time of diagnosis. Short-interval follow-up of a small (< 1 cm), well-circumscribed mass that has a low probability of malignancy is a reasonable method to avoid unnecessary biopsies.

If the mass has any other sonographic characteristics, then it is category 4 or 5. Examples of these lesions include (1) solid masses within cysts, (2) masses that have any other shape or that are microlobulated, (3) lesions that exhibit heterogeneous echogenicity or that present as a focal area of intense shadowing, (4) tumors with either completely or partially ill-defined margins, and (5) masses associated with other sonographic abnormalities such as architectural distortion.

Masses with microlobulations or other shapes that cannot be classified as circumscribed should be considered irregular in shape (see Chapters 7 and 8). Although benign etiologies may produce an irregular mammographic mass, all mammographically irregular masses should be pathologically examined unless the lesion is a benign scar. Scars resulting from previous surgery may appear similar to malignancies. A careful patient history with a map of the scar is necessary to correlate the mammographic abnormality with the clinical information. If this information is sufficient, previous films commonly document either stability or reduction of the lesion density and size. Occasionally, sonography may be necessary to differentiate scar from malignancy. In these cases, sonography may confidently exclude malignancy if only hyperechoic architectural distortion is present without mass. Furthermore, sonographically, scars change in appearance with different transducer positions. Even if there is a wide area of severe shadowing in one view, the orthogonal view will demonstrate only a thin line of architectural distortion characteristic of scar. Because scar attenuates high-frequency more than low-frequency ultrasound, commonly low-frequency sonography is more effective in characterizing scar (see Case 28.4).

Besides scar, other benign entities produce irregular masses. These lesions include fat necrosis, sclerosing adenosis, focal fibrosis, hematoma, abscess, and benign neoplasms such as fibroadenomas and papillary lesions. However, unless the patient has a clinical history or symptoms suggesting recent trauma, surgery, or infection, these lesions cannot be differentiated from the malignancy and should be biopsied. When clinical information suggests that a hematoma or abscess may be responsible for the mammographic abnormality, then sonography is useful to identify these processes.

Finally, radial scars also produce irregular masses. The mammographic characteristics of radial scars include (1) change in appearance from one mammographic projection to another, (2) no dense central mass, (3) the radiating lines are long and thin, (4) the radiating structures are commonly dominated by radiolucent linear lines, (5) no skin thickening, and (6) very little palpable abnormality. Although radial scars may be differentiated from malignancy, they are commonly associated with malignant neoplasms and therefore should be excised.

Asymmetries

Analysis of an asymmetry should start with a close evaluation of the entire mammographic examination. It is important to initially define if the asymmetry diffusely involves a large area of the breast or a small area (see Chapters 20 and 21). If the asymmetry is diffuse, then the skin should be carefully examined. If the asymmetry is only due to increased fibroglandular tissue, then a physiologic or pharmacologic etiology may be responsible. Heterogeneous or extremely dense parenchymal composition is more common in younger premenopausal women but is also common in older women, especially those with fibrocystic changes. Medications such as estrogen replacement therapy sometimes increase the overall mammographic parenchymal density.

If skin thickening is present, then the etiologies include axillary lymphatic obstruction, lymphatic spread of breast cancer, inflammation, and systemic fluid overload. Axillary lymphatic drainage may be blocked by ipsilateral breast cancer metastases or hematologic malignancies (e.g., lymphomas). Lymphatic spread of breast cancer to the contralateral breast will block lymphatic channels and produce lymphedema. Inflammation and abscess will thicken the skin and produce increased density, particularly around the areola. In this situation, the axillary portion of the breast is relatively spared. Finally, any condition that produces systemic fluid overload such as heart failure will produce breast lymphedema.

If the asymmetry involves a small area, you should carefully examine the area to determine if the asymmetry represents a mass, normal asymmetric fibroglandular tissue, or overlap of normal parenchymal tissue. A focal asymmetry is an asymmetry that cannot be reliably identified on more than one view. If the asymmetry is only visible on the craniocaudal (CC) view, a 90-degree mediolateral (ML) view may demonstrate the mass better than the mediolateral oblique (MLO) view. Spot compression of an asymmetry may clarify the shape of the mass, but sometimes malignancies such as lobular carcinoma may compress and blend into the normal breast parenchymal background. For small or less dense lesions, consider using rolled or oblique views to confirm the presence of the mass (**Fig. 1.3**). Normal fibroglandular tissue will blend into the adjacent tissue with oblique views. The tissue will not exhibit any architectural distortion. If you cannot distinguish between a mass and normal fibroglandular tissue, then sonography may be useful. However, to adequately perform this

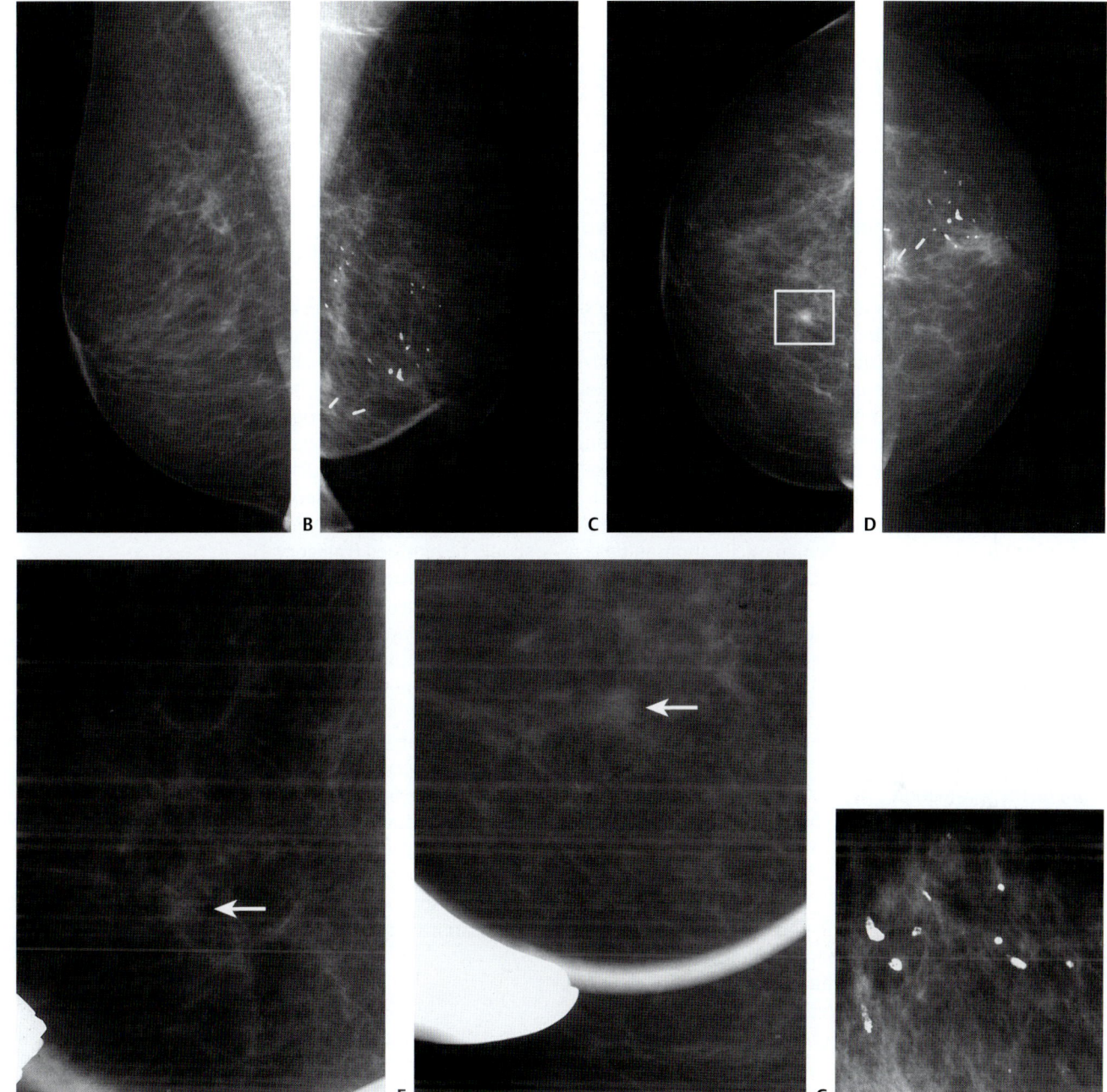

Fig. 1.3 (**A**) Right MLO digital mammogram. (**B**) Left MLO digital mammogram. (**C**) Right CC digital mammogram. (**D**) Left CC digital mammogram. (**E**) Right MLO spot compression mammogram (*arrow* points to mass). (**F**) Right CC spot compression mammogram. (**G**) Left lateromedial (LM) digital mammogram (close-up). (**A–G**) The patient had left lumpectomy and radiation therapy 7 years ago. (**B,D,G**) The left breast demonstrates stable scarring and benign calcifications from fat necrosis. In the right breast there is an asymmetric density (*square*) that is initially visible only on the CC view. (**E,F**) However, spot compression views demonstrate that it is an ill-defined mass (*arrow*). This mass is infiltrating ductal carcinoma.

differentiation, you must have high resolution and high frequency, be familiar with the normal sonographic appearance of breast parenchyma, and be comfortable with cross-correlating mammography with sonography (see Chapter 2). If the patient is high risk for malignancy, and high-frequency sonography is negative or unavailable, then magnetic resonance is a reasonable method to clarify the etiology of a worrisome asymmetry.

Calcifications

There are a wide variety of breast calcifications (see Chapters 9 through 19). Analysis of calcifications should start with excluding calcifications that are characteristic for benign lesions. If the calcification does not fit in these obviously benign categories, then the shape of the calcification should be analyzed and placed into patterns that can be related to the American College of Radiology BI-RADS assessment categories.

Calcifications or densities simulating calcifications that may be excluded from further work-up include technical artifacts, substances on the skin (e.g., lotions, deodorants), and calcifications that are pathognomonic for benign entities. Processor artifacts and dirty screens may produce tiny dots or irregularities that are confused with calcifications. These artifacts are generally whiter than calcifications and have unusual shapes. Constant evaluation of processing is critical to avoid these problems. Materials on the skin may also initially appear as calcifications. However, these densities are unusual in configuration and are commonly located in the axilla. Thorough cleansing of the skin prior to reevaluation generally removes these particles. Educating patients to avoid using these materials prior to mammography will also reduce the chance of encountering this problem. Certain calcifications are pathognomonic for benign entities. These include oil cysts; dermal, vascular, and secretory calcifications; and milk of calcium calcifications (**Fig. 1.3B,D,G**). By reviewing these characteristic benign calcifications in texts or teaching files, one can confidently identify them.

If calcifications or densities are not included in the above categories, then further analysis is necessary. The first characteristic to examine is size. If the calcifications are large, then they are benign. Malignant calcifications are generally smaller than 0.5 mm. The smallest thickness or diameter of a benign calcification is more than 1 to 2 mm. These large calcifications may be confidently excluded from further evaluation.

If the calcification is small, you should study the shape of the calcification. The shape of calcifications can be categorized into four patterns: (1) round or punctate; (2) amorphous or indistinct; (3) heterogeneous or pleomorphic; and (4) fine linear, branching, or casting calcifications. If the calcifications are round or punctate, determine whether they are scattered, which means they are benign (category 2). If they are clustered but have been stable for 3 years, then they are benign (category 2). If they are new or on a baseline mammogram, then they are probably benign (category 3) and should be followed by 6-month examinations for a total of 1 year and then yearly evaluations for a total of 3 years. If these calcifications change into a more suspicious shape or increase in number, then biopsy is warranted (category 4). The reason that new clustered punctate calcifications should be followed is that ductal carcinoma occasionally may present with punctate clustered calcifications. These calcifications may represent either a variant of the malignant amorphous pattern (see below) or cancerization of lobules (see Cases 16.6 and 16.9).

If the calcifications are amorphous in shape, they should be biopsied (category 4). Amorphous calcifications are commonly round, but they are hazy in appearance and do not have sharp, smooth edges. Malignant amorphous calcifications are generally clustered, but occasionally these calcifications may cover a larger area, such as a segment or quadrant of the breast. Malignant amorphous calcifications are the result of superimposition of numerous tiny calcifications within the mucin secreted by cells of ductal carcinoma in situ. Sometimes amorphous calcifications may overlap in appearance with the round, punctate pattern. Very early, tiny amorphous calcifications may appear punctate. If they are initially misidentified, this error would be discovered as long as the calcifications are closely followed.

Heterogeneous or pleomorphic calcifications are irregular in shape. Furthermore, they also vary in size and density (**Fig. 1.4**). These calcifications have also been described as resembling crushed stones or granulated sugar. The larger calcifications are commonly larger than amorphous calcifications, but they are still smaller than 0.5 mm in size. Malignant heterogeneous calcifications generally present in a cluster unless the patient presents with advanced disease. These calcifications are commonly the result of necrosis from intermediate- or lower-grade ductal carcinoma in situ. Therefore, heterogeneous calcifications should be biopsied (category 4).

Like heterogeneous calcifications, fine linear and branching calcifications are irregular calcifications that vary in size and density. However, unlike heterogeneous calcifications, these calcifications form thin, irregular lines that occasionally branch. These calcifications are generally clustered, but extensive disease will present with a segmental distribution. These calcifications should be biopsied (category 4). High-grade ductal carcinoma in situ produces extensive calcified necrosis that fills the ducts. The configuration and alignment of these calcifications mirror the intraductal spread of malignancy. When a large number of these calcifications are present, they are extremely suspicious, and in those cases, assessment of these calcifications may be upgraded to category 5.

Architectural Distortion

Generally, mammographers easily recognize asymmetries or calcifications unless these findings are small or partially obscured by normal fibroglandular tissue. However, perception of architectural distortion is more difficult because parenchymal patterns vary with different individuals. Perception and characterization of architectural distortion are aided by recognizing normal parenchymal anatomy. The breast parenchymal pattern consists of thin, curvilinear lines that are directed toward the nipple. This radiating pattern is broken only by blood vessels. Adjacent to the subcutaneous fat, the Cooper's ligaments form a scalloped parenchymal edge. The parenchymal edge generally thins out into the axilla and chest wall. These areas commonly form ill-defined curvilinear, feathery borders in patients with scattered or heterogeneous dense breasts. In patients with extremely dense breasts, these borders tend to be well defined. However, the contours are still curvilinear. With heterogeneously dense and extremely dense breasts, the superior corner of the MLO view and the

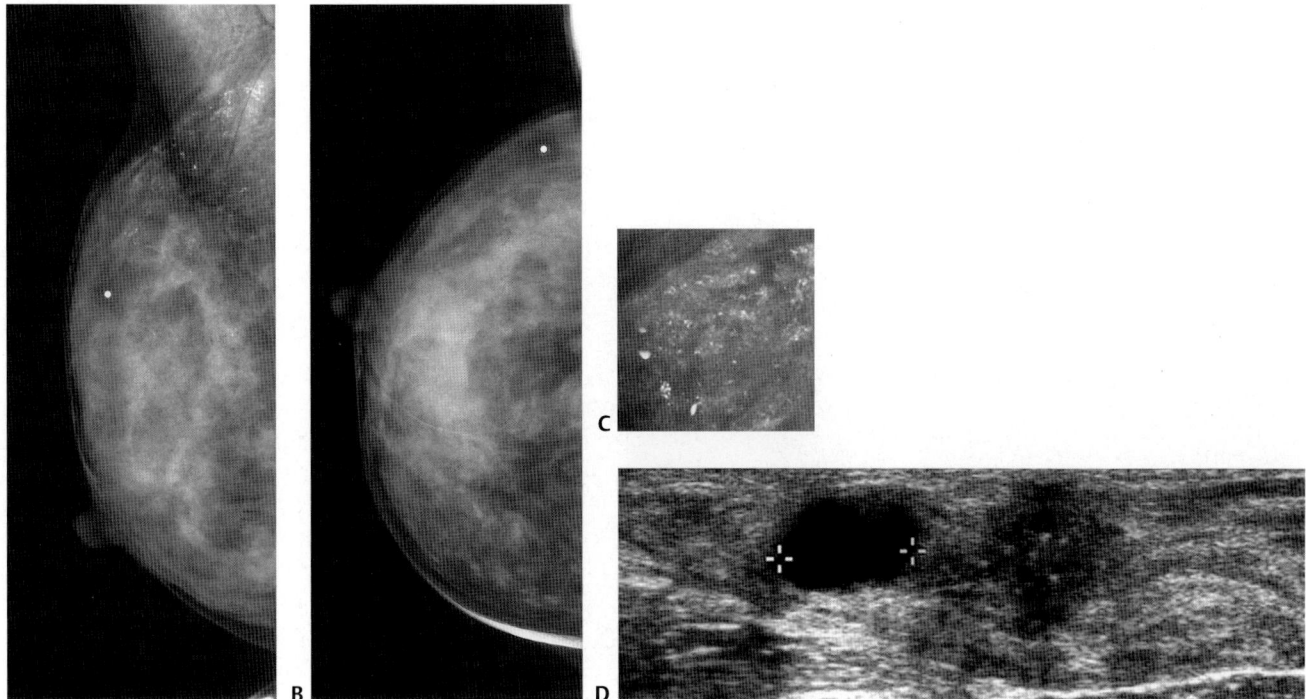

Fig. 1.4 (**A**) Right MLO digital mammogram. (**B**) Right CC digital mammogram. (**C**) Right MLO digital mammogram (close-up). (**A–C**) In the upper outer quadrant of the right breast, there is a palpable lump that is labeled with a radiopaque dot. Just distal to the dot are extensive heterogeneous calcifications. (**D**) Right antiradial breast sonogram: the palpable mass corresponds to a combination of a cyst and a spiculated hypoechoic mass with punctate calcifications. Mastectomy specimen shows that this sonographic mass and the mammographic calcifications are mixed infiltrating lobular and ductal carcinoma with an extensive intraductal component.

medial and lateral corners of the CC view are also generally curvilinear or rounded.

Architectural distortion may be either central or peripheral (see Chapters 22 and 23). Central distortion results when the ductal and trabecular lines deviate from the nipple. This distortion is commonly due to a spiculated lesion producing straight lines that point to the center of the abnormality. Commonly, these abnormal spiculations are thicker than normal trabecular lines (**Fig. 1.5**).

Abnormalities that affect the edge of the parenchyma cause peripheral architectural distortion. Lesions may cause retraction, flattening, straightening, or bulging of the parenchymal contours (**Fig. 1.6**). When the density in the superior parenchymal edge of the MLO view is affected, it may form a sharp triangular corner. Although some women normally have sharply angulated parenchymal corners, if there is asymmetry between the corners, or if there has been a change in configuration, you should search for a subtle spiculated lesion (**Fig. 1.7**). Retraction of the posterior edge of the parenchyma has been labeled the "tent sign," as the retraction produces a biconvex V-shaped border resembling the peak of a tent (**Fig. 1.8**).

When architectural distortion is present, the breast imager should perform additional mammographic views to identify a mass. Spot compression views may demonstrate a spiculated mass. Oblique views may clarify the location of architectural distortion that is initially visible only on one view. Magnification views may be useful to identify associated malignant calcifications.

Causes of architectural distortion include focal fibrosis, sclerosing adenosis, fat necrosis, scar, radial scar, and malignancy. The breast imager identifies surgical scars and fat necrosis by correlating regions of previous surgery or trauma with the architectural distortion. Radial scars usually have thin spiculations and a radiolucent center. Neoplasms usually produce architectural distortion that is evident on two orthogonal views and is associated with a dense central mass. Occasionally, malignancies demonstrate very little central density. Therefore, if architectural distortion is not due to a surgical scar, it should be biopsied (category 4).

If the lesion is small or the breast composition is dense, the architectural distortion may be visible on only one view. In these cases, sonography may be useful to demonstrate a mass and localize biopsy. Sonographically, normal fibroglandular tissue and fibrosis will be uniformly hyperechoic. Fat necrosis may be either heterogeneous or hyperechoic echogenicity. Both surgical and radial scars strongly attenuate the sonographic beam, so shadowing may be the predominant feature. If heavy shadowing is present, a lower-frequency examination may penetrate the scar and demonstrate no mass. However, in some cases, surgical scars cannot be differentiated from neoplasms, and biopsy is necessary. If radial scar is suspected, then ex-

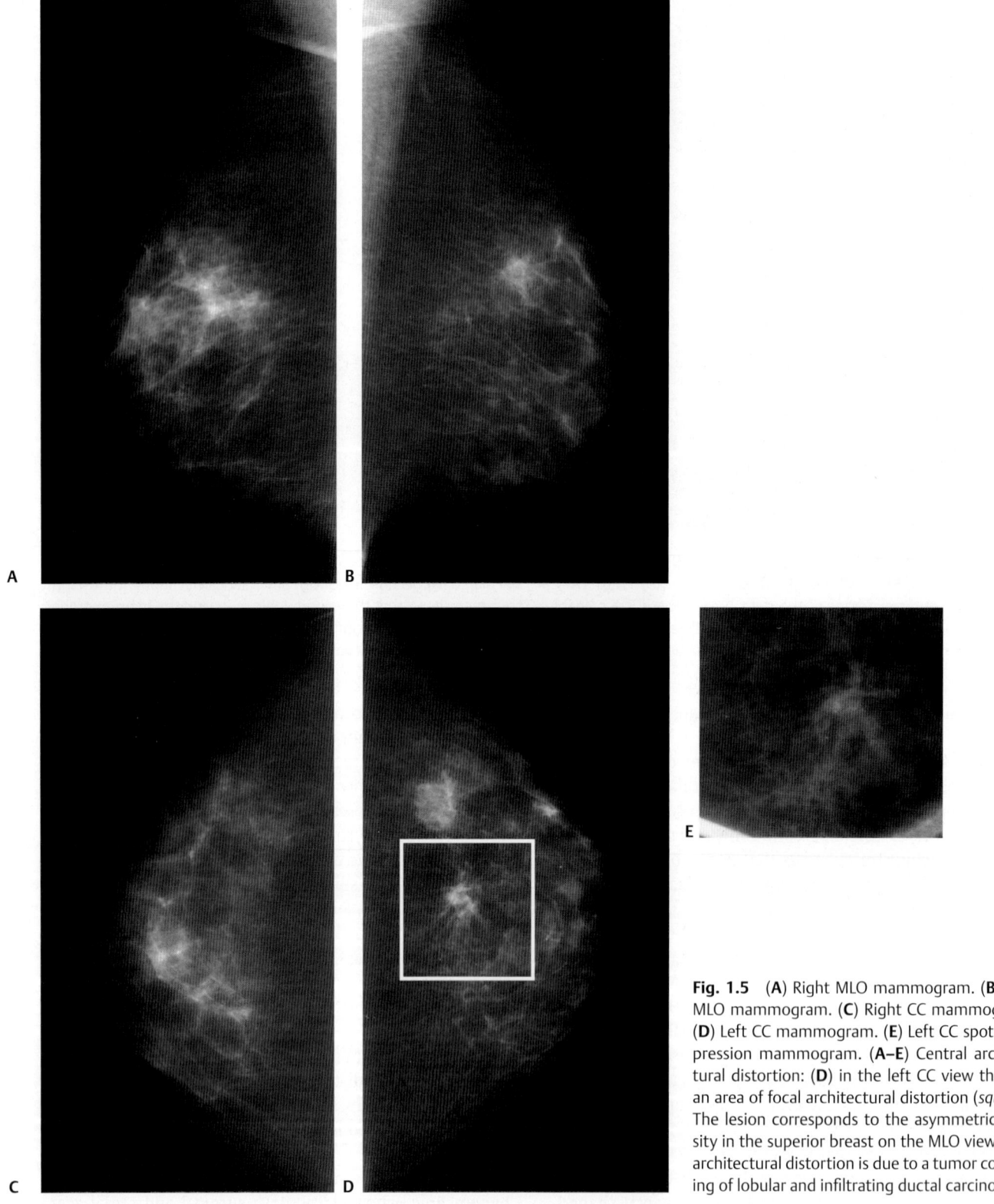

Fig. 1.5 (**A**) Right MLO mammogram. (**B**) Left MLO mammogram. (**C**) Right CC mammogram. (**D**) Left CC mammogram. (**E**) Left CC spot compression mammogram. (**A–E**) Central architectural distortion: (**D**) in the left CC view there is an area of focal architectural distortion (*square*). The lesion corresponds to the asymmetric density in the superior breast on the MLO view. This architectural distortion is due to a tumor consisting of lobular and infiltrating ductal carcinoma.

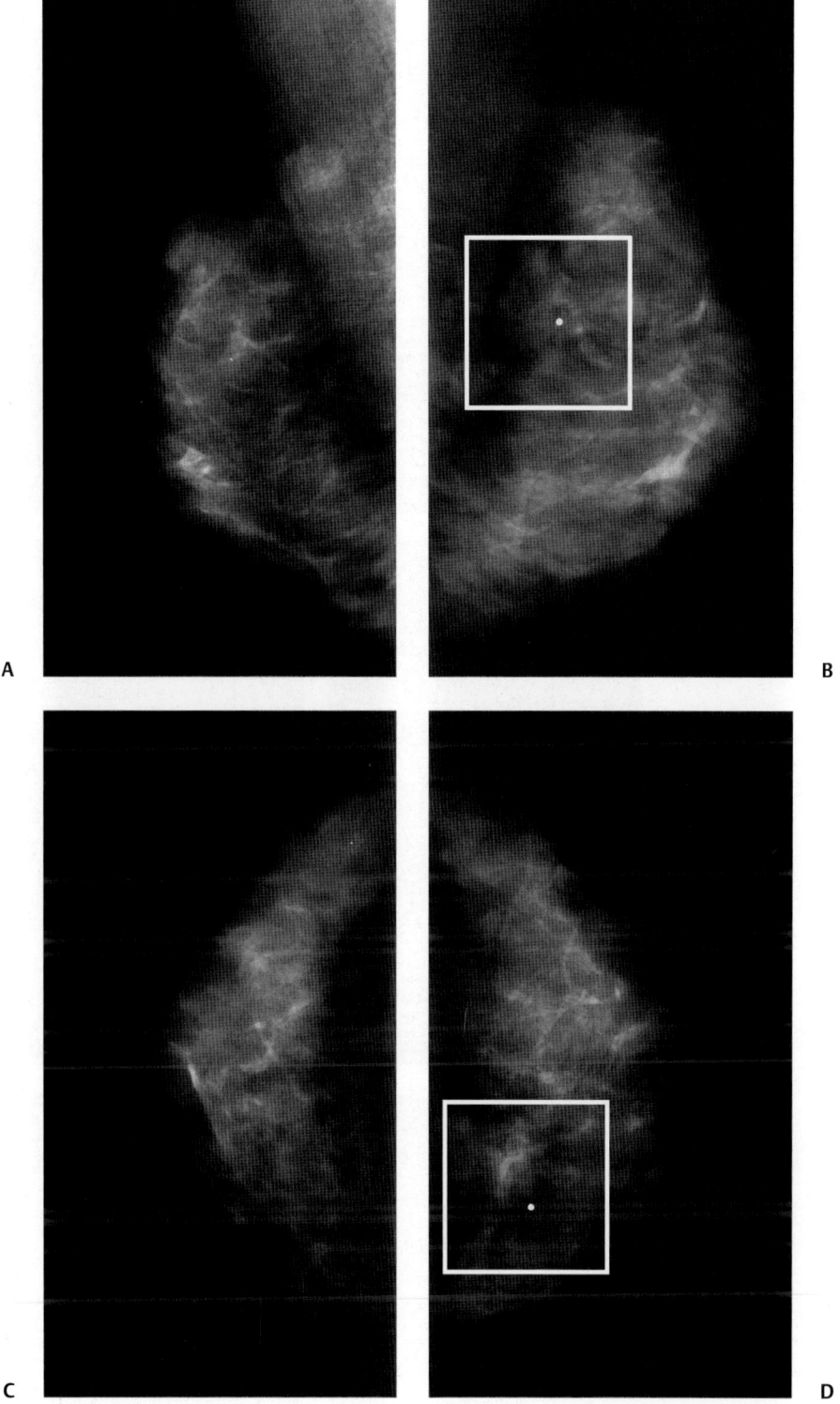

Fig. 1.6 (**A**) Right MLO mammogram. (**B**) Left MLO mammogram. (**C**) Right CC mammogram. (**D**) Left CC mammogram. (**A–D**) Peripheral architectural distortion: a lobulated mass extends outside the posterior border of the fibroglandular border (*square*). This mass corresponds to an infiltrating ductal tumor.

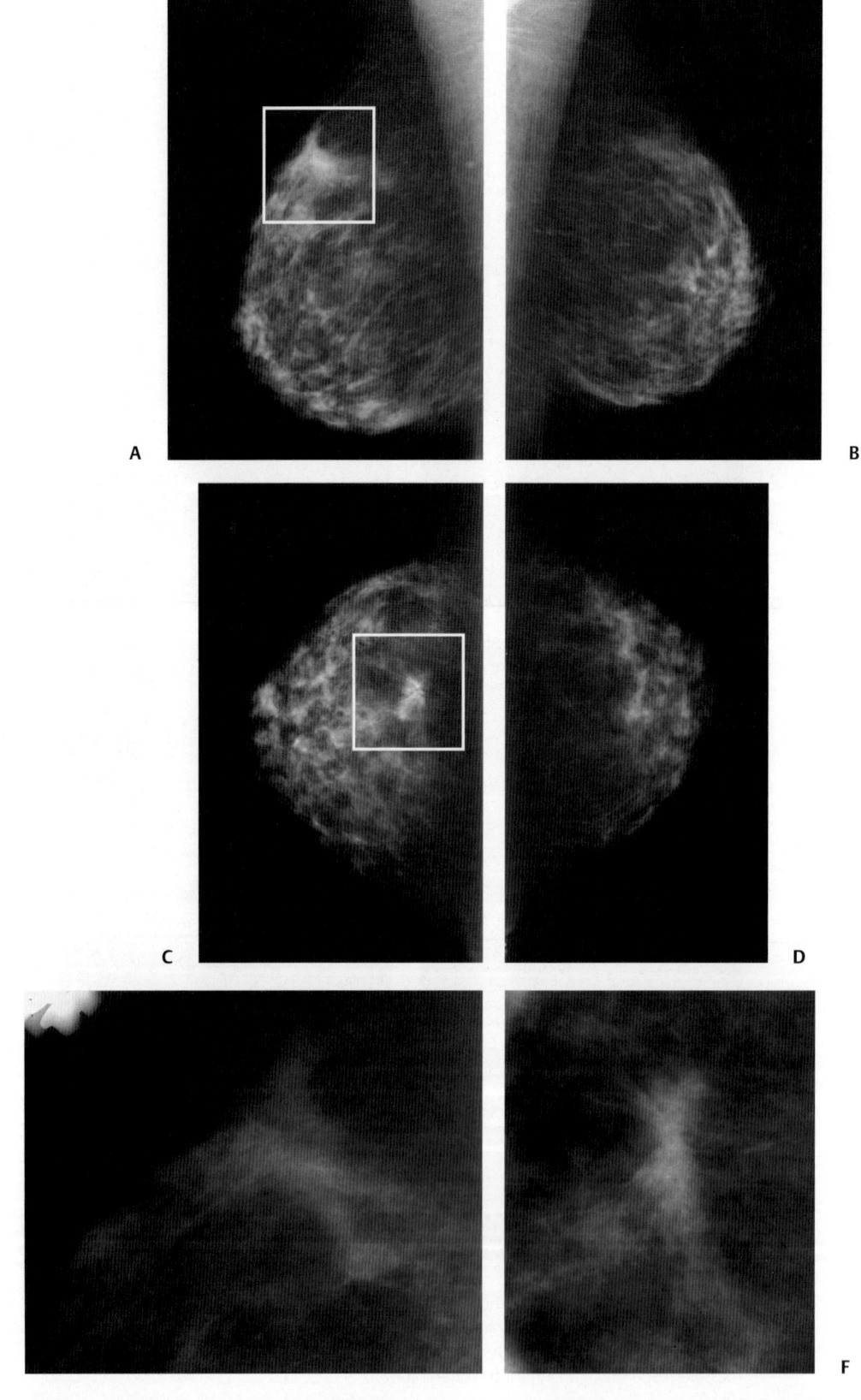

Fig. 1.7 (**A**) Right MLO mammogram. (**B**) Left MLO mammogram. (**C**) Right CC mammogram. (**D**) Left CC mammogram. (**E**) Left MLO spot magnification mammogram. (**F**) Left CC spot magnification mammogram. (**A–F**) Superior peripheral architectural distortion: an irregular mass (marked by a *square*) at the 12 o'clock position produces a sharp angulation of the superior parenchymal corner (**A**) in the right MLO view. This mass represents tubular carcinoma.

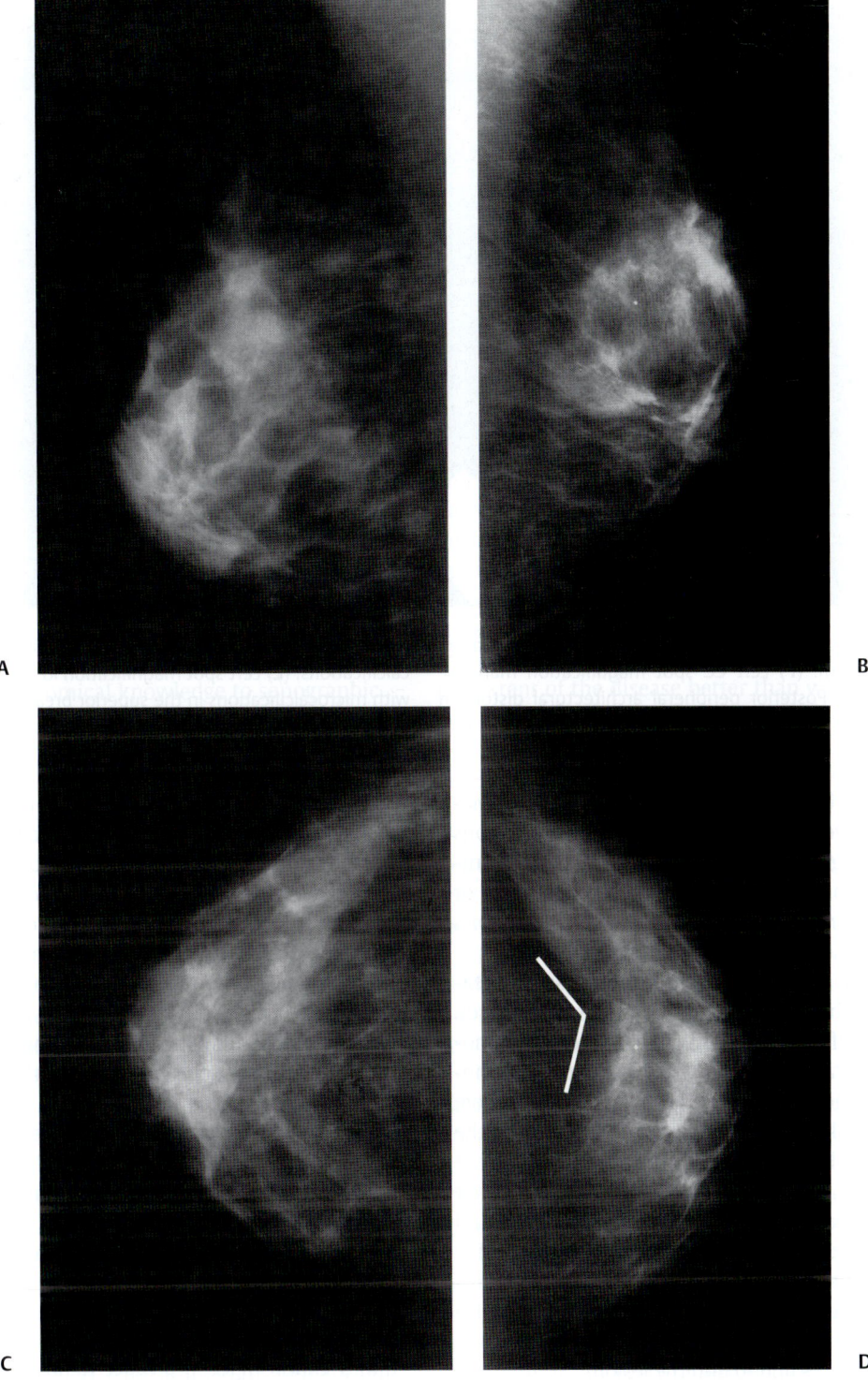

Fig. 1.8 (**A**) Right MLO mammogram. (**B**) Left MLO mammogram. (**C**) Right CC mammogram. (**D**) Left CC mammogram. (**A–D**) Posterior peripheral architectural distortion (tent sign). (**D**) In the left CC view, the posterior parenchymal border exhibits retraction (marked with a *white bracket*), (**B**) although the abnormality is difficult to identify in the left MLO view. *(continued on page 14)*

Sonographic Technique and Cross-Correlation with Mammography

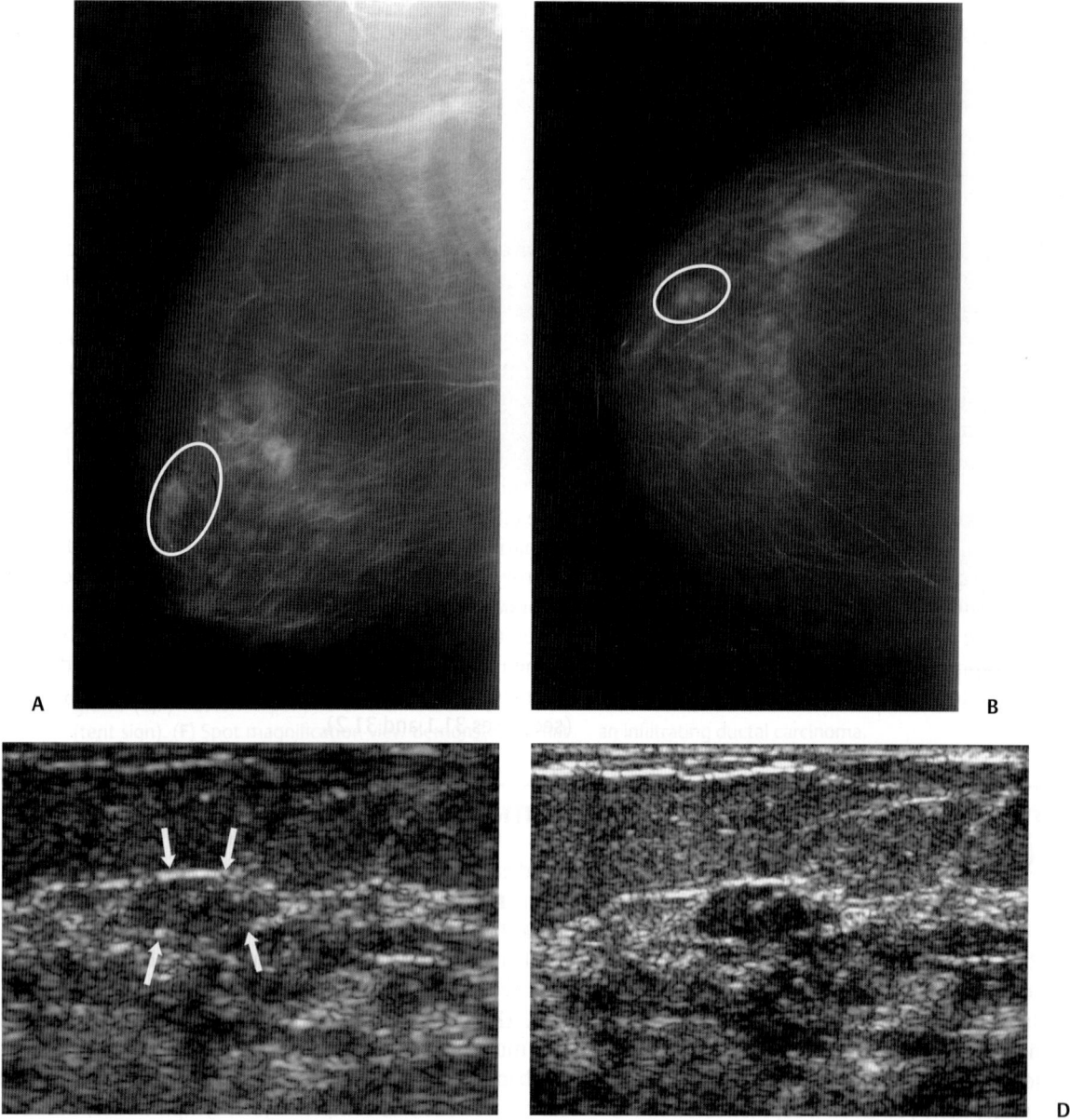

Fig. 2.1 (**A**) Right mediolateral oblique (MLO) mammogram. (**B**) Right craniocaudal (CC) mammogram. (**A,B**) In the upper outer right breast, there is a lobulated density (*circle*). (**C**) Right radial breast sonogram: a 5 MHz transducer does not clearly demonstrate the lobulated mass (*arrows*). The inadequate size and contrast resolution result in poor definition of the mass. (**D**) Right radial breast sonogram: an 8 MHz transducer improves the definition of the mass. This result allows an observer to confidently localize the mass. This mass is a fibroadenoma.

of the equipment to learn which imaging techniques are available (**Fig. 2.2**; also see Case 6.11).

Besides adjusting image contrast, you should be aware of software methods to optimize resolution. These methods include increasing the line density of the image, increasing the persistence, and adjusting the focal zones. The main disadvantage of these methods is a slower frame rate. If you are merely characterizing a lesion, a slower frame rate may not be a problem. However, the slower frame rate may be disconcerting with real-time imaging of interventional procedures.

Color or power Doppler is a useful method to quickly assess vascularity. Breast vascularity is low, so you should be aware of methods to optimize the color or power Doppler. Generally, this means that you are using a color or power Doppler frequency slightly lower than the gray scale frequency and the focal zone adjusted at the correct depth. The filter and scale should be low. The Doppler gain is optimized by initially increasing the gain until the entire screen is filled with color and then by slowly reducing the gain until the color appears only within pulsating vascular structures. If no color is detected using these methods,

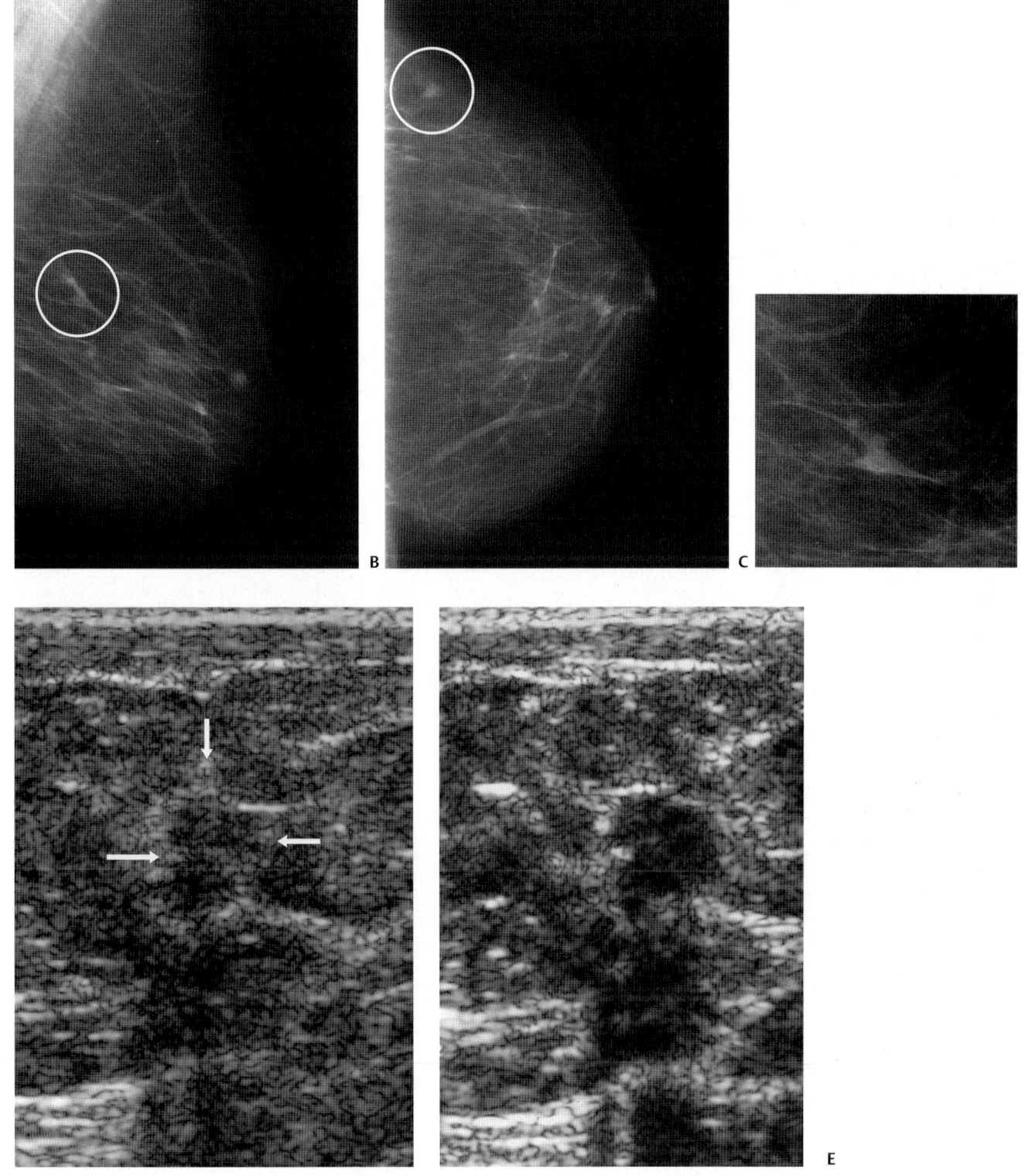

Fig. 2.2 (**A**) Left MLO mammogram. (**B**) Left CC mammogram. (**C**) Left MLO spot magnification mammogram. (**A–C**) In the left upper outer quadrant, there is a small, irregular mass (*circle*). (**D**) Left antiradial (8 MHz) breast sonogram: sonographic examination of the mammographic mass with a low-contrast technique poorly demonstrates the mass (*arrows*). The hypoechogenicity of the mass blends into the surrounding fat. (**E**) Left antiradial (8 MHz) breast sonogram: sonographic examination of the same location as (**D**) with high-contrast technique greatly improves the conspicuity of the mass. This mass is a mucinous carcinoma.

then the sample volume size should be increased. Increasing the sample volume size reduces color resolution. The color may "bleed" and be demonstrated outside the vessel walls. Color or power Doppler is useful to delineate vessels or highly vascular structures such as arteriovenous malformations. This Doppler technique is also useful to clarify whether a hypoechoic or anechoic mass is cystic or solid (**Fig. 2.3**; also see Case 6.25).

Dynamic clips are useful to document vascularity and to demonstrate the spatial relationship of multiple lesions. Dynamic clips are the ideal method to show color flow in pseudoaneurysms or intravenous contrast enhancement of solid masses. Until high-resolution three-dimensional (3D) imaging is universally available, dynamic clips are an excellent way to demonstrate the relationship of multiple cysts to a solid mass or to show debris or calcifications moving within a complex cyst.

Wide field-of-view compound imaging is sometimes useful to document larger masses or the relationship of multiple masses in the same plane. The wider field of view provides observers with more landmarks, so cross-correlation with mammography and magnetic resonance imaging (MRI) may be easier.

Newer sonographic techniques that may have more applications in the future are 3D imaging and harmonic imaging. Like compound imaging, 3D imaging may produce a wide field of view that would be similar to a mammogram or MRI. In the future, 3D imaging may also allow surgeons and patients to better appreciate the location and size of sonographic findings and facilitate surgical planning.

Harmonic imaging may improve image resolution and increase both gray scale and color Doppler sensitivity for intravenous sonographic contrast agents. These contrast agents may improve both vascular and gray scale characterization of masses.

■ Approach to a Palpable Mass

In many breast centers, palpable masses are the most common reason for a breast sonogram. Therefore, it is important that sonographic breast imagers learn how to palpate breasts. Usually, the patient will be able to identify the palpable lump. When the patient locates the lump, the breast imager should confirm the presence of the lump by palpating the area identified by the patient. Even if the lump is obvious, the imager should scan the lump and reconfirm the location of the lump by moving a finger into the scan plane. If the imager cannot detect the lump, or if the patient is not sure of the exact location of the lump, then palpation of the entire quadrant is useful. By palpating a larger area, the imager is able to detect asymmetries within the region. Finally, if palpating the quadrant is not helpful, palpating the comparable area in the opposite breast is helpful. Commonly, the parenchymal pattern of patients is symmetric, so the physical exam is also symmetric. By palpating the

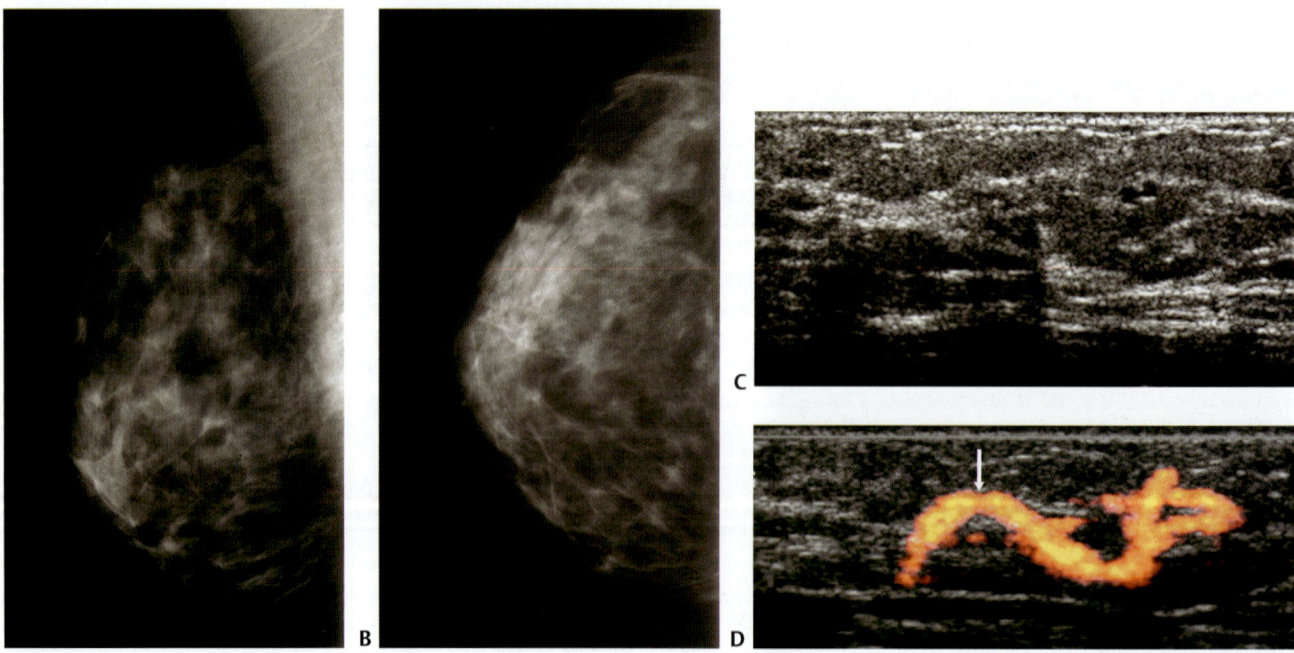

Fig. 2.3 (**A**) Right MLO mammogram. (**B**) Right CC mammogram. (**A,B**) The patient and the breast surgeon have identified some small, palpable lumps at the 9 o'clock position of the right breast. The lumps are arranged in a linear pattern. The left breast has similar lumps that are less conspicuous. Bilateral mammograms are normal. (**C**) Right radial breast sonogram: gray scale sonographic examination of the palpable lumps shows normal tissue. (**D**) Right radial breast sonogram: color Doppler examination of the palpable lumps demonstrates that the lumps are due to the lateral blood vessels of the breast. Each lump corresponds to the superficial curve of the blood vessel (*arrows*).

corresponding contralateral quadrant, you can detect abnormal asymmetries. This technique is particularly useful with malignancies that are commonly difficult to feel, such as lobular carcinoma.

■ Cross-Correlation of Sonographic and Mammographic Image

To accurately, efficiently, and confidently identify a mammographic abnormality sonographically, the technician who performs the breast sonographic examination should be familiar with mammographic imaging. Furthermore, the ultrasound examiner should be able to review the mammogram and identify internal landmarks that can be cross-correlated with the ultrasound. Finally, by confirming the mammographic landmarks sonographically, the examiner should be able to pinpoint the location of the mammographic abnormality in the breast with ultrasound and consequently be able to explain the etiology of the puzzling mammographic finding.

Unfortunately, sometimes the ultrasound examiner does not attempt to closely cross-correlate anatomically the ultrasound examination with the mammogram. Some examiners do not attempt to correlate the exams because they do not routinely interpret mammograms and are uncomfortable reviewing mammograms. However, more common reasons for lack of close cross-correlation include the following: (1) The sonographic image has a small field of view compared with the mammographic global field of view. (2) The patient position for an ultrasound examination is completely different from the position for the mammographic examination. Therefore, the position of a breast mass for these exams appears extremely different. (3) Even if the examiner places the patient in the same position, the difference in technology between ultrasound and mammography creates different orientations of tissue visualization. (4) Unlike other organs, the breast does not have a uniform or constant normal anatomy. The breasts of different individuals have different breast architecture. Furthermore, some individuals have a right breast that exhibits a pattern different from the left breast. Finally, the breasts of many individuals change with age.

For these reasons, ultrasound examiners commonly ignore internal breast anatomical landmarks and estimate the location of the mammographic abnormality using external landmarks. The most commonly used systems are the "o'clock" method and the quadrant method. The o'clock method views the breast as a circular clock with the nipple in the center circle: 12 o'clock is directly above the nipple, 3 o'clock is to the left of the nipple, 6 o'clock is below the nipple, and 9 o'clock is to the right of the nipple. The quadrant method divides the breast into four parts or quadrants. These quadrants are defined by drawing a horizontal and a vertical line through the nipple. The quadrants label four regions of the breast: upper outer quadrant, upper inner quadrant, lower outer quadrant, and lower inner quadrant.

There are several problems with using external anatomical landmarks for locating mammographic abnormalities: (1) mammographic estimation of location is not accurate and may be difficult to determine if the abnormality is only on one view, (2) the change in patient position between the mammogram and the ultrasound commonly results in changes in the relative position of internal breast structures compared with external landmarks, and (3) the external breast position of a handheld transducer does not correlate with a specific internal imaging position.

Estimating location on a mammogram is commonly inaccurate, as the standard mammographic views are the craniocaudal (horizontal) and mediolateral oblique views. The greatest source of error is related to the mediolateral oblique view because this view is not oriented 90 degrees to the craniocaudal view. Furthermore, this view's long axis angle varies with the anatomy of the patient. For example, a mass that is deep to the nipple on the craniocaudal view and directly above the nipple in the mediolateral oblique view may be identified as being located at the 12 o'clock position but may actually be located between 11:30 and 9:30.

Even if the location of a lesion is accurately identified by the mammogram, its relative position may change when the patient changes position for the ultrasound. Usually the mammogram is performed with the patient in the upright position, and the ultrasound is performed with the patient in the supine position. Because the breast is a flexible structure, it changes its shape from one position to the other. In the upright position, the position of the breast drops due to gravity, whereas in the supine position, the breast flattens against the chest wall. Compared with other external landmarks, the nipple may be lower in the upright position compared with the supine position. Therefore, a lesion above the nipple in the upright position may shift to the same level as the nipple in the supine position. For example, a 10:00 lesion in the upright position may become a 9:00 lesion in the supine position. The larger the breast, the greater the movement of the breast.

Finally, the external position of the handheld transducer does not necessarily correlate with the internal position of the lesion. Even if a linear transducer is used, the examiner commonly uses a variety of angles and hand pressures to optimally visualize the abnormality. Even slight angulation will produce a discrepancy between the position of the sonographic transducer and the actual position of the lesion. Furthermore, transducer pressure may cause the lesion to shift position relative to the nipple. Both of these factors may produce a discrepancy between the mammographic position and the sonographic position.

Because external landmarks are not reliable in cross-correlating mammographic/sonographic abnormalities, you should use internal landmarks. However, you must use a technique that addresses the problems listed earlier:

(1) limited sonographic field of view compared with mammography, (2) differences between mammographic and sonographic patient position and technical orientation, and (3) nonuniformity of breast anatomy both between individuals and within the same individual.

By using internal breast anatomical landmarks, you immediately address the first two problems. If you identify location by the internal anatomy of an organ, then relating the position of a focal abnormality from the limited sonographic field of view to a wide field of view modality is not a problem. Furthermore, unlike external landmarks, internal landmarks do not shift with body position. For example, in the abdomen, examiners are commonly challenged with the problem of sonographically deciding whether a small liver lesion previously identified on a computed tomography (CT) scan is cystic or solid. Even though the CT scan is a wide field-of-view modality, experienced examiners easily localize the position of the CT lesion sonographically. These examiners are able to confidently localize the lesion because they relate the lesion to the internal anatomy of the liver as displayed on the CT and then sonographically find the same hepatic location using the same internal hepatic landmarks. Furthermore, this process of anatomical cross-correlation would not be different even if the patient were lying prone because, unlike external landmarks, internal anatomical landmarks do not change relative to each other.

Even though internal landmarks solve the problems of limited sonographic field of view and positional changes, many examiners are inhibited from using internal breast landmarks, as there is great anatomical variation between different breasts. However, whenever you perform a breast sonogram to identify a mammographic abnormality, you should always have the corresponding mammogram. The mammogram provides an anatomical map to the patient's breast. If you are able to cross-correlate mammographic structures with sonographic structures, then you may use the mammogram as a sonographic guide to locating the lesion. Therefore, ideally sonographic examiners should be able to sonographically interpret the mammographic image.

To systematically cross-correlate sonography with mammography, you should be familiar with normal breast anatomy. There are mainly seven sonographically different structures in the breast and chest wall of the average normal 45-year-old woman. These structures, from superficial to deep, are the following (**Fig. 2.4**):

1. *Skin:* The skin is a hyperechoic 3 mm layer on the surface of the breast.
2. *Subcutaneous fatty layer:* This structure lies under the skin and appears as an anterior hypoechoic layer of tissue, which tends to thicken at the periphery of the breast and is more prominent in the medial portion of the breast.
3. *Superficial fascia:* The superficial and deep layers of the fascia envelop the breast. The superficial layer is an undulating hyperechoic line within the subcutaneous fat that parallels the skin. The deep layer is a hyperechoic line within the retromammary fat that parallels the anterior chest wall muscles.
4. *Cooper's ligaments:* The ligaments are curved hyperechoic lines within the subcutaneous fat that extend from the superficial fascia to the deeper adjacent tissue.
5. *Glandular tissue:* Normal glandular tissue consists of hyperechoic glandular lobes that are in a radial arrangement around the nipple. Each lobe is in the shape of a prolate ellipse and is surrounded anteriorly by the subcutaneous fat and posteriorly by the retromammary fat. Within the lobes, main ducts originate from the nipple and end in a series of terminal duct lobular units.
6. *Anterior chest wall muscles:* This layer is formed by the pectoralis minor and major muscles and appears as a hypoechoic solid layer posterior to the retromammary fat.
7. *Chest wall:* This structure consists of ribs connected by intercostal muscles and covered on the deep surface by the pleura.

Most of these anatomical structures are also generally identifiable mammographically.

Rules of Cross-Correlation

Once you are familiar with normal sonographic and mammographic breast anatomy, you will be able to anatomically cross-correlate the two modalities. If you are not familiar with cross-correlation of these modalities, you should not be intimidated by the task of cross-correlating sonographic and mammographic structures. A simple way to start is to remember two basic imaging rules. The first rule is that the background breast tissue appearance is similar on the two modalities. This means that normal fibroglandular parenchyma is white (or dense) on mammography and white (or hyperechoic) on sonography. Furthermore, fat appears dark (or lucent) on mammography and dark (or hypoechoic) on sonography (**Fig. 2.5**). The main exception to this rule is the presence of dilated ducts that are sonographically dark (hypoechoic) and mammographically white (dense). When the breast tissue is filled with dilated ducts, such as in ductal ectasias, the breast tissue appears white (dense) on mammography but has numerous linear dark structures (dilated ducts) on sonography.

When you are aware of the appearance of breast tissue with the two modalities, then when you review a mammogram you should be able to predict the sonographic appearance of the breast. For example, a mammographically fatty, lucent breast will be sonographically hypoechoic. Conversely, a mammographically dense breast usually sonographically exhibits diffusely hyperechoic fibroglandular parenchyma.

Generally, the breasts of most women are not completely dense or lucent. This system of pattern recognition is even more valuable in these breasts. When a breast has a mixture

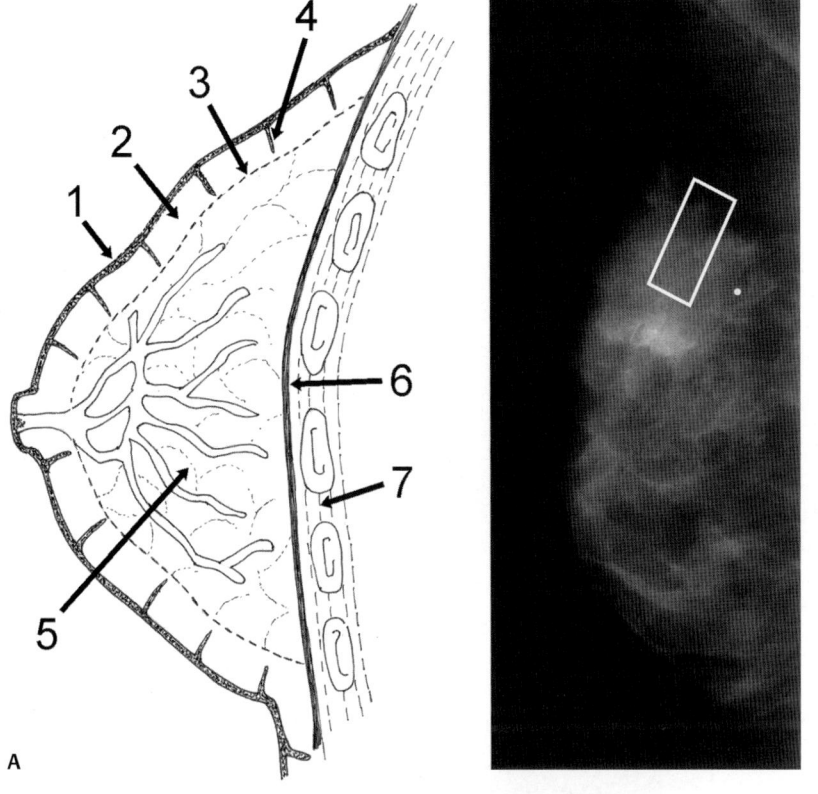

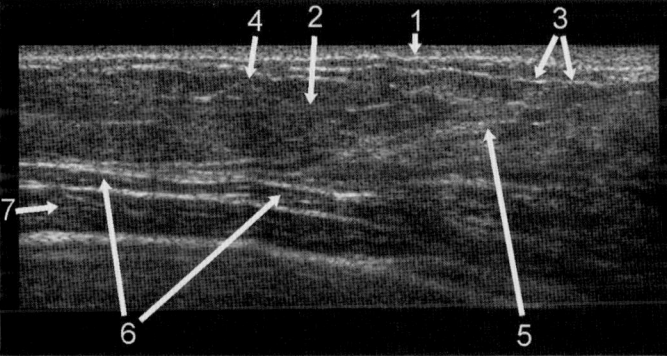

Fig. 2.4 (**A**) A schematic diagram showing the normal structures of the breast: skin (1), subcutaneous fatty layer (2), superficial fascia (3), Cooper's ligaments (4), glandular tissue (5), anterior chest wall muscles (6), chest wall (7). (**B**) Radial breast sonogram (10 o'clock position): sonographic image demonstrates the normal anatomical structures of the breast (same as above). (**C**) Right MLO mammogram: this is the mammogram of the patient whose sonogram is seen in **Fig. 2.2**. In the upper outer quadrant, the sonographic image corresponds to the outer edge of the patient's fibroglandular density. Box denotes location of transducer.

of tissues, these tissues form unique mammographic structural patterns that may be sonographically reproduced. For example, commonly the mammogram exhibits dense parenchymal tissue primarily in the upper outer quadrant. Sonographically, you can also outline this tissue by noticing the junction between the hyperechoic parenchyma and the adjacent hypoechoic fat. Furthermore, if the medial aspect of the mammogram is lucent, then the corresponding sonographic examination should display hypoechoic fat.

The second cross-correlation imaging rule is that most focal breast masses have dissimilar appearances on the two modalities. For example, lymph nodes, cysts, and fibroadenomas appear white (dense) on mammography but dark (hypoechoic) on sonography. Neoplasms appear white (dense) on mammography but dark (hypoechoic or heterogeneous echogenicity) on sonography. The main common exceptions to this rule are benign scars, radial scars, and occasionally fat necrosis. These lesions are sonographically hyperechoic (white).

If you are familiar with the mammographic and sonographic appearance of breast structures, then you will be able to sonographically localize a focal mammographic abnormality using internal anatomical landmarks. The steps that I use when faced with an anatomically difficult breast problem are the following:

1. Review the mammogram and identify the abnormality. Notice the parenchymal pattern between the nipple and the lesion. Also, study the pattern of the breast tissue surrounding the abnormality. Estimate the general location of the abnormality (i.e., quadrant and finger breadths from nipple).

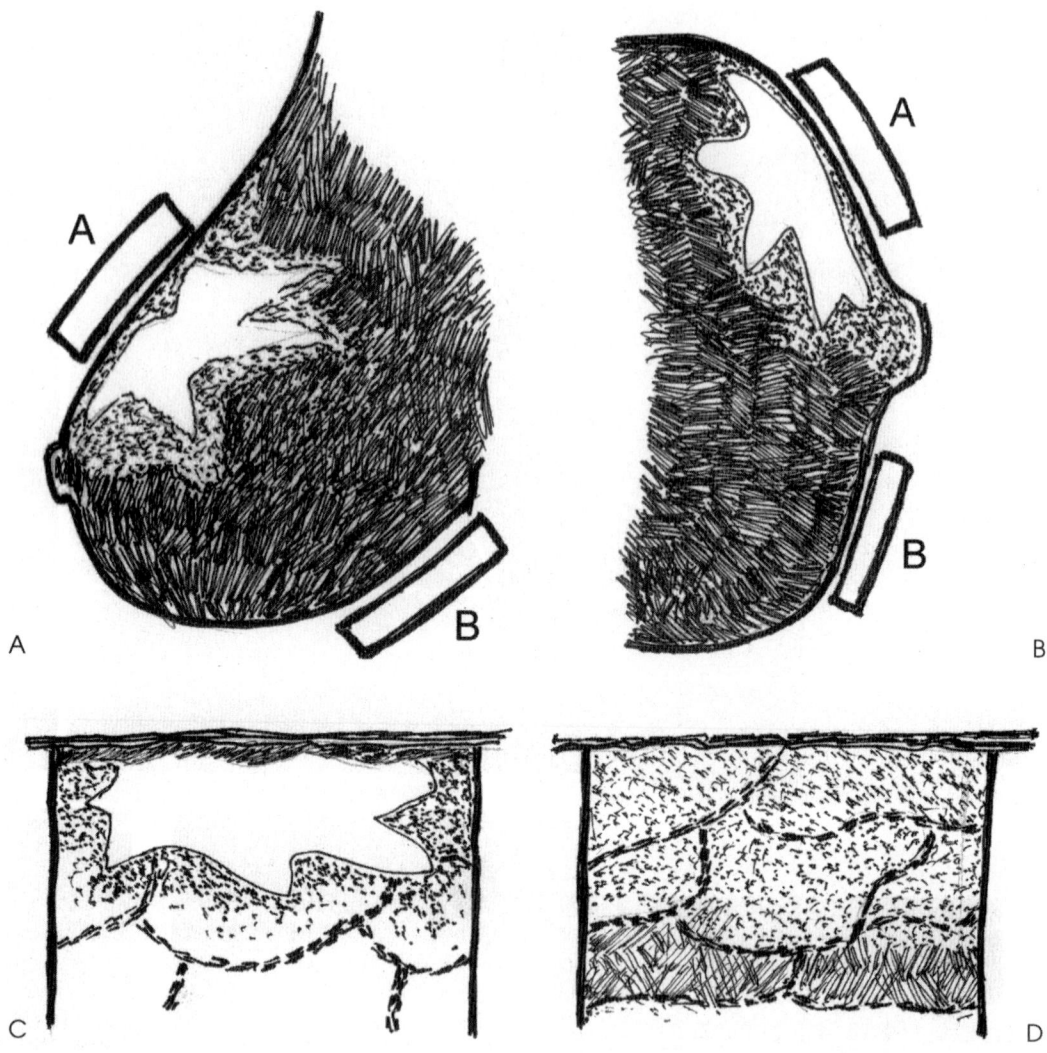

Fig. 2.5 These schematic diagrams illustrate the anatomical cross-correlation between mammography and sonography. In this patient, transducer A is positioned over the dense fibroglandular tissue in the upper outer quadrant. Sonographically, this tissue is hyperechoic (labeled C). Transducer B demonstrates the fatty parenchyma in the inferior inner quadrant that is sonographically hypoechoic (labeled D). (**A**) Schematic image of an MLO mammogram shows two transducers, labeled A and B. (**B**) Schematic image of a CC mammogram showing the position of transducers A and B. (**C**) Schematic image of a breast sonogram that corresponds to tissue imaged by transducer A. (**D**) Schematic image of a breast sonogram that corresponds to tissue imaged by transducer B.

2. Place the transducer with one edge at the nipple and sonographically examine the breast in a radial orientation. Look for the same parenchymal patterns that you noticed on the mammogram. When you recognize the parenchymal landmarks that surround the abnormality, sonographically focus the examination in this area.
3. Characterize the lesion sonographically (**Fig. 2.6**). Using this method, you would first approach finding the mass in **Fig. 2.6** by noting the general mammographic location of the lesion near the left 9 o'clock position. The irregular mass is surrounded by fatty density but linked to the subareolar density by linear densities (**Fig. 2.6A–C**). You would initially place the transducer near the nipple and confirm the presence of dense (hyperechoic) subareolar tissue. In the inner breast you would extend the transducer away from the nipple. This "trail" of hyperechoic tissue will lead to the hypoechoic shadowing mass (**Fig. 2.6D**) that corresponds to the mammographic mass.

This method is particularly useful when the mammographic abnormality is not easily visualized. Case 21.2 demonstrates an asymmetric density that is visible in only one mammographic view. In this case, the abnormal density is at the distal border of the fibroglandular density. Therefore, to find this type of lesion, you should start near the nipple and confirm the presence of diffuse hyperechoic fibroglandular tissue. You should then move the

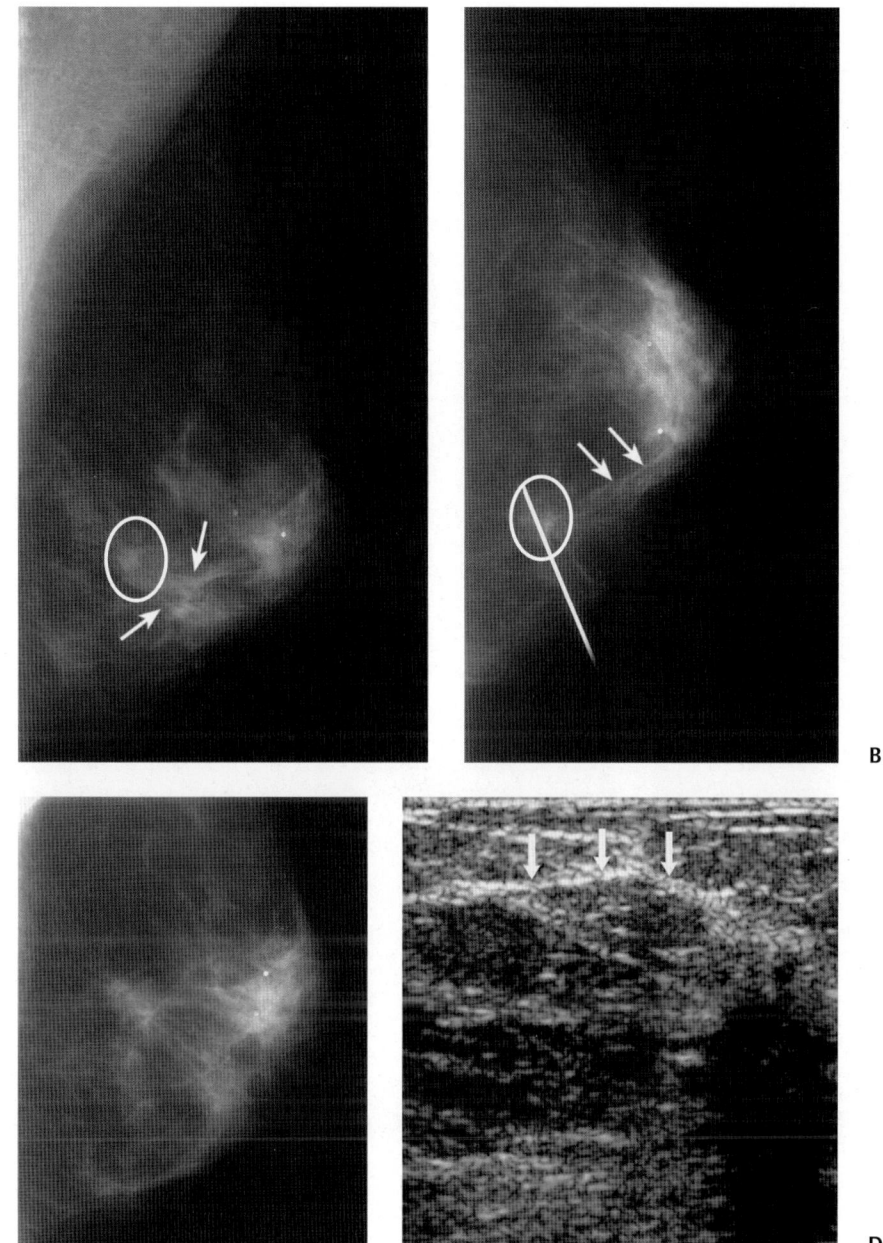

Fig. 2.6 (**A**) Left MLO mammogram. (**B**) Left CC mammogram. (**C**) Left lateromedial (LM) spot compression mammogram. (**A–C**) At the 9 o'clock position of the left breast, there is an irregular mass (*circle*). This mass is primarily surrounded by fatty density but is linked with dense spiculations (*arrows*) to the main subareolar fibroglandular density. (**D**) Left radial breast sonogram: the mammographic irregular density corresponds to a heavily shadowing focal mass. These mammographic spiculations correspond to the hyperechoic curvilinear tissue (*arrows*). This mass is infiltrating ductal carcinoma.

transducer toward the outer breast until you visualize fatty hypoechoic tissue. Then, you should scan only the border between the hyperechoic and hypoechoic tissue. You will then discover the hypoechoic malignant mass.

When evaluating the location of a lesion from the mammogram, the internal parenchymal landmarks that you should notice are (1) the location of the edge of the parenchyma—many lesions are at the border of the fibroglandular (white) tissue and the fat (dark); (2) the configuration of the fibroglandular tissue—the lesion may be linked to the largest area of this tissue; (3) adjacent masses—the mammogram may demonstrate another mass next to the questionable lesion. By cross-correlating these mammographic landmarks on the breast sonogram, you will be more successful in identifying mammographic lesions (**Fig. 2.7**).

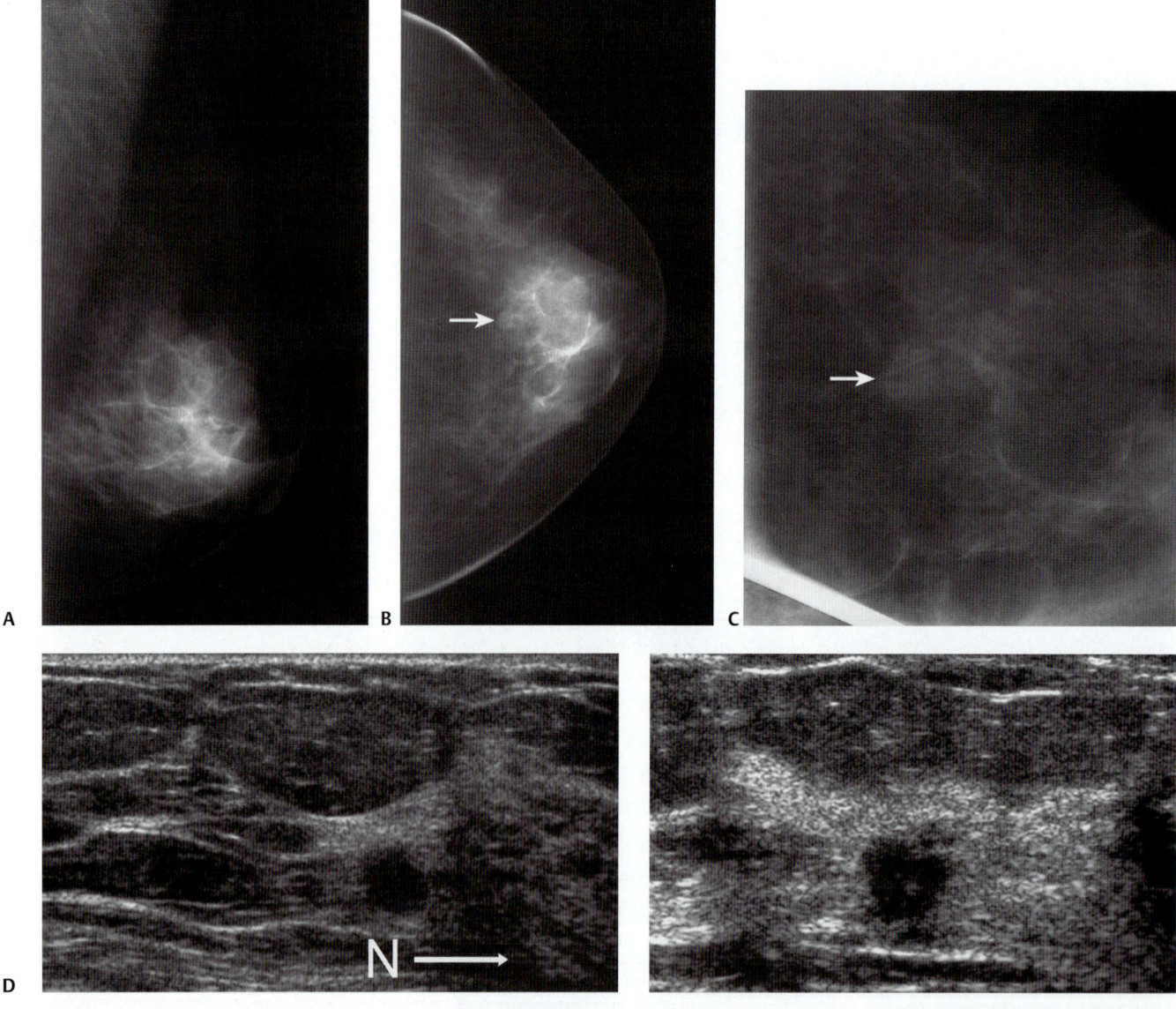

Fig. 2.7 (A) Left MLO digital mammogram. (B) Left CC digital mammogram. (C) Left CC spot magnification mammogram. (A–C) A partially obscured oval density (*arrow*) is visible in the central area of the CC view. This density is not visible on the MLO view. In the CC view, the density is at the distal edge of the fibroglandular density. (D) Left radial breast sonogram: a hypoechoic mass is present at the 12 o'clock position of the breast. In this view, the parenchymal anatomy matches the mammographic anatomy of the CC view. On the side closest to the nipple, the tissue is white fibroglandular parenchyma. On the side away from the nipple, the tissue is hypoechoic fat. N, arrow points toward the direction of the nipple. (E) Left antiradial breast sonogram: the antiradial view demonstrates irregularity of the margins of the mass. This mass is a mixed infiltrating ductal and lobular carcinoma.

Special Sonographic Problems

Shadowing

One difficulty in cross-correlating mammography with sonography is sonographic shadowing. Shadowing is confusing. It is a nonspecific finding because it is associated with both benign and malignant entities. Shadowing is particularly a problem for those who use high-frequency equipment, as all tissues more readily attenuate high frequencies, and therefore shadowing is more frequent. To analyze shadowing, you should be familiar with the etiologies of shadowing. If the shadow hides the lesion, reduce or eliminate the shadow. Also, characterize the tissue that causes the shadow.

The etiologies of shadowing can be divided into two main categories: reflection and absorption. Reflection of sound is affected by two factors: acoustic impedance and angle of incidence. Acoustic impedance is a fundamental property of matter and is related to the density of the material and the speed of sound in the material. A portion of a sound wave is reflected whenever the wave strikes an interface between two substances with different acoustic impedances. This principle is the basis for diagnostic sonography. The reflected sound is received by the ultrasound machine and transformed into visual information. The amount of reflection is dependent on the difference in acoustic impedance between the substances. If the difference is great, then a large percentage of the sound wave is reflected. Acoustic impedance differences between most tissues within the breast such as fat and fibroglandular tissue are very small, so generally less than 1% of the sound wave is reflected. However, air and bone have acoustic impedances that are very different from breast tissue. When the sound wave strikes a rib, approximately 90% of the sound is reflected, and when the wave strikes the lung, over 99% of the wave is reflected.

The second factor that affects the amount of reflected sound is the angle of incidence, or the angle at which the sound strikes an object. The closer the sound beam is to a right angle (or perpendicular to the surface of the object), the less the reflection. The proportion of reflected sound increases with decreasing angles. When the sound beam strikes the object at an extremely acute angle (i.e., critical angle), all of the sound is reflected. This phenomenon is evident when sound hits the side of a curved mass such as a cyst. In this situation, the reflected sound produces thin shadows at the edge of the cyst.

Besides reflection, shadowing is caused by absorption. Absorption is the conversion of sound into heat. A shadow results if the material completely absorbs the sound beam. In the body, absorption is directly proportional to transducer frequency. Therefore, absorption is double for 14 MHz compared with 7 MHz. This increased absorption is the main reason that high-frequency sonography is associated with more shadowing than lower-frequency sonography.

Upon encountering a confusing shadow, a breast imager should initially judge whether the shadow is due to reflection or absorption. After making this decision, you should eliminate or reduce the shadow. If the shadow is due to reflection, then the shadow is due to either the acoustic impedance of the material or the angle of the sound beam. If the shadowing is due to acoustic impedance, you cannot eliminate the shadow but you would have a short list of materials that would produce this shadowing (i.e., air, bone, metal). However, if the shadow is due to the angle of the sound beam, then changing the position of the transducer can eliminate the shadow. Many structures within the breast are curved and create this type of shadow. Pseudomasses may be created by several of these shadows that are close together. To distinguish a true mass from an artificial one, you should routinely study the mass from multiple transducer angles (**Figs. 2.8** and **2.9**).

If the shadow results from absorption, then you should decrease the frequency of the transducer. This technique is useful to better characterize lesions associated with severe shadowing. Both benign and malignant masses appear as areas of focal shadowing. By lowering the transducer frequency, you may reduce or eliminate the shadowing and be able to visualize the lesion causing the shadow. This technique is useful to differentiate scars or highly absorbing fibroglandular tissue from masses. With lower frequency, no mass will be evident with scars or fibroglandular tissue. The main problem associated with this technique is that lower-frequency imaging still has the disadvantages of relatively poor resolution and contrast. You may miss masses because they may blend into the surrounding fibroglandular tissue. Margins and architectural distortion are poorly defined. To avoid missing masses, you should have a high degree of suspicion. Closely examine the area for subtle inhomogeneity and echogenicity (see Cases 6.5 and 7.7).

Even after lowering the frequency, shadowing sometimes persists. In this situation, you should first attempt to discover whether the shadowing is caused by a mass or results from the patient's dense fibroglandular tissue. To differentiate shadowing from these sources, compare the region of interest with normal fibroglandular tissue of the same breast or the opposite breast. Most women have symmetric fibroglandular tissue. Therefore, if the region

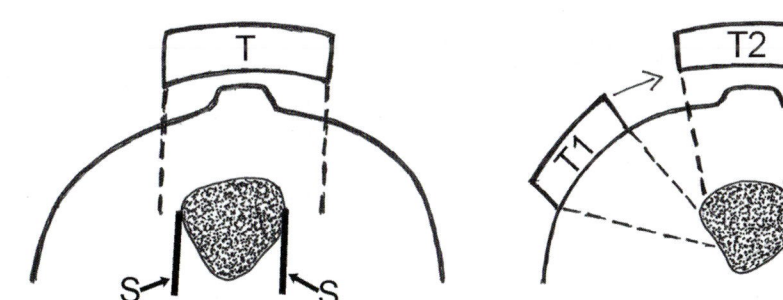

Fig. 2.8 (**A**) Schematic of breast sonogram: when a transducer (T) is positioned over a curved object, the sound at the edges of the object is reflected, so shadowing (S) is produced at the edges of the mass. (**B**) Schematic of breast sonogram: when the transducer (T1–T3) is repositioned around the curved object, shadowing is reduced.

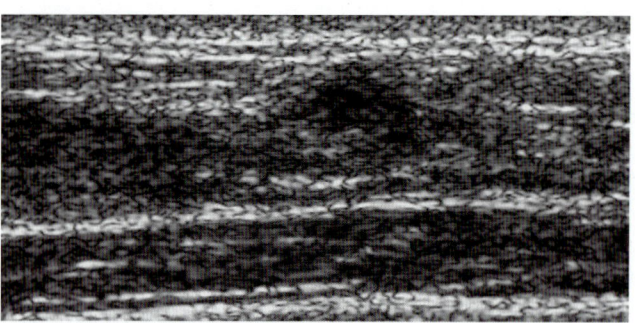 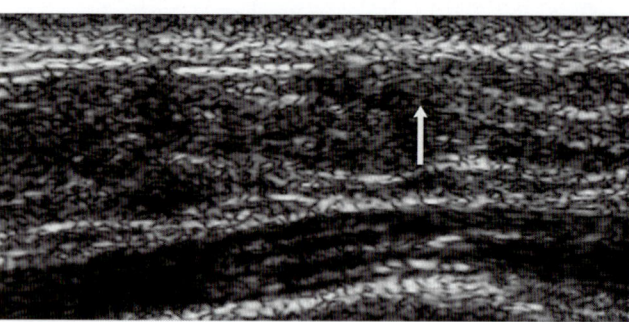

Fig. 2.9 (**A**) This 35-year-old woman presents with a palpable lump. Sonographically, the lump has been found to be an ill-defined hypoechoic mass. The mass is considered suspicious, and biopsy is recommended. The patient returns 2 days later for the biopsy. When the patient returns, the original hypoechoic area is identified (**A**), but by slightly changing the angle of the transducer, the hypoechoic area disappears (**B**). The hypoechoic "mass" represents unusual shadowing from a Cooper's ligament attachment. This attachment is also the etiology of the small, superficial, palpable lump. (**A**) Left radial breast sonogram of a hypoechoic "mass." (**B**) Left radial breast sonogram of the same area as (**A**): pressure on the transducer has slightly changed the sonographic angle. Cooper's ligament attachment (*arrow*).

of interest is in the right upper outer quadrant, then compare this area with the left upper outer quadrant. Or if the patient's mammogram is completely white, compare the region of interest with another area of the same breast. If the normal fibroglandular tissue does not shadow, you should be suspicious that the shadowing represents an active process. If the patient's normal fibroglandular tissue does shadow, try to use a lower frequency in which the fibroglandular tissue appears hyperechoic. You may then use this new lower frequency to evaluate the region of interest.

Finally, if shadowing persists, you should evaluate the appearance of the shadow. Is it focal? Does it persist consistently in multiple angles? Masses that shadow have borders. Therefore, if the shadow has edges that define a focal area, then the shadowing should be considered a suspicious mass.

■ Architectural Distortion and Focal Asymmetric Density

Mammographic architectural distortion and asymmetric density are difficult problems to correlate sonographically. When these findings are present without a mass, they are extremely subtle and commonly visible only in one mammographic view. Because obvious architectural distortion or asymmetry generally may be well characterized with mammography alone, sonography is most valuable when the mammographic findings are uncertain. Therefore, if you are using sonography for this purpose, you should use only high-resolution equipment and be experienced in cross-correlating cases.

The principles for cross-correlating architectural distortion and focal asymmetric density are the same as for a mass. You should match the internal sonographic landmarks to the mammogram. If the area of architectural distortion or focal asymmetry is dark sonographically, suspect a mass (**Fig. 2.10**). Otherwise, the area will appear to be white fibroglandular tissue.

Generally, the sonographic findings are complementary to the mammographic information, so you can be more confident about the final recommendation. However, occasionally, the sonographic and mammographic findings are discordant. In this case, if one of the modalities has information indicating malignancy, then you should recommend biopsy of the abnormality (American College of Radiology Breast Imaging and Data System categories 4 and 5).

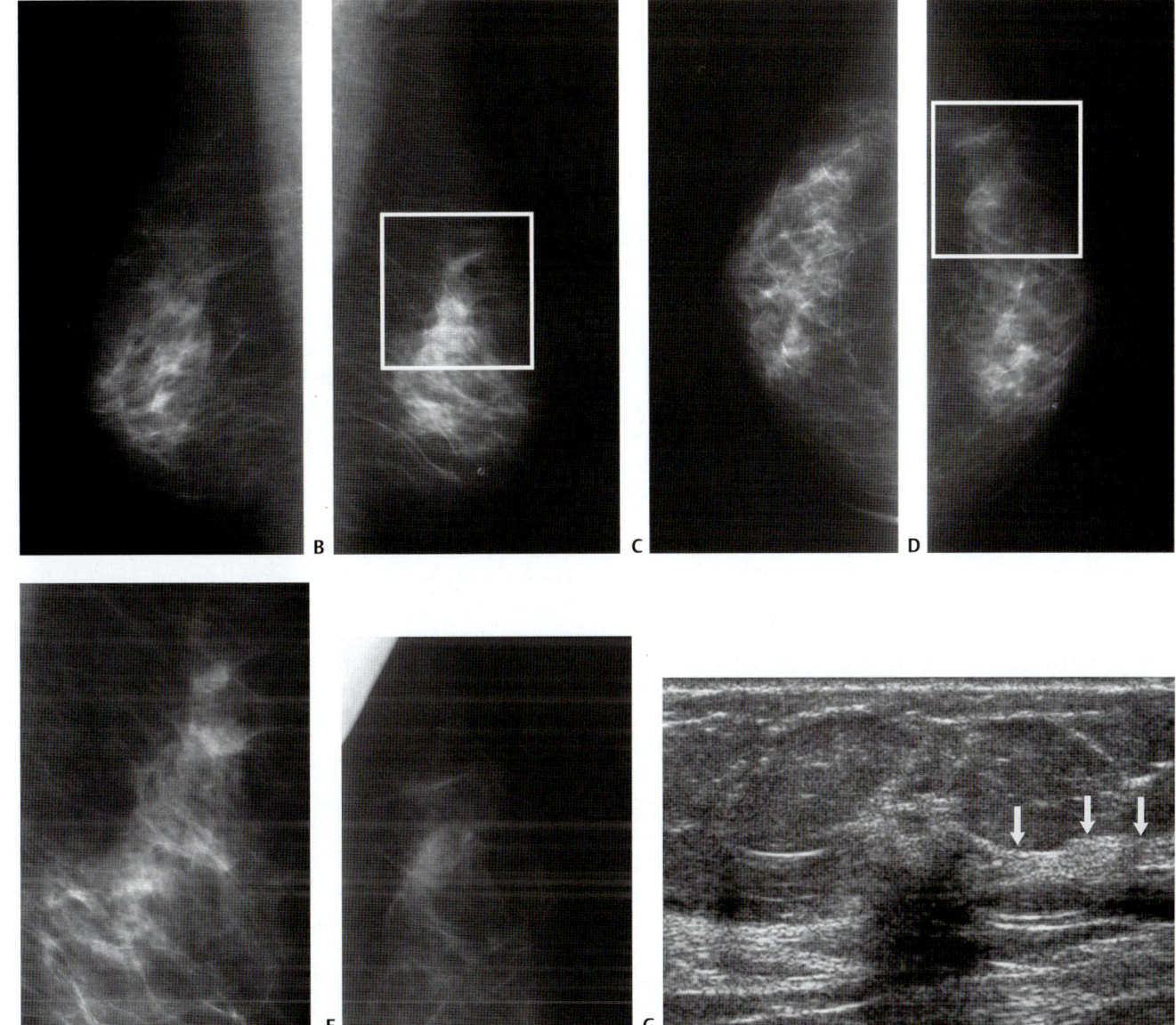

Fig. 2.10 (**A**) Right MLO mammogram. (**B**) Left MLO mammogram. (**C**) Right CC mammogram. (**D**) Left CC mammogram. (**E**) Left MLO spot compression mammogram. (**F**) Left CC spot compression mammogram. (**A–F**) Subtle architectural distortion (*square*) is present in the left upper outer quadrant. The architectural distortion blends into the normal central white fibroglandular density. (**G**) Left radial breast sonogram: sonographic examination of the left upper outer quadrant demonstrates that the architectural distortion corresponds to an irregular hypoechoic mass with shadowing. The mass is connected to hyperechoic tissue (*arrows*) that corresponds to the central mammographic fibroglandular density. The mass is a lobular carcinoma.

3 Approach to Magnetic Resonance Imaging

■ Analyzing the Breast Magnetic Resonance Imaging Scan

Identifying Suspicious Lesions

Similar to mammography, effective evaluation of breast magnetic resonance imaging (MRI) requires an organized approach. The first step involves identifying all possible suspicious lesions. Because suspicious lesions exhibit contrast enhancement, you should review MRI sequences that are produced after contrast injection. Depending on the MRI protocol, these sequences may be T1 fat-suppressed images, maximum intensity projection (MIP) images, or T1 subtracted images in which the image results from subtracting the precontrast image from the postcontrast image. Various MRI computer-aided detection (CAD) systems may also aid in quickly demonstrating potentially suspicious enhancing lesions. Upon identifying suspicious enhancement, you face the first diagnostic decision: does the lesion represent a mass, non-mass enhancement, or a focus? Whereas a mass is a space-occupying lesion, non-mass enhancement represents a pattern of enhancement that does not have a defined three-dimensional shape. In contrast to the mass, the focus represents punctuate enhancement that is too small to be characterized.

If the lesion is a mass, then the next step is to assess if it is benign (American College of Radiology [ACR] Breast Imaging Reporting and Data System [BI-RADS] category 2). The easiest lesions to characterize as benign are masses such as lymph nodes and cysts. If these masses are suspected, review T2 images without fat suppression to search for the fatty hilum of the lymph node and the fluid composition of the cyst. If the mass is not clearly benign, analyze the shape and margin of the mass, preferably on high-resolution images that are produced soon after contrast injection. These characteristics are best identified when the mass reaches maximal enhancement; as the enhancement fades, the margins of the mass may be distorted or indistinct.

Masses with irregular shape or irregular or spiculated margins are either suspicious or highly suspicious (ACR BI-RADS category 4 or 5). Enhancement patterns that increase the suspicious nature of the mass include enhancing septations and central enhancement. Rim enhancement is also a suspicious finding. The most common benign entities that may exhibit rim enhancement are an inflamed cyst and fat necrosis. These abnormalities may be differentiated from malignancy by the appearance of cyst fluid or fat on the T2 non–fat-suppressed image. Masses that exhibit suspicious or highly suspicious morphology should be biopsied no matter what type of kinetic curve the mass exhibits (**Table 3.1**).

For those masses that are not clearly suspicious, kinetic curve analysis is important in determining the final assessment of the mass. Masses that require kinetic curve analysis include those that have round, oval, or lobulated shapes as well as smooth contours. There are three main types of kinetic curves: type I, persistent; type II, plateau; and type III, washout. Type I curves show enhancement that increases throughout the entire observed time course. Type II curves exhibit an early rise in enhancement, then reach a steady state. Type III curves initially demonstrate a rapid increase, reach a peak, then decrease in enhancement (**Fig. 3.1**). Benign lesions tend to exhibit type I curves, and malignant entities commonly demonstrate type II (30%) or III (60%) curves. If the round, oval, lobulated mass with smooth contours exhibits a type I curve, then the mass is assessed as probably benign, and short interval follow-up MRI is recommended (ACR category 3). However, if the mass has a type II or III curve, then the mass is suspicious, and biopsy is recommended (ACR category 4).

If the lesion is not a mass, then the lesion is either a focus or exhibits non-mass enhancement. A focus is generally ≤ 5 mm in size. When there are multiple foci, the pattern of the foci is important. Multiple diffusely scattered, bilateral foci are generally benign. This pattern is most commonly due to fibrocystic changes but is sometimes related to hormonal effects. If foci are distributed in a linear or segmental pattern, the foci may be due to ductal carcinoma in situ. Furthermore, if the multiple foci are close to a dominant malignancy, then these foci are likely to be satellite malignancies.

Single foci are more worrisome than multiple foci. Although these foci are most likely benign (< 3% in one series), if they exhibit a suspicious kinetic curve, they should be biopsied. The differential diagnosis of foci include hormonal enhancement (either physiologic or due to exogenous hormone replacement), fibrocystic change, fibroadenoma, papilloma, radial scar, atypical ductal hyperplasia, lobular carcinoma in situ, ductal carcinoma in situ, and invasive lobular or ductal carcinoma.

Of the non–mass-enhancing descriptions, the most suspicious are ductal and clumped enhancement. Ductal enhancement is linear enhancement that is oriented toward the nipple and conforms to a duct. Clumped enhancement in a focal location looks like a bunch of grapes or, when linear, looks like a string of pearls. When clumped enhancement involves larger areas of the breast, this enhancement pattern looks like cobblestones.

Table 3.1 Summary of the American College of Radiology Breast Imaging Reporting and Data System (BI-RADS) Assessments for MRI Mass or Non-Mass Findings

BI-RADS Assessment	Definition	Examples MRI Findings
Category 2	Benign finding	1. Cyst 2. Fat necrosis 3. Lymph node 4. Mass: oval, round, lobulated shape, and smooth margin with dark septation (fibroadenoma)
Category 3	Probably benign finding; initial short-term interval follow-up suggested	Mass: oval, round, or lobulated shape and smooth margins and homogeneous enhancement and benign kinetic curve (e.g., persistent time course)
Category 4	Suspicious abnormality; biopsy should be considered	1. Mass: oval, round, or lobulated shape and smooth margins and homogeneous enhancement and suspicious kinetic curve (e.g., plateau or washout time course) 2. Mass: irregular shape, irregular margin, persistent kinetic curves 3. Non-mass: segmental enhancement with clumped or ductal enhancement and either persistent or plateau kinetic curves
Category 5	Highly suspicious for malignancy	1. Mass: irregular shape, spiculated margin, and any kinetic curve 2. Mass: irregular shape, irregular margin, and any of the following enhancement patterns: rim (first, rule out fat necrosis and inflammatory cyst), enhancing septations, or central enhancement 3. Mass: irregular shape, irregular margin with rapid enhancement and washout 4. Non-mass: segmental with clumped or ductal internal enhancement with rapid enhancement and washout

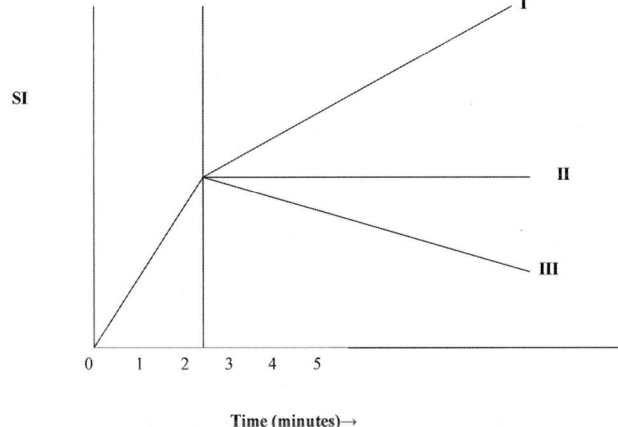

Fig. 3.1 Schematic diagram of contrast enhancement kinetic curves. The diagram illustrates the three types of kinetic curves exhibited by breast masses. Type I is the persistent curve that exhibits increasing enhancement. Type II is the plateau curve that initially increases and then reaches a stable level. Type III is the washout curve that initially increases, reaches a peak level between 2 and 3 minutes, then decreases. Type I curves tend to characterize benign lesions. Malignant masses most commonly produce type II and III curves. SI, signal intensity.

Ductal and clumped enhancements are suspicious because ductal carcinoma in situ commonly presents with these enhancement patterns. Whereas 65 to 70% of MRI detected ductal carcinoma in situ presents as non-mass enhancement, the majority of these non-mass lesions appear as ductal or clumped enhancement. The ductal enhancement may be solitary or in a segmental distribution, and the clumped enhancement may be solitary, linear, ductal, or segmental. Besides ductal carcinoma in situ, the differential diagnosis of clumped enhancement includes fibrocystic change, chronic inflammation, ruptured duct, hemangiomas, papillomas, lobular carcinoma in situ, atypical ductal hyperplasia, and invasive ductal or lobular carcinoma. If invasive malignancy is present, there is commonly an extensive intraductal component.

Technique for "Second Look" Ultrasound on Suspicious Lesions

When a suspicious lesion is identified on MRI, biopsy is required. Because sonographically guided biopsies are less cumbersome and less expensive than MRI-guided biopsies, sonographic evaluation of the breast is commonly performed to identify and biopsy the MRI finding. Because sonography is operator dependent, the results of "second look" ultrasound varies greatly; investigators report success rates of 23 to 100% in sonographically identifying MRI lesions.

The approach of sonographically finding an MRI lesion is similar to the method of cross-correlating sonography and mammography. First, the imager studies the location of the MRI finding and identifies the general quadrant and distance of the abnormality from the nipple. Second, the radiologist reviews non–fat-suppressed images to identify the relationship of the MRI lesion within the fibroglandular parenchyma. Commonly, the lesions are located on the edge of the glandular tissue or are adjacent to other identifiable masses such as cysts or the known malignancy. Finally, the breast radiologist analyzes the MRI findings and determines the most likely sonographic appearance. If the MRI abnormality is a mass, then the sonographic finding will probably be a mass (**Fig. 3.2**). If the MRI lesion is non-

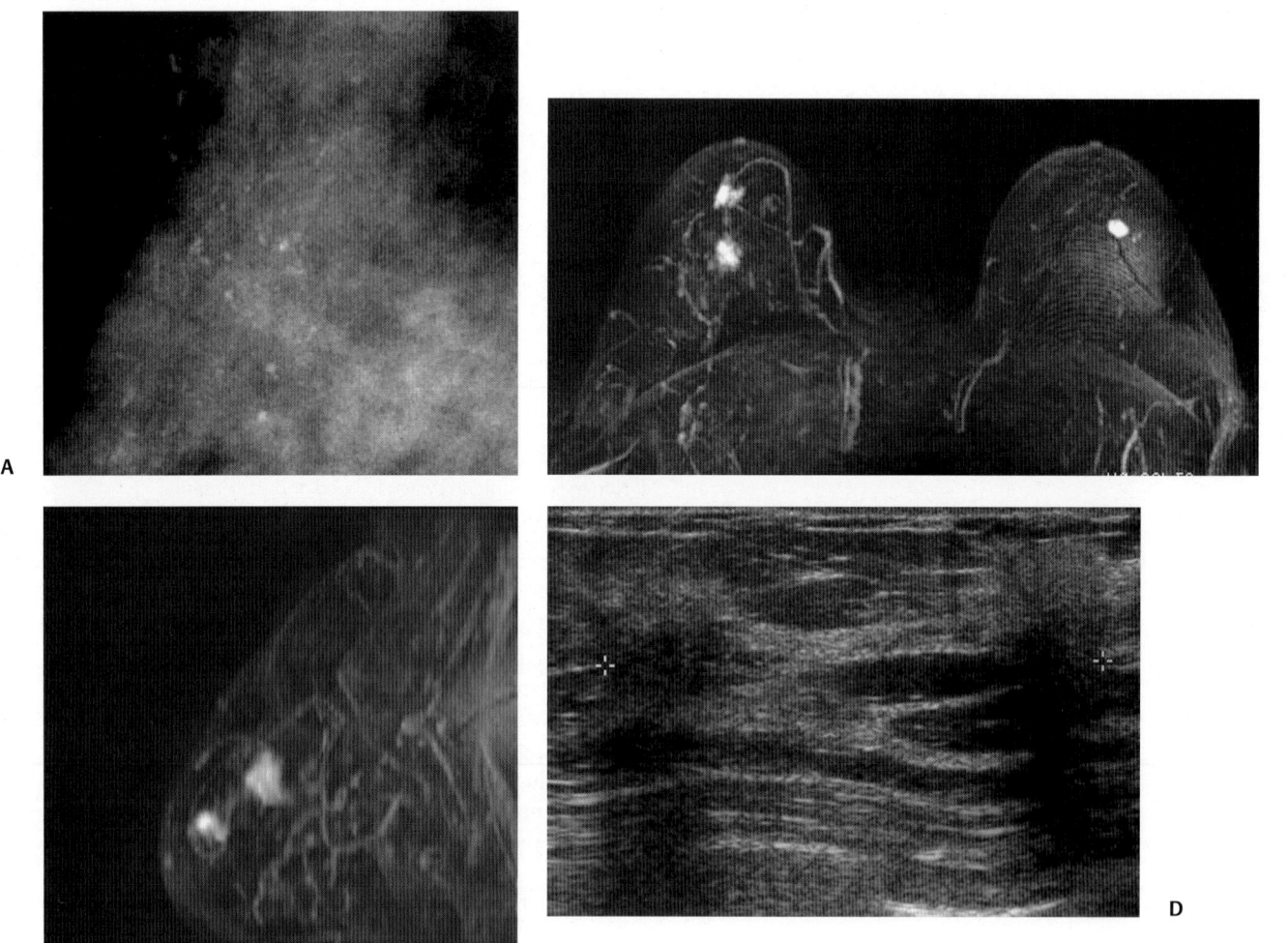

Fig. 3.2 A 47-year-old woman presents for screening mammogram. (**A**) Her right breast mammogram demonstrates a highly suspicious cluster of pleomorphic calcifications at the 12 o'clock position that are found to be due to invasive ductal carcinoma. (**B,C**) She undergoes bilateral breast MRI, which reveals that besides the right known malignancy at the 12 o'clock position, she has two other highly suspicious enhancing MRI masses in the right subareolar region as well as in the left 6 o'clock position. These two additional masses are mammographically occult. (**D,E**) Sonographic examination identifies all three masses. The mammographically occult masses are both invasive ductal carcinoma. This case illustrates the usefulness of MRI in identifying unsuspected right multifocal and contralateral malignancies that altered the treatment of this patient. Furthermore, the sonographic evaluation of the MRI masses resulted in sonographically guided biopsies that are faster and less expensive compared with MRI-guided biopsies. (**A**) Right mediolateral (ML) magnification mammogram. (**B**) Contrast-enhanced axial bilateral breast MRI maximum projection intensity (MIP) image. (**C**) Contrast-enhanced sagittal right breast MRI MIP image. (**D**) Right radial breast sonogram. (**E**) Left radial breast sonogram.

mass enhancement, then the imager searches for ductal carcinoma in situ. Sonographically, ductal carcinoma in situ appears as a solid or cystic mass, abnormal ducts (diffusely or focally dilated ducts, thick-walled ducts, ducts with mass, debris, or calcifications) (see Cases 34.6 and 39.1), or as normal glandular tissue (see Cases 28.14 and 31.3). Color Doppler sometimes aids in identifying the location of the MRI lesion when the glandular tissue appears "normal." If the imager is not confident that the MRI-suspicious abnormality has been identified sonographically, then the lesion must be localized by MRI and biopsied or excised.

Applications of Breast Magnetic Resonance Imaging

Screening High-Risk Women

The American Cancer Society (ACS) has recommended that women with a lifetime risk of greater than 20 to 25% be screened with MRI. On the basis of published studies, patients who meet this criterion include those with a proven *BRCA* mutation, an untested first-degree relative of a *BRCA* carrier, or a woman with a risk assessment calculated from standard clinical programs such as the Gail, Claus, and Tyrer-Cusick models. These clinical models are useful to assess patients with strong family histories but no documented genetic mutation. The ACS consensus expert panel also recommends that other high-risk groups should also be included in MRI screening: women who have had chest radiation between the ages of 10 and 30 years, women with Li-Fraumeni syndrome or first-degree relatives with the syndrome, and women with Cowden and Bannayan-Riley-Ruvalcaba syndromes or first-degree relatives with the syndromes. The Li-Fraumeni syndrome is an autosomal dominant disease associated with increased risk of sarcoma and breast and brain cancers. Cowden and Bannayan-Riley-Ruvalcaba syndromes are genetically related autosomal dominant diseases with increased risk of breast, thyroid, and skin cancers.

Define the Extent of Disease

Once a patient has been found to have breast cancer, MRI has been shown to be a better method to define the extent of disease compared with mammography. In the ipsilateral breast, studies have found that MRI identifies 6 to 34% additional malignant sites that are occult to mammography and physical exam. Furthermore, MRI demonstrates 1 to 20% additional malignant sites in the same quadrant as the known primary malignancy and 2 to 24% more tumors in quadrants other than the known primary (**Fig. 3.2**).

MRI is particularly useful for lobular cancer because this malignancy has been found to be associated with multicentric disease more often than is invasive ductal cancer. Memorial Sloan-Kettering Cancer Center reported that of 62 patients with lobular cancer, MRI identified 11 additional malignancies in the ipsilateral breast and 5 malignancies in the contralateral breast. The improved MRI identification of additional malignancies has been shown to alter treatment of lobular cancer.

Identifying Residual or Recurrent Disease

Immediately after breast conservation surgery, the lumpectomy site normally exhibits a smooth enhancing wall that is generally ≤ 4 mm in thickness. Factors that increase the risk of residual disease include microscopic close or positive margins, young age, and extensive intraductal component. Investigators have found that MRI has an accuracy of 88% in identifying residual disease. Because postoperative changes may mask residual disease, the optimum time for MRI examination is approximately 1 month after the surgical procedure. Usually a normal MRI 18 months after the surgical procedure appears to exclude recurrence because new enhancement only rarely occurs after that time.

Assessing Response to Therapy

MRI is an excellent method to determine response to neoadjuvant therapy. Although early articles indicated that MRI underestimates tumor size and therefore overestimates response to treatment, more recent studies have shown excellent correlation between MRI tumor size and microscopic examination. Tumor size correlation coefficients between MRI and histology are reported between 0.89 and 0.97. Belli and coworkers[1] report that MRI sensitivity and specificity for detecting residual disease are 90.5 and 100%, respectively. The difference between these recent reports and other reports is that these researchers have relaxed the criteria for determining malignancy on posttreatment MRI studies compared with pretreatment exams. For posttreatment lesions, residual malignancy is defined as any tissue, within the region of previous tumor, with enhancement greater than normal parenchyma. This alteration in diagnostic criteria is in response to the observation that malignant tissue that is altered by chemotherapy exhibits less rapid and lower peak enhancement compared with untreated malignancy. When posttreatment malignancies are measured using the same criteria as pretreatment tumors, MRI overestimates the number of patients with complete response.

Identifying an Unknown Primary

MRI may be useful in identifying a primary breast malignancy for women who present with metastatic adenopathy and no detectable mammographic malignancy. Although conclusive identification of the primary malignancy is helpful for tailoring treatment in patients with advanced stage IV disease, diagnosis is particularly important if the patient has stage II disease and is a candidate for breast

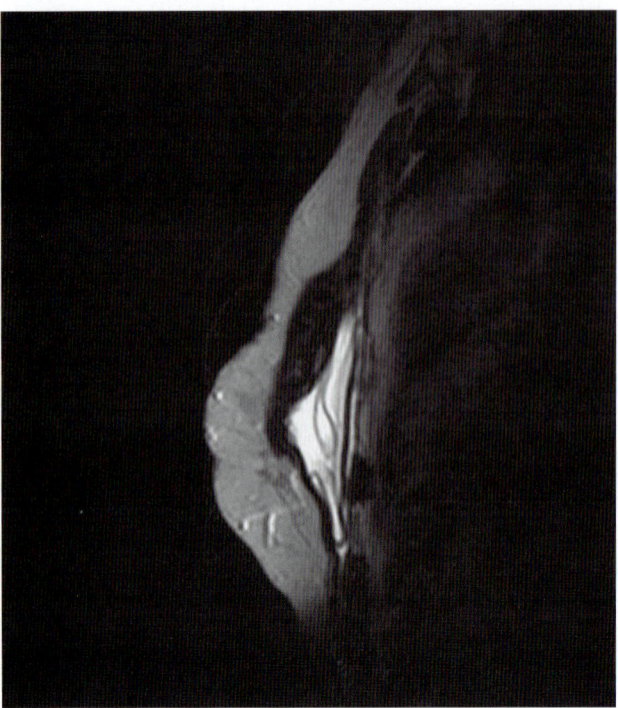

Fig. 3.3 T2-weighted left sagittal breast MRI. A 51-year-old woman is 16 years status post–left partial mastectomy for breast cancer with reconstruction using a subpectoral implant. Her left breast has now decreased in size. Left breast MRI demonstrates that the implant has ruptured and the elastomeric shell has collapsed and formed the linguini sign.

conservation. Because this clinical circumstance is rare, reported studies are small or only in abstract form. Sloan-Kettering reported 69 patients with primary breast cancer that was occult to mammography and physical exam. Of these patients, 55 had metastatic axillary adenopathy (stage II disease), and 14 presented with stage IV disease.

MRI correctly identified the primary malignancy in 26/55 (47%) with stage II and 7/14 (50%) with stage IV disease.

Identifying Breast Implant Rupture

Identification of breast implant rupture is one of the oldest applications of MRI. MRI has been shown to be superior to mammography, sonography, and computed tomography (CT) in demonstrating implant rupture, with sensitivities of 72 to 94% and specificities of 85 to 100%. The most reliable MRI findings of implant rupture are the "linguini" sign, which represents collapse of the gel-filled implant (**Fig. 3.3**), and free silicone, which occurs when the fibrous capsule ruptures.

Since the 1960s, there have been at least three generations of silicone gel implants. Each of these generations presents with slightly different MRI findings. The first- and second-generation implants manufactured from 1960 to the late-1980s present commonly with either the linguini sign or the "teardrop" sign. The teardrop sign results when the elastomeric shell is torn but does not collapse. Silicone leaks outside this shell and fills the space around a radial fold. Third-generation implants, used since the late 1980s, have a multilayer shell and thick silicone gel. These implant shells generally do not collapse, so they generally do not present with the linguini sign. Instead, they generally present with the teardrop sign.

■ Conclusion

The volume of breast MRI examinations has greatly increased due to expansion of MRI clinical applications. These additional applications challenge breast imagers to develop efficient, accurate approaches to identifying and assessing MRI lesions. Familiarity with MRI findings is the key to successfully handling these complex cases.

Reference

1. Belli P, Costantini M, Malaspina C, Magistrelli A, Latorre G, Bonomo L. MRI accuracy in residual disease evaluation in breast cancer patients treated with neoadjuvant chemotherapy. Clin Radiol 2006; 61:946–953

Suggested Reading

American College of Radiology (ACR). ACR Breast Imaging Reporting and Data System (BI-RADS)—magnetic resonance imaging. In: Breast Imaging Reporting and Data System, Breast Imaging Atlas. Reston, VA: American College of Radiology; 2003

Berg WA, Caskey CI, Hamper UM, et al. Diagnosing breast implant rupture with MR imaging, US, and mammography. Radiographics 1993;13:1323–1336

Berg WA, Caskey CI, Hamper UM, et al. Single- and double-lumen silicone breast implant integrity: prospective evaluation of MR and US criteria. Radiology 1995;197:45–52

Berg WA, Nguyen TK, Middleton MS, Soo MS, Pennello G, Brown SL. MR imaging of extracapsular silicone from breast implants: diagnostic pitfalls. AJR Am J Roentgenol 2002;178:465–472

Buchanan CL, Morris EA, Dorn PL, Borgen PI, Van Zee KJ. Utility of breast magnetic resonance imaging in patients with occult primary breast cancer. Ann Surg Oncol 2005;12:1045–1053

Gökalp G, Topal U. MR imaging in probably benign lesions (BI-RADS category 3) of the breast. Eur J Radiol 2006;57:436–444

Gorczyca DP, Gorczyca SM, Gorczyca KL. The diagnosis of silicone breast implant rupture. Plast Reconstr Surg 2007;120(7, Suppl 1):49S–61S

Hashimoto BE, Morgan GN, Kramer DJ, Lee ME. Systematic approach to difficult problems in breast sonography. Ultrasound Q 2008;24:31–38

Ikeda DM, Hylton NM, Kinkel K, et al. Development, standardization, and testing of a lexicon for reporting contrast-enhanced breast magnetic resonance imaging studies. J Magn Reson Imaging 2001;13:889–895

Kim SJ, Morris EA, Liberman L, et al. Observer variability and applicability of BI-RADS terminology for breast MR imaging: invasive carcinomas as focal masses. AJR Am J Roentgenol 2001;177:551–557

Kinkel K, Helbich TH, Esserman LJ, et al. Dynamic high-spatial-resolution MR imaging of suspicious breast lesions: diagnostic criteria and interobserver variability. AJR Am J Roentgenol 2000;175:35–43

Kuhl CK. Dynamic breast magnetic resonance imaging. In: Morris EA, Liberman L, eds. Breast MRI Diagnosis and Intervention. New York: Springer; 2005:79–139

Kuhl CK, Mielcareck P, Klaschik S, et al. Dynamic breast MR imaging: are signal intensity time course data useful for differential diagnosis of enhancing lesions? Radiology 1999;211:101–110

Lee CH, Smith RC, Levine JA, Troiano RN, Tocino I. Clinical usefulness of MR imaging of the breast in the evaluation of the problematic mammogram. AJR Am J Roentgenol 1999;173:1323–1329

Liberman L, Morris EA, Benton CL, Abramson AF, Dershaw DD. Probably benign lesions at breast magnetic resonance imaging: preliminary experience in high-risk women. Cancer 2003;98:377–388

Liberman L, Morris EA, Dershaw DD, Abramson AF, Tan LK. Ductal enhancement on MR imaging of the breast. AJR Am J Roentgenol 2003;181:519–525

Liberman L, Morris EA, Lee MJ-Y, et al. Breast lesions detected on MR imaging: features and positive predictive value. AJR Am J Roentgenol 2002;179:171–178

Macura KJ, Ouwerkerk R, Jacobs MA, Bluemke DA. Patterns of enhancement on breast MR images: interpretation and imaging pitfalls. Radiographics 2006;26:1719–1734, quiz 1719

Morris EA. Breast cancer imaging with MRI. Radiol Clin North Am 2002;40:443–466

Morris EA, Schwartz LH, Dershaw DD, van Zee KJ, Abramson AF, Liberman L. MR imaging of the breast in patients with occult primary breast carcinoma. Radiology 1997;205:437–440

Nunes LW, Schnall MD, Orel SG, et al. Breast MR imaging: interpretation model. Radiology 1997;202:833–841

Nunes LW, Schnall MD, Siegelman ES, et al. Diagnostic performance characteristics of architectural features revealed by high spatial-resolution MR imaging of the breast. AJR Am J Roentgenol 1997;169:409–415

Orel SG, Schnall MD, LiVolsi VA, Troupin RH. Suspicious breast lesions: MR imaging with radiologic-pathologic correlation. Radiology 1994;190:485–493

Partridge SC, Gibbs JE, Lu Y, Esserman LJ, Sudilovsky D, Hylton NM. Accuracy of MR imaging for revealing residual breast cancer in patients who have undergone neoadjuvant chemotherapy. AJR Am J Roentgenol 2002;179:1193–1199

Rieber A, Brambs H-J, Gabelmann A, Heilmann V, Kreienberg R, Kühn T. Breast MRI for monitoring response of primary breast cancer to neoadjuvant chemotherapy. Eur Radiol 2002;12:1711–1719

Rieber A, Zeitler H, Rosenthal H, et al. MRI of breast cancer: influence of chemotherapy on sensitivity. Br J Radiol 1997;70:452–458

Saslow D, Boetes C, Burke W, et al; American Cancer Society Breast Cancer Advisory Group. American Cancer Society guidelines for breast screening with MRI as an adjunct to mammography. CA Cancer J Clin 2007;57:75–89

Schnall MD, Blume J, Bluemke DA, et al. Diagnostic architectural and dynamic features at breast MR imaging: multicenter study. Radiology 2006;238:42–53

Sherif H, Mahfouz A-E, Oellinger H, et al. Peripheral washout sign on contrast-enhanced MR images of the breast. Radiology 1997;205:209–213

Tozaki M, Igarashi T, Matsushima S, Fukuda K. High-spatial-resolution MR imaging of focal breast masses: interpretation model based on kinetic and morphological parameters. Radiat Med 2005;23:43–50

Weatherall PT, Evans GF, Metzger GJ, Saborrian MH, Leitch AM. MRI vs. histologic measurement of breast cancer following chemotherapy: comparison with x-ray mammography and palpation. J Magn Reson Imaging 2001;13:868–875

Wedegärtner U, Bick U, Wörtler K, Rummeny E, Bongartz G. Differentiation between benign and malignant findings on MR-mammography: usefulness of morphological criteria. Eur Radiol 2001;11:1645–1650

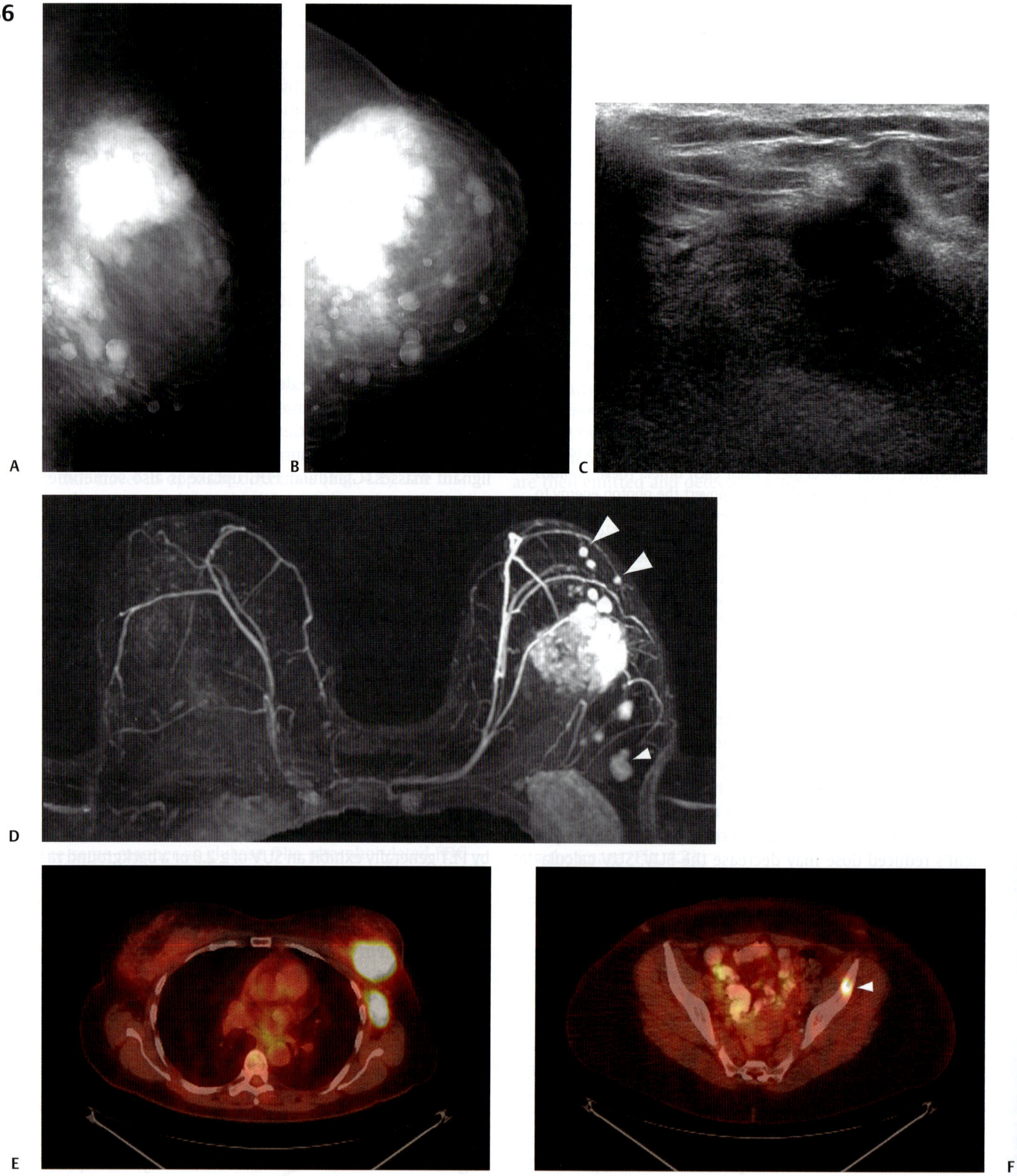

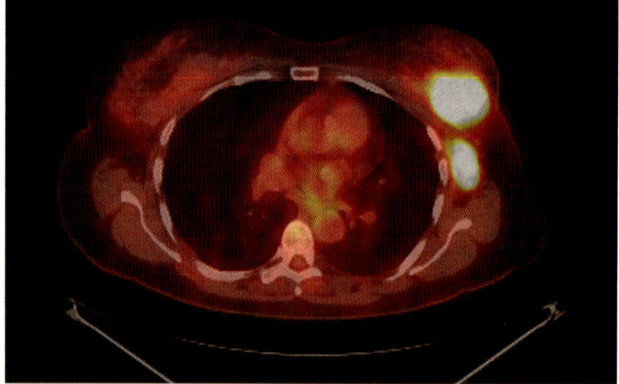

Fig. 4.3 PET-CT staging breast cancer. A 65-year-old woman presents with a palpable left breast lump. Forty years earlier she had silicone injections for breast augmentation. Her left mammograms (**A,B**) and ultrasound (**C**) demonstrate extensive free silicone with a large irregular mass that corresponds to the palpable lump. This mass is biopsied and is invasive ductal carcinoma. (**D**) Bilateral breast MRI shows left axillary adenopathy and multiple highly suspicious satellite masses associated with the large irregular known malignancy. PET-CT is performed to identify any distant metastases. (**E**) Besides the large breast malignancy and axillary adenopathy, PET-CT reveals abnormal uptake in the left iliac wing (**F**), which subsequent biopsy demonstrates is metastatic adenocarcinoma. After 6 months of chemotherapy, the patient has left mastectomy and axillary dissection, which demonstrates a residual 5 cm invasive ductal cancer with metastatic disease to 6 of 16 axillary nodes. (**A**) Left mediolateral oblique (MLO) mammogram. (**B**) Left craniocaudal (CC) mammogram. (**C**) Left breast ultrasound. (**D**) Bilateral contrast-enhanced breast MRI maximum projection intensity (MIP) image (*large arrowheads*, satellite masses; *small arrowhead*, axillary adenopathy). (**E**) Axial PET-CT of the chest. (**F**) Axial PET-CT of the pelvis (*large arrowhead*, iliac metastasis).

Identification of Recurrent Malignancy

PET is useful when a patient is suspected of having recurrent breast cancer (**Figs. 4.4** and **4.5**). PET is better than CT or MRI in differentiating local recurrence from postoperative changes. Furthermore, PET identifies metastatic disease to the axillary, supraclavicular, mediastinal, and internal mammary nodes. In patients with locally advanced disease, PET has been shown to identify distant metastatic disease better than does conventional imaging involving chest x-ray, bone scan, liver ultrasound, or CT. Eight percent of patients with distant metastases were identified by PET but not with conventional imaging.

Response to Therapy

PET provides valuable prognostic information for patients being treated for breast cancer. Patients with a primary breast tumor with an SUV ≥ 3.0 are found to have poor prognosis for survival. When PET is used to follow response to chemotherapy, an SUV reduction of ≥ 55% after the first cycle of chemotherapy has been associated with a good response to therapy.

Pitfalls and Limitations

To understand the role of PET in breast cancer imaging, one must be aware of the limitations of this modality. The main limitations include poor size resolution, nonspecific FDG uptake, relative insensitivity to certain breast histologies, lower sensitivity compared with other techniques for selective metastatic locations, and benign conditions that increase FDG uptake. PET is not sensitive for malignancies < 1 cm, and PET generally does not identify breast cancers < 0.5 cm. Therefore, this modality is not a good tool to screen for breast cancer, and it may miss small malignant breast satellite lesions. Furthermore, PET is less sensitive than MRI for multifocal disease. Therefore, PET is less useful to stage patients with small T1 primary tumors because they have a small chance of additional bulky disease.

Because increased FDG is associated with any condition that increases glucose metabolism, FDG is not specific for neoplasm. Inflammatory or infectious conditions such as mastitis or traumatic breast injury result in increased FDG uptake. Furthermore, benign tumors such as duct adenomas and occasionally fibroadenomas may exhibit increased FDG activity. In general, fibroadenomas usually do not exhibit increased FDG uptake.

For staging, PET is not as sensitive as other methods in identifying certain types of metastatic disease. For example, PET is not as sensitive as axillary lymph node dissection in identifying metastatic axillary malignancy, so this modality cannot replace lymph node dissection for staging. Overall, PET has similar sensitivity and specificity to bone scan for all metastatic bone disease. However, whereas PET is more sensitive than bone scan for osteolytic metastases, bone scan is more sensitive for osteoblastic metastases.

Finally, certain nonmalignant conditions produce increased FDG uptake. One confusing normal variant is FDG uptake in brown fat (see Case 40.3). The body has two types of fat: white fat and brown fat. White fat stores energy, and brown fat produces heat. FDG uptake in brown fat can appear similar to metastatic adenopathy. Although the SUV may be very high within brown fat, the observer can usually identify the benign etiology by the pattern of uptake. PET-CT is particularly useful in this situation because no

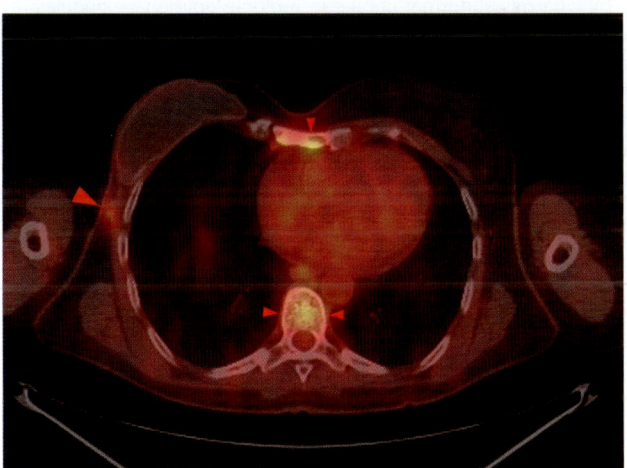

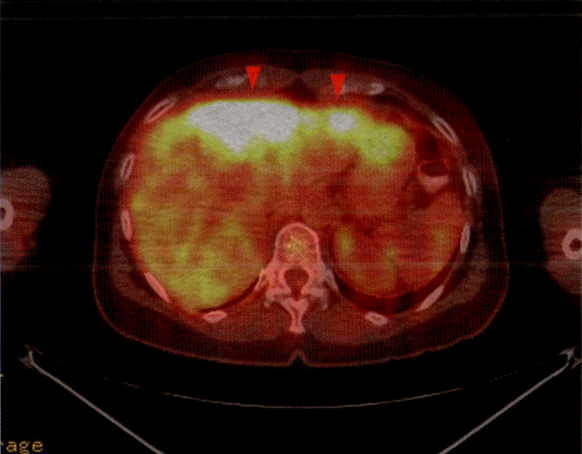

Fig. 4.4 PET-CT for recurrent cancer. A 54-year-old woman presents with left arm pain. Eight years earlier, she had a right mastectomy and axillary for stage II breast cancer with two positive axillary nodes. A bone scan shows abnormal humeral and sternal uptake. PET-CT demonstrates abnormal uptake in the sternum, thoracic spine, right axilla, and liver. In this case, PET-CT is more helpful than bone scan because PET-CT reveals metastatic disease in a wider variety of sites. (**A**) Axial PET-CT of the chest (*large arrowhead*, axillary node; *single small arrowhead*, abnormal sternal uptake; *double small arrowheads*, abnormal thoracic spine uptake). (**B**) Axial PET-CT of abdomen (*arrowheads*, liver metastases).

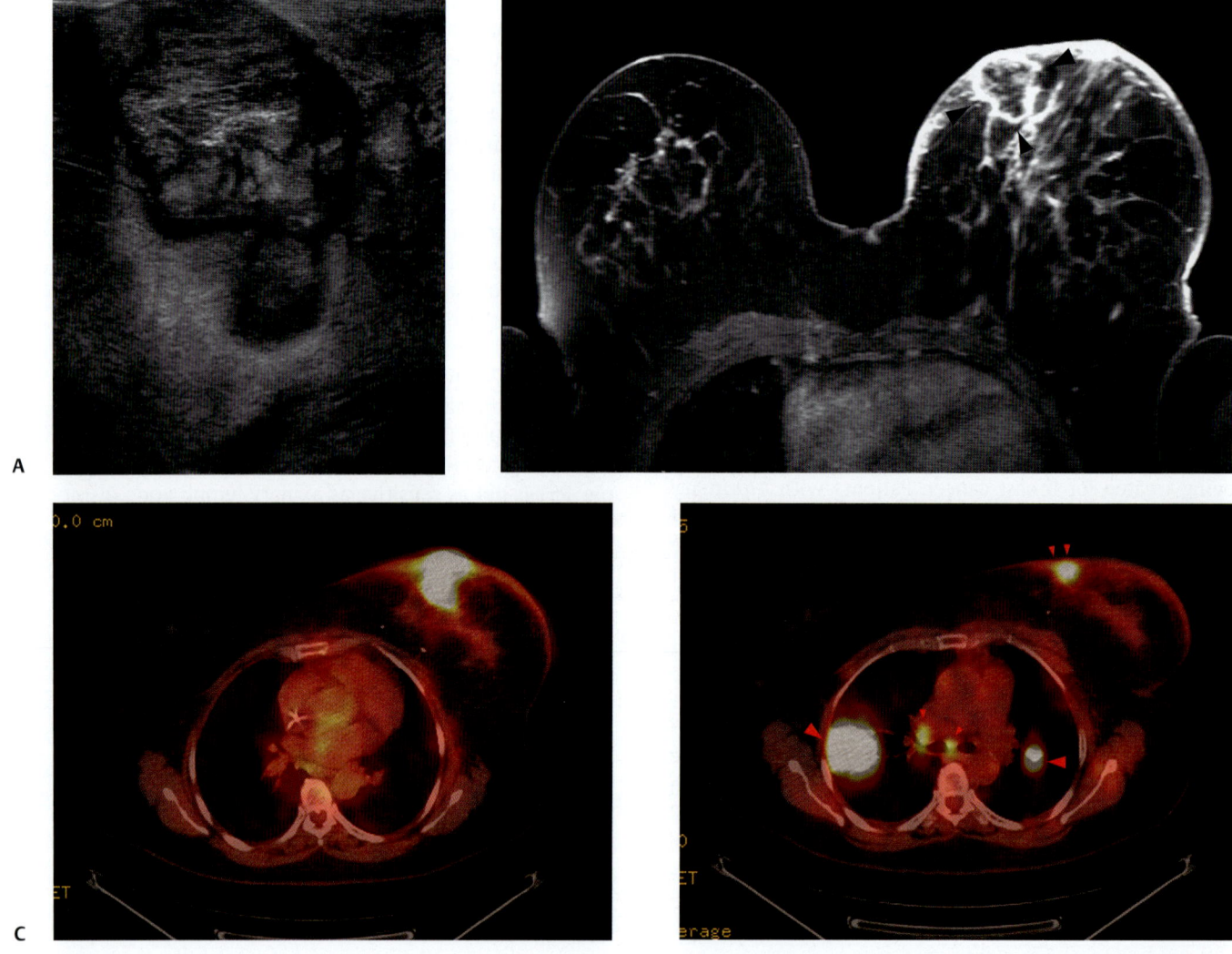

Fig. 4.5 PET-CT for recurrent cancer. A 56-year-old woman presents with increasing pain in her lumpectomy site. Three months earlier, she had a partial mastectomy with widely clear margins for a 4 cm high-grade invasive ductal cancer with three positive axillary nodes. (**A**) Sonographic examination of the lumpectomy site demonstrates a heterogeneous mass, which was biopsied and found to be malignant. (**B**) Clinically, the patient appears to have inflammatory breast recurrence. MRI shows a malignant rim-enhancing mass with edema associated with trabecular thickening, reticular, dendritic enhancement, and enhancing skin. (**C**) Besides the breast mass and skin thickening, (**D**) PET-CT reveals abnormal uptake in multiple pulmonary nodules, as well as hilar and mediastinal nodes. (**A**) Left breast sonogram. (**B**) Bilateral contrast-enhanced axial breast high-resolution MRI (*arrowheads*, rim-enhancing mass). (**C**) Axial PET-CT of the chest demonstrating the inflammatory left breast malignancy. (**D**) Axial PET-CT of the chest (*large arrowhead*, pulmonary nodules; *small arrowheads*, mediastinal and hilar adenopathy; *double small arrowheads*, breast malignancy).

adenopathy will be present on the CT. Another nonmalignant cause for increased uptake is treatment with granulocyte colony-stimulating factors (see Case 40.4). This therapy causes an increase in bone marrow production of cells, which increases the uptake of FDG in the skeleton. This increased activity simulates diffuse bone metastases.

■ Conclusion

PET-CT is a valuable tool for breast cancer imaging. Even though PET-CT is less sensitive to small malignancies, PET-CT is valuable for staging patients with larger primary tumors who have a high risk of metastatic malignancy and for following patients during chemotherapy. In addition, FDG activity provides valuable physiologic information that is not available from the other anatomical imaging modalities, such as mammography, ultrasound, and MRI. This physiologic information results in PET-CT's ability to differentiate malignant recurrence from surgical scar.

Suggested Reading

Avril N, Rosé CA, Schelling M, et al. Breast imaging with positron emission tomography and fluorine-18 fluorodeoxyglucose: use and limitations. J Clin Oncol 2000;18:3495–3502

Hicks RJ, Binns D, Stabin MG. Pattern of uptake and excretion of (18)F-FDG in the lactating breast. J Nucl Med 2001;42:1238–1242

Hollinger EF, Alibazoglu H, Ali A, Green A, Lamonica G. Hematopoietic cytokine-mediated FDG uptake simulates the appearance of diffuse metastatic disease on whole-body PET imaging. Clin Nucl Med 1998;23:93–98

Kostakoglu L, Goldsmith SJ. 18F-FDG PET evaluation of the response to therapy for lymphoma and for breast, lung, and colorectal carcinoma. J Nucl Med 2003;44:224–239

Lin EC, Abass A. Patient preparation. In: Lin EC, Abass A, eds. PET and PET/CT. New York: Thieme; 2005:23–27

Lin EC, Abass A, Lee M. Breast cancer. In: Lin EC, Abass A, eds. PET and PET/CT. New York: Thieme; 2005:112–121

Mason NS, Lin EC. In: Lin EC, Abass A, eds. PET and PET/CT. New York: Thieme; 2005:15–20

Nakai T, Okuyama C, Kubota T, et al. Pitfalls of FDG-PET for the diagnosis of osteoblastic bone metastases in patients with breast cancer. Eur J Nucl Med Mol Imaging 2005;32:1253–1258

Schmitz R, Allessio A, Kinahan P. The physics of PET/CT scanners. In: Lin EC, Abass A, eds. PET and PET/CT. New York: Thieme; 2005:15–20

Thie JA. Understanding the standardized uptake value, its methods, and implications for usage. J Nucl Med 2004;45:1431–1434

Truong MT, Erasmus JJ, Munden RF, et al. Focal FDG uptake in mediastinal brown fat mimicking malignancy: a potential pitfall resolved on PET/CT. AJR Am J Roentgenol 2004;183:1127–1132

van der Hoeven JJM, Krak NC, Hoekstra OS, et al. 18F-2-fluoro-2-deoxy-D-glucose positron emission tomography in staging of locally advanced breast cancer. J Clin Oncol 2004;22:1253–1259

Vranjesevic D, Schiepers C, Silverman DH, et al. Relationship between 18F-FDG uptake and breast density in women with normal breast tissue. J Nucl Med 2003;44:1238–1242

Wahl RL, Siegel BA, Coleman RE, Gatsonis CG; PET Study Group. Prospective multicenter study of axillary nodal staging by positron emission tomography in breast cancer: a report of the staging breast cancer with PET Study Group. J Clin Oncol 2004;22:277–285

Yeung HW, Grewal RK, Gonen M, Schöder H, Larson SM. Patterns of (18)F-FDG uptake in adipose tissue and muscle: a potential source of false-positives for PET. J Nucl Med 2003;44:1789–1796

Zimny M, Siggelkow W. Positron emission tomography scanning in gynecologic and breast cancers. Curr Opin Obstet Gynecol 2003;15:69–75

Circumscribed Masses

This is a schematic diagram of the diagnostic approach to mammographic circumscribed masses. For further discussion, see Chapter 1.

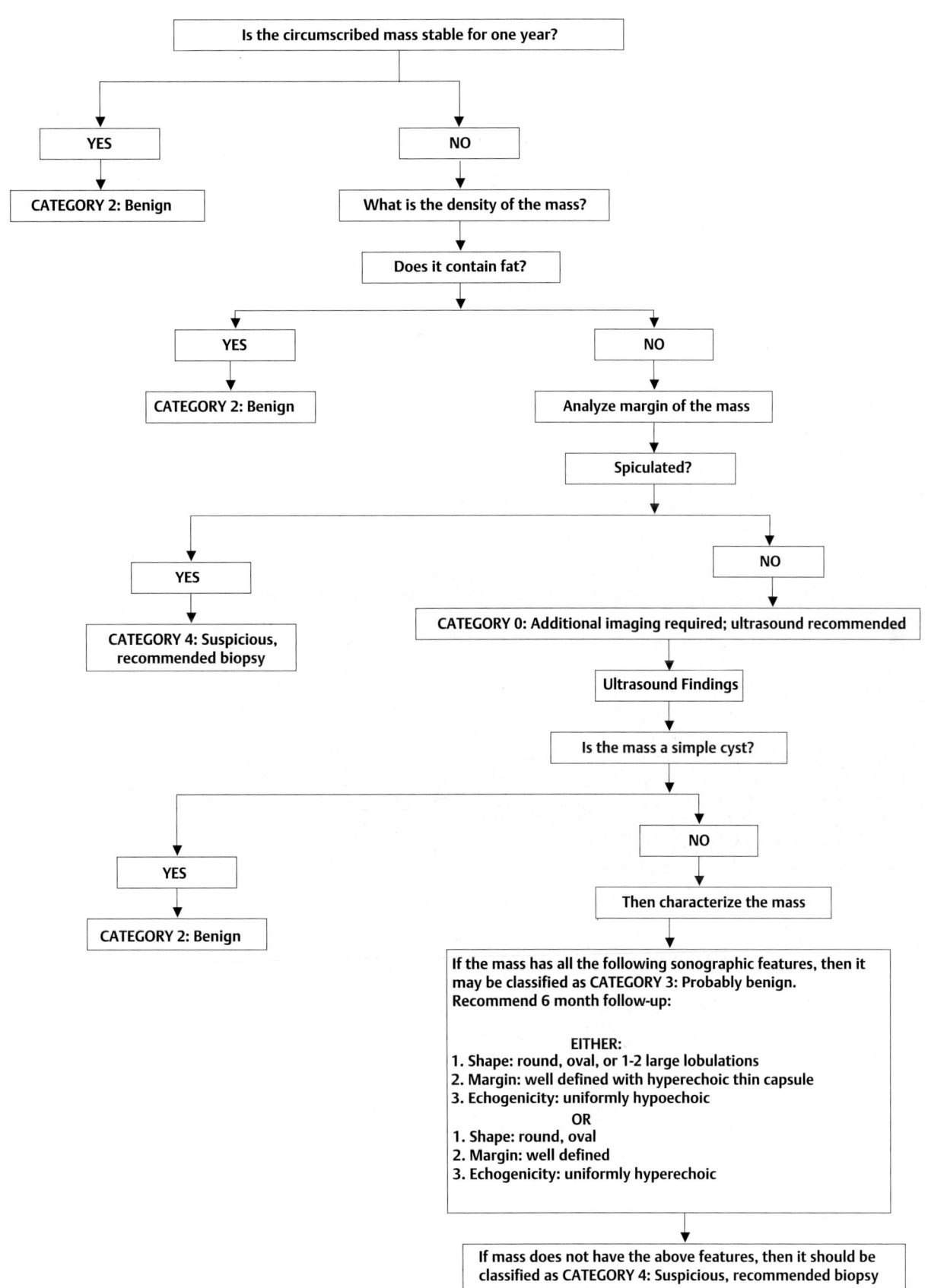

5 Circumscribed Masses: Fat-Containing Masses

■ Case 5.1 Galactocele

Case History

A 39-year-old woman has just stopped breast-feeding her 10-month-old infant and now finds a new breast lump.

Physical Examination

- Left breast: 3 cm lump in the upper outer quadrant
- Right breast: normal exam

Mammogram

Mass (Fig. 5.1)
- Margin: circumscribed
- Shape: oval
- Density: fat-containing

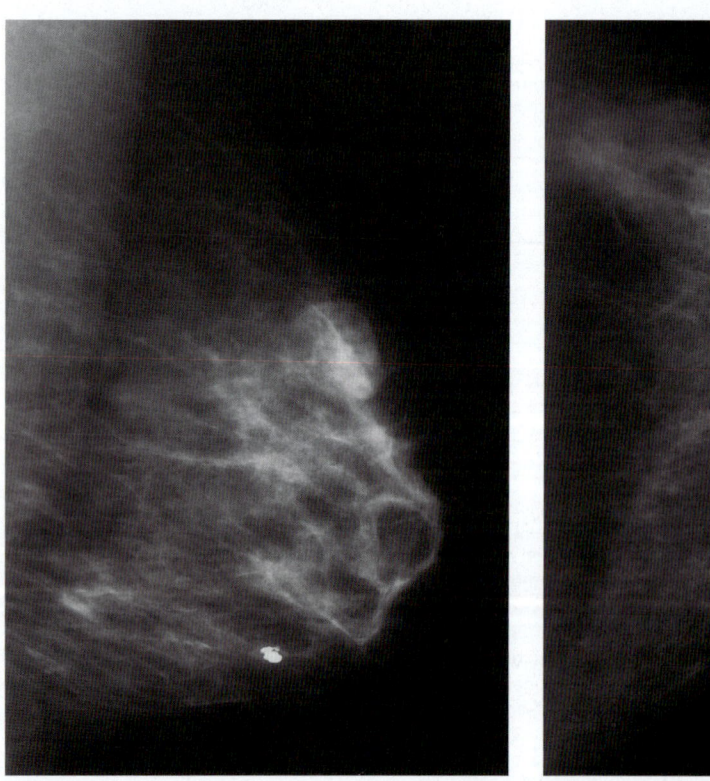
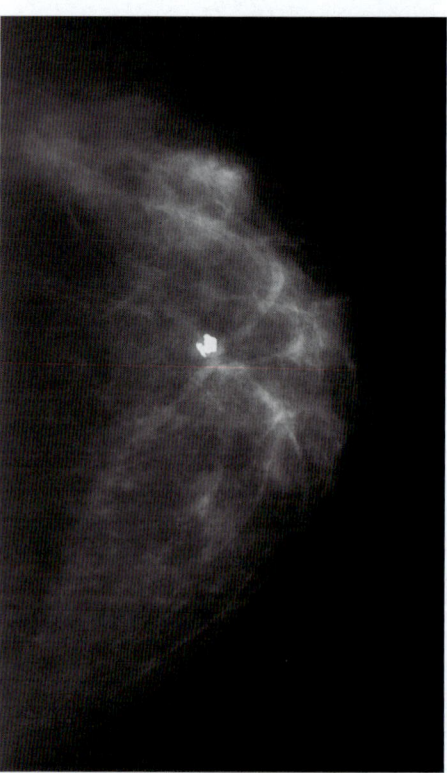

Fig. 5.1 In the upper outer quadrant of the left breast, there is a well-defined oval mass. (**A**) Left mediolateral oblique (MLO) mammogram. (**B**) Left craniocaudal (CC) mammogram.

Ultrasound

Frequency
- 10 MHz

Mass
- Margin: well defined
- Echogenicity: isoechoic
- Retrotumoral acoustic appearance: single edge shadowing
- Shape: ellipsoid (**Fig. 5.2**)

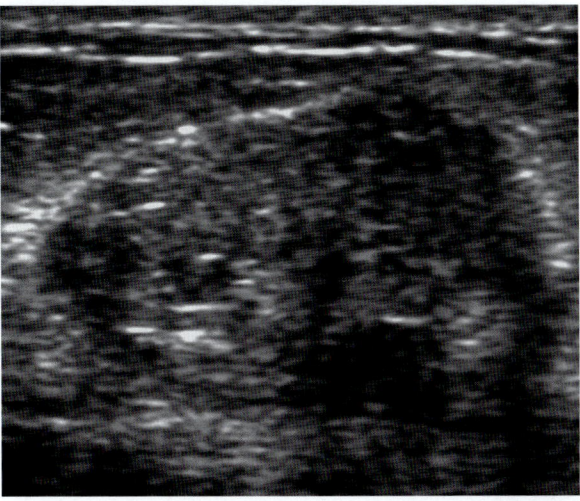

Fig. 5.2 Left radial breast sonogram. The mammographic mass identified in **Fig. 5.1** corresponds to a well-defined mass with heterogeneous echogenicity. Milky fluid was aspirated from this mass.

Pathology
- Galactocele

Management
- Breast Imaging Reporting and Data System (BI-RADS) assessment category 2, benign finding

Pearls and Pitfalls
- Galactoceles are benign milk-filled cysts. This lesion is generally discovered either during or shortly after lactation. Mammographically, galactoceles are well-defined and oval and may appear to be completely fat density, heterogeneous density, or equal density to glandular parenchyma.
- Sonographically, galactoceles are hypoechoic, isoechoic, or heterogeneous in echogenicity. Fluid debris levels may be present.

Suggested Reading
Jackson VP, Jahan R, Fu YS. Benign breast lesions. In: Bassett LW, Jackson VP, Jahan R, Fu YS, Gold RH, eds. Diagnosis of Diseases of the Breast. Philadelphia: WB Saunders; 1997:357–443

Salvador R, Salvador M, Jimenez JA, Martinez M, Casas L. Galactocele of the breast: radiologic and ultrasonographic findings. Br J Radiol 1990;63:140–142

Case 5.2 Hamartoma

Case History

A 39-year-old woman presents with a new left breast lump. Left breast sonography is initially performed. As a result of the sonogram, a mammogram has been done.

Physical Examination
- Left breast: 5 cm palpable lump in the upper inner quadrant
- Right breast: normal exam

Mammogram

Mass (Fig. 5.3)
- Margin: circumscribed
- Shape: oval
- Density: fat-containing

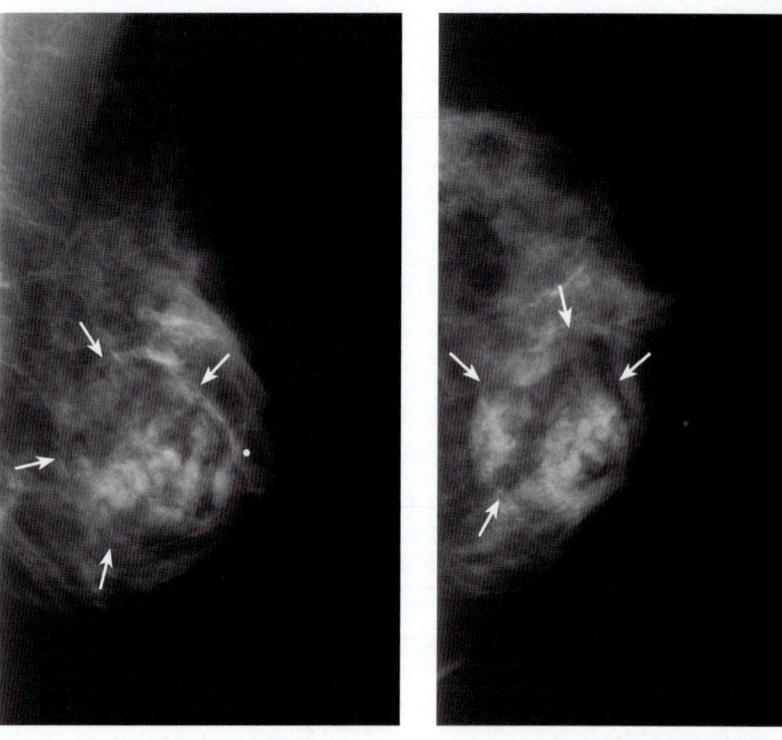

Fig. 5.3 At the 9 o'clock position of the left breast, there is a well-defined, oval, fat-containing mass with heterogeneous density (*arrows*). (**A**) Left MLO mammogram. (**B**) Left CC mammogram.

Ultrasound

Frequency
- 10 MHz

Mass (Fig. 5.4)
- Margin: well defined
- Echogenicity: heterogeneous
- Retrotumoral acoustic appearance: no shadowing
- Shape: ellipsoid

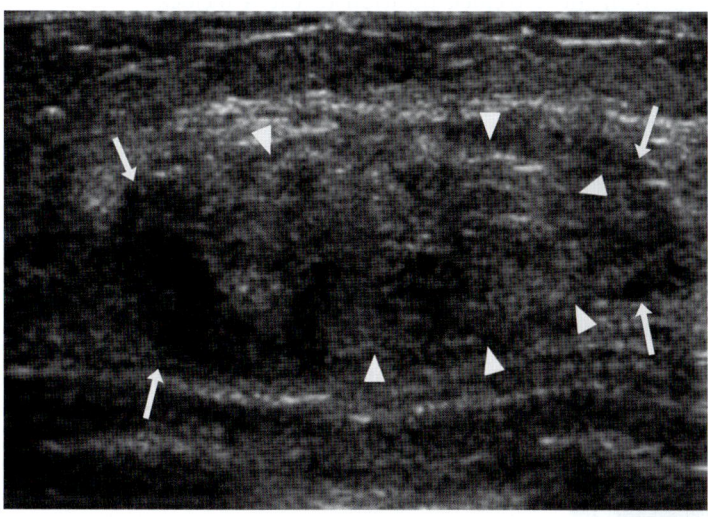

Fig. 5.4 Left radial breast sonogram. The palpable lump corresponds to a well-defined, oval, solid mass of heterogeneous echogenicity. The peripheral portion of this mass is isoechoic to fat (*arrows*), and the central portion is hyperechoic (*arrowheads*). This mass corresponds to the lesion identified in **Fig. 5.3**.

Pathology
- Hamartoma

Management
- BI-RADS assessment category 2, benign finding

Pearls and Pitfalls

- Hamartoma is a benign tumor that consists of mature tissues normally present in the breast. However, usually one element dominates the mass. Mammographically, the mass is well defined, but the density of the mass varies with its composition. If the mass does not have much fat, then it may be completely radiopaque. However, if the mass is a mixture of fat and other soft tissues, then it will be mixed density, as in this case. If the mass is completely radiopaque, then the differential diagnosis is fibroadenoma, cyst, or carcinoma. If the mass has mixed density, then the mammogram is diagnostic of hamartoma.
- Sonographically, hamartoma has a variety of appearances. The individual components of the tumor should sonographically match their corresponding normal elements within the breast. The fatty component is isoechoic to fat, and the fibroglandular elements are hyperechoic to fat.

Suggested Reading

Adler DD, Jeffries DO, Helvie MA. Sonographic features of breast hamartomas. J Ultrasound Med 1990;9:85–90

Anderson I, Hildell J, Linell F, et al. Mammary hamartomas. Acta Radiol 1979;20:712–720

Beatty SM, Orel SG, McCarthy DM, et al. Breast hamartomas: MR appearance. Breast Dis 1995;8: 275–281

Cooper RA, Johnson MS, Laissue J-A. Juvenile hypertrophy presenting as a discrete breast mass. Can Assoc Radiol J 1992;43:218–220

Crothers JG, Butler NF, Fortt RW, Gravelle IH. Fibroadenolipoma of the breast. Br J Radiol 1985;58:191–202

Evers K, Yeh I-T, Troupin RH, et al. Mammary hamartomas: the importance of radiologic-pathologic correlation. Breast Dis 1992;5:35–43

Case 5.4 Lipoma

Case History

A 73-year-old woman presents for a screening mammogram. She has a history of a soft mass in the upper outer left breast for more than 20 years.

Physical Examination
- Left breast: very soft area of asymmetry in the upper outer quadrant
- Right breast: normal exam

Mammogram

Mass (Fig. 5.7)
- Margin: circumscribed
- Shape: round
- Density: fat-containing

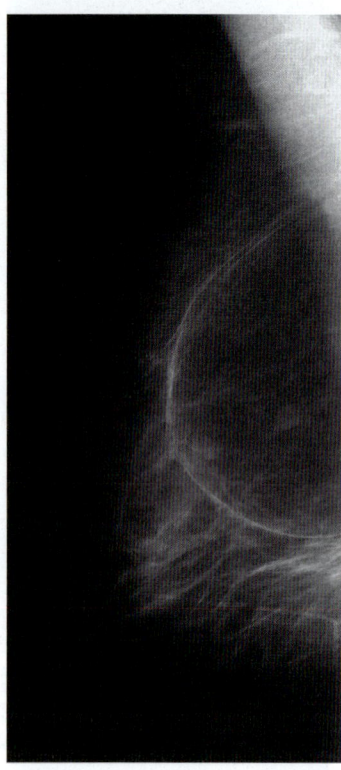

Fig. 5.7 Right MLO mammogram. There is a large, well-defined radiolucent lipoma. The small nodule that projects in the center of the mass is a lymph node located just medial to the lipoma on the CC view.

Ultrasound

Frequency
- 11.5 MHz

Mass (Figs. 5.8 and 5.9)
- Margin: well defined
- Echogenicity: isoechoic
- Retrotumoral acoustic appearance: no shadowing
- Shape: ellipsoid

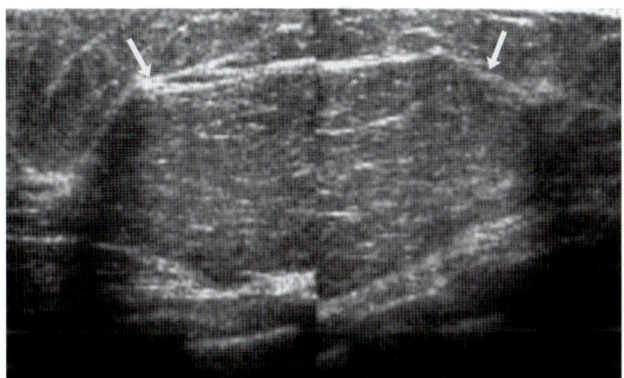

Fig. 5.8 Left radial breast sonogram. Combined images of the upper outer quadrant show the margins of the lipoma (*arrows*). The mass created by the lipoma pushes the thin hyperechoic parenchymal lines (representing lobular regression) superiorly.

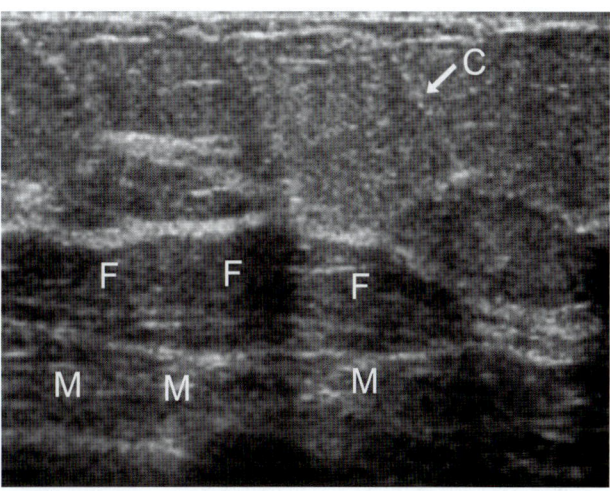

Fig. 5.9 Left radial breast sonogram. Sonogram is in a normal portion of the same breast as **Fig. 5.8**. This image is intended to demonstrate the normal architecture of the fatty breast parenchyma. F, fatty breast parenchyma; C, Cooper's ligaments; M, chest wall muscle.

Pathology
- Lipoma

Management
- BI-RADS assessment category 2, benign finding

Pearls and Pitfalls

- Mammographic fat-containing masses are benign, so sonographic examination is generally not necessary. However, occasionally, a patient is referred for sonography for a palpable fatty mass that has not been mammographically characterized. In these cases it is important to be familiar with the sonographic appearance of fatty masses and recommend mammography to confirm the benign identity of the mass.
- Sonographically, lipomas are generally oval and well defined. They are hypoechoic, isoechoic, hyperechoic, or heterogeneous in echogenicity. In a fatty breast, isoechoic tumors are sometimes difficult to identify. However, this case emphasizes that lipomas do not have the same internal architecture as normal fatty parenchyma. The echogenic lines within the lipoma do not follow a normal pattern of lobular regression.

Suggested Reading
Fornage BD, Tassin GB. Sonographic appearances of superficial soft tissue lipomas. J Clin Ultrasound 1991;19:215–220

Case 5.5 Lipoma

Case History
A 73-year-old woman presents for screening mammogram.

Physical Examination
- Normal exam

Mammogram

Mass (Fig. 5.10)
- Margin: circumscribed
- Shape: oval
- Density: fat-containing

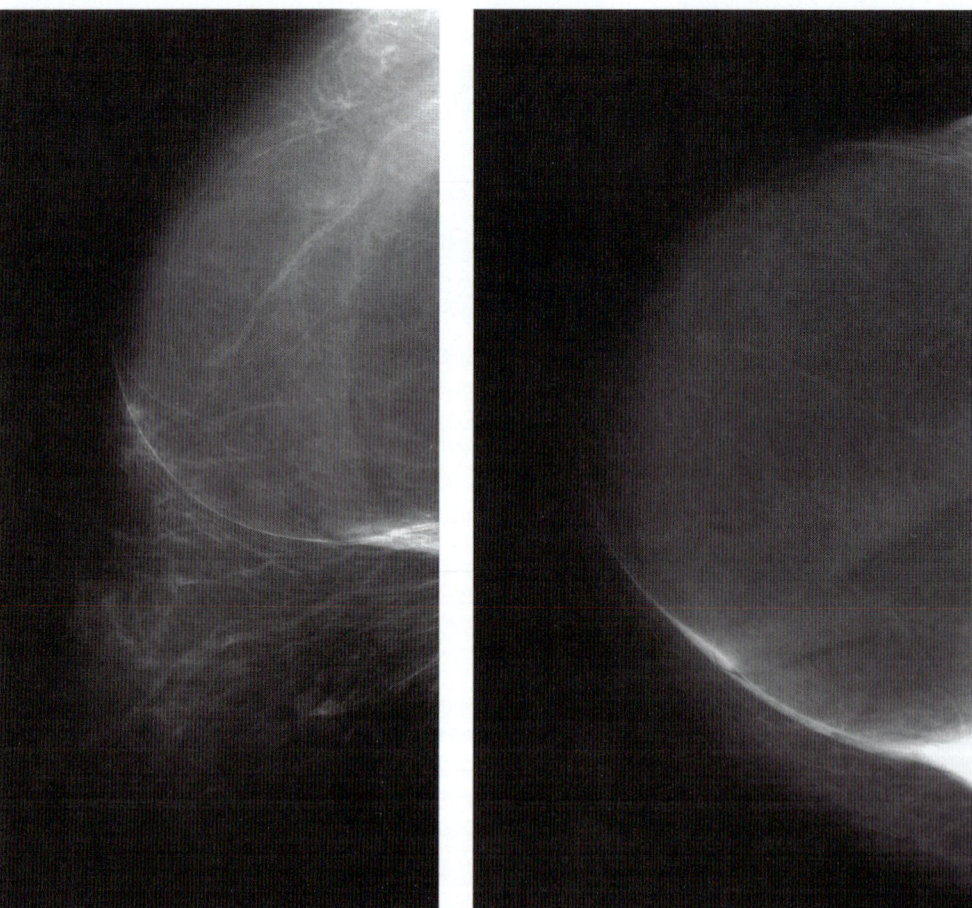

Fig. 5.10 The right breast is dominated by a fat density mass. This mammographic appearance is diagnostic of a lipoma. (**A**) Right MLO mammogram. (**B**) Right CC mammogram.

Pathology
- Lipoma

Management
- BI-RADS assessment category 2, benign finding

Fat-Containing Masses

> **Pearls and Pitfalls**
>
> - Lipomas are common benign breast masses. The average age of presentation is in the late 40s or early 50s. Generally, these tumors are unilateral. In 3% of cases, bilateral lipomas are present. Histologically, these tumors are composed of mature lipocytes surrounded by a capsule.

Suggested Reading

Tavassoli FA. Mesenchymal lesions. In: Tavassoli FA, Fattaneh A, eds. Pathology of the Breast, 2nd ed. Stamford: Appleton and Lange; 1999: 675–729

Case 5.6 Oil Cyst/Fat Necrosis

Case History

A 48-year-old woman presents status postlumpectomy 16 months ago. She now has a small palpable lump in her lumpectomy site. She is initially studied sonographically. Upon discovery of a sonographic nodule, mammographic examination has been performed.

Physical Examination

- Left breast: 8 mm lump at the 6 o'clock position within the scar of the lumpectomy site
- Right breast: normal exam

Mammogram

Mass (Fig. 5.11)
- Margin: circumscribed
- Shape: oval
- Density: fat-containing

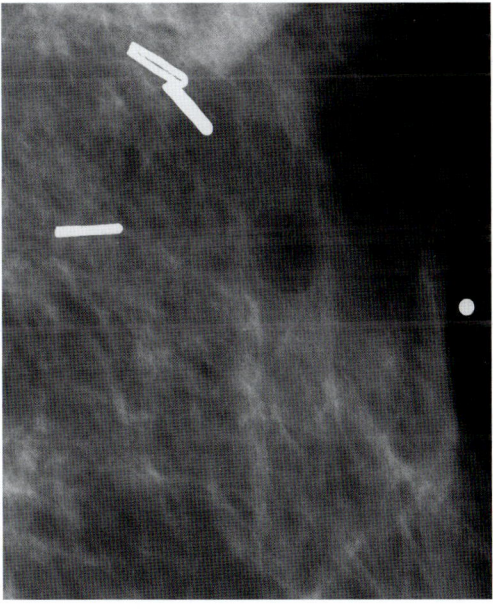

Fig. 5.11 Left MLO magnification spot mammogram. In the region of the patient's lumpectomy site, there is an oval radiolucent nodule.

Ultrasound

Frequency
- 13 MHz

Mass (Fig. 5.12)
- Margin: well defined
- Echogenicity: hypoechoic
- Retrotumoral acoustic appearance: no shadowing
- Shape: ellipsoid

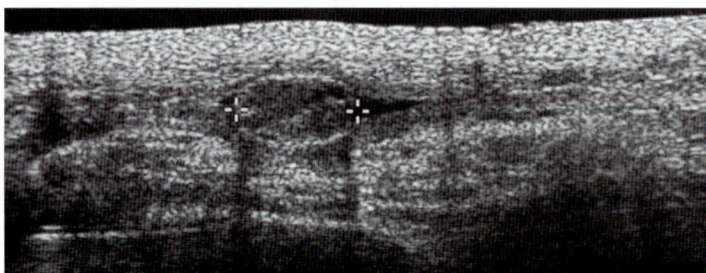

Fig. 5.12 Left antiradial breast sonogram. A well-defined oval nodule corresponds to the palpable lump and the oval mammographic lucency. The nodule has a thin hyperechoic rim and a hypoechoic center.

Pathology
- Oil cyst

Management
- BI-RADS assessment category 2, benign finding

Pearls and Pitfalls
- The ultrasound nodule is consistent with either an organizing hematoma or an oil cyst. However, the mammographic fat density of the nodule is diagnostic of an oil cyst.

Suggested Reading

Tohno D, Cosgrove DO, Sloane JP. Benign processes: trauma and iatrogenic conditions. In: Tohno D, Cosgrove DO, Sloane JP, eds. Ultrasound Diagnosis of Breast Diseases. New York: Churchill Livingstone; 1996:139–155

Case 5.7 Oil Cyst/Fat Necrosis

Case History
A 54-year-old woman is status post–replacement of a left breast implant and now has a new mass on her screening mammogram.

Physical Examination
- Normal exam

Mammogram

Mass (Fig. 5.13)
- Margin: circumscribed
- Shape: oval
- Density: fat-containing

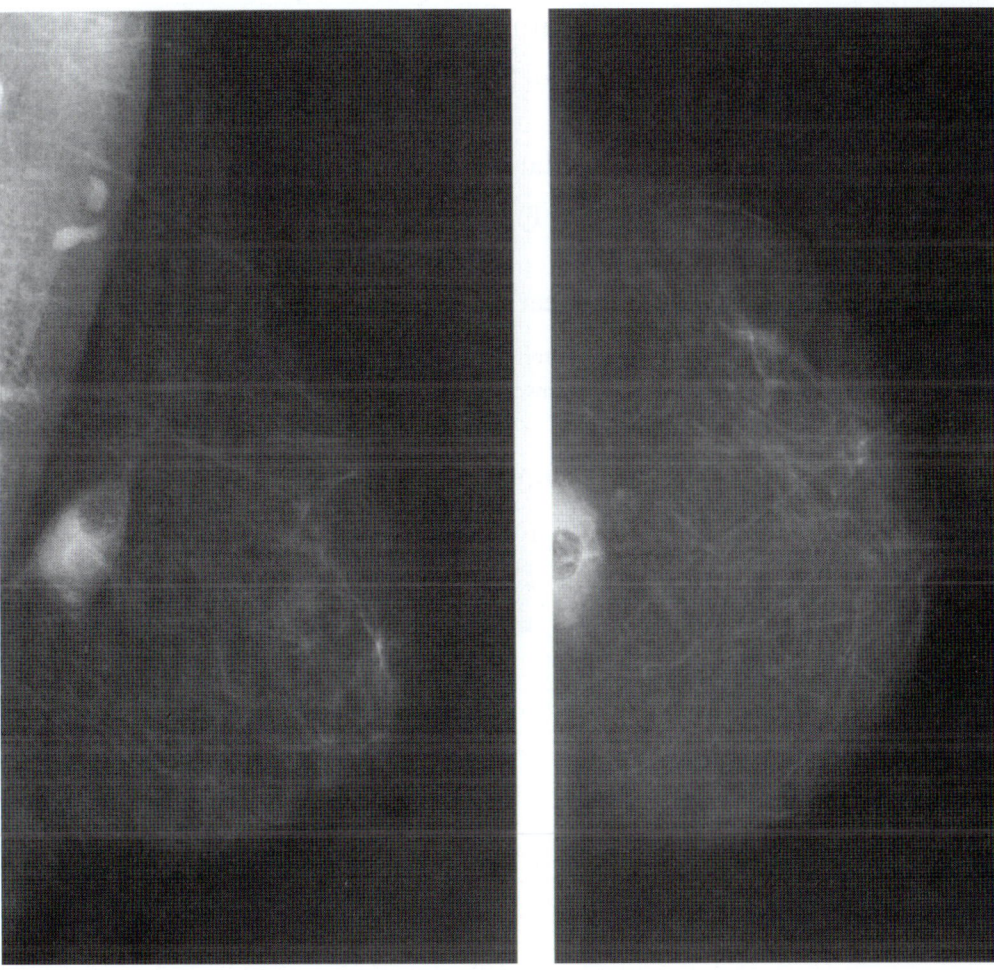

Fig. 5.13 Deep to the nipple in the posterior third of the left breast is a well-defined oval mass that contains a round lucent mass. (**A**) Left MLO mammogram. (**B**) Left CC mammogram.

54 Circumscribed Masses

Ultrasound

Frequency
- 7.5 MHz

Mass (Fig. 5.14)
- Margin: well defined
- Echogenicity: heterogeneous
- Retrotumoral acoustic appearance: enhanced acoustic transmission
- Shape: ellipsoid

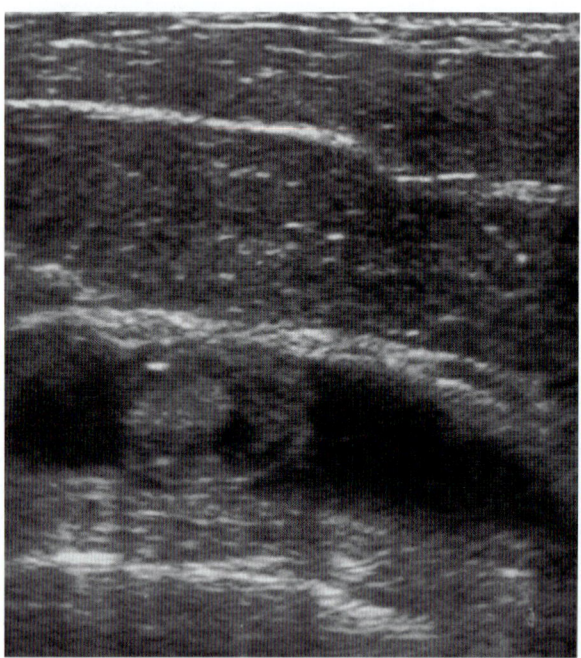

Fig. 5.14 Left transverse breast sonogram. The mass identified in **Fig. 5.13** corresponds to an anechoic fluid-filled cyst that contains a round heterogeneous mass, which represents the lucent mammographic mass. In real time this heterogeneous mass moves with changes in patient position and floats to the top of the fluid.

Pathology
- Oil cyst

Management
- BI-RADS assessment category 2, benign finding

Pearls and Pitfalls

- The mammographic mass corresponds to an oil cyst that is floating within a water density cyst. The oil cyst represents fat necrosis that resulted from removal of the previous implant.
- Sonographically, oil cysts are generally round or oval, hypoechoic, isoechoic, heterogeneous, or less commonly hyperechoic compared with fat. When the oil cyst is not calcified, sound transmission is generally increased or unchanged. As in this case, the identity of the oil cyst is clarified by the mammogram.

Suggested Reading

Heywang-Kobrunner SH, Schreer I, Dershaw DD. Post-traumatic, post-surgical and post-therapeutic changes. In: Heywang-Kobrunner SH, Schreer I, Dershaw DD. Diagnostic Breast Imaging. New York: Thieme; 1997:280–316

6 Circumscribed Masses: Medium- or High-Density Masses

Case 6.1: Benign—Angiolipoma

Case History
A 68-year-old woman presents with a new mass on her left screening mammogram.

Physical Examination
- Normal exam

Mammogram

Mass (Fig. 6.1)
- Margin: circumscribed
- Shape: oval
- Density: equal density

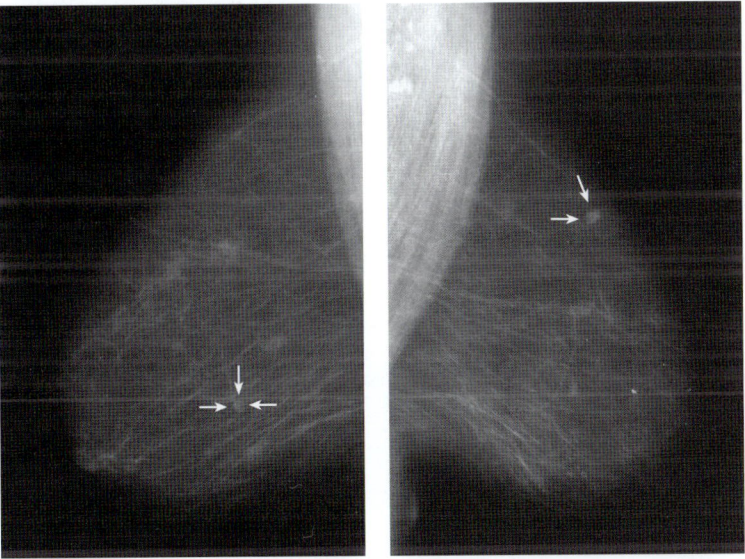
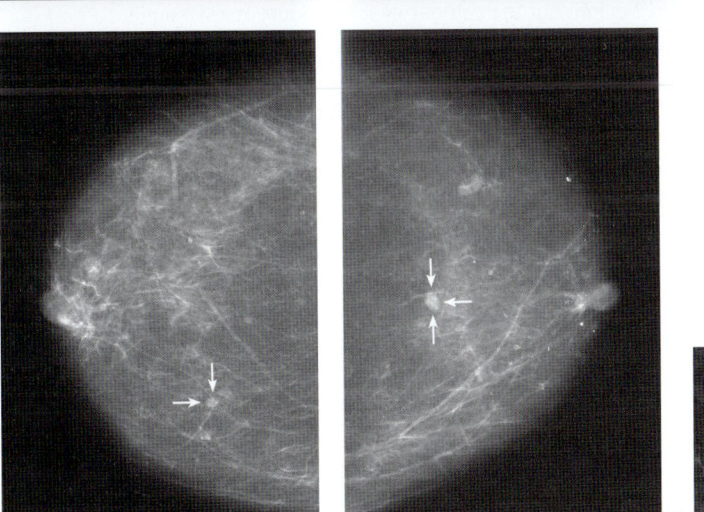
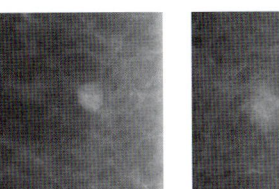
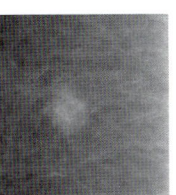

Fig. 6.1 At the 12 o'clock position of the left breast and the 3 o'clock position of the right breast, there are two oval masses (*arrows*). The spot compression views demonstrate that the margins of the right mass are well defined, and the margins of the left mass are ill defined. (**A**) Right MLO mammogram. (**B**) Left MLO mammogram. (**C**) Right CC mammogram. (**D**) Left CC mammogram. (**E**) Right CC spot compression mammogram. (**F**) Left CC spot compression mammogram.

Ultrasound

Frequency
- 10 MHz

Mass (Figs. 6.2 and 6.3)
- Margin: ill defined
- Echogenicity: hyperechoic
- Retrotumoral acoustic appearance: no shadowing
- Shape: ellipsoid

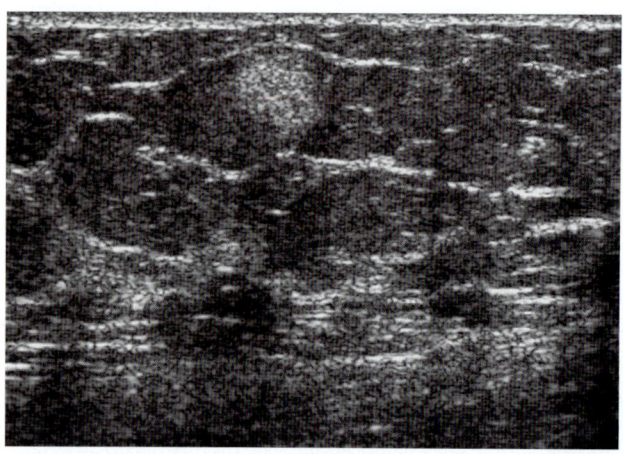 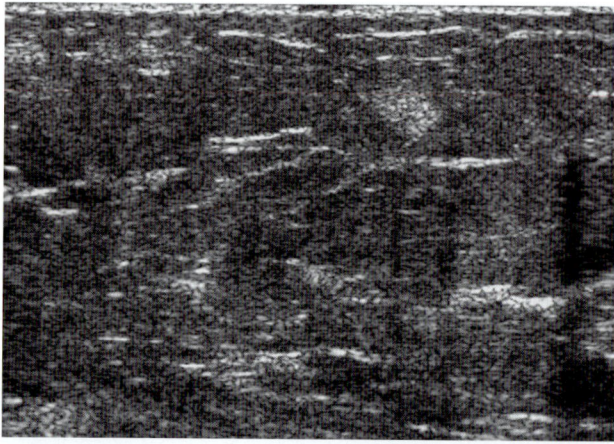

Fig. 6.2 Right radial breast sonogram. The right mammographic mass identified in **Fig. 6.1** corresponds to an oval, well-defined, hyperechoic mass.

Fig. 6.3 Left radial breast sonogram. The left mammographic mass identified in **Fig. 6.1** corresponds to a hyperechoic mass similar to the right breast mass.

Pathology
- Angiolipoma

Management
- BI-RADS assessment category 4, suspicious; biopsy should be considered.

Pearls and Pitfalls

- Uniformly hyperechoic sonographic masses are generally benign, but the category 4 (suspicious) assessment is based upon the information that the masses are new and the left mass is mildly ill-defined mammographically.
- Clinically, angiolipomas resemble lipomas. Over 75% of patients are older than 50 years. Angiolipomas in other sites of the body generally are associated with pain. However, breast angiolipomas are generally painless. Microscopically, the mass consists of mature lipocytes associated with an extensive vascular network. Microthrombi are a prominent feature of the lesion. This mass is benign and does not recur.

Suggested Reading

Brown RW, Bhathal PS, Scott PR. Multiple bilateral angiolipomas of the breast: a case report. Aust N Z J Surg 1982;52:614–616

Fleishman JS, Schwartz RA. Angiolipoma presenting as a breast mass. Ariz Med 1980;37:403–404

Sibala JL, Chang CH, Lin F, Thomas JH. CT of angiolipoma of the breast. AJR Am J Roentgenol 1980;134:840–841

Case 6.2: Benign—Cyst

Case History
A 43-year-old woman presents for screening mammogram.

Physical Examination
- Bilateral lumpy breasts; no new lumps

Mammogram

Mass (Fig. 6.4)
- Margin: circumscribed
- Shape: oval
- Density: equal density

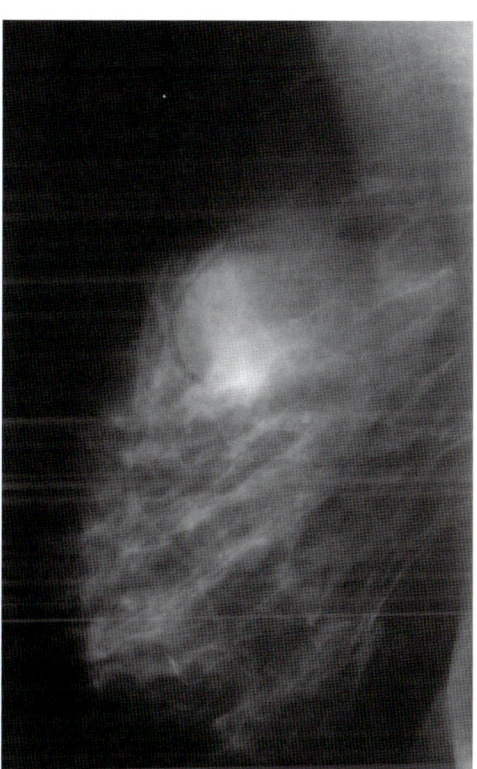 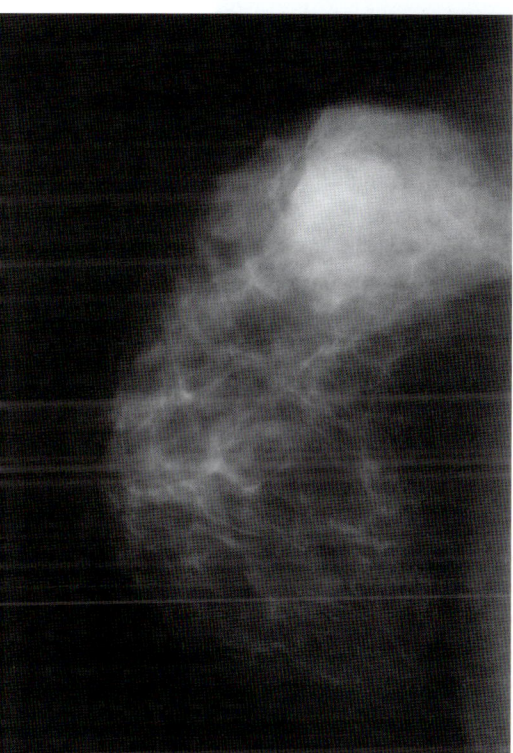

Fig. 6.4 In the upper outer quadrant of the right breast, there is an oval mass. Part of its margin is obscured by surrounding dense tissue, and part of the margin is associated with a lucent halo. (**A**) Right MLO mammogram. (**B**) Right CC mammogram.

Ultrasound

Frequency
- 10 MHz

Mass (Fig. 6.5)
- Margin: well defined
- Echogenicity: anechoic
- Retrotumoral acoustic appearance: increased acoustic transmission
- Shape: ellipsoid

Circumscribed Masses

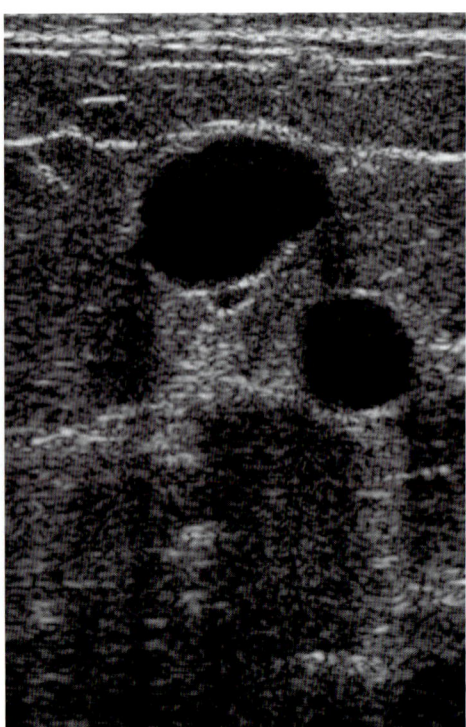

Fig. 6.7 Right transverse breast sonogram. The two mammographic masses correspond to two cysts. The fluid collections are anechoic; have well-defined, thin, hyperechoic walls; and have increased acoustic transmission.

Pathology
- Cysts

Management
- BI-RADS assessment category 2, benign finding

Pearls and Pitfalls

- Cysts are a component of fibrocystic change. This process has been identified clinically in about one third of women between 20 and 45 years of age. Autopsy studies have found approximately 54% of normal breasts have histologic evidence of cystic changes.

Suggested Reading

Frantz VK, Pickren JW, Melcher GW, Auchincloss H Jr. Incidence of chronic cystic disease in so-called normal breasts: a study based on 225 postmortem examinations. Cancer 1951;4:762–783

Jones BM, Bradbeer JW. The presentation and progress of macroscopic breast cysts. Br J Surg 1980;67:669–671

Leis HP Jr. Fibrocystic disease of the breast. J Med Assoc State Ala 1962;32:97–104

Leis HP Jr, Kwon CS. Fibrocystic disease of the breast. J Reprod Med 1979;22:291–296

Love SM, Gelman RS, Silen W. Sounding board. Fibrocystic "disease" of the breast—a nondisease? N Engl J Med 1982;307:1010–1014

Case 6.4: Benign—Cyst

Case History
A 48-year-old woman presents for screening mammogram.

Physical Examination
- No new breast lumps; both breasts normally lumpy

Mammogram

Mass (Fig. 6.8)
- Margin: circumscribed
- Shape: oval
- Density: equal density

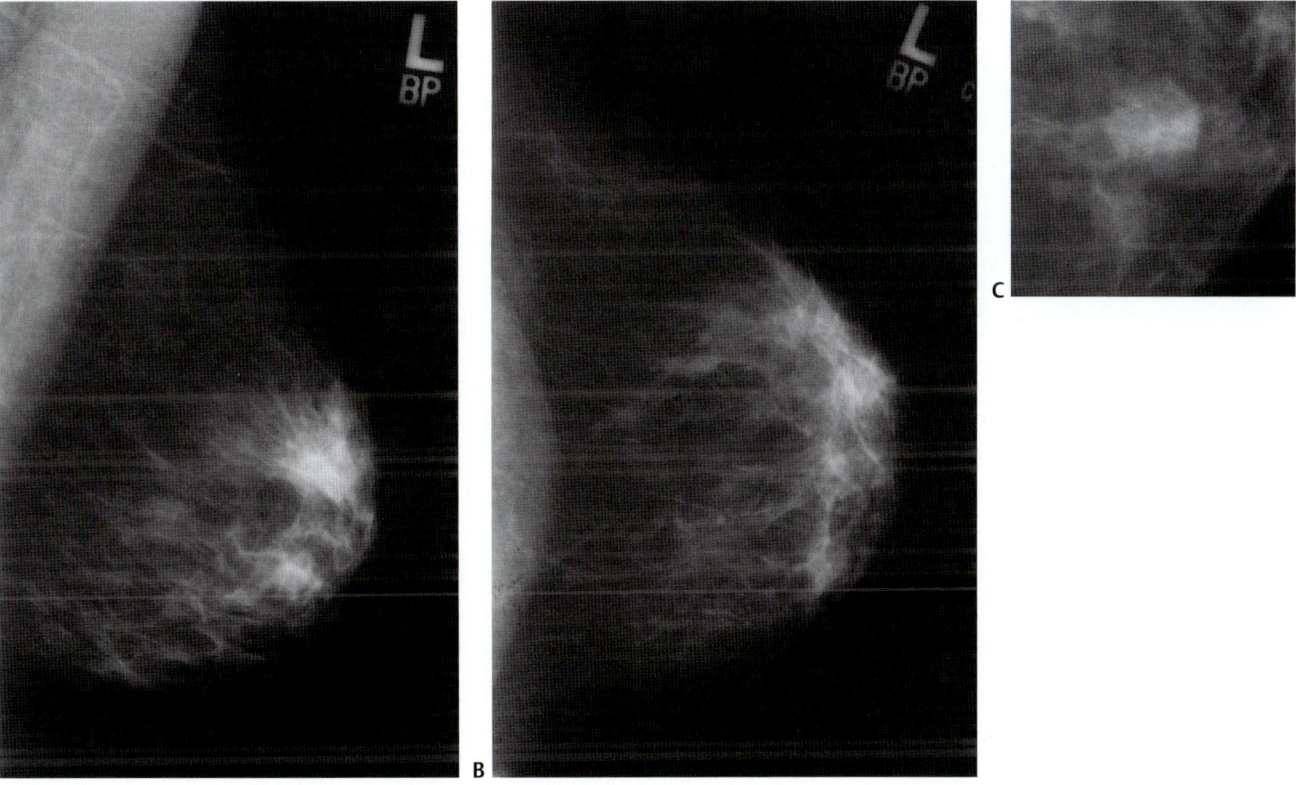

Fig. 6.8 In the left inferior inner quadrant, there is a circumscribed mass. This mass was new compared with previous exams. (**A**) Left MLO mammogram. (**B**) Left CC mammogram. (**C**) Left CC spot compression mammogram.

Ultrasound

Frequency
- 7.5 MHz

Mass (Fig. 6.9)
- Margin: well defined
- Echogenicity: heterogeneous
- Retrotumoral acoustic appearance: bilateral edge shadowing
- Shape: ellipsoid

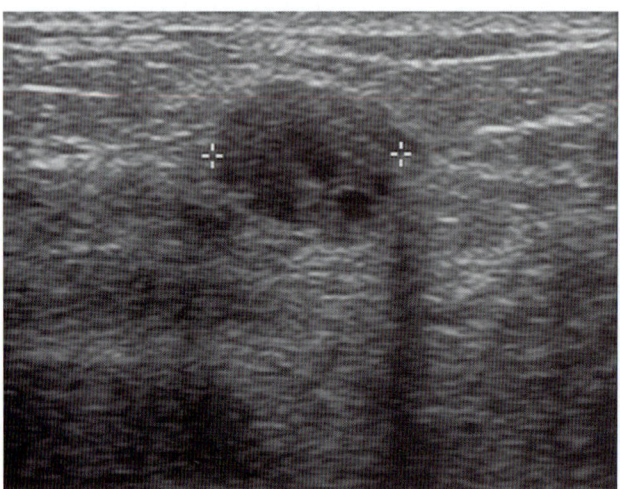

Fig. 6.9 Left longitudinal breast sonogram. The mammographic mass corresponds to a well-defined sonographic mass that is predominantly isoechoic to fat with a few anechoic oval lucencies within it. This mass was biopsied and found to be a complex benign cyst.

Pathology
- Cyst

Management
- BI-RADS assessment category 4, suspicious; biopsy should be considered.

Pearls and Pitfalls

- Sonography usually is successful in identifying benign cysts. However, occasionally, cysts exhibit internal echoes. These echoes may be caused by poor sonographic technique (e.g., gain settings too high), artifact (e.g., reverberation), proteinaceous debris, hemorrhage, infected debris, or cholesterol crystals. If the material completely moves, then the cyst is probably benign. However, if the material does not move, then an intracystic mass should be considered. In these cases, either aspiration or biopsy should be performed to identify intracystic tumors; 75% of solid intracystic masses are benign (mostly papillomas), 20% are malignant, and 5% are phyllodes tumors.

Suggested Reading

Khaleghian R. Breast cysts: pitfalls in sonographic diagnosis. Australas Radiol 1993;37:192–194

Sohn C, Blohmer J-U, Hamper UM. Fibrocystic changes and breast cysts. In: Sohn C, Blohmer J-U, Hamper UM, eds. Breast Ultrasound. New York: Thieme; 1999:75–90

Stavros AT, Dennis MA. The ultrasound of breast pathology. In: Parker SH, Jobe WE, eds. Percutaneous Breast Biopsy. New York: Raven Press; 1993:111–127

Case 6.5: Benign—Diabetic Fibrous Mastopathy

Case History
A 32-year-old woman presents with a new left breast lump. She is diabetic and has been insulin dependent since childhood.

Physical Examination
- Left breast: large hard mass at the 3 o'clock position
- Right breast: normal exam

Mammogram

Mass (Fig. 6.10)
- Margin: circumscribed
- Shape: oval
- Density: high density

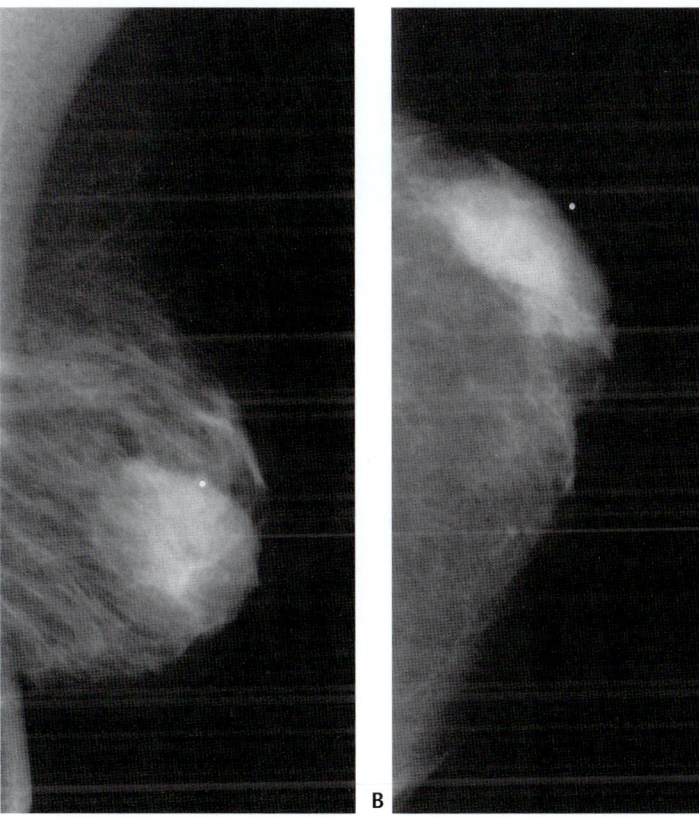

Fig. 6.10 In the 3 o'clock to 4 o'clock position of the left breast, there is a circumscribed oval mass that corresponds to the palpable mass designated by the metallic marker. (**A**) Left MLO mammogram. (**B**) Left CC mammogram.

Circumscribed Masses

Ultrasound

Low Frequency

Frequency
- 8 MHz

Mass (Fig. 6.11)
- Margin: ill defined
- Echogenicity: hypoechoic
- Retrotumoral acoustic appearance: severe shadowing, mass completely obscured
- Shape: irregular

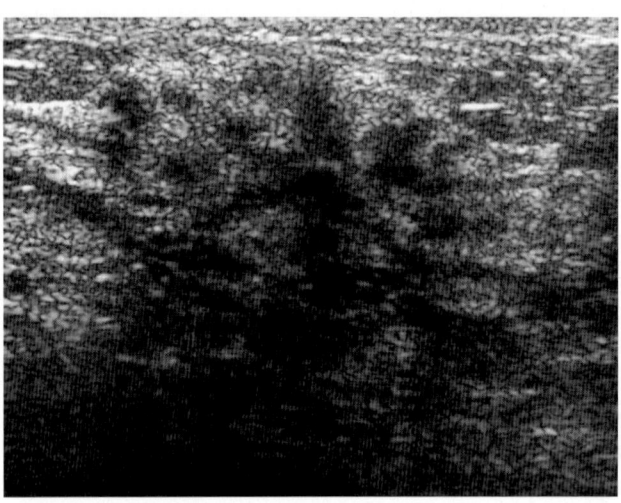

Fig. 6.11 Low-frequency left radial breast sonogram. (Same mass as **Fig. 6.12**.) As the frequency decreases, the mass attenuates the sound less, so the internal details of the mass become more apparent. The mass has a predominantly hyperechoic periphery with multiple linear lucencies centrally.

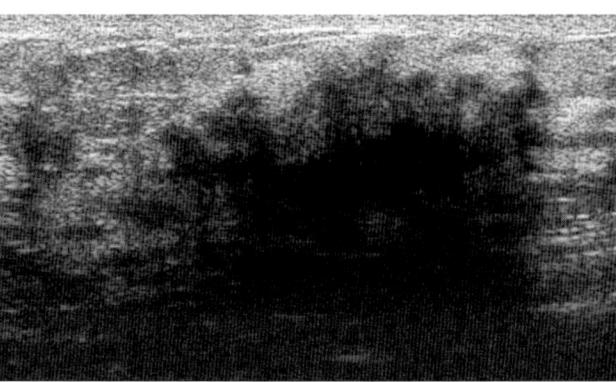

Fig. 6.12 High-frequency left radial breast sonogram. With high frequency, the palpable mass attenuates the sound so only a heavily shadowing area is evident.

High Frequency

Frequency
- 13 MHz

Associated Findings
- Lower frequency is more informative than high frequency for masses that severely attenuate sound because the internal architecture of the shadowing lesion is better displayed with the lower frequency (**Fig. 6.11**).
- With high frequency, the palpable mass attenuates the sound so only a heavily shadowing area is evident (**Fig. 6.12**).

Pathology
- Diabetic mastopathy

Management
- BI-RADS assessment category 4, suspicious; biopsy should be considered.

Pearls and Pitfalls

- Occasionally, diabetes will affect the breast, causing diabetic mastopathy. Microscopically, diabetic mastopathy consists of perivasculitis, keloidlike fibrosis, and ductitis or lobulitis. Clinically, this abnormality presents as a hard breast mass. The palpable mass cannot be distinguished from malignancy. However, this presentation in a young woman who has had long-term insulin dependence should be a strong clue to the diagnosis.
- The mammographic findings of diabetic mastopathy include a diffusely dense breast, asymmetric focal density, an irregular mass, and less commonly a circumscribed mass.
- Sonographically, the fibrosis strongly attenuates sound, so usually only shadowing is evident. With very low frequencies, the internal architecture of the mass is identified.

Suggested Reading

Boullu S, Andrac L, Piana L, Darmon P, Dutour A, Oliver C. Diabetic mastopathy, complication of type 1 diabetes mellitus: report of two cases and a review of the literature. Diabetes Metab 1998;24:448–454

Byrd BF Jr, Hartmann WH, Graham LS, Hogle HH. Mastopathy in insulin-dependent diabetics. Ann Surg 1987;205:529–532

Hunfeld KP, Bässler R. Lymphocytic mastitis and fibrosis of the breast in long-standing insulin-dependent diabetics: a histopathologic study on diabetic mastopathy and report of ten cases. Gen Diagn Pathol 1997;143:49–58

Pluchinotta AM, Talenti E, Lodovichetti G, Tiso E, Biral M. Diabetic fibrous breast disease: a clinical entity that mimics cancer. Eur J Surg Oncol 1995;21:207–209

Seidman JD, Schnaper LA, Phillips LE. Mastopathy in insulin-requiring diabetes mellitus. Hum Pathol 1994;25:819–824

Case 6.6: Fibroadenoma

Case History
A 40-year-old woman presents with a palpable left breast lump.

Physical Examination
- Left breast: palpable lump in left lateral breast
- Right breast: normal exam

Mammogram

Mass (Fig. 6.13)
- Margin: well defined
- Shape: oval
- Density: equal

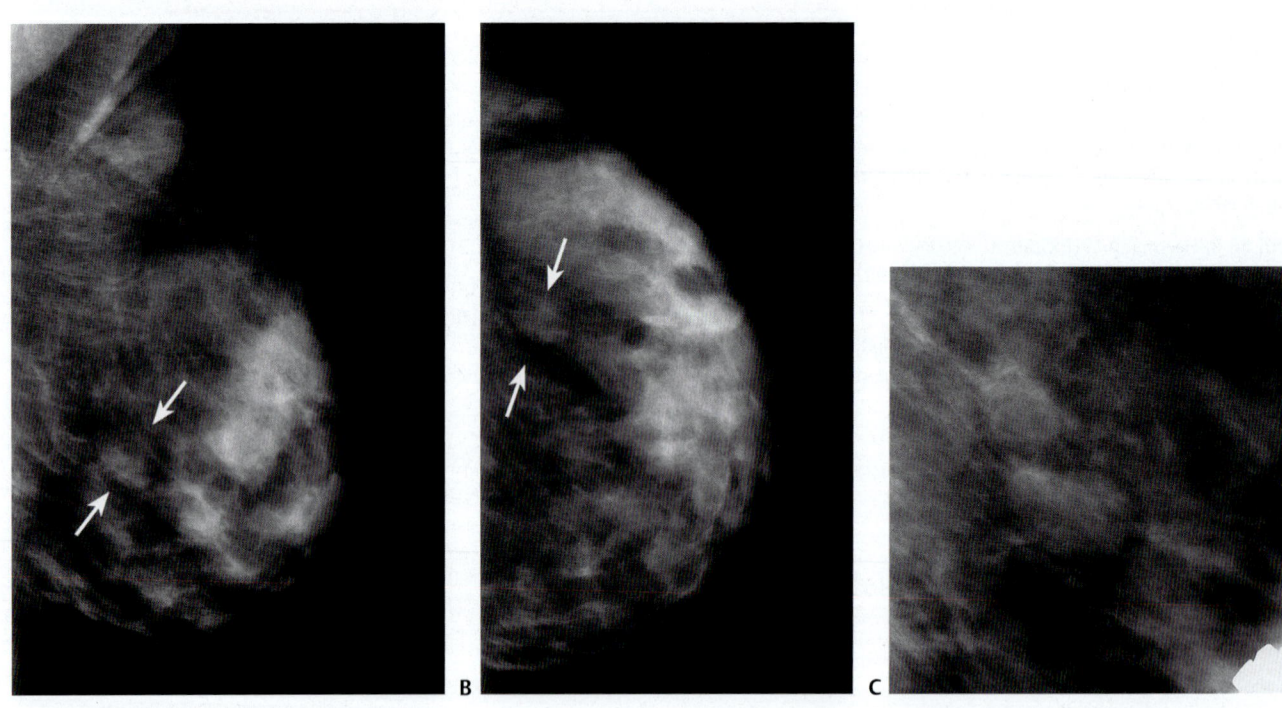

Fig. 6.13 At the 3 o'clock position of the left breast, there is an oval mass (*arrows*). The spot compression view demonstrates that the mass has well-defined margins and a lucent halo around part of the border. (**A**) Left MLO mammogram. (**B**) Left CC mammogram. (**C**) Left MLO spot compression mammogram.

Ultrasound

Frequency
- 10 MHz

Mass (Fig. 6.14)
- Margin: well defined
- Echogenicity: hypoechoic
- Retrotumoral acoustic appearance: no shadowing
- Shape: oval

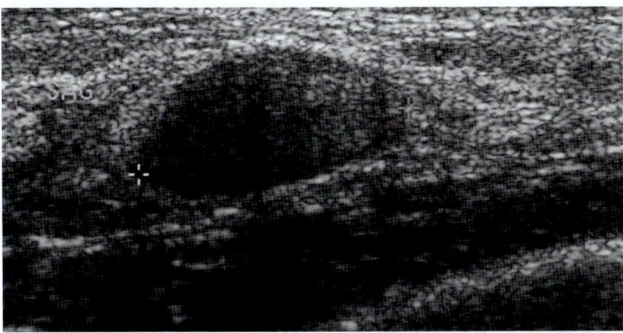

Fig. 6.14 Left radial breast sonogram. The oval mammographic density identified in **Fig. 6.13** corresponds to a well-defined, hypoechoic solid mass.

Pathology
- Fibroadenoma

Management
- BI-RADS assessment category 3, probably benign; short-interval follow-up

Pearls and Pitfalls

- Sonographically, if the mass has a well-defined margin, a hyperechoic, thin capsule, and no shadowing and is also homogeneously hypoechoic, then the chances of malignancy are very low (< 5%). Even though this lump was palpable, we chose short term follow up since the mass appeared sonographically to probably be benign.

Suggested Reading

Cole-Beuglet C, Soriano RZ, Kurtz AB, Goldberg BB. Fibroadenoma of the breast: sonomammography correlated with pathology in 122 patients. AJR Am J Roentgenol 1983;140:369–375

Fornage BD, Lorigan JG, Andry E. Fibroadenoma of the breast: sonographic appearance. Radiology 1989;172:671–675

Jackson VP, Rothschild PA, Kreipke DL, Mail JT, Holden RW. The spectrum of sonographic findings of fibroadenoma of the breast. Invest Radiol 1986;21:34–40

Stavros AT, Thickman D, Rapp CL, Dennis MA, Parker SH, Sisney GA. Solid breast nodules: use of sonography to distinguish between benign and malignant lesions. Radiology 1995;196:123–134

Case 6.7: Benign—Fibrocystic Change

Case History
A 48-year-old woman presents with a new palpable right lump.

Physical Examination
- Right breast: palpable lump at the 10 o'clock position
- Left breast: normal exam

Mammogram

Mass (Fig. 6.15)
- Margin: obscured
- Shape: oval
- Density: equal density

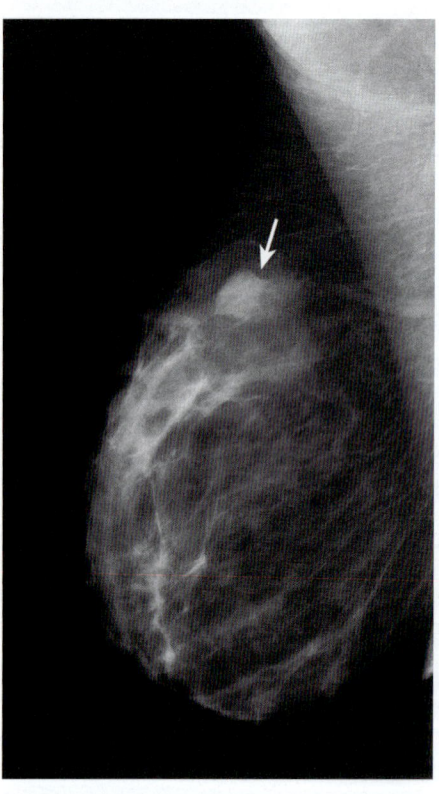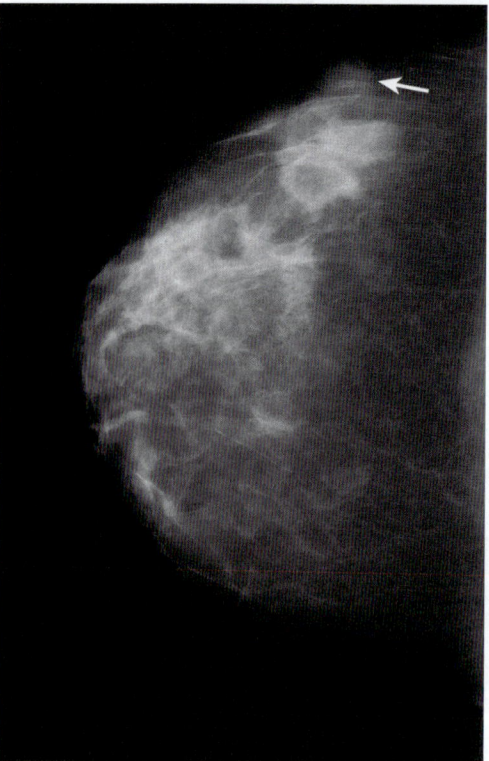

Fig. 6.15 In the right upper outer quadrant, there is an oval mass (*arrow*) with obscured margins, which corresponds to the palpable lump demarcated with a metallic marker. (**A**) Right MLO mammogram. (**B**) Right CC mammogram.

Ultrasound

Frequency
- 13 MHz

Mass (Fig. 6.16)
- Margin: well defined
- Echogenicity: hypoechoic
- Retrotumoral acoustic appearance: single edge shadowing
- Shape: lobulated

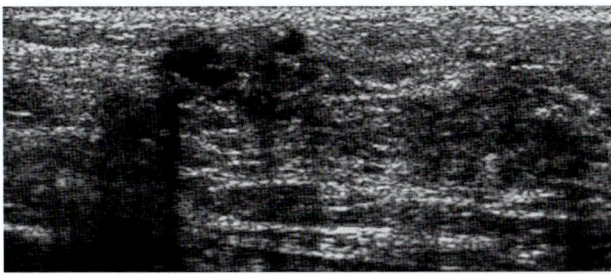

Fig. 6.16 Right antiradial breast sonogram. At the 10 o'clock position, there is a hypoechoic, lobulated mass that corresponds to the mass identified in **Fig. 6.15**.

Pathology
- Fibrocystic changes
- Stromal hyalinization, microscopic cysts, and apocrine metaplasia

Management
- BI-RADS assessment category 4, suspicious; biopsy should be considered.

Pearls and Pitfalls

- In retrospect, the sonographic appearance of the mass correlates well with the histology as small cysts are evident within the lesion.
- Fibrocystic changes generally cause symptoms in premenopausal women. About 75% of affected women are in the fourth or fifth decade. Three clinical stages have been described. Initially, women note premenstrual breast swelling or pain. Later, they develop breast lumps. Finally, the period of breast tenderness becomes continuous throughout the menstrual cycle. After menopause, the symptoms wane. Although at autopsy 25% of women have fibrocystic changes, only 10% of women older than 60 years have symptoms.

Suggested Reading

Leis HP Jr, Kwon CS. Fibrocystic disease of the breast. J Reprod Med 1979;22:291–296

Tavassoli FA. Benign lesions. In: Tavasolli FA, Fattaneh A, eds. Pathology of the Breast. 2nd ed. Stamford: Appleton and Lange; 1999:115–204

Vorherr H. Fibrocystic breast disease: pathophysiology, pathomorphology, clinical picture, and management. Am J Obstet Gynecol 1986;154:161–179

Case 6.8: Benign—Fibrocystic Change

Case History
A 65-year-old woman presents for her first mammogram.

Physical Examination
- Normal exam

Mammogram

Mass (Fig. 6.17)
- Margin: circumscribed
- Shape: oval
- Density: equal density

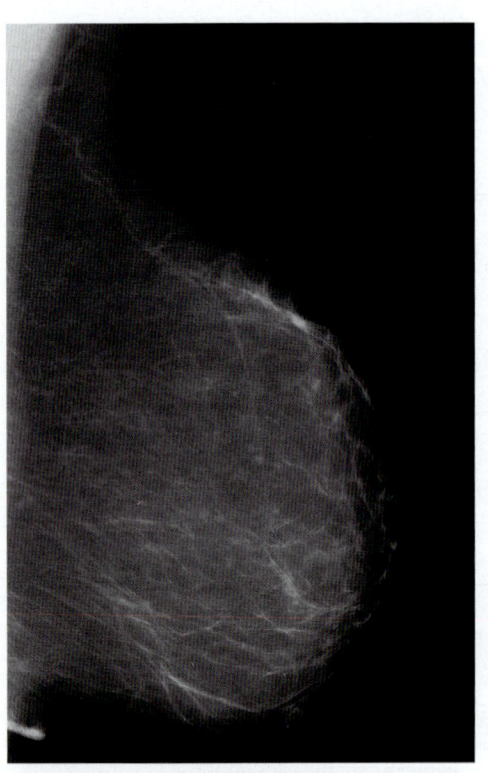
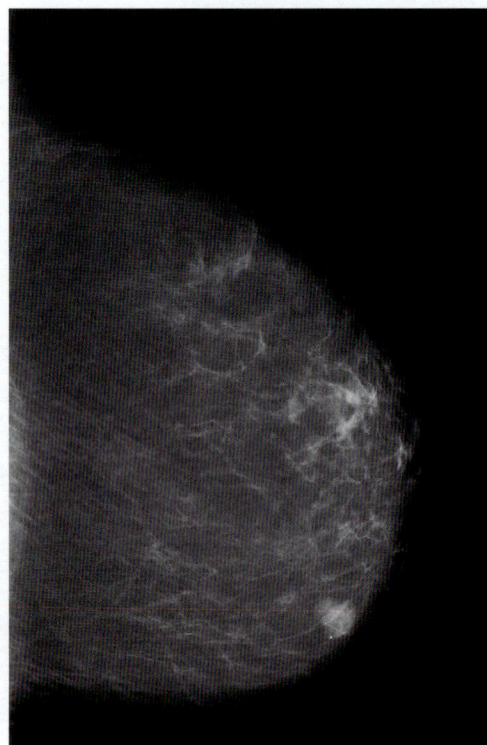
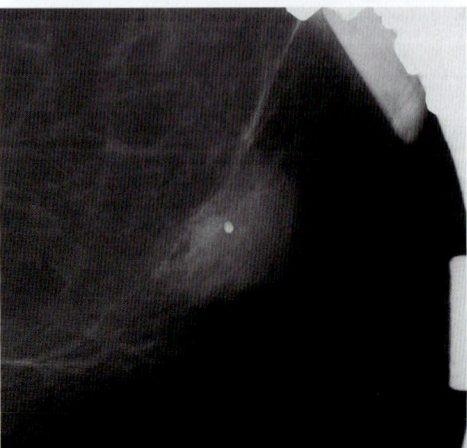

Fig. 6.17 In the inferior medial left breast, there is an oval mass with a single round calcification. The spot compression view suggests that the margins are ill defined. (**A**) Left MLO mammogram. (**B**) Left CC mammogram. (**C**) Left MLO spot compression mammogram.

Ultrasound

Frequency
- 7.5 MHz

Mass (Fig. 6.18)
- Margin: well defined
- Echogenicity: heterogeneous
- Retrotumoral acoustic appearance: posterior shadowing distal to mass
- Shape: ellipsoid

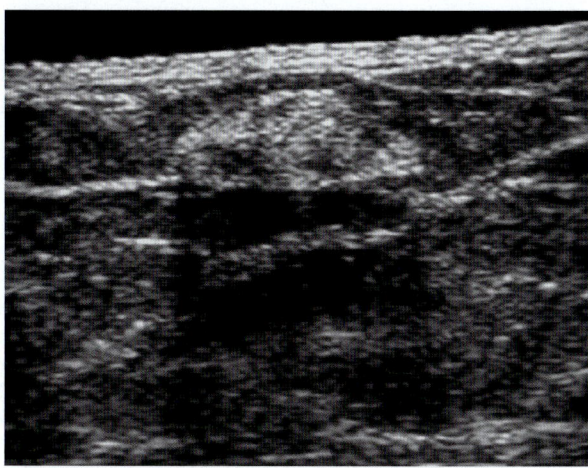

Fig. 6.18 Left radial breast sonogram. At the 8 o'clock position of the left breast there is a well-defined oval mass of heterogeneous (predominantly hyperechoic) echogenicity.

Pathology
- Fibrocystic change
- Hyalin sclerosis (fibrosis)

Management
- BI-RADS assessment category 4, suspicious; biopsy should be considered.

Pearls and Pitfalls

- The recommendation for biopsy is based on the mildly ill-defined mammographic margins and the mildly heterogeneous sonographic echogenicity.
- When fibrocystic changes produce a circumscribed mammographic mass, the sonographic findings correspond to either a cyst or a focal solid mass. The sonographic appearance of a solid mass is variable and biopsy is generally required. The sonographic fibrocystic masses may be either well or ill defined. They may be hyperechoic, hypoechoic, or heterogeneous echogenicity.

Suggested Reading

Love SM, Gelman RS, Silen W. Sounding board. Fibrocystic "disease" of the breast—a nondisease? N Engl J Med 1982;307:1010–1014

Teboul M, Halliwell M. Atlas of Ultrasound and Ductal Echography of the Breast, 2nd ed. Cambridge: Blackwell Science;1996:106–110, 180–185

Tohno D, Cosgrove DO, Sloane JP. Benign breast change. In: Tohno D, Cosgrove DO, Sloane JP, eds. Ultrasound Diagnosis of Breast Diseases. New York: Churchill Livingstone, 1996:121–130

Case 6.9: Benign—Hematoma

Case History
A 53-year-old woman presents with a new area of bruising in the right upper breast. She does not remember any trauma. She feels a lump under the bruise.

Physical Examination
- Right breast: ecchymosis associated with a palpable nodule in the upper breast at approximately the 12 o'clock position
- Left breast: normal exam

Mammogram

Mass (Fig. 6.19)
- Margin: circumscribed
- Shape: lobular
- Density: equal density

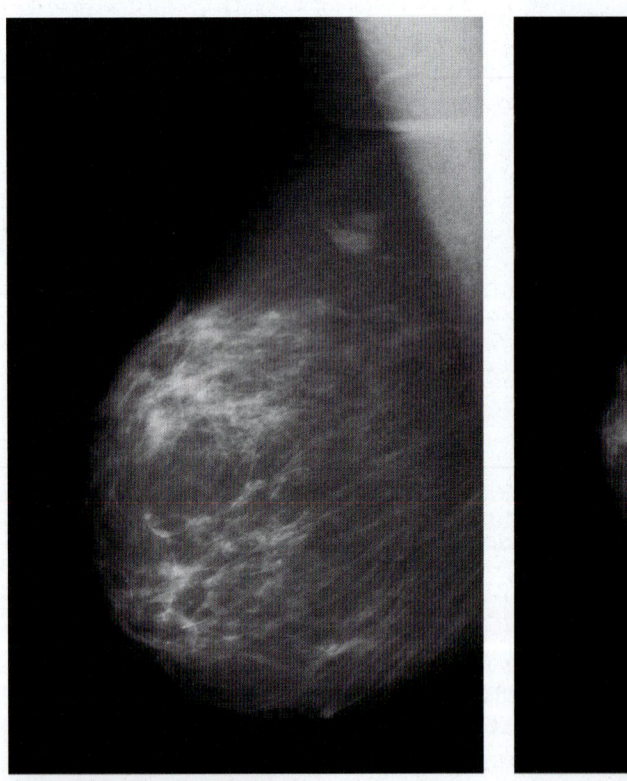
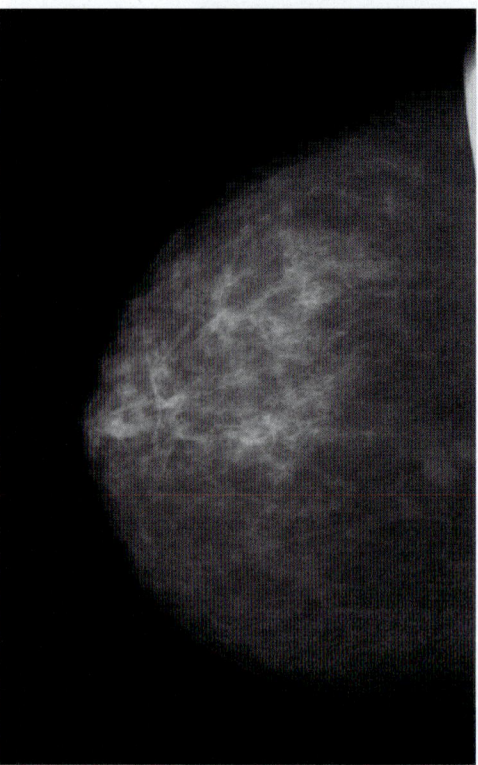

Fig. 6.19 At the 12 o'clock position of the right breast, there is a lobulated density. (**A**) Right MLO mammogram. (**B**) Right CC mammogram. (**C**) Right CC spot compression mammogram.

Ultrasound

Frequency
- 7 MHz

Mass (Fig. 6.20)
- Margin: well defined
- Echogenicity: heterogeneous
- Retrotumoral acoustic appearance: bilateral edge shadowing
- Shape: ellipsoid

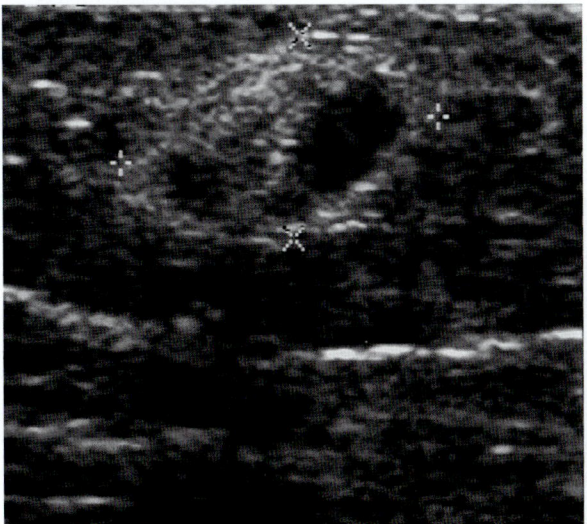 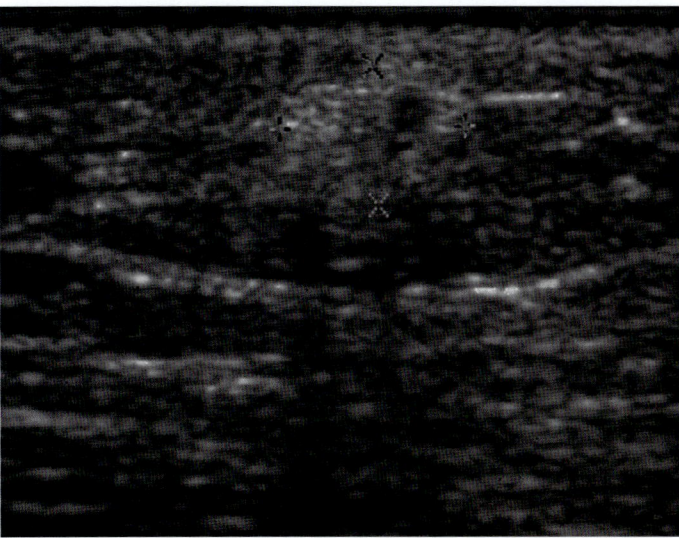

Fig. 6.20 (A) Right radial breast sonogram. The mammographic density identified in **Fig. 6.19** corresponds to an oval mass of heterogeneous echogenicity with a hyperechoic rim. (B) Right radial breast sonogram. One month after the sonogram performed in **A**, the sonographic mass is smaller and has changed in appearance to an oval, predominantly hyperechoic mass. This change in size and appearance is consistent with a healing hematoma.

Pathology
- Hematoma

Management
- BI-RADS assessment category 3, probably benign; short-interval follow-up

Pearls and Pitfalls

- Mammographically, acute hematomas are ill-defined or, less frequently, well-defined masses. As the hematoma resolves, a seroma or oil cyst may form, producing a well-defined round or oval mass. Finally, as the hematoma becomes fibrotic, the scar produces an irregular density or architectural distortion. The diagnosis of a breast hematoma rarely requires imaging, because there is usually a clear history of trauma or surgery. In this case, a mammogram 2 years later demonstrates complete resolution of the hematoma.
- Sonographically, hematomas are uniformly hypoechoic or mixed echogenicity. They should demonstrate no internal flow with color Doppler and should decrease in size on subsequent exams.

Suggested Reading

Harlow CL, Schackmuth EM, Bregman PS, Zeligman BE, Coffin CT. Sonographic detection of hematomas and fluid after imaging guided core breast biopsy. J Ultrasound Med 1994;13:877–882

Stigers KB, King JG, Davey DD, Stelling CB. Abnormalities of the breast caused by biopsy: spectrum of mammographic findings. AJR Am J Roentgenol 1991;156:287–291

Case 6.10: Benign—Leiomyoma

Case History
A 67-year-old woman presents with an enlarging left breast mass.

Physical Examination
- Left breast: multiple stable lumps; enlarging mass cannot be palpated
- Right breast: normal exam

Mammogram

Mass (Fig. 6.21)
- Margin: obscured
- Shape: oval
- Density: equal density

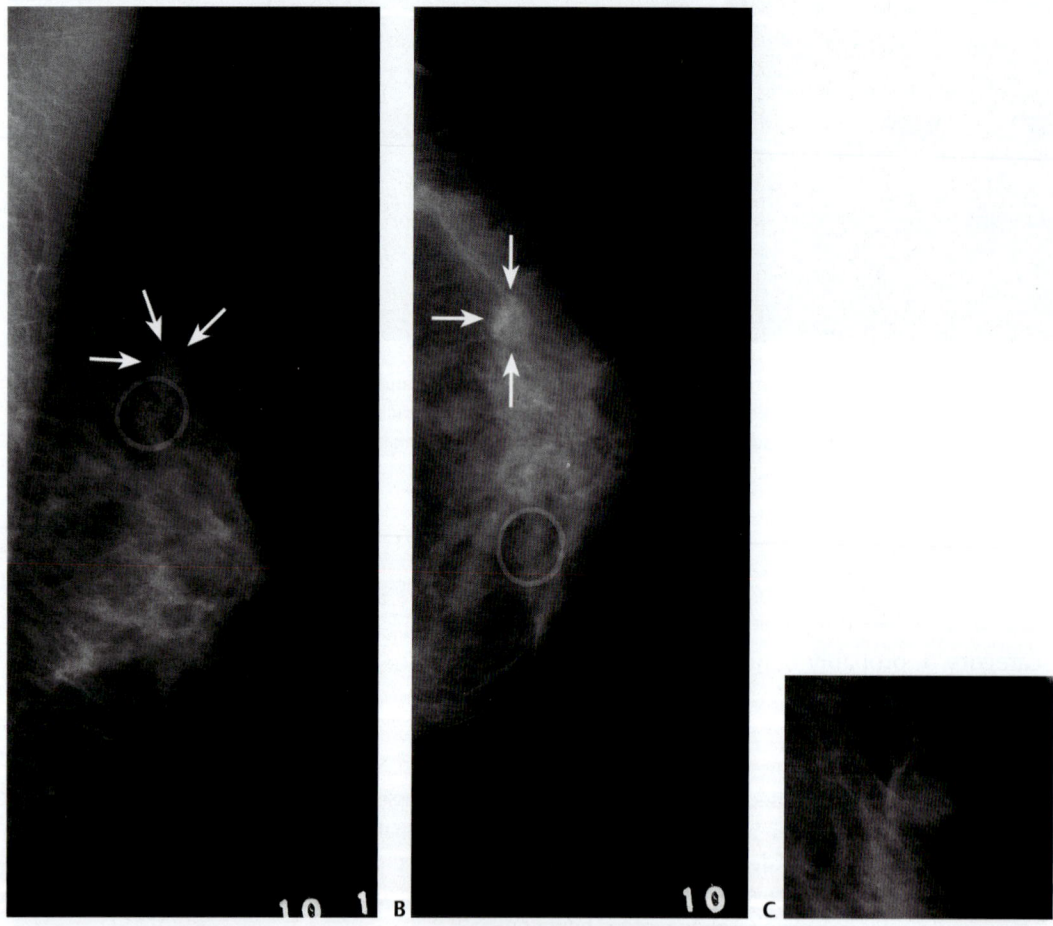

Fig. 6.21 In the left upper outer quadrant, there is an oval mass (*arrows*) with obscured margins. The radiopaque circle and dot markers denote a skin lesion in the upper inner breast. (**A**) Left MLO mammogram. (**B**) Left CC mammogram. (**C**) Left MLO spot compression mammogram.

Ultrasound

Frequency
- 13 MHz

Mass (Fig. 6.22)
- Margin: well defined
- Echogenicity: hypoechoic
- Retrotumoral acoustic appearance: single edge shadowing
- Shape: lobulated

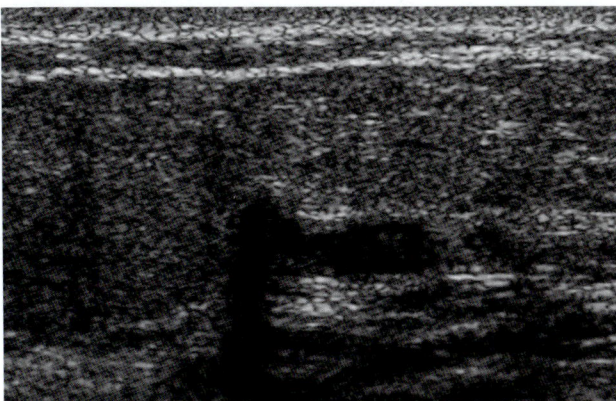 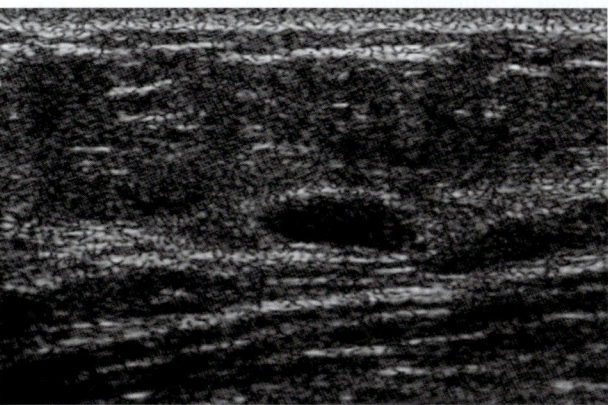

Fig. 6.22 The mammographic mass identified in **Fig. 6.21** corresponds sonographically to a well-defined, lobulated, hypoechoic mass. (**A**) Left radial breast sonogram. (**B**) Left antiradial breast sonogram.

Pathology
- Leiomyoma

Management
- BI-RADS assessment category 4, suspicious; biopsy should be considered.

Pearls and Pitfalls

- Leiomyomas (smooth muscle) of the breast are extremely rare. They originate from the nipple or subareolar region, or within the breast parenchyma. They present as well-defined solid masses. In this case, the management assessment is based on the progressive growth of the lesion and the inability to mammographically display well-defined margins.

Suggested Reading

Diaz-Arias AA, Hurt MA, Loy TS, Seeger RM, Bickel JT. Leiomyoma of the breast. Hum Pathol 1989;20:396–399

Nascimento AG, Karas M, Rosen PP, Caron AG. Leiomyoma of the nipple. Am J Surg Pathol 1979;3:151–154

Tavassoli FA. Mesenchymal lesions. In: Tavasolli FA, Fattaneh A, eds. Pathology of the Breast. 2nd ed. Stamford: Appleton and Lange; 1999:675–729

76 Circumscribed Masses

Case 6.11: Benign—Lymph Node

Case History
A 48-year-old woman presents for screening mammogram.

Physical Examination
- Normal exam

Mammogram

Mass (Fig. 6.23)
- Margin: circumscribed
- Shape: oval
- Density: equal density

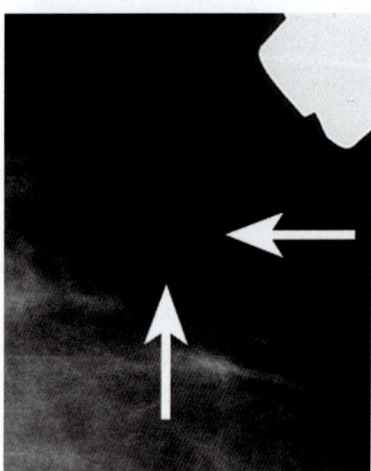

Fig. 6.23 Left CC spot compression mammogram. In the outer breast, there is an oval mass (*arrows*).

Ultrasound

Low Frequency

Frequency
- 7.5 MHz

Mass (Fig. 6.24)
- Margin: well defined
- Echogenicity: heterogeneous
- Retrotumoral acoustic appearance: single edge shadowing
- Shape: ellipsoid

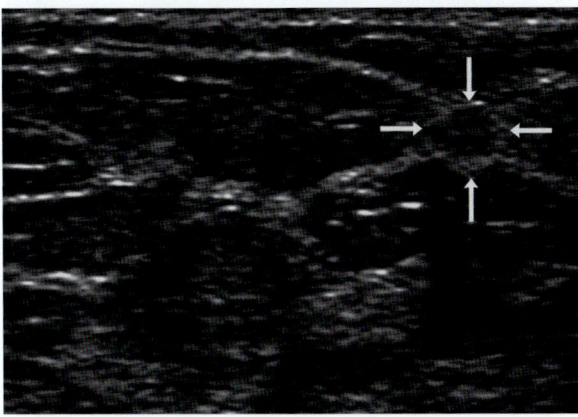

Fig. 6.24 Left radial breast sonogram. Using a lower-frequency transducer, the mass (*arrows*) is difficult to identify.

High Frequency

Frequency
- 11.5 MHz

Associated Findings

In this case, a benign mass is originally missed with the lower-frequency examination. The mass is missed for two reasons: (1) the echogenicity of the mass matches the surrounding tissues because the dynamic range of the imaging program is too high, and (2) the internal architecture of the mass cannot be resolved due to poor resolution from the lower frequency. The higher-frequency study not only localizes the mammographic mass but also clearly identifies the benign nature of the mass (**Figs. 6.25** and **6.26**).

78 Circumscribed Masses

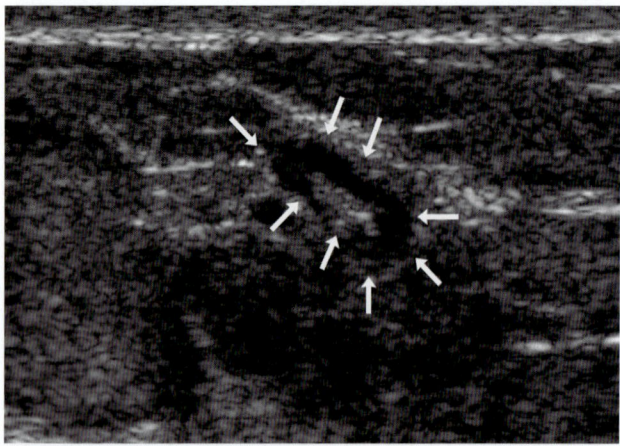

Fig. 6.25 Left antiradial breast sonogram. Higher-frequency examination of the same area as **Fig. 6.24** demonstrates that the mammographic mass is a normal lymph node (*arrows*).

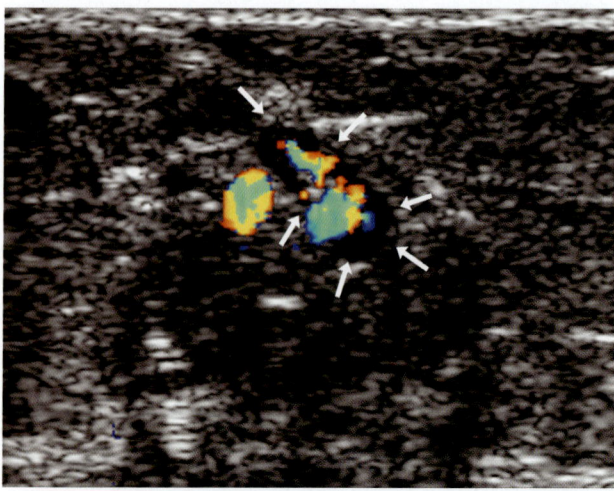

Fig. 6.26 Left antiradial color Doppler breast sonogram. Color flow high-frequency images confirm the normal pattern of blood flow through the center of the lymph node (*arrows*).

Pathology
- Lymph node

Management
- BI-RADS assessment category 2, benign finding

Pearls and Pitfalls

- Masses may be missed with lower-frequency sonography because the lower resolution provides fewer visual clues to characterize masses. In this case, the hyperechoic center of the lymph node could not be identified with the lower frequency.

Suggested Reading

Leucht D, Madjar H. Axillary, supraclavicular and infraclavicular lymph nodes. In: Leucht D, ed. Teaching Atlas of Breast Ultrasound. New York: Thieme; 1996:181–188

Sohn C, Blohmer J-U, Hamper UM. Sonography of the axilla. In: Sohn C, Blohmer J-U, Hamper UM, eds. Breast Ultrasound. New York: Thieme; 1999:94–97

Case 6.12: Benign—Nipple Out of Profile

Case History

A 53-year-old woman presents for screening mammogram.

Physical Examination
- Normal exam

Mammogram

Mass (Figs. 6.27 and 6.28)
- Margin: indistinct
- Shape: oval
- Density: equal density

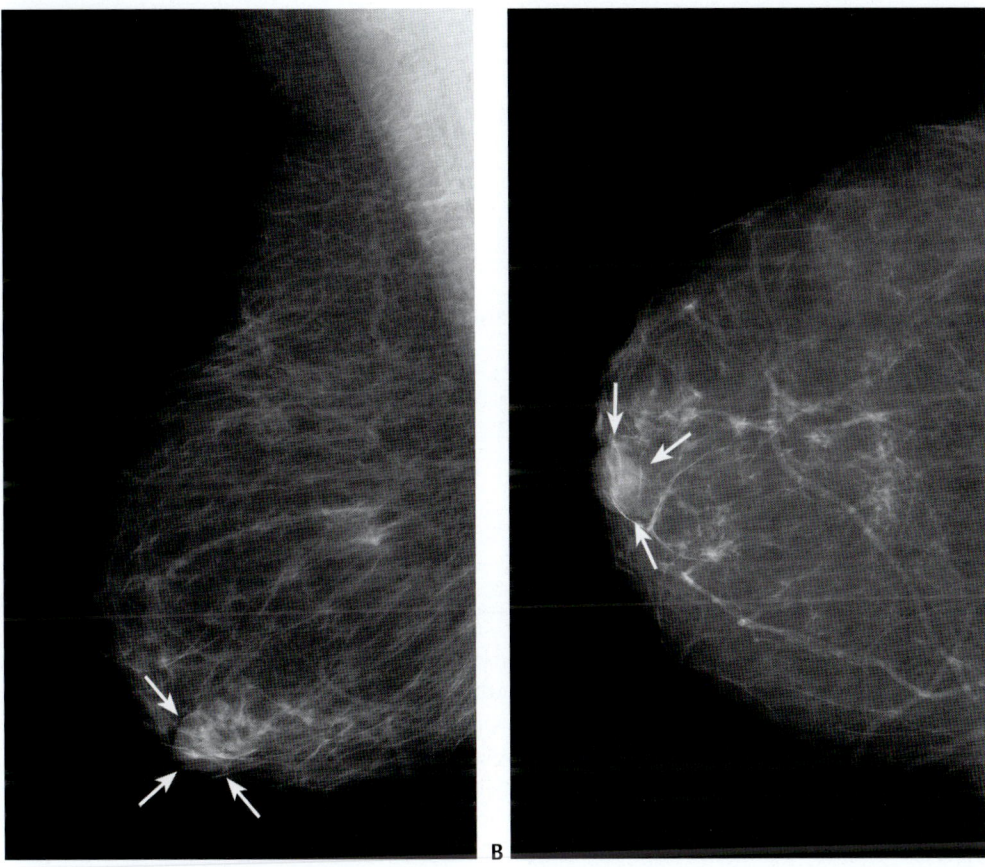

Fig. 6.27 In the subareolar region, there is an oval density (*arrows*). (**A**) Right MLO mammogram. (**B**) Right CC mammogram.

Circumscribed Masses

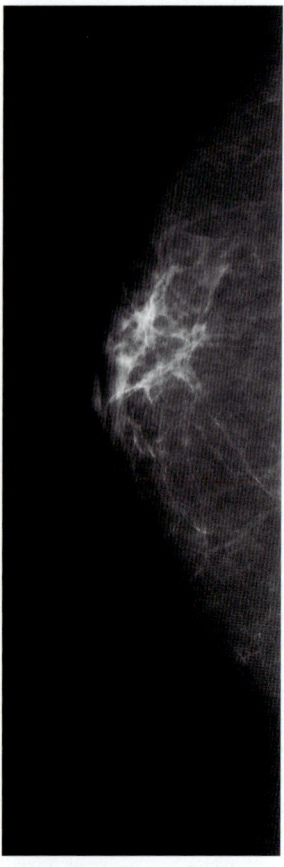

Fig. 6.28 Right CC nipple profile mammogram. The oval density corresponds to the nipple.

Pathology
- Nipple

Management
- BI-RADS assessment category 2, benign finding

Pearls and Pitfalls

- If the nipple is inverted or the breast is asymmetric, the nipple may be difficult to place in profile on the routine screening views. Besides being a requirement for good technique, placing the nipple in profile eliminates the mistake of confusing the nipple with an intramammary mass and optimizes the evaluation of the subareolar region. This visualization is necessary to exclude malignant causes for nipple displacement. A nipple profile view may be necessary to image the subareolar area.

Suggested Reading

American College of Radiology Committee on Quality Assurance in Mammography. Mammography Quality Control Manual. Reston: ACR; 1999:23–112

Bassett LW, Hirbawi IA, DeBruhl N, Hayes MK. Mammographic positioning: evaluation from the view box. Radiology 1993;188:803–806

Right Breast 1:00 Mass (Fig. 6.52 and 6.53)

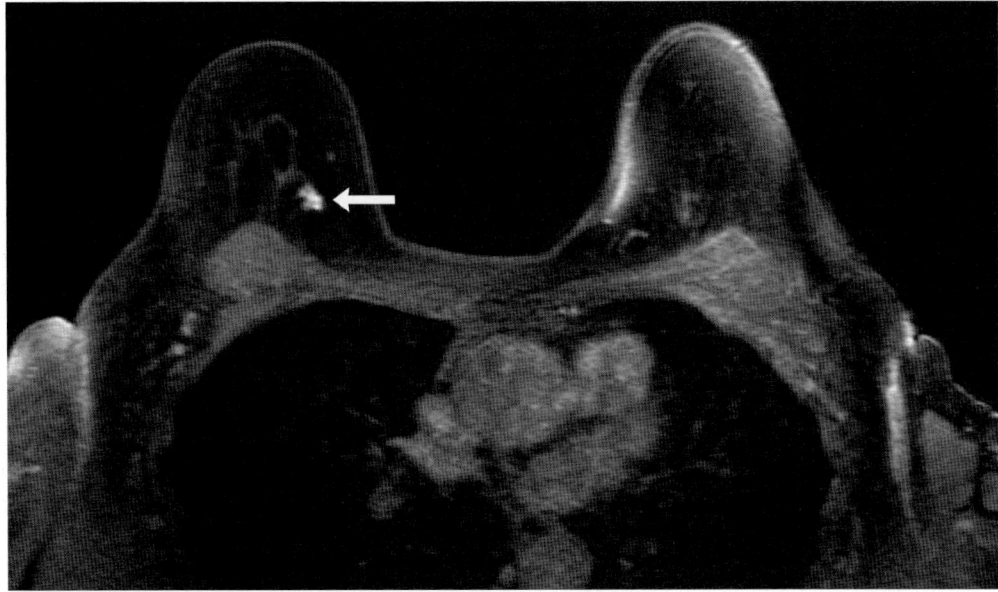

Fig. 6.52 Bilateral contrast-enhanced axial breast high-resolution MRI, delayed image. The MRI identifies a mammographically occult right breast 10 mm rapidly enhancing irregular mass (*arrow*) near the 1 o'clock position.

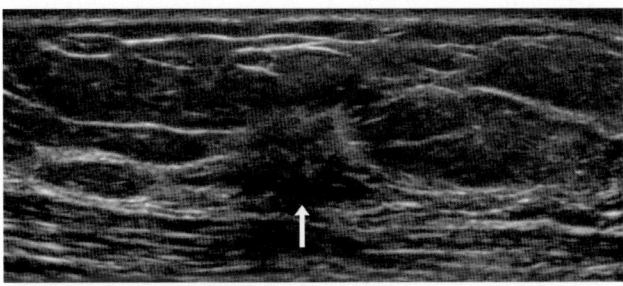

Fig. 6.53 Right antiradial breast sonogram at the 1 o'clock position. Sonogram is performed to identify the MRI mass for sonographic biopsy. The mammographically occult MRI mass in the upper inner quadrant corresponds to an irregular hypoechoic solid mass (*arrow*).

Right Breast 8:00 Mass (Fig. 6.54 and 6.55)

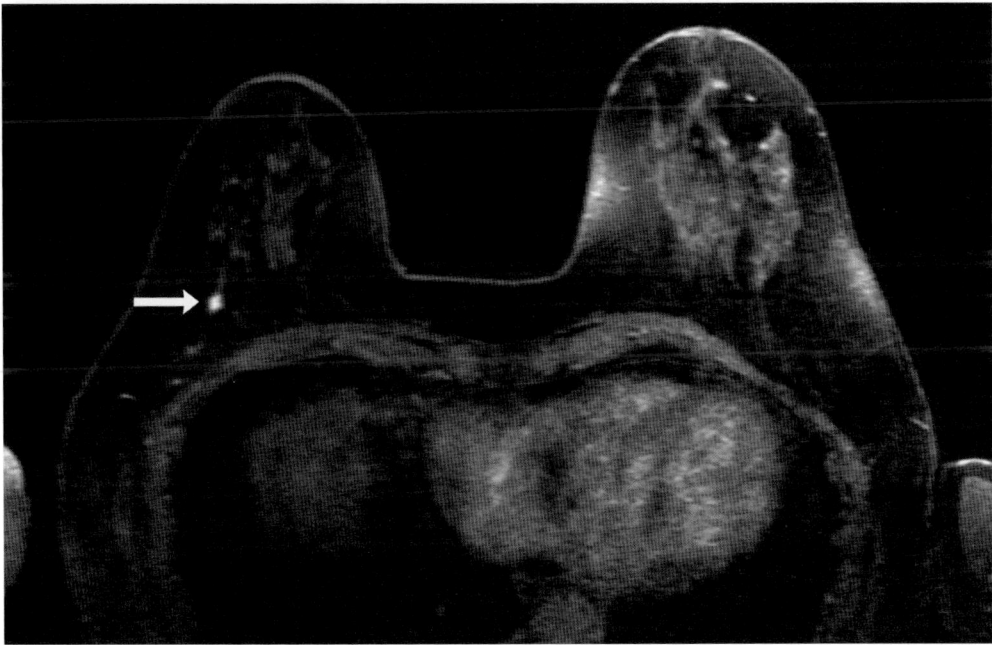

Fig. 6.54 Bilateral contrast-enhanced axial breast high-resolution MRI, delayed image. The MRI identifies a mammographically occult right breast 5 mm rapidly enhancing irregular focus (*arrow*) near the 8 o'clock position. Notice that the focus is at the edge of the lower outer parenchyma.

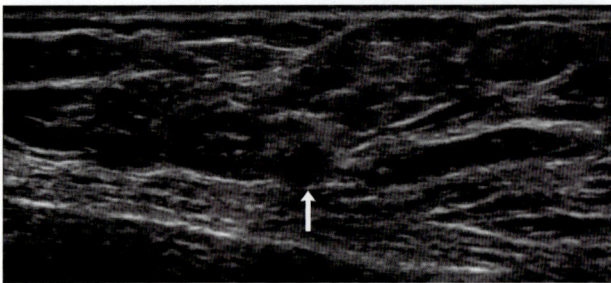

Fig. 6.55 Right antiradial breast sonogram at the 8 o'clock position. Sonogram is performed to identify the MRI focus for sonographic biopsy. The mammographically occult MRI focus in the lower outer quadrant corresponds to an irregular hypoechoic solid mass (*arrow*).

Pathology
- Left breast: invasive ductal carcinoma
- Right breast, 1 o'clock position: invasive carcinoma with ductal and lobular features
- Right breast, 8 o'clock position: invasive lobular carcinoma

Management
- Right breast MRI and sonographic mass at the 1 o'clock position: BI-RADS assessment category 5, highly suggestive of malignancy.
- Right breast MRI focus and sonographic mass at the 8 o'clock position: BI-RADS assessment category 4, suspicious; biopsy should be considered.

Pearls and Pitfalls

- Because sonographic biopsy is generally faster and less expensive than MRI-guided biopsy, sonographic breast evaluation of MRI lesions has become an accepted routine. However, sonographic identification of MRI masses is operator dependent. The literature reports that busy centers may identify only 23% of MRI lesions. To improve identification of MRI lesions, cross-correlate the MRI and sonogram. Besides recognizing the general location of the lesion (i.e., quadrant or o'clock), study the MRI for internal landmarks that would aid recognition. In this case, the 8 o'clock focus was initially missed because it is extremely small and subtle. However, when the focus is at the inferior outer parenchymal edge on the MRI, the general location of this focus can be identified with greater diagnostic confidence. To sonographically find this lesion, identify the hyperechoic parenchymal strands that extend into the inferior outer breast, and then closely examine the distal edge of these strands.

Suggested Reading
Hashimoto BE, Morgan GN, Kramer DJ, Lee ME. Systematic approach to difficult problems in breast sonography. Ultrasound Q 2008;24: 31–38

Case 6.24: Malignant or Locally Recurrent—Infiltrating Ductal Carcinoma

Case History
A 79-year-old woman presents with enlarging left breast nodule.

Physical Examination
- Normal exam

Mammogram

Mass (Fig. 6.56)
- Margin: circumscribed
- Shape: oval
- Density: equal density

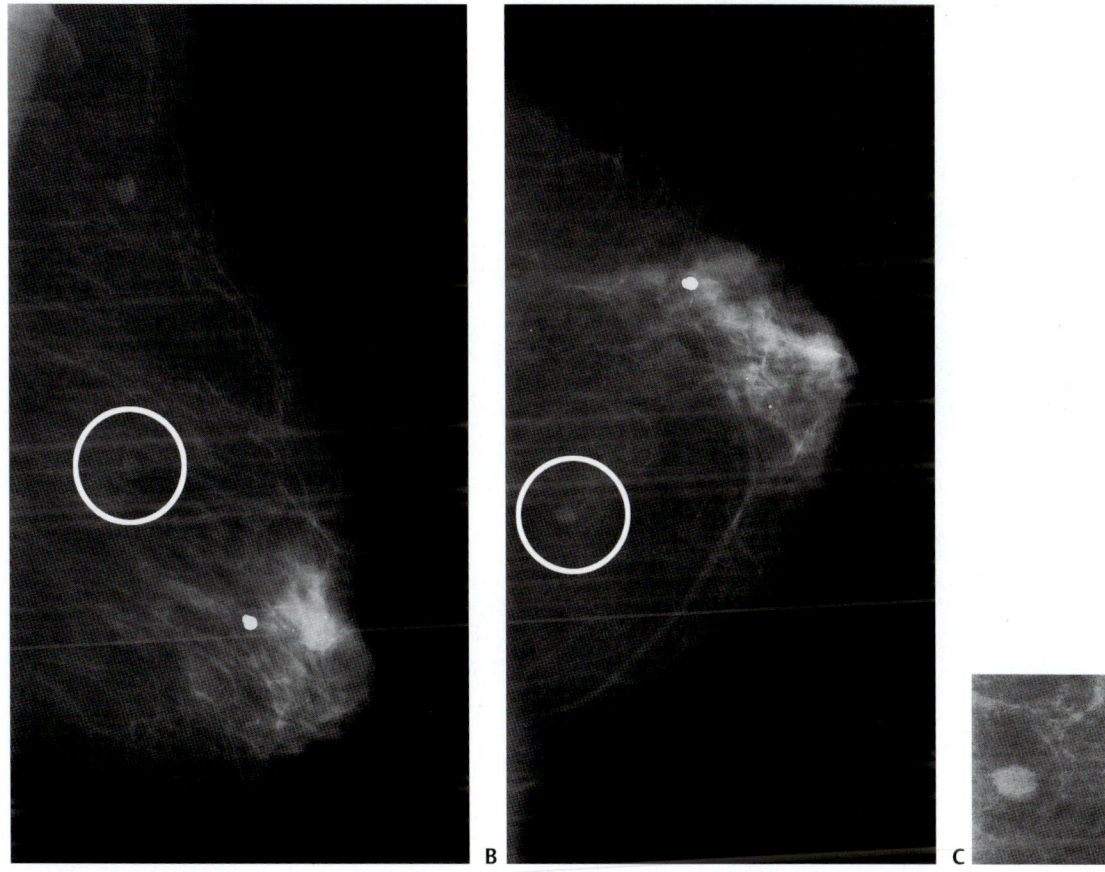

Fig. 6.56 In the upper inner left breast, there is a circumscribed oval mass. This mass has increased in size since the patient's prior exam. (**A**) Left MLO mammogram. (**B**) Left CC mammogram. (**C**) Left MLO spot mammogram.

Circumscribed Masses

Ultrasound

Low Frequency

Frequency
- 7 MHz

Mass (Fig. 6.57)
- Margin: ill defined
- Echogenicity: hypoechoic
- Retrotumoral acoustic appearance: posterior shadowing distal to mass
- Shape: lobulated

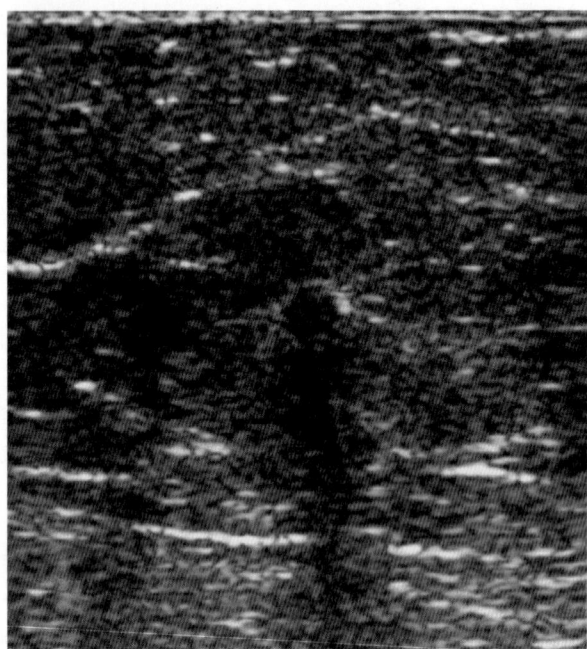

Fig. 6.57 Left radial breast sonogram. The mass identified in **Fig. 6.56** corresponds to a round, hypoechoic mass with acoustic shadowing.

High Frequency

Frequency
- 11.5 MHz

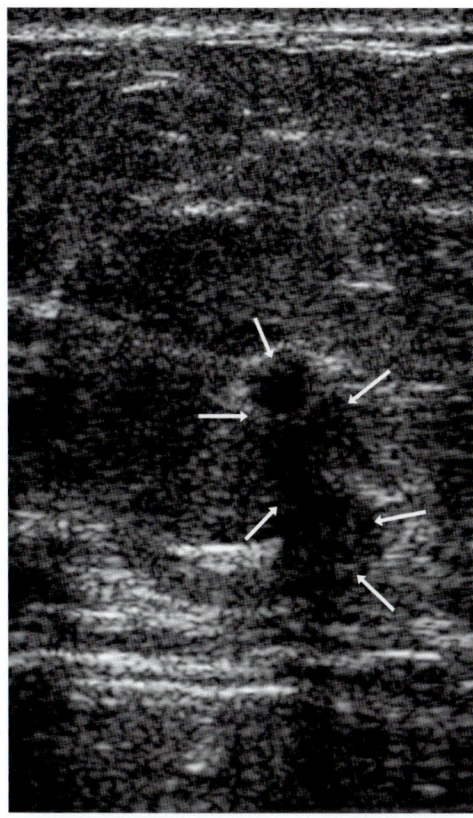

Fig. 6.58 Left radial breast sonogram. The mass identified in **Fig. 6.57** corresponds to an irregular, ill-defined mass (*arrows*) with posterior acoustic shadowing.

Associated Findings

The higher-frequency exam improves the definition of the mass. With the lower frequency, the mass may be mistaken for a benign round cyst or fibroadenoma with a fibrotic wall causing the shadowing. The higher frequency displays the irregular shape of the mass (**Fig. 6.58**).

Pathology

- Infiltrating ductal carcinoma

Management

- BI-RADS assessment category 4, suspicious; biopsy should be considered.

Pearls and Pitfalls

- This case illustrates that higher frequency sonography improves delineation of masses. If you wish to use sonographic information to determine management assessment, initially use the highest ultrasound that adequately penetrates the mass.

Suggested Reading

Marsteller LP, Shaw de Paredes EKK. Well-defined masses in the breast. Radiographics 1989;9:13–37

Moskowitz M. The predictive value of certain mammographic signs in screening for breast cancer. Cancer 1983;51:1007–1011

Sickles EA. Mammographic features of 300 consecutive nonpalpable breast cancers. AJR Am J Roentgenol 1986;146:661–663

Case 6.25: Malignant or Locally Recurrent—Invasive Papillary Carcinoma

Case History
A 51-year-old woman presents with a new left breast lump.

Physical Examination
- Left breast: palpable lump in the left breast at the 2 o'clock position
- Right breast: normal exam

Mammogram

Mass (Fig. 6.59)
- Margin: circumscribed
- Shape: oval
- Density: high

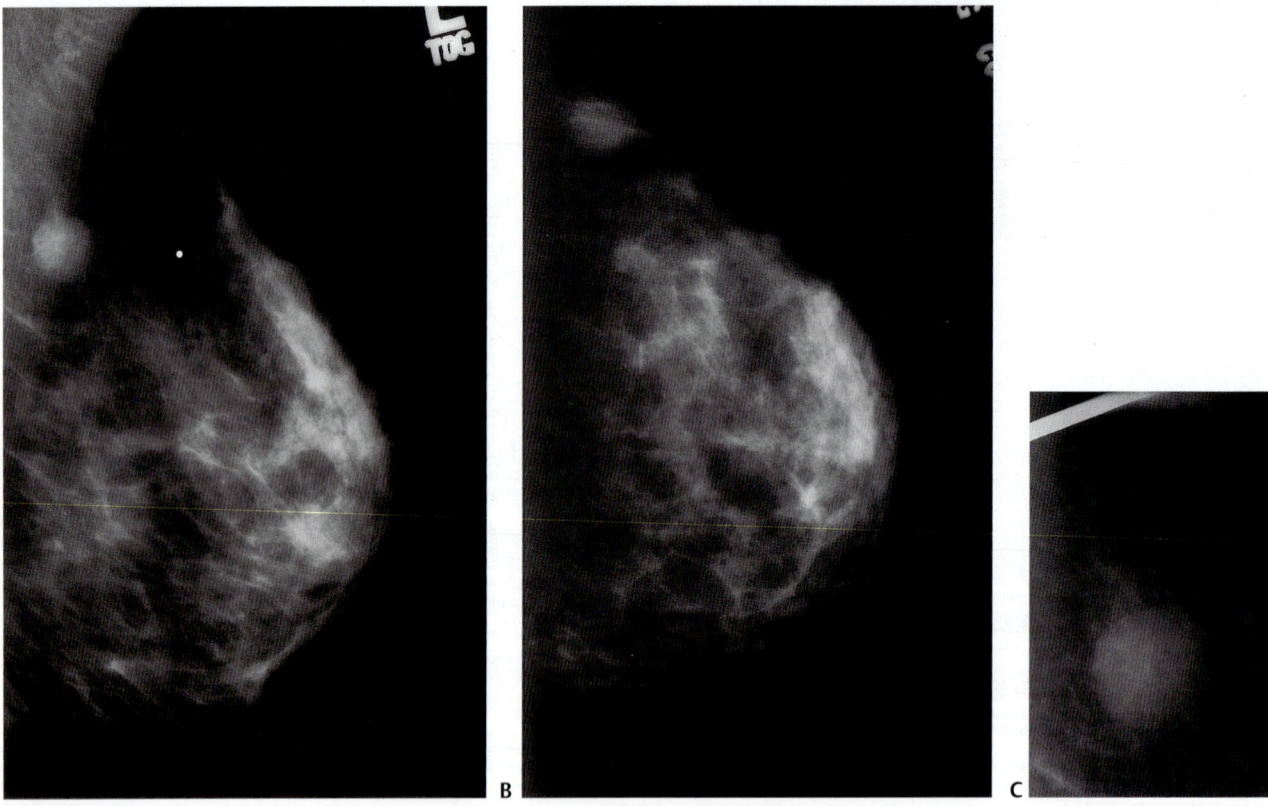

Fig. 6.59 There is a well-circumscribed oval density in the left upper outer breast. This mass corresponds to a palpable lump and is new since the screening mammogram of the previous year. A small segment of the margin is indistinct even with spot compression views. (**A**) Left MLO mammogram. (**B**) Left CC mammogram. (**C**) Left MLO spot compression view.

Ultrasound

Frequency
- 11.5 MHz

Mass (Figs. 6.60 and 6.61)
- Margin: well defined
- Echogenicity: hypoechoic
- Retrotumoral acoustic appearance: retrotumoral enhancement present
- Shape: ellipsoid

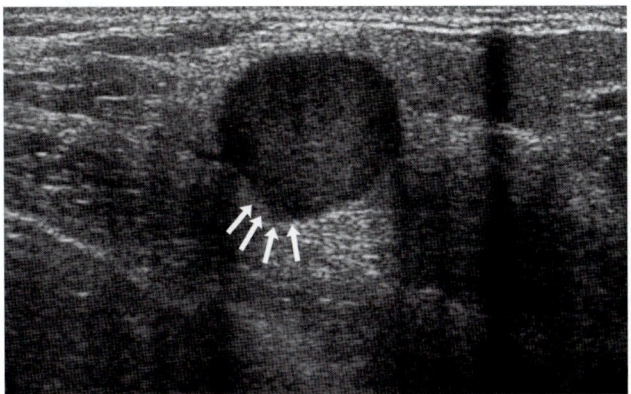

Fig. 6.60 Left antiradial breast sonogram. The nodule identified in **Fig. 6.59** sonographically corresponds to a well-defined hypoechoic, oval mass with increased posterior acoustic enhancement. Although the margin is well defined, there is slight flattening and angularity of the deep margin of the mass (*arrows*). A solid or complex cystic mass may produce this appearance.

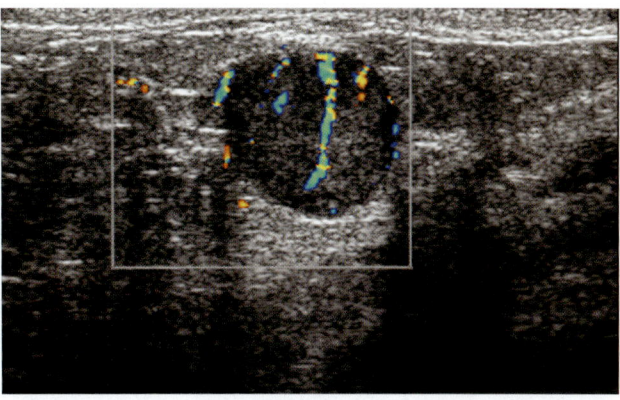

Fig. 6.61 Left antiradial color Doppler breast sonogram. Color Doppler demonstrates blood flow throughout the mass, indicating that this nodule is solid.

Pathology
- Invasive papillary carcinoma

Management
- BI-RADS assessment category 4, suspicious abnormality; biopsy should be considered

Pearls and Pitfalls

- Papillary carcinoma represents approximately 2% of breast cancers. Most patients are between 40 and 60 years old. About 90% of central papillary carcinomas present with a palpable mass, and most patients notice bloody nipple discharge.
- Mammographically, there are two common presentations of papillary carcinomas. One type is central in location and well circumscribed. The second type presents as nonpalpable multifocal peripheral cancers. This second type of papillary carcinoma behaves like the usual ductal carcinoma in situ. Mammographically, this peripheral papillary carcinoma appears as clustered calcifications.
- Sonographically, the first type of papillary carcinoma appears as an oval or round, well-defined mass that is commonly within a cyst or duct. In this case, the shape of the mass and the ill-defined mammographic margins result in a suspicious assessment. Even if this mass displayed sonographically benign characteristics, it should be biopsied because it is increasing in size and has a mammographically suspicious appearance.

Suggested Reading

Denehy AS, Sanders LM, Titus JM, Kalisher L. Breast imaging case of the day: invasive papillary carcinoma. Radiographics 1997;17:1607–1610

Merchant TE, Kievit HC, Beijerink D, van der Putte SC, de Graaf PW. MRI appearance of multiple papilloma of the breast. Breast Cancer Res Treat 1991;19:63–67

Schneider JA. Invasive papillary breast carcinoma: mammographic and sonographic appearance. Radiology 1989;171:377–379

Soo MS, Williford ME, Walsh R, Bentley RC, Kornguth PJ. Papillary carcinoma of the breast: imaging findings. AJR Am J Roentgenol 1995;164:321–326

112 Circumscribed Masses

Case 6.26: Lobular Carcinoma

Case History

A 68-year-old woman presents with mammographic enlargement of a left breast nodule.

Physical Examination
- Normal exam

Mammogram

Mass (Fig. 6.62)
- Margin: obscured
- Shape: oval
- Density: equal

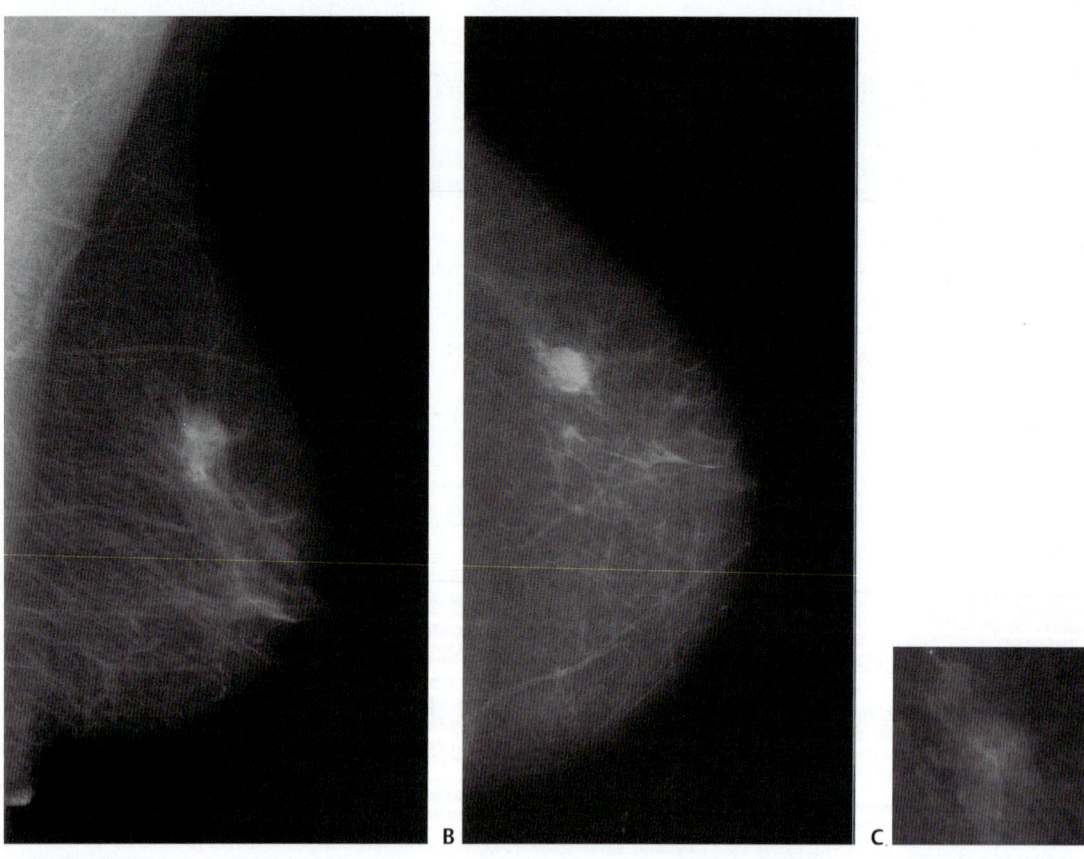

Fig. 6.62 An oval, circumscribed nodule with obscured margins is present in the upper outer breast. (**A**) Left MLO mammogram. (**B**) Left CC mammogram. (**C**) Left ML spot compression mammogram.

Ultrasound

Frequency
- 10 MHz

Mass (Fig. 6.63)
- Margin: spiculation/architectural distortion
- Echogenicity: isoechoic to fat
- Retrotumoral acoustic appearance: bilateral edge shadowing
- Shape: ellipsoid

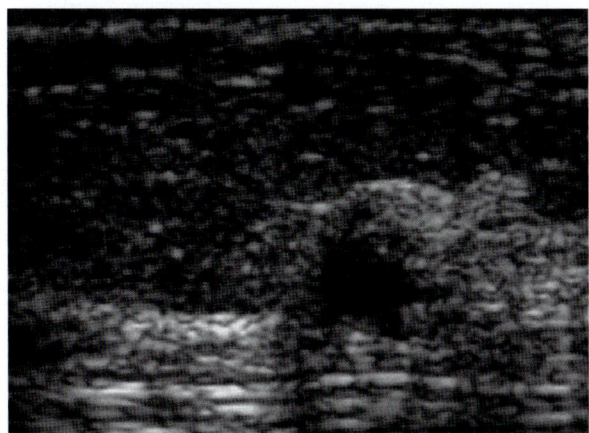

Fig. 6.63 Left longitudinal breast sonogram. The mammographic nodule identified in **Fig. 6.62** corresponds to a mass with hypoechoic spiculations extending into the surrounding hyperechoic breast tissue.

Pathology
- Invasive lobular carcinoma

Management
- BI-RADS assessment category 4, suspicious; biopsy should be considered.

Pearls and Pitfalls

- Mammographically, 50 to 70% of lobular carcinomas appear as spiculated or ill-defined masses. This tumor rarely (< 5% of cases) appears as a circumscribed mass.
- Sonographically, lobular carcinoma has the following appearances: a heterogeneous or hypoechoic irregular mass with ill-defined margins (60–85% of cases), a well-circumscribed mass (12–15%), or an area of severe shadowing that obscures the mass (15%).

Suggested Reading

Butler RS, Venta LA, Wiley EL, Ellis RL, Dempsey PJ, Rubin E. Sonographic evaluation of infiltrating lobular carcinoma. AJR Am J Roentgenol 1999;172:325–330

Cornford EJ, Wilson AR, Athanassiou E, et al. Mammographic features of invasive lobular and invasive ductal carcinoma of the breast: a comparative analysis. Br J Radiol 1995;68:450–453

Hilleren DJ, Andersson IT, Lindholm K, Linnell FS. Invasive lobular carcinoma: mammographic findings in a 10-year experience. Radiology 1991;178:149–154

Krecke KN, Gisvold JJ. Invasive lobular carcinoma of the breast: mammographic findings and extent of disease at diagnosis in 184 patients. AJR Am J Roentgenol 1993;61:957–960

Mendelson EB, Harris KM, Doshi N, Tobon H. Infiltrating lobular carcinoma: mammographic patterns with pathologic correlation. AJR Am J Roentgenol 1989;153:265–271

Paramagul CP, Helvie MA, Adler DD. Invasive lobular carcinoma: sonographic appearance and role of sonography in improving diagnostic sensitivity. Radiology 1995;195:231–234

Yeh C, Titus JM, Kalisher L. Breast imaging case of the day: infiltrating lobular carcinoma (ILC). Radiographics 1997;17:1328–1332

Case 6.27: Malignant or Locally Recurrent—Lymph Nodes

Case History
A 59-year-old woman presents with palpable left axillary nodes. Biopsy of one of the nodes is consistent with breast cancer.

Physical Examination
- Left breast: enlarged axillary node; no other palpable masses
- Right breast: normal exam

Mammogram

Mass (Fig. 6.64)
- Margin: circumscribed
- Shape: lymph node
- Density: high density

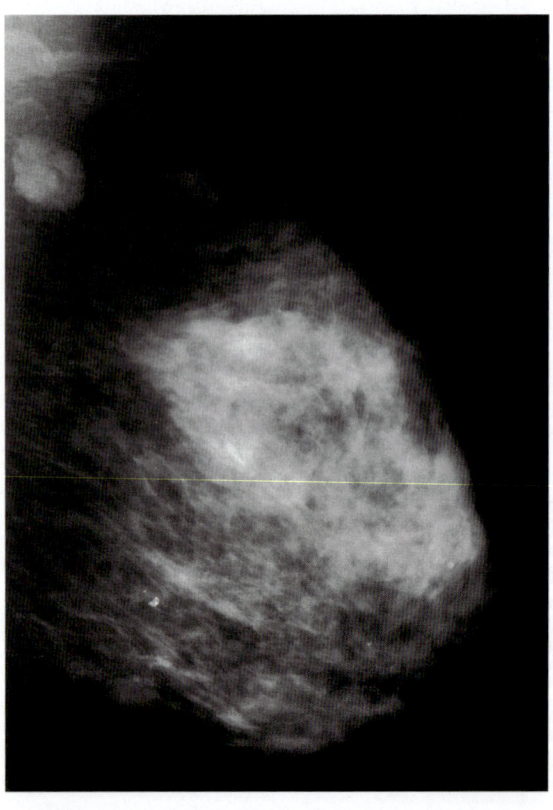
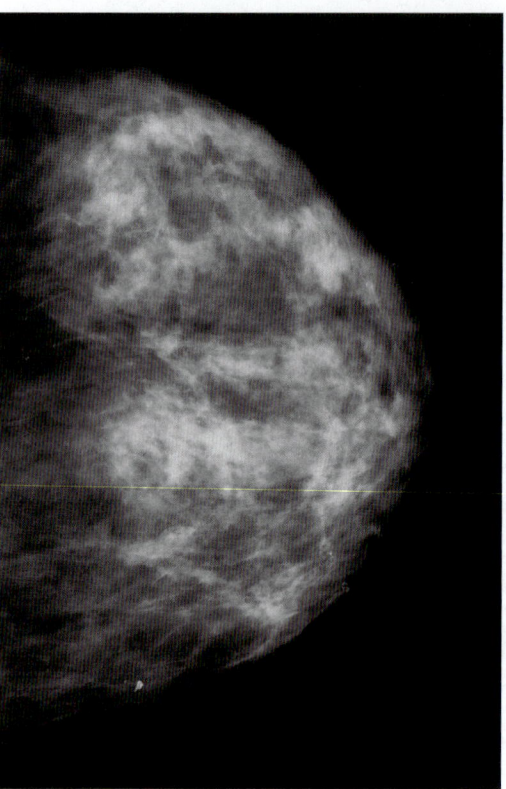

Fig. 6.64 In the left axilla, there are multiple enlarged axillary nodes. No suspicious mammographic masses or calcifications are present. (**A**) Left MLO mammogram. (**B**) Left CC mammogram.

Ultrasound

Frequency
- 11.5 MHz

Mass (Fig. 6.65)
- Margin: ill defined
- Echogenicity: hypoechoic
- Retrotumoral acoustic appearance: posterior shadowing distal to mass
- Shape: irregular

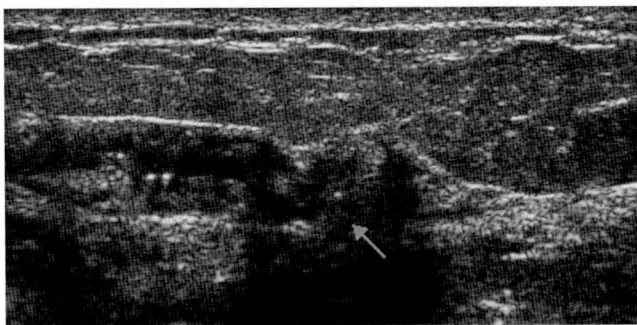
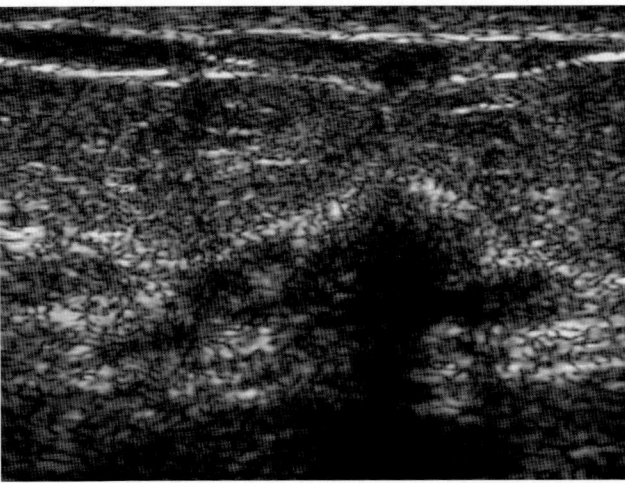

Fig. 6.65 At the 6 o'clock position of the left breast, there is a hypoechoic, irregular mass. This area appears to best correlate with the area of abnormal MRI contrast enhancement (**Fig. 6.66**). However, percutaneous sonographic-guided biopsy of this area was benign. (**A**) Left radial breast sonogram. (**B**) Left antiradial breast sonogram.

Other Modalities: MRI (Fig. 6.66)

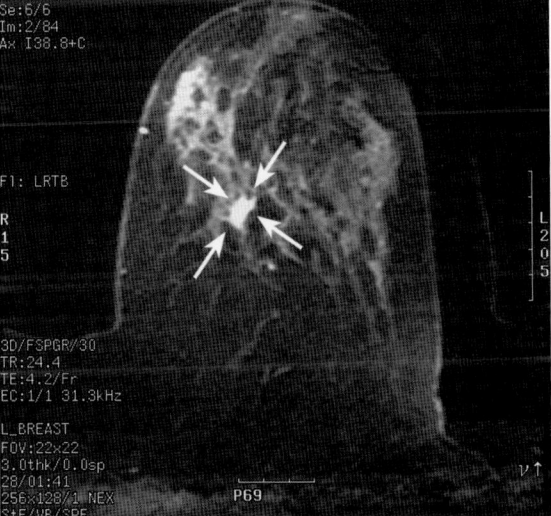

Fig. 6.66 Left transverse dynamic bolus 3D volume gradient breast MRI. In the inferior breast, there is an irregular contrast-enhancing spiculated mass (*arrows*).

Pathology
- Invasive ductal carcinoma

Management
- BI-RADS assessment category 4, suspicious; biopsy should be considered.

Pearls and Pitfalls

- This case illustrates a tumor that is detectable only with MRI. Mastectomy specimen demonstrates that the MRI mass corresponds to a 1.5 cm infiltrating ductal carcinoma. No other tumors are detected within the breast. One of 12 axillary nodes is positive for metastatic disease.
- Breast cancer presents as axillary adenopathy in 0.3 to 1% of reported series. Besides breast cancer, metastatic disease from other distant primaries may present in this manner. The most common primary is melanoma. If the adenopathy is due to breast cancer and the mammogram is normal, then the primary tumors are generally less than 2 cm. In over half of the cases, the breast tumor is in the upper outer quadrant.

Suggested Reading

Ashikari R, Rosen PP, Urban JA, Senoo T. Breast cancer presenting as an axillary mass. Ann Surg 1976;183:415–417

Feuerman L, Attie JN, Rosenberg B. Carcinoma in axillary lymph nodes as an indicator of breast cancer. Surg Gynecol Obstet 1962;114:5–8

Fitts WT, Steiner GC, Enterline HT. Prognosis of occult carcinoma of the breast. Am J Surg 1963;106:460–463

Leibman AJ, Kossoff MB I. Mammography in women with axillary lymphadenopathy and normal breasts on physical examination: value in detecting occult breast carcinoma. AJR Am J Roentgenol 1992;159:493–495

Merson M, Andreola S, Galimberti V, Bufalino R, Marchini S, Veronesi U. Breast carcinoma presenting as axillary metastases without evidence of a primary tumor. Cancer 1992; 70:504–508

Owen HW, Dockerty MB, Gray HK. Occult carcinoma of the breast. Surg Gynecol Obstet 1954;98:302–308

Rosen PP. Axillary lymph node metastases in patients with occult noninvasive breast carcinoma. Cancer 1980;46:1298–1306

Vilcoq JR, Calle R, Ferme F, Veith F. Conservative treatment of axillary adenopathy due to probable subclinical breast cancer. Arch Surg 1982;117:1136–1138

Case 6.28: Malignant or Locally Recurrent—Medullary Carcinoma

Case History
A 72-year-old woman presents with a new density on her screening mammogram.

Physical Examination
- Normal exam

Mammogram

Mass (Fig. 6.67)
- Margin: indistinct
- Shape: oval
- Density: equal density

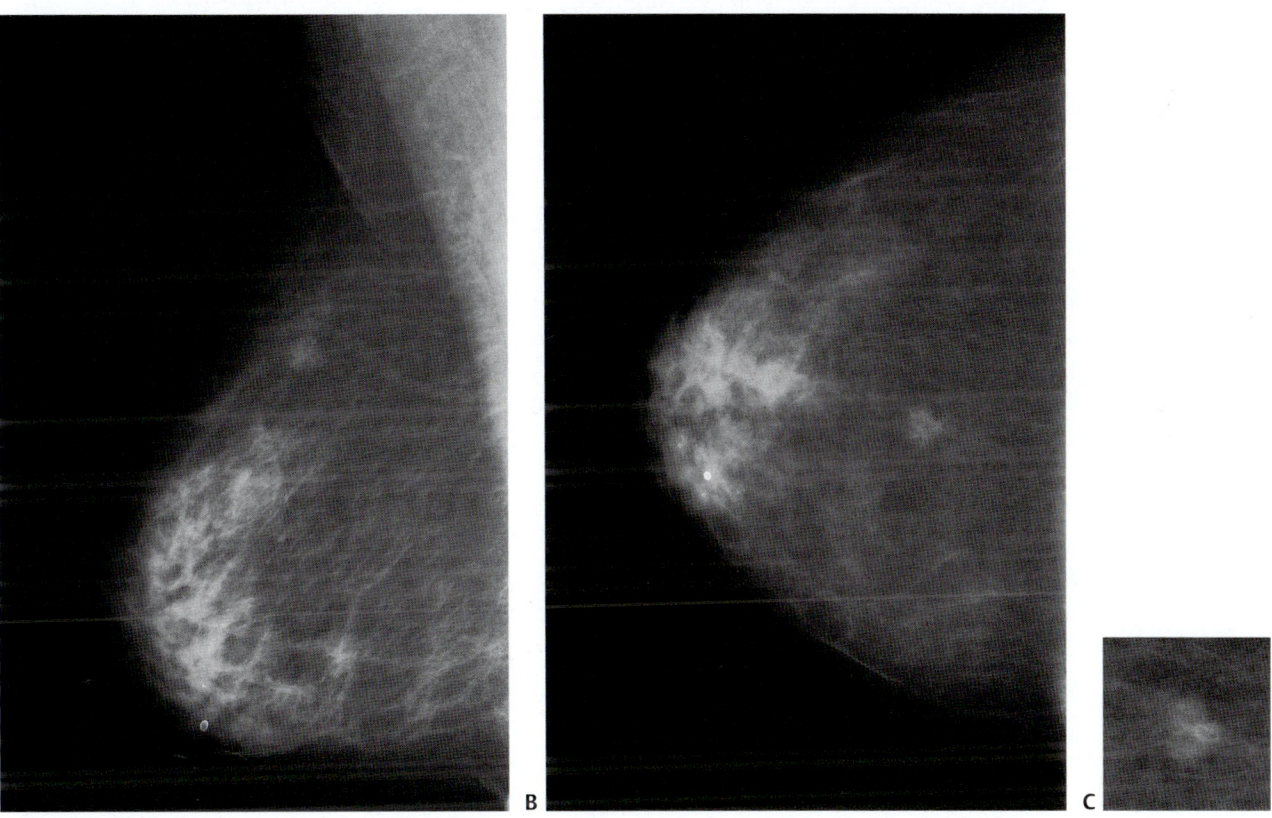

Fig. 6.67 At the 12 o'clock position, there is an oval mass. Spot compression view demonstrates that the mass is mildly lobulated and has an ill-defined margin. (**A**) Right MLO mammogram. (**B**) Right CC mammogram. (**C**) Right CC spot compression.

Pathology
- Medullary carcinoma

Management
- BI-RADS assessment category 4, suspicious abnormality; biopsy should be considered.

> **Pearls and Pitfalls**
>
> - Medullary carcinoma represents between 5 and 7% of all breast cancers. The mean patient age is 50 years.
> - Series that describe medullary carcinoma commonly include both typical and atypical medullary carcinomas. Typical medullary carcinoma (TMC) is an uncalcified mass with either well-defined or ill-defined margins. Atypical medullary carcinoma (AMC) generally presents with ill-defined margins. Histologically, AMC is commonly mistaken for TMC.
> - Whereas TMC has a favorable prognosis (5-year survival rate of 75%), AMC prognosis is similar to infiltrating ductal cancer (5-year survival rate of 66%).

Suggested Reading

Bloom HJG, Richardson WW, Field JR. Host resistance and survival in carcinoma of breast: a study of 104 cases of medullary carcinoma in a series of 1,411 cases of breast cancer followed for 20 years. BMJ 1970;3:181–188

Hoge AF, Asal N, Owen W, Anderson P. Histologic and staging classification of breast cancer: implications for therapy. South Med J 1982;75):1329–1334

Jensen ML, Kiaer H, Andersen J, Jensen V, Melsen F. Prognostic comparison of three classifications for medullary carcinomas of the breast. Histopathology 1997;30:523–532

Liberman L, LaTrenta LR, Samli B, Morris EA, Abramson AF, Dershaw DD. Overdiagnosis of medullary carcinoma: a mammographic-pathologic correlative study. Radiology 1996;201:443–446

Maier WP, Rosemond GP, Goldman LI, Kaplan GF, Tyson RR. A ten-year study of medullary carcinoma of the breast. Surg Gynecol Obstet 1977;144:695–698

Richardson WW. Medullary carcinoma of the breast; a distinctive tumour type with a relatively good prognosis following radical mastectomy. Br J Cancer 1956;10:415–423

Ridolfi RL, Rosen PP, Port A, Kinne D, Miké V. Medullary carcinoma of the breast: a clinicopathologic study with 10-year follow-up. Cancer 1977;40:1365–1385

Case 6.29: Malignant or Locally Recurrent—Metaplastic Carcinoma

Case History
A 28-year-old woman presents with a palpable right breast lump.

Physical Examination
- Right breast: palpable lump at the 11 o'clock position of the right breast
- Left breast: normal exam

Mammogram

Mass (Fig. 6.68)
- Margin: obscured
- Shape: oval
- Density: equal density

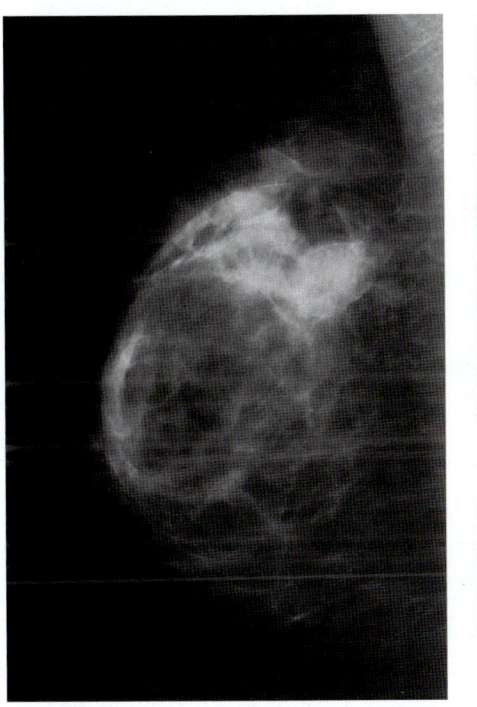
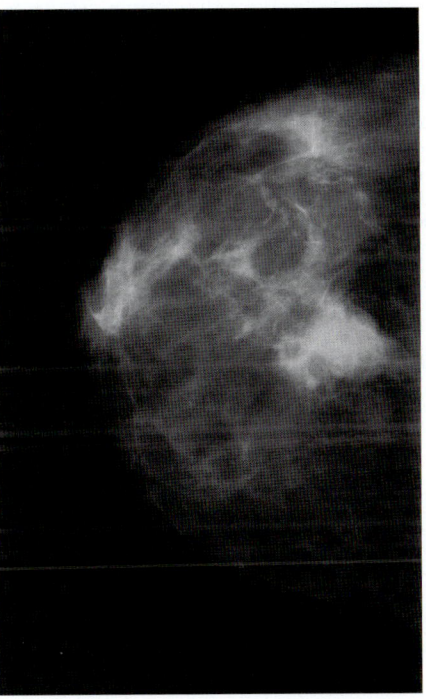

Fig. 6.68 At the 11 o'clock position of the right breast, there is an oval mass with partially obscured margins. This mass corresponds to the palpable mass. (**A**) Right MLO mammogram. (**B**) Right CC mammogram.

Ultrasound

Frequency
- 11.5 MHz

Mass (Fig. 6.69)
- Margin: well defined
- Echogenicity: hypoechoic
- Retrotumoral acoustic appearance: bilateral edge shadowing
- Shape: ellipsoid

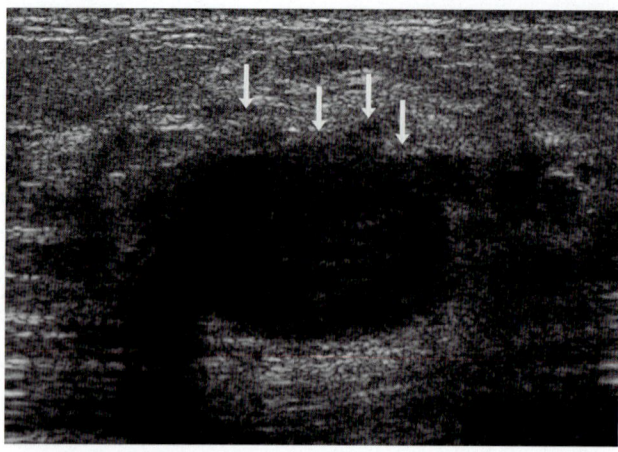

Fig. 6.69 Right radial breast sonogram. The palpable lump corresponds to a hypoechoic oval mass. Most of the margin is well defined, but mild irregularity and lobulation of the superficial margin are present (*arrows*).

Other Modalities: Lymphoscintigraphy (Fig. 6.70)

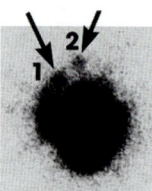

Fig. 6.70 Right breast lymphoscintigraphy. Two sentinel lymph nodes (*arrows*) are identified after injection around the tumor illustrated in **Fig. 6.69**. Both of these nodes were removed, and no metastatic disease was identified histologically.

Pathology
- Metaplastic carcinoma
- Combination of high-grade infiltrating ductal carcinoma and metaplastic changes of benign osteoclastic cells, cartilage, and osteoid

Management
- BI-RADS assessment category 4, suspicious; biopsy should be considered.

Pearls and Pitfalls

- Metaplastic carcinoma is a combination of adenocarcinoma (such as invasive ductal) and a second epithelial (e.g., squamous, spindle) or mesenchymal (chondroid, osseous) cell type.
- Mammographically, these tumors appear as circumscribed lobular, oval, or round masses. If there is a significant invasive ductal component, then the margins may be ill defined or spiculated.
- Carcinomas with chondroid and osseous differentiation appear to have a better prognosis than those with infiltrating ductal carcinoma in a small series.

Suggested Reading

Brenner RJ, Turner RR, Schiller V, Arndt RD, Giuliano A. Metaplastic carcinoma of the breast: report of three cases. Cancer 1998;82:1082–1087

Chhieng C, Cranor M, Lesser ME, Rosen PP. Metaplastic carcinoma of the breast with osteocartilaginous heterologous elements. Am J Surg Pathol 1998;22:188–194

Patterson SK, Tworek JA, Roubidoux MA, Helvie MA, Oberman HA. Metaplastic carcinoma of the breast: mammographic appearance with pathologic correlation. AJR Am J Roentgenol 1997;169:709–712

Tavasoli PA. Metaplastic carcinoma. In: Pathology of the Breast. Stamford: Appleton and Lange; 1999:481–504

Case 6.30: Malignant or Locally Recurrent—Metastases

Case History
A 50-year-old woman presents with a newly discovered lump in her left breast.

Physical Examination
- Left breast: palpable 1 cm mass at the 12 o'clock position
- Right breast: normal exam

Mammogram

Mass (Fig. 6.71)
- Margin: indistinct
- Shape: oval
- Density: high density

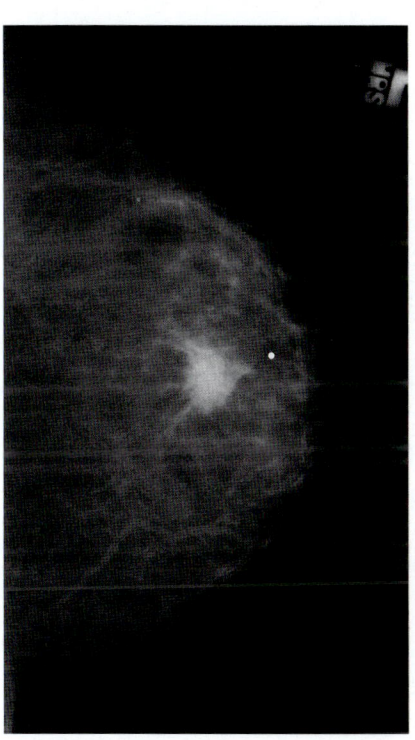
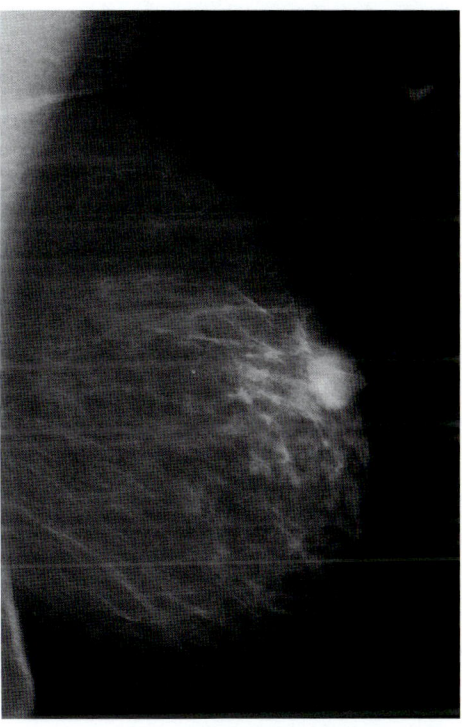

Fig. 6.71 At the 12 o'clock position of the left breast, there is an ill-defined oval mass that corresponds to the palpable lump. (**A**) Left MLO mammogram. (**B**) Left CC mammogram.

Ultrasound

Frequency
- 10 MHz

Mass (Fig. 6.72)
- Margin: ill defined
- Echogenicity: hypoechoic
- Retrotumoral acoustic appearance: increased acoustic transmission
- Shape: lobulated

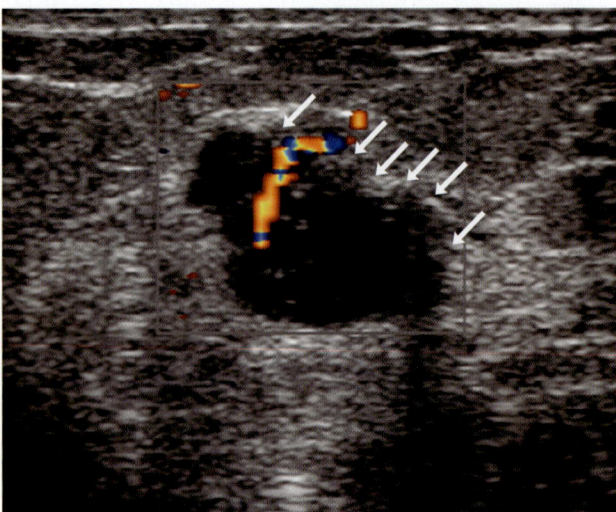

Fig. 6.72 Left transverse color Doppler breast sonogram. At the 12 o'clock position, there is a lobulated multicystic mass. The septations within the mass have color flow, and the edge of the mass consists of solid tissue that forms an ill-defined margin (arrows).

Pathology
- Metastases: metastatic melanoma

Management
- BI-RADS assessment category 4, suspicious; biopsy should be considered.

Pearls and Pitfalls

- Extramammary metastases to the breast represent approximately 1% of all clinically detected breast malignancies.
- Excluding lymphomas and leukemias, the most common extramammary types of metastases to the breast are (in decreasing order of frequency) melanoma, lung, prostate, ovary, gastrointestinal, and cervix.
- Mammographically, metastases to the breast are noncalcified round or oval masses with either well-defined or ill-defined margins. They are generally superficial and commonly palpable.
- Sonographically, metastases are most commonly hypoechoic solid round, oval, or lobulated masses with either well-defined or ill-defined margins. Posterior acoustic shadowing is generally not present. Melanoma has increased color flow compared with normal breast parenchyma.

Suggested Reading

Bohman LG, Bassett LW, Gold RH, Voet R. Breast metastases from extramammary malignancies. Radiology 1982;144:309–312

Derchi LE, Rizzatto G, Giuseppetti GM, Dini G, Garaventa A. Metastatic tumors in the breast: sonographic findings. J Ultrasound Med 1985;4:69–74

McCrea ES, Johnston C, Haney PJ. Metastases to the breast. AJR Am J Roentgenol 1983;141:685–690

Moncada R, Cooper RA, Garces M, Badrinath K. Calcified metastases from malignant ovarian neoplasm: review of the literature. Radiology 1974;113:31–35

Paulus DD, Libshitz HI. Metastasis to the breast. Radiol Clin North Am 1982;20:561–568

Tavassoli FA. Metastatic carcinoma. In: Tavassoli FA, Fattaneh A. Pathology of the Breast. 2nd ed. Stamford: Appleton and Lange; 1999:551–555

Tohno E, Cosgrove DO, Sloane JP. Metastases to the Breast. In: Tohno D, Cosgrove DO, Sloane JP, eds. Ultrasound Diagnosis of Breast Diseases. New York: Churchill Livingstone; 1994:185–186

Toombs BD, Kalisher L. Metastatic disease to the breast: clinical, pathologic, and radiographic features. AJR Am J Roentgenol 1977;129:673–676

Case 6.31: Malignant or Locally Recurrent—Mucinous Carcinoma

Case History
A 39-year-old woman presents with a new left breast lump.

Physical Examination
- Left breast: palpable mass at the 4 o'clock position; a second mammographic mass is not palpable
- Right breast: normal exam

Mammogram

Mass (Fig. 6.73)
- Margin: circumscribed
- Shape: oval
- Density: high density

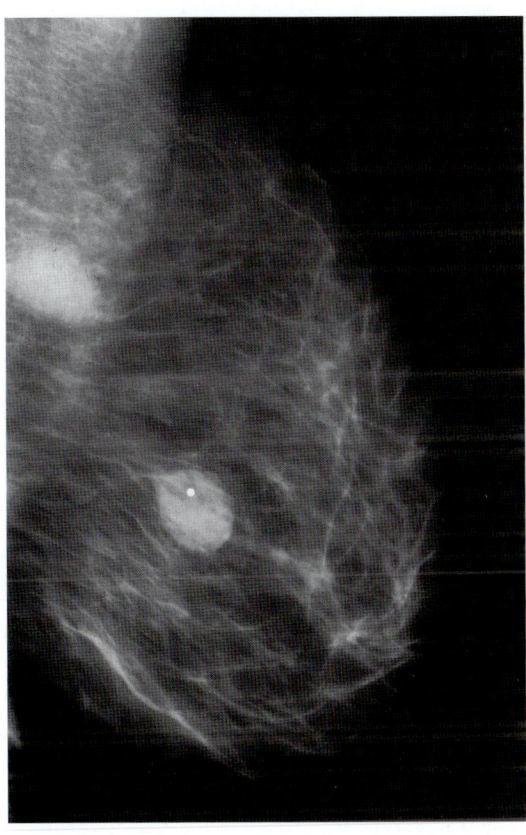
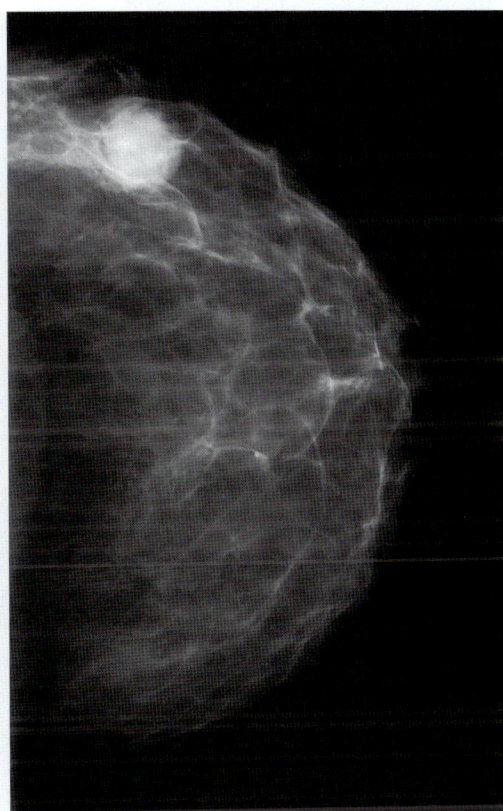

Fig. 6.73 Two similar circumscribed oval masses are present in the left breast. One mass is in the upper outer quadrant, and the other is in the outer inferior quadrant. These masses are new since the patient's baseline mammogram 3 years ago. (**A**) Left MLO mammogram. (**B**) Left CC mammogram.

124 Circumscribed Masses

Ultrasound

Frequency
- 11.5 MHz

Mass (Figs. 6.74 and 6.75)
- Margin: well defined
- Echogenicity: hypoechoic
- Retrotumoral acoustic appearance: bilateral edge shadowing
- Shape: ellipsoid

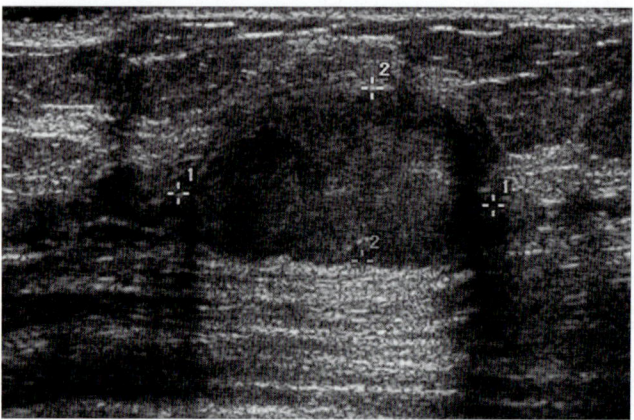

Fig. 6.74 Left radial breast sonogram at the 2 o'clock position. The mammographic mass in the left upper outer quadrant (**Fig. 6.73**) corresponds to a well-defined, oval, hypoechoic mass with posterior acoustic enhancement.

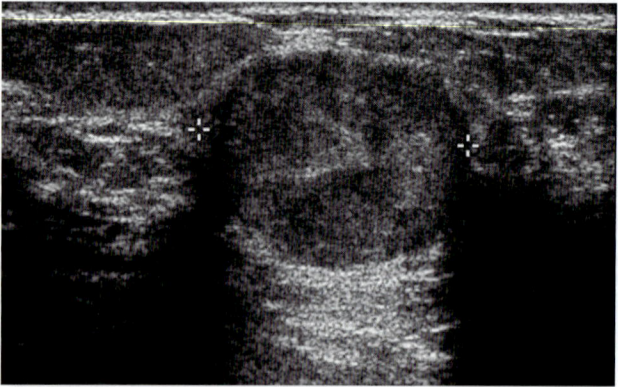

Fig. 6.75 Left radial breast sonogram at the 4 o'clock position. The mammographic mass in the inferior outer quadrant (**Fig. 6.73**) corresponds to a well-defined, oval, hypoechoic mass with increased acoustic enhancement. The appearance of this mass is similar to the mass at the 2 o'clock position (**Fig. 6.74**).

Pathology
- Mucinous carcinoma

Management
- BI-RADS assessment category 4, suspicious; biopsy should be considered

Pearls and Pitfalls
- Mucinous carcinoma accounts for 1 to 7% of all breast cancers. The mean age of patients is in the seventh decade.
- Mammographically, mucinous cancers are oval or lobulated and may have either ill-defined or well-defined margins. Low-grade, pure mucinous tumors tend to have well-defined margins.
- Sonographically, mucinous neoplasms appear as well-defined, lobulated or oval hypoechoic masses with a thin hyperechoic capsule. They may exhibit decreased, equal, or increased acoustic transmission.

Suggested Reading

Cardenosa G, Doudna C, Eklund GW. Mucinous (colloid) breast cancer: clinical and mammographic findings in 10 patients. AJR Am J Roentgenol 1994;162:1077–1079

Chopra S, Evans AJ, Pinder SE, et al. Pure mucinous breast cancer—mammographic and ultrasound findings. Clin Radiol 1996;51:421–424

Conant EF, Dillon RL, Palazzo J, Ehrlich SM, Feig SA. Imaging findings in mucin-containing carcinomas of the breast: correlation with pathologic features. AJR Am J Roentgenol 1994;163:821–824

Ruggieri AM, Scola FH, Schepps B, et al. Mucinous carcinoma of the breast: mammographic findings. Breast Dis 1995;8:353–361

Wilson TE, Helvie MA, Oberman HA, Joynt LK. Pure and mixed mucinous carcinoma of the breast: pathologic basis for differences in mammographic appearance. AJR Am J Roentgenol 1995;165:285–289

Case 6.32: Malignant or Locally Recurrent—Phyllodes Tumor

Case History
A 43-year-old woman presents with a palpable lump. The lump was first detected 1 year ago and had been found to be sonographically solid.

Physical Examination
- Left breast: 2 to 3 cm mass at the 1 o'clock position
- Right breast: normal exam

Mammogram

Mass (Fig. 6.76)
- Margin: circumscribed
- Shape: oval
- Density: equal density

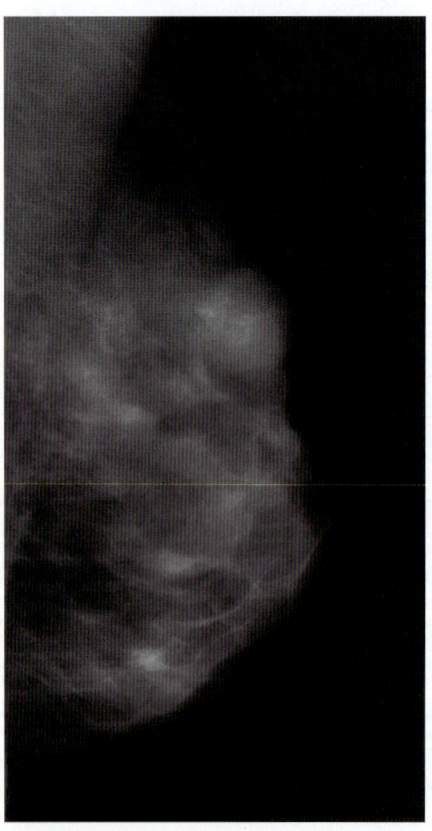
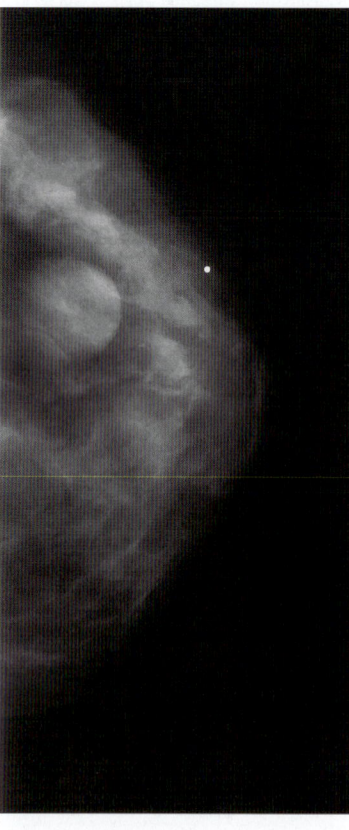

Fig. 6.76 At the 1 o'clock position of the left breast there is a predominantly circumscribed oval mass that corresponds to the patient's palpable lump. (**A**) Left MLO mammogram. (**B**) Left CC mammogram.

Ultrasound

Frequency
- 7.5 MHz

Mass (Fig. 6.77)
- Margin: well defined
- Echogenicity: heterogeneous (mixed)
- Retrotumoral acoustic appearance: retrotumoral enhancement present
- Shape: ellipsoid

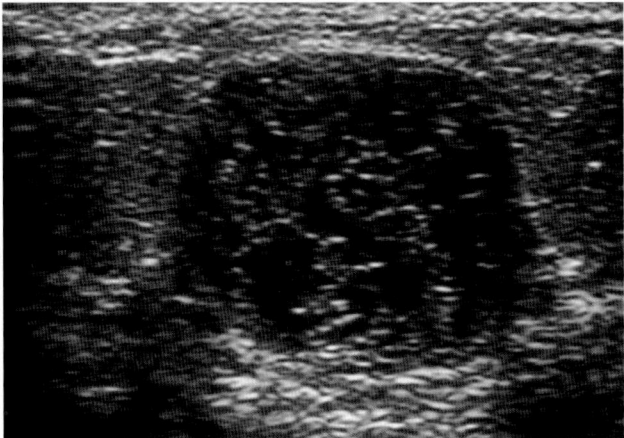

Fig. 6.77 Left longitudinal breast sonogram. The palpable mass corresponds to a well-defined, oval solid mass with heterogeneous echogenicity and increased acoustic transmission. Irregular cystic spaces are present throughout the mass. Since the previous sonogram (1 year prior), the mass has doubled in size.

Pathology
- Phyllodes tumor (cystosarcoma phyllodes)

Management
- BI-RADS assessment category 4, suspicious abnormality; biopsy should be considered.

Pearls and Pitfalls
- Phyllodes tumors constitute 0.3% of all breast tumors. Women with this tumor are generally older than women with fibroadenomas. The average age is 45. About 30% of phyllodes tumors recur, and 10% metastasize. This tumor most frequently metastasizes to lungs (66%), skeleton (28%), and lymph nodes (15%).
- Mammographically, phyllodes tumors are generally well defined, uncalcified, and lobulated, round, or oval. They are similar to fibroadenomas, but they should be considered if the mass is > 6 to 8 cm or is rapidly growing.
- Sonographically, these masses are hypoechoic or heterogeneous echogenicity with posterior acoustic enhancement. Unlike fibroadenomas, phyllodes tumors commonly have thin, irregular cystic spaces within them.

Suggested Reading

Buchberger W, Strasser K, Heim K, Müller E, Schröcksnadel H. Phylloides tumor: findings on mammography, sonography, and aspiration cytology in 10 cases. AJR Am J Roentgenol 1991;157:715–719

Czum JM, Sanders LM, Titus JM, Kalisher L. Breast imaging case of the day: benign phyllodes tumor. Radiographics 1997;17:548–551

Liberman L, Bonaccio E, Hamele-Bena D, Abramson AF, Cohen MA, Dershaw DD. Benign and malignant phyllodes tumors: mammographic and sonographic findings. Radiology 1996;198:121–124

Tavassoli FA, Fattaneh A. Pathology of the Breast, 2nd ed. Stamford: Appleton and Lange; 1999:598–631

Case 6.33: Granular Cell Tumor

Case History
A 45-year-old woman presents for screening mammogram.

Physical Examination
- Normal exam

Mammogram

Mass (Fig. 6.78)
- Margin: indistinct
- Shape: oval
- Density: high density

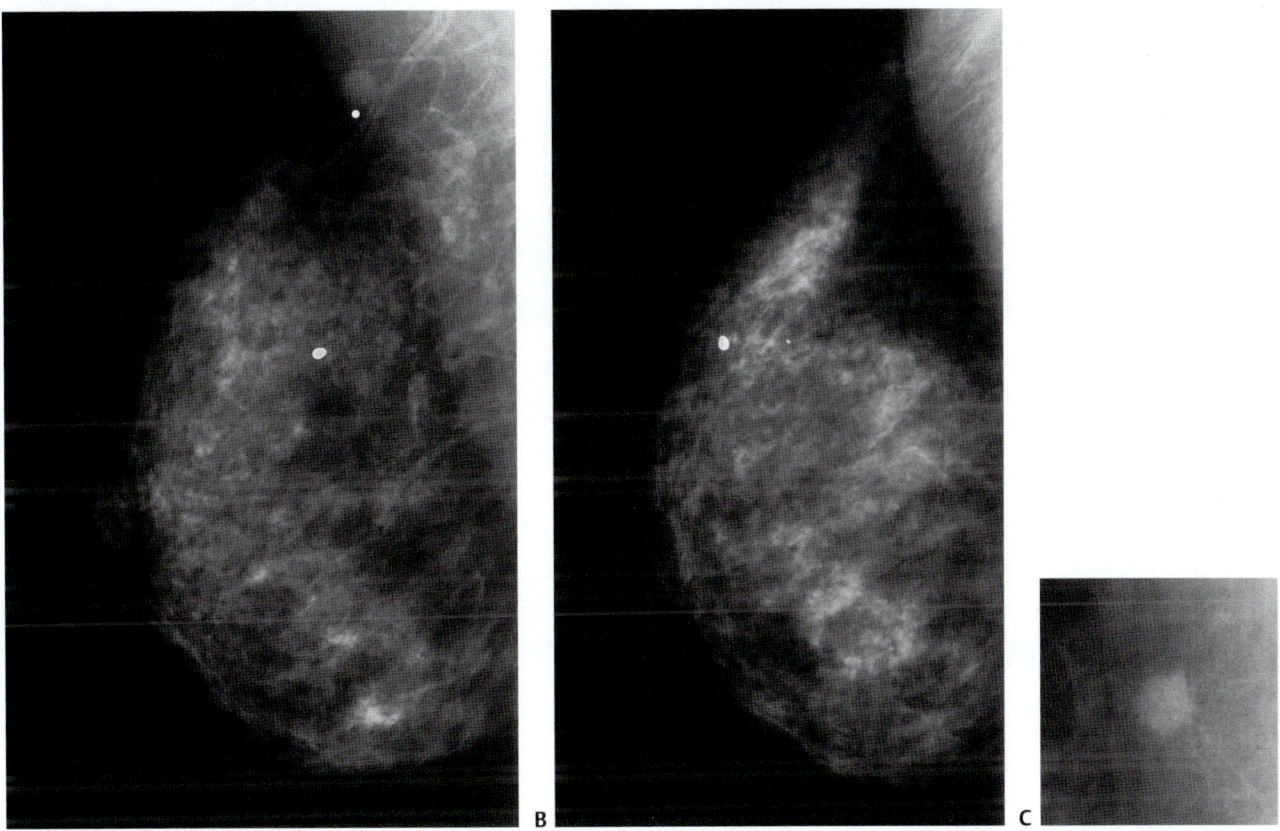

Fig. 6.78 In the right upper outer quadrant, there is an ill-defined oval mass. (**A**) Right MLO mammogram. (**B**) Right exaggerated CC mammogram. (**C**) Right MLO spot compression mammogram.

Ultrasound

Frequency
- 13 MHz

Mass (Figs. 6.79 and 6.80)
- Margin: ill defined
- Echogenicity: hypoechoic
- Retrotumoral acoustic appearance: bilateral edge shadowing
- Shape: ellipsoid

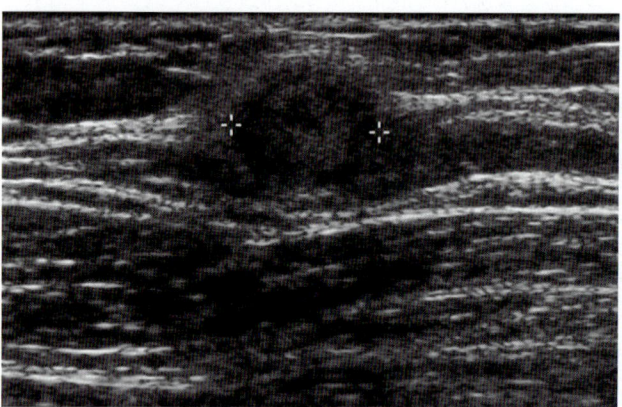

Fig. 6.79 Right radial breast sonogram. The mammographic mass corresponds to an oval, hypoechoic solid mass. In this view, the mass has a subtle hyperechoic, irregular halo.

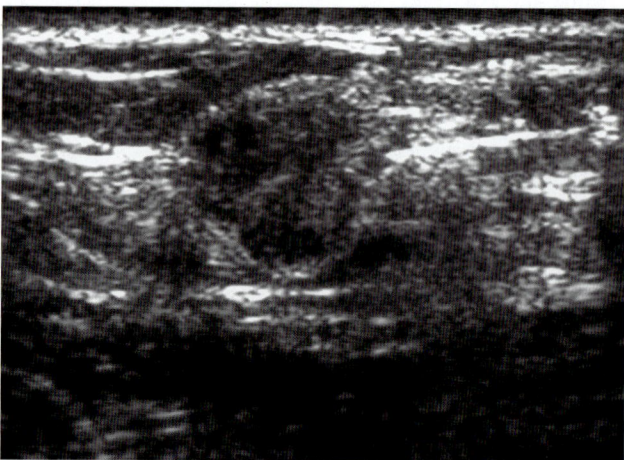

Fig. 6.80 Right antiradial breast sonogram. The irregular margin of the mass is better demonstrated in this view.

Pathology
- Granular cell tumor

Management
- BI-RADS assessment category 4, suspicious; biopsy should be considered.

> **Pearls and Pitfalls**
>
> - Granular cell tumors represent < 0.1% of breast lesions. Although the tumor has been reported in a wide age range (17 to 75 years), it tends to present in younger women (average age in the 30s).
> - Mammographically and sonographically, this tumor presents as an oval or round mass with ill-defined or spiculated margins.
> - Although this mass may simulate carcinoma, it rarely metastasizes. It may be infiltrative, so local excision is required.

Suggested Reading

Bassett LW, Cove HC. Myoblastoma of the breast. AJR Am J Roentgenol 1979;132:122–123

Baum JK, Robins JR, Schnitt S, Houlihan MJ. The ultrasound appearance of granular cell tumor of the breast: a case report. Breast Dis 1994;7:281–285

Ilkhanipour ZS, Harris KM, Kanbour AI. Granular cell tumor of the breast: two case reports mimicking carcinoma. Breast Dis 1993;6:221–225

Tavassoli FA, Fattaneh A. Pathology of the Breast. 2nd ed. Stamford: Appleton and Lange; 1999:697

Irregular Masses

This is an outline of the approach to mammographic irregular masses. For further discussion, see Chapter 1.

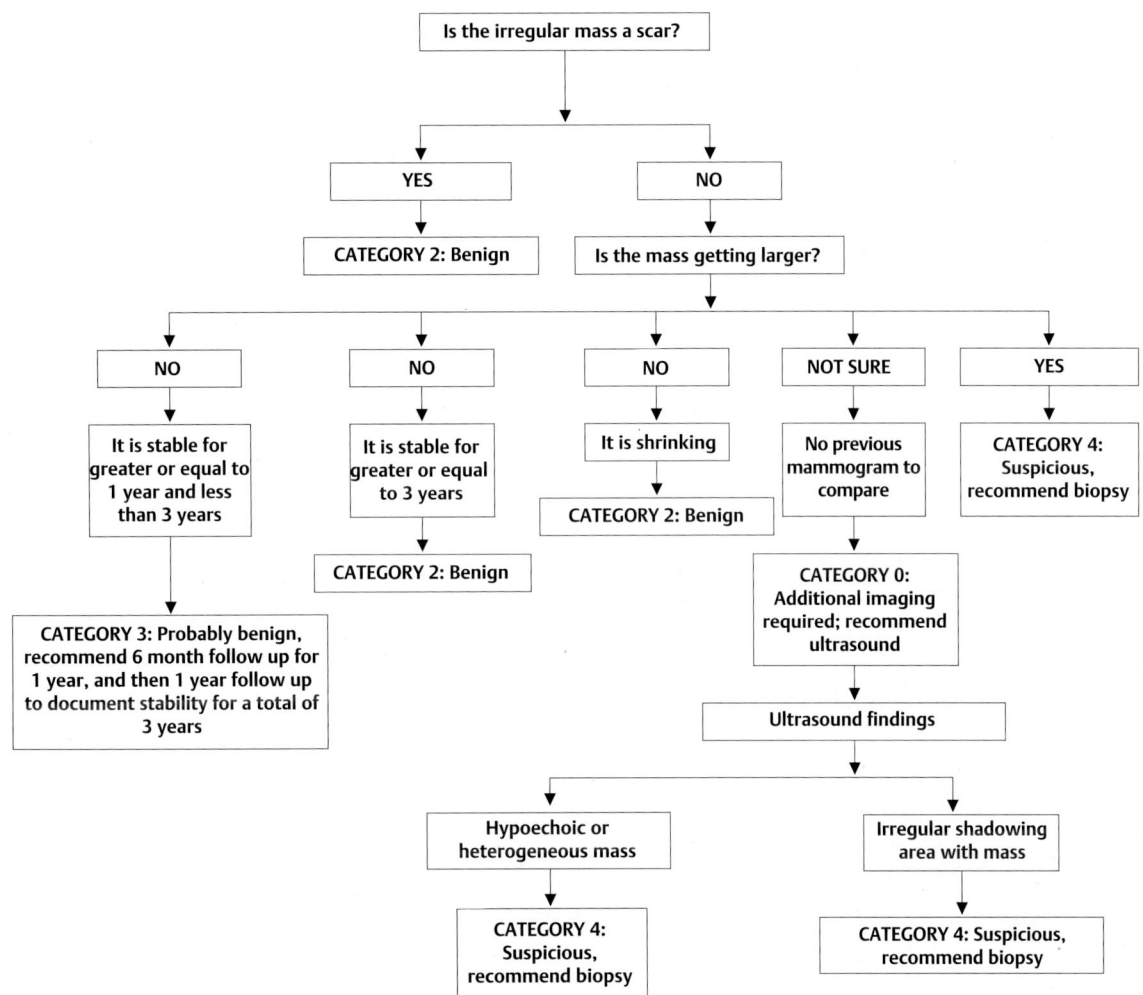

7 Irregular Masses: Benign Masses

Case 7.1: Adenosis

Case History

An 86-year-old woman presents with a new left breast palpable lump.

Physical Examination
- Left breast: palpable lump in upper outer quadrant
- Right breast: normal exam

Mammogram

Mass (Fig. 7.1)
- Margin: indistinct
- Shape: irregular
- Density: equal density

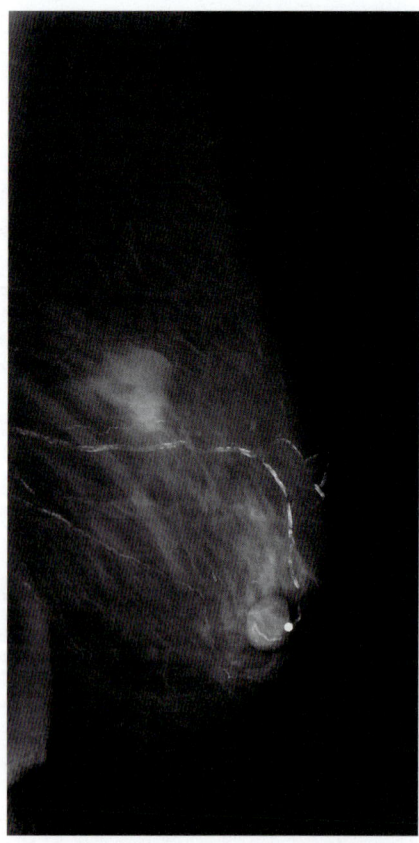
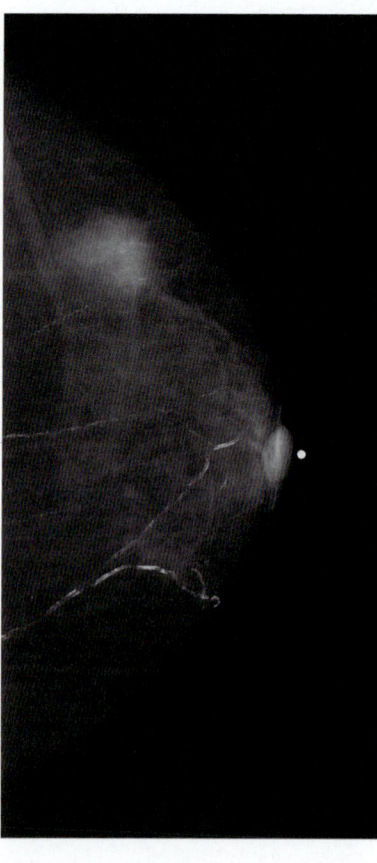

Fig. 7.1 In the left upper outer quadrant, there is an irregular mass that corresponds to the palpable lump. (**A**) Left MLO mammogram. (**B**) Left CC mammogram.

Ultrasound

Frequency
- 8 MHz

Mass (Fig. 7.2)
- Margin: ill defined
- Echogenicity: hyperechoic
- Retrotumoral acoustic appearance: posterior shadowing distal to mass
- Shape: ellipsoid

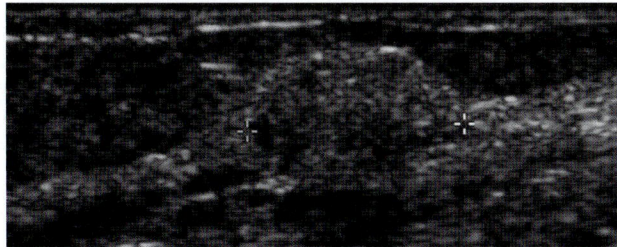

Fig. 7.2 Left radial breast sonogram. The palpable mammographic mass corresponds to a hyperechoic oval mass, which has a partially ill-defined margin.

Pathology
- Microglandular adenosis

Management
- BI-RADS assessment category 4, suspicious; biopsy should be considered.

Pearls and Pitfalls

- Microglandular adenosis is a rare type of adenosis. Most patients present with a palpable lump.
- There are no specific radiographic or sonographic patterns for this disease due to its rarity.
- Microglandular adenosis has been associated with infiltrating carcinoma, so lesions that increase in size should be critically reevaluated.

Suggested Reading

James BA, Cranor ML, Rosen PP. Carcinoma of the breast arising in microglandular adenosis. Am J Clin Pathol 1993;100:507–513

Rosen PP. Microglandular adenosis. A benign lesion simulating invasive mammary carcinoma. Am J Surg Pathol 1983;7:137–144

Rosenblum MK, Purrazzella R, Rosen PP. Is microglandular adenosis a precancerous disease? A study of carcinoma arising therein. Am J Surg Pathol 1986;10:237–245

Tavassoli FA. Benign lesions. In: Tavasolli FA, Fattaneh A, eds. Pathology of the Breast. 2nd ed. Stamford: Appleton and Lange; 1999:115–204

Case 7.2: Fat Necrosis

Case History
A 60-year-old woman presents with a new right breast lump. She has no previous trauma, breast surgery, or biopsy.

Physical Examination
- Right breast: palpable lump at the 11 o'clock position
- Left breast: normal exam

Mammogram

Mass (Fig. 7.3)
- Margin: indistinct
- Shape: irregular
- Density: equal density

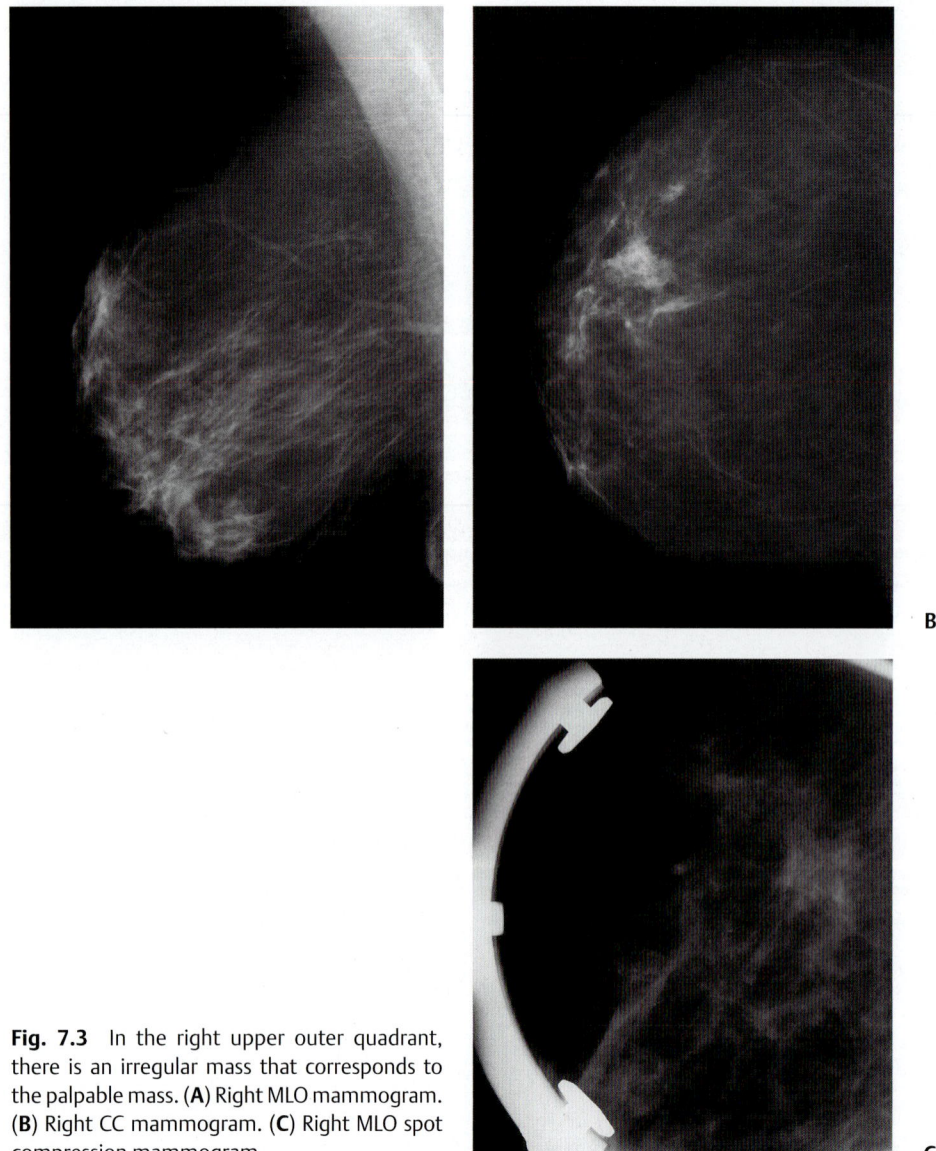

Fig. 7.3 In the right upper outer quadrant, there is an irregular mass that corresponds to the palpable mass. (**A**) Right MLO mammogram. (**B**) Right CC mammogram. (**C**) Right MLO spot compression mammogram.

Ultrasound

Frequency
- 11.5 MHz

Mass (Fig. 7.4)
- Margin: ill defined
- Echogenicity: heterogeneous
- Retrotumoral acoustic appearance: posterior shadowing distal to mass
- Shape: irregular

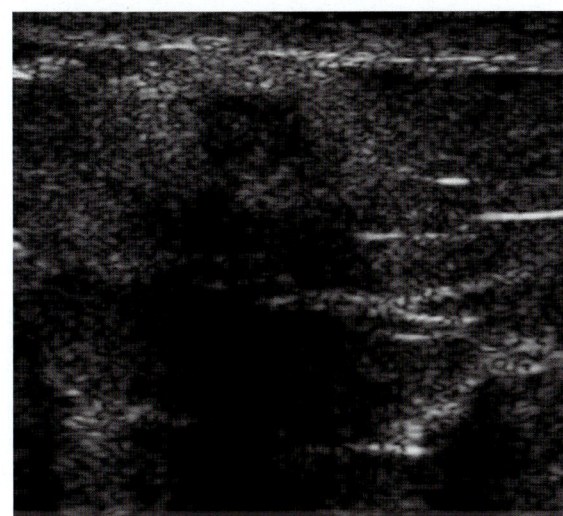

Fig. 7.4 Right radial breast sonogram. The palpable mammographic mass corresponds to an ill-defined irregular mass with a hyperechoic rim and hypoechoic center. The mass exhibits severe acoustic shadowing.

Pathology
- Fat necrosis

Management
- BI-RADS assessment category 4, suspicious; biopsy should be considered.

Pearls and Pitfalls

- Although only 40% of patients with fat necrosis have a history of previous breast injury, this lesion has a traumatic origin. Fat necrosis has two different appearances. In some patients, the fat necrosis causes a fibrotic response that results in an irregular solid mass (illustrated in this case), which may be associated with skin thickening and nipple retraction. This mass cannot be distinguished mammographically or sonographically from carcinoma. Besides producing an irregular mass, fat necrosis may also produce a lipid collection without an inflammatory response. This second type of fat necrosis results in a round or oval nodule (oil cyst) that is either calcium or fat density mammographically.

Suggested Reading

Bassett LW, Gold RH, Cove HC. Mammographic spectrum of traumatic fat necrosis: the fallibility of "pathognomonic" signs of carcinoma. AJR Am J Roentgenol 1978;130:119–122

Evers K, Troupin RH. Lipid cyst: classic and atypical appearances. AJR Am J Roentgenol 1991;157:271–273

Orson LW, Cigtay OS. Fat necrosis of the breast: characteristic xeromammographic appearance. Radiology 1983;146:35–38

Case 7.3: Fat Necrosis

Case History
A 72-year-old woman status-post right lumpectomy and radiation therapy has developed a new mammographic finding near the surgical site. This is the same patient as Case 7.9.

Physical Examination
- Right breast: subareolar scar
- Left breast: normal exam

Mammogram

Mass (Fig. 7.5)
- Margin: spiculated
- Shape: irregular
- Density: equal density

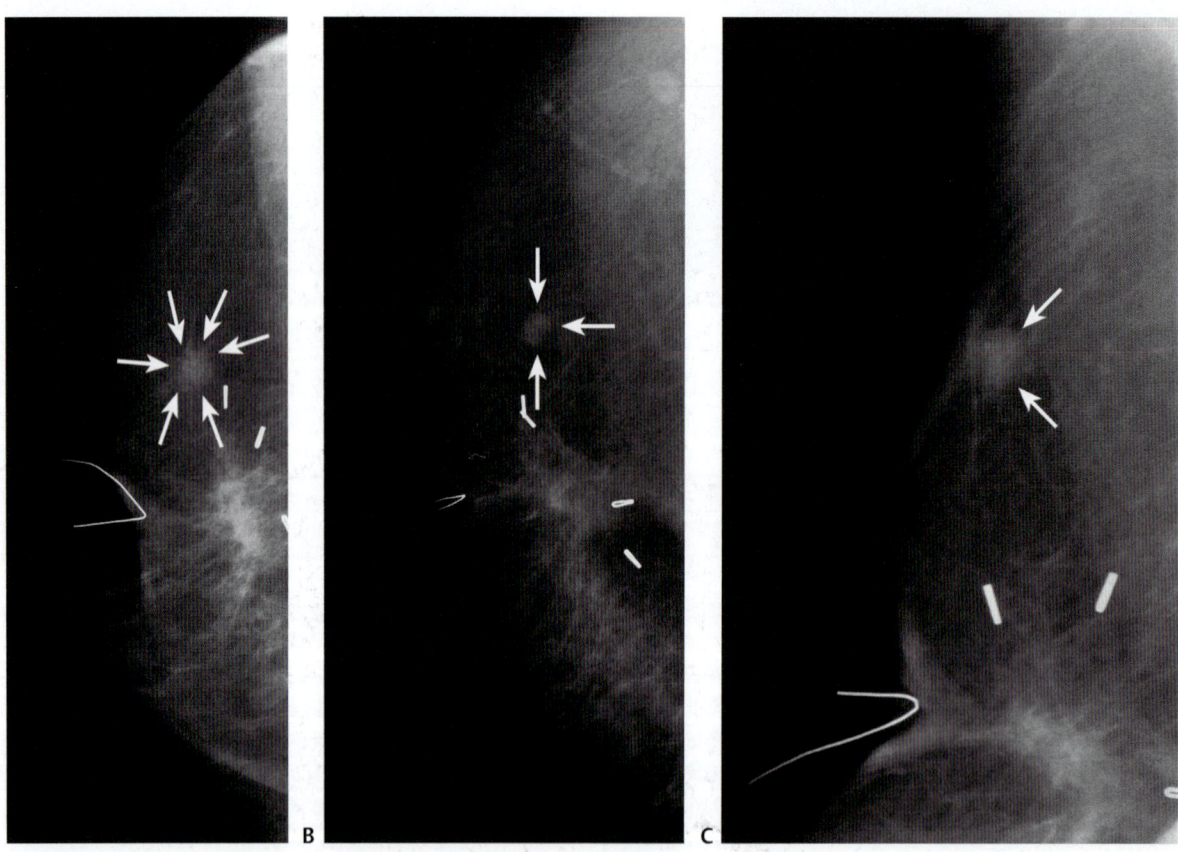

Fig. 7.5 There is a spiculated density deep to the right nipple. This density corresponds to the scar from the patient's lumpectomy. In the upper outer breast, there is a spiculated mass (*arrows*), which is separate from the main scar. This spiculated mass is new since the patient's previous exam. (**A**) Right LM mammogram. (**B**) Right CC mammogram. (**C**) Right mammogram tangential to spiculated mass (*arrows*).

Ultrasound

Frequency
- 10 MHz

Mass (Fig. 7.6)
- Margin: ill defined
- Echogenicity: hypoechoic
- Retrotumoral acoustic appearance: severe shadowing
- Shape: irregular

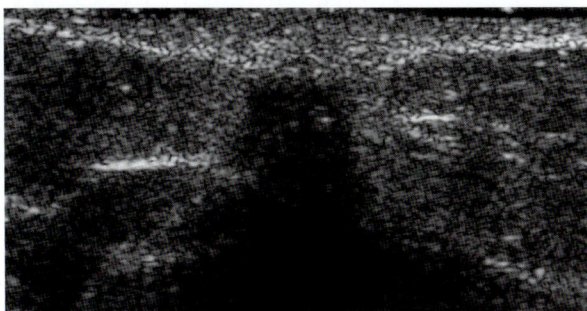

Fig. 7.6 Right radial breast sonogram. In the upper outer quadrant, the new small spiculated mammographic mass corresponds to an ill-defined hypoechoic shadowing mass. The hyperechoic halo around the mass corresponds to the mammographic spiculations.

Pathology
- Fat necrosis: the new spiculated mass in the right upper outer quadrant corresponded to fat necrosis.

Management
- BI-RADS assessment category 4, suspicious; biopsy should be considered.

Pearls and Pitfalls
- When fat necrosis causes new irregular masses in the area of a lumpectomy site, this abnormality cannot be distinguished from malignancy mammographically or sonographically.

Suggested Reading

Sohn C, Blohmer J-U, Hamper UM. Sonography in the follow-up of breast cancer. In: Sohn C, Blohmer J-U, Hamper UM, eds. Breast Ultrasound. New York: Thieme; 1999:98–102

Tohno E, Cosgrove DO, Sloane JP. Postoperative scarring. In: Tohno D, Cosgrove DO, Sloane JP, eds. Ultrasound Diagnosis of Breast Diseases. New York: Churchill Livingstone; 1994:146–147

138 Irregular Masses

Case 7.4: Fibroadenoma

Case History

A 49-year-old woman presents with a new density on her right screening mammogram.

Physical Examination
- Normal exam

Mammogram

Mass (Fig. 7.7)
- Margin: indistinct
- Shape: irregular
- Density: equal density

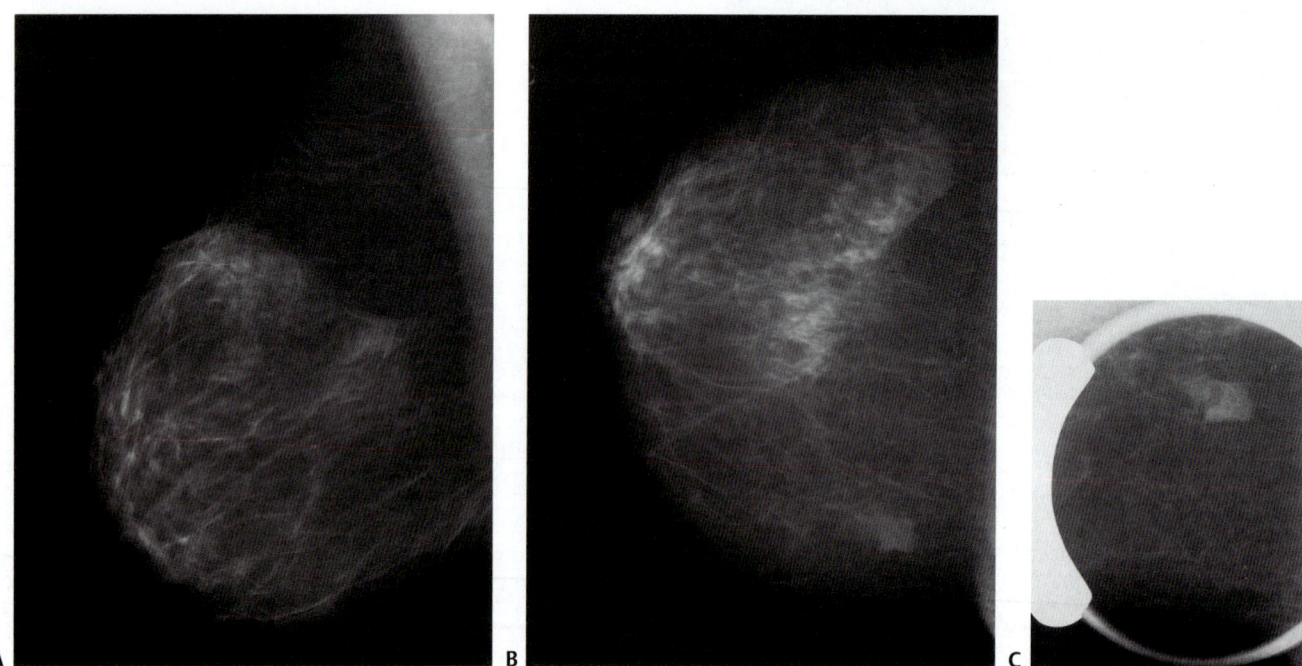

Fig. 7.7 In the right upper medial breast, there is an irregular mass that is partially obscured by the dense overlapping breast tissue. (**A**) Right MLO mammogram. (**B**) Right CC mammogram. (**C**) Right CC spot compression mammogram.

Ultrasound

Frequency
- 7.5 MHz

Mass (Fig. 7.8)
- Margin: ill defined
- Echogenicity: hyperechoic
- Retrotumoral acoustic appearance: posterior shadowing distal to mass
- Shape: irregular

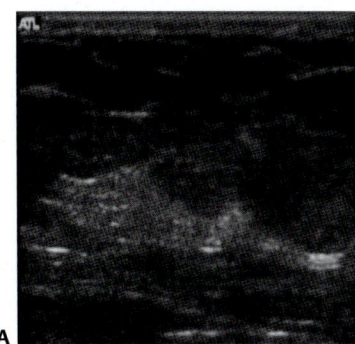 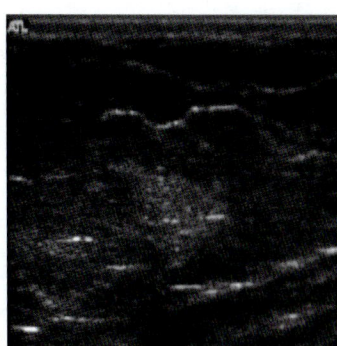

Fig. 7.8 Right breast sonogram. The irregular density identified in **Fig. 7.7** corresponds to a homogeneously hyperechoic irregular mass. (**A**) Right radial breast sonogram. (**B**) Right radial breast sonogram.

Pathology
- Fibroadenoma

Management
- BI-RADS assessment category 4, suspicious; biopsy should be considered.

Pearls and Pitfalls

- Fibroadenomas are the most common mass in women younger than 40 years of age. Researchers have reported that these masses are present in 9 to 25% of autopsy cases. The highest incidence of fibroadenomas is in women younger than 25 years of age.
- Mammographically, fibroadenomas are most commonly oval, round, or lobular circumscribed masses. Sometimes they appear irregular, as in this case. Fibroadenomas may have large "popcorn" calcifications. Rarely, their calcifications simulate malignant microcalcifications.
- Sonographically, these masses are generally oval, round, or lobular, well-defined solid masses. Less than one third of fibroadenomas have irregular margins. Echogenicity of fibroadenomas is generally hypoechoic (92%). Less commonly, they are hyperechoic (4%), heterogeneous (2%), or anechoic (1%).

Suggested Reading

Cole-Beuglet C, Soriano RZ, Kurtz AB, Goldberg BB. Fibroadenoma of the breast: sonomammography correlated with pathology in 122 patients. AJR Am J Roentgenol 1983;140:369–375

Fornage BD, Lorigan JG, Andry E. Fibroadenoma of the breast: sonographic appearance. Radiology 1989;172:671–675

Frantz VK, Pickren JW, Melcher GW, Auchincloss H Jr. Incidence of chronic cystic disease in so-called normal breasts: a study based on 225 postmortem examinations. Cancer 1951; 4:762–783

Jackson VP, Rothschild PA, Kreipke DL, Mail JT, Holden RW. The spectrum of sonographic findings of fibroadenoma of the breast. Invest Radiol 1986;21:34–40

Meyer JE, Frenna TH, Polger M, Sonnenfeld MR, Shaffer K. Enlarging occult fibroadenomas. Radiology 1992;183:639–641

140 Irregular Masses

Case 7.5: Fibroadenoma

Case History

An 84-year-old woman presents for screening mammogram.

Physical Examination

- Normal exam

Mammogram

Mass (Fig. 7.9)
- Margin: indistinct
- Shape: irregular
- Density: equal density

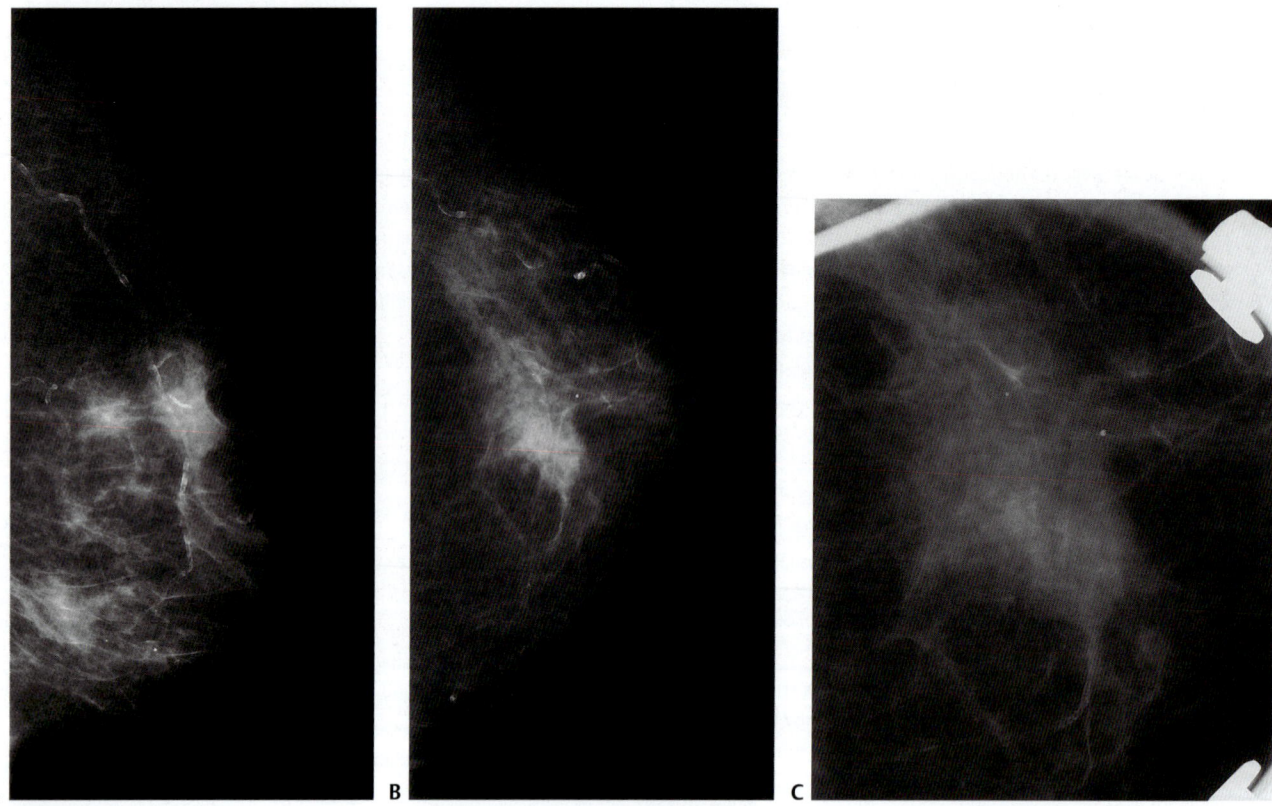

Fig. 7.9 In the left upper inner breast, there is an ill-defined mass. (**A**) Left ML mammogram. (**B**) Left CC mammogram. (**C**) Left CC spot compression mammogram.

Ultrasound

Frequency
- 10 MHz

Mass (Fig. 7.10)
- Margin: ill defined
- Echogenicity: hypoechoic
- Retrotumoral acoustic appearance: posterior shadowing distal to mass
- Shape: irregular

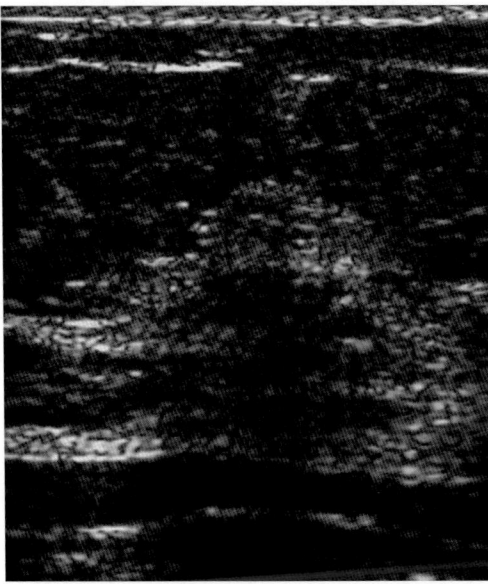

Fig. 7.10 Left radial breast sonogram. The mammographic mass in **Fig. 7.9** corresponds to a solid hypoechoic irregular mass with posterior acoustic shadowing.

Other Modalities (Fig. 7.11)

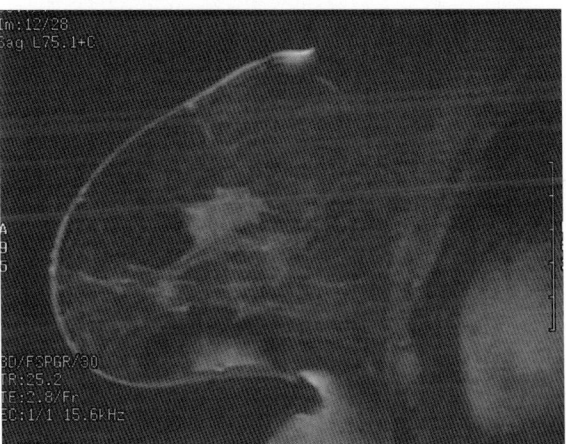

Fig. 7.11 Left sagittal dynamic bolus three-dimensional (3D) volume gradient series breast MRI. The mass does not exhibit early contrast enhancement and cannot be separated from the surrounding breast parenchyma.

Pathology
- Fibroadenoma

Management
- BI-RADS assessment category 4, suspicious; biopsy should be considered.

Pearls and Pitfalls

- In this case, the MRI was the most helpful test in predicting the benign nature of the mass. Although the mass has an irregular shape, the fibroadenoma did not exhibit early gadolinium contrast enhancement, which is characteristic of malignancies.

Suggested Reading

Hochman MG, Orel SG, Powell CM, Schnall MD, Reynolds CA, White LN. Fibroadenomas: MR imaging appearances with radiologic-histopathologic correlation. Radiology 1997; 204:123–129

Kvistad KA, Rydland J, Vainio J, et al. Breast lesions: evaluation with dynamic contrast-enhanced T1-weighted MR imaging and with $T2^*$-weighted first-pass perfusion MR imaging. Radiology 2000;216:545–553

Stelling CB, Powell DE, Mattingly SS. Fibroadenomas: histopathologic and MR imaging features. Radiology 1987;162: 399–407

Case 7.6: Hematoma

Case History
A 42-year-old woman has a bruised right breast from a recent seat belt injury.

Physical Examination
- Right breast: large ecchymosis, covering the upper outer quadrant, that is associated with a 3 cm palpable mass
- Left breast: normal exam

Mammogram

Mass (Fig. 7.12)
- Margin: indistinct
- Shape: irregular
- Density: high density

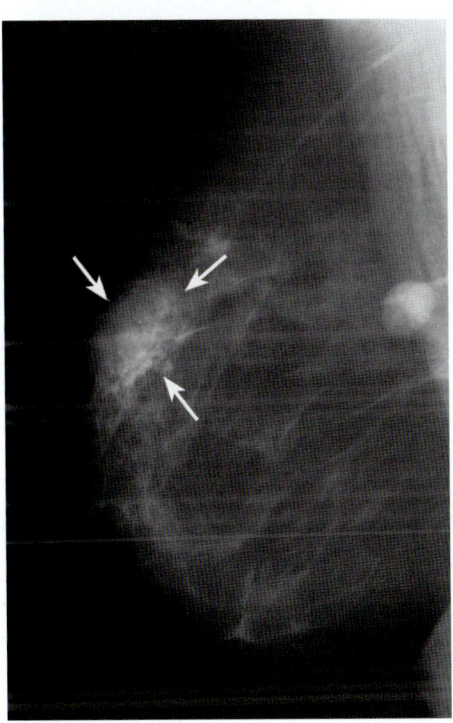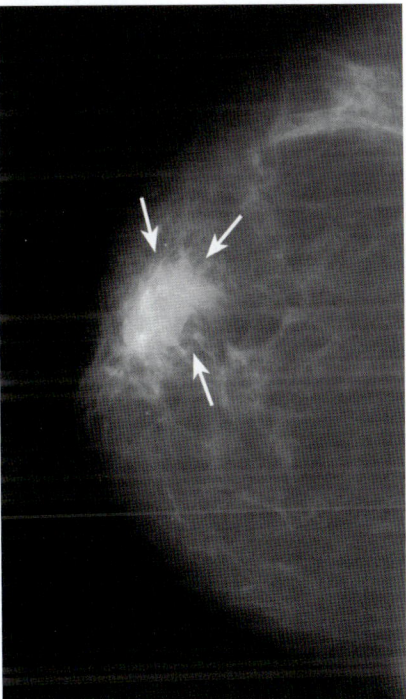

Fig. 7.12 In the anterior upper outer quadrant of the right breast, there is an ill-defined mass (*arrows*), which is in the same position as the ecchymosis and palpable lump. The well-defined oval mass in the posterior upper outer quadrant is a benign fibroadenoma. (**A**) Right MLO mammogram. (**B**) Right CC mammogram.

Ultrasound

Frequency
- 7 MHz

Mass (Figs. 7.13 and 7.14)
- Margin: well defined
- Echogenicity: hypoechoic
- Retrotumoral acoustic appearance: increased acoustic transmission
- Shape: ellipsoid

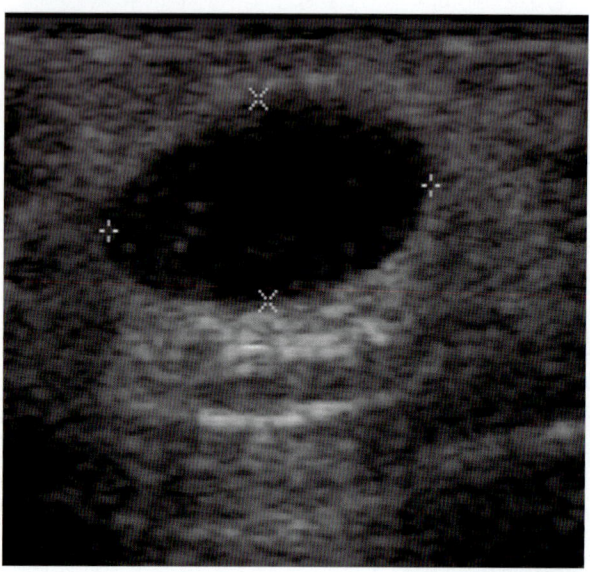

Fig. 7.13 Right longitudinal breast sonogram. The palpable lump associated with the ecchymosis is a well-defined, hypoechoic, complex fluid collection.

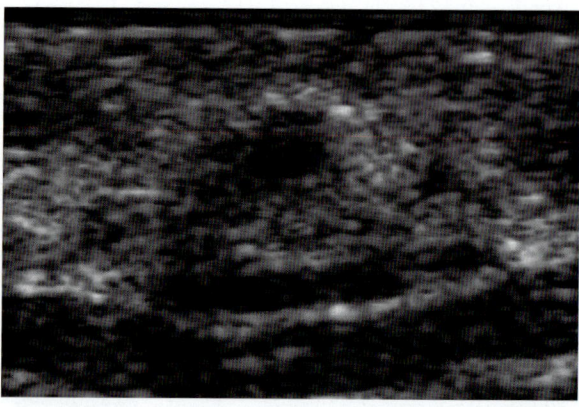

Fig. 7.14 Right longitudinal breast sonogram. Two months after the first sonogram (**Fig. 7.14**), the palpable lump is smaller and corresponds to a heterogeneous solid mass. This change in appearance is consistent with a hematoma.

Pathology
- Hematoma

Management
- BI-RADS assessment category 3, probably benign; short-interval follow-up

Pearls and Pitfalls

- Mammographically, acute hematomas present as either ill-defined or circumscribed masses.
- Sonographically, hematomas are usually anechoic or hypoechoic. Rarely, a hematoma is uniformly hyperechoic or has echogenic debris, which either has layers or adheres to one wall. Inflamed tissues around the hematoma may produce a hyperechoic halo. The differential diagnosis of a hematoma is abscess. If adherent debris is present, then intracystic neoplasm should be considered.

Suggested Reading

Jackson VP, Jahan R, Fu YS. Benign breast lesions. In: Bassett LW, Jackson VP, Jahan R, Fu YS, Gold RH, eds. Diagnosis of Diseases of the Breast. Philadelphia: WB Saunders, 1997:357–443

Kopans DB. Ultrasound and breast evaluation. In: Kopans DB. Breast Imaging. 2nd ed. Philadelphia: Lippincott-Raven; 1998:409–443

Tohno E, Cosgrove DO, Sloane JP. Haematoma. In: Tohno D, Cosgrove DO, Sloane JP, eds. Ultrasound Diagnosis of Breast Diseases. New York: Churchill Livingstone; 1994:144–145

Benign Masses | **145**

Case 7.7: Papillary Lesions

Case History
A 46-year-old woman presents for screening mammogram. After mammogram is done, patient's physician detects a palpable lump in the same area as the mammographic abnormality.

Physical Examination
- Left breast: palpable lump in the upper outer quadrant
- Right breast: normal exam

Mammogram

Mass (Fig. 7.15)
- Margin: indistinct
- Shape: irregular
- Density: equal density

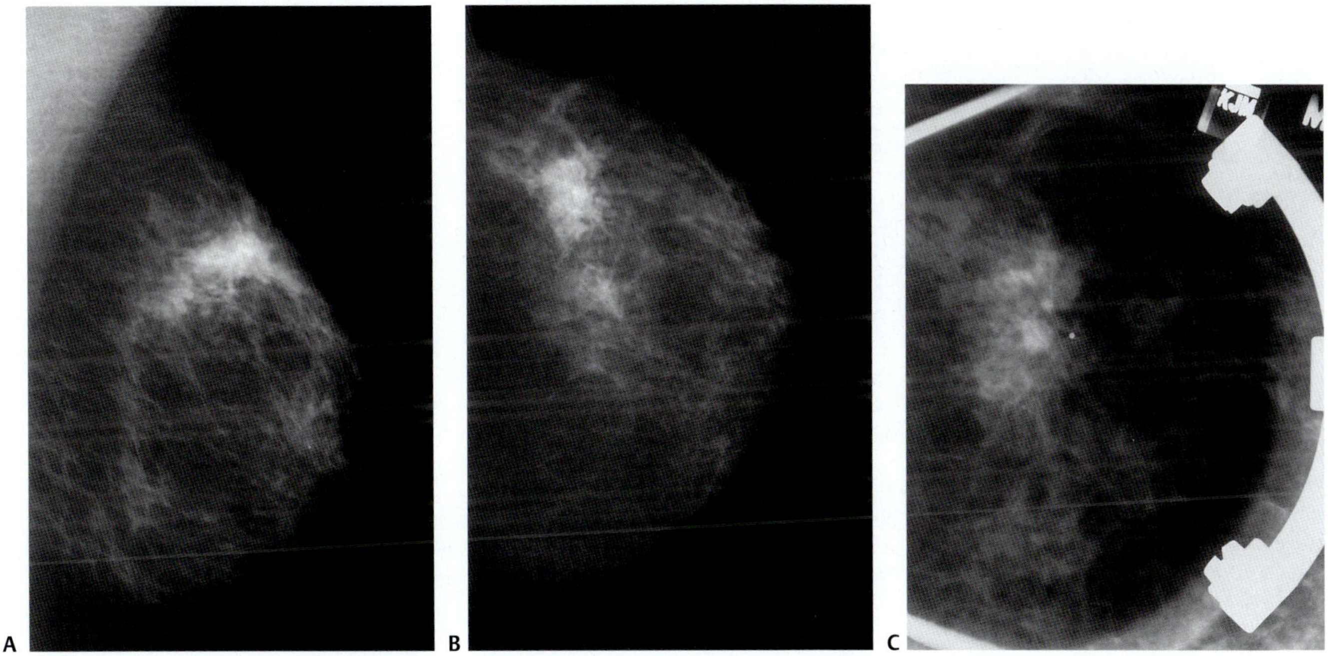

Fig. 7.15 In the upper outer quadrant of the left breast, there is an irregular mass with architectural distortion. (**A**) Left MLO mammogram. (**B**) Left CC mammogram. (**C**) Left CC spot mammogram.

Ultrasound

Low Frequency

Frequency
- 6 MHz

Mass (Fig. 7.16)
- Margin: ill defined
- Echogenicity: hypoechoic
- Retrotumoral acoustic appearance: severe shadowing, mass completely obscured
- Shape: irregular

High Frequency

Frequency
- 10 MHz

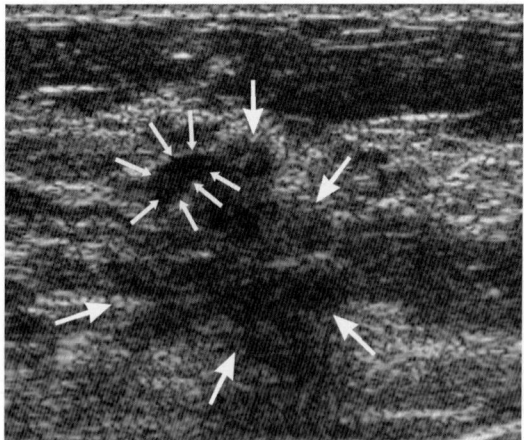

Fig. 7.16 Left radial breast sonogram. Lower-frequency examination demonstrates that the lesion identified in **Fig. 7.17** corresponds to a mass (*larger arrows*) that consists of a collection of multiple short tubular structures. The *smaller arrows* outline one tubular structure.

Associated Findings (Fig. 7.17)

In this case, the higher frequency is less useful because the fibrotic tissue around the thick walled ducts produces severe shadowing, so the internal structures cannot be identified.

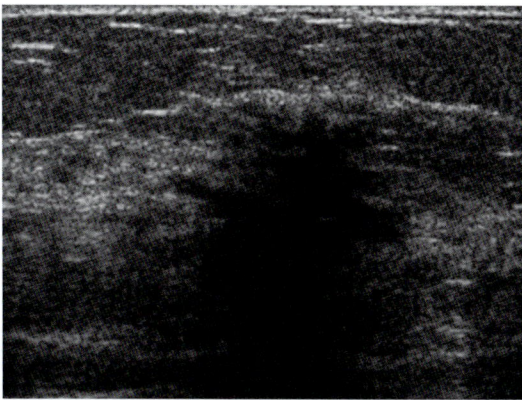

Fig. 7.17 Left radial breast sonogram. Higher frequency sonogram of same mass as **Fig. 7.16** demonstrates that the palpable lump corresponding to the mammographic mass is hypoechoic with severe shadowing.

Pathology
- Papilloma (multiple fibrous walled ducts surrounding sclerosing papillomas)

Management
- BI-RADS assessment category 4, suspicious; biopsy should be considered.

Pearls and Pitfalls

- Papillomas may develop sclerosis. Microscopically, these sclerosing papillomas generally do not appear as intracystic masses. The sclerotic papillomas are surrounded by thickened duct walls.
- Sclerosing papillomas produce a palpable lump. These lesions are rarely associated with nipple discharge or pain.
- Mammographically, sclerosing papillomas present as a circumscribed mass or as an ill-defined mass with spiculation and architectural distortion.
- Sonographically, this lesion presents as an ill-defined, hypoechoic, shadowing mass. This lesion consists of several sclerotic papillomas that appear as short tubular structures.

Suggested Reading

Fenoglio C, Lattes R. Sclerosing papillary proliferations in the female breast: a benign lesion often mistaken for carcinoma. Cancer 1974;33:691–700

Tavasoli FA. Papillary lesions. In: Tavassoli FA, Fattaneh A. Pathology of the Breast. 2nd ed. Stamford: Appleton and Lange; 1999:325–371

Pathology
- Radial sclerosing lesion (radial scar)

Management
- BI-RADS assessment category 4, suspicious; biopsy should be considered.

Pearls and Pitfalls
- Radial scars are common lesions. They have been identified in 28% of autopsied women. Women with radial scars have about twice the risk of malignancy compared with those without this lesion. Therefore, radial scars should be completely excised for thorough pathologic examination.
- Mammographically, radial scars exhibit spiculations and architectural distortion. The center is less dense than the usual carcinoma. Spot compression reveals multiple oval and linear lucencies within the central area. Commonly, this lesion is either only visible or much better identified on one view.
- Sonographically, the radial scar is an irregular hypoechoic mass associated with architectural distortion and severe shadowing with high frequencies. With low frequencies (< 7 MHz), the radial scar may be an irregular, hyperechoic area with little or no shadowing. Sonographically, this lesion cannot be differentiated from either a surgical scar or a malignant mass.
- On MRI, radial scars may enhance in a pattern similar to malignancies.

Suggested Reading

Cohen MA, Sferlazza SJ. Role of sonography in evaluation of radial scars of the breast. AJR Am J Roentgenol 2000;174:1075–1078

Jacobs TW, Byrne C, Colditz G, Connolly JL, Schnitt SJ. Radial scars in benign breast-biopsy specimens and the risk of breast cancer. N Engl J Med 1999;340:430–436

Tabar L, Dean PB. Stellate/spiculated lesions. In: Tabar L, Dean PB. Teaching Atlas of Mammography. 3rd ed. New York: Thieme; 2001:93–147

Weissman BN, Wong M, Smith DN. Image interpretation session: 1996. Tracheal amyloidoma. Radiographics 1997;17:243–246

Case 7.9: Scar

Case History
A 72-year-old woman status post–right lumpectomy and radiation therapy has developed a new mammographic finding near the surgical site.

Physical Examination
- Right breast: subareolar scar
- Left breast: normal exam

Mammogram

Mass (Fig. 7.21)
- Margin: spiculated
- Shape: irregular
- Density: equal density

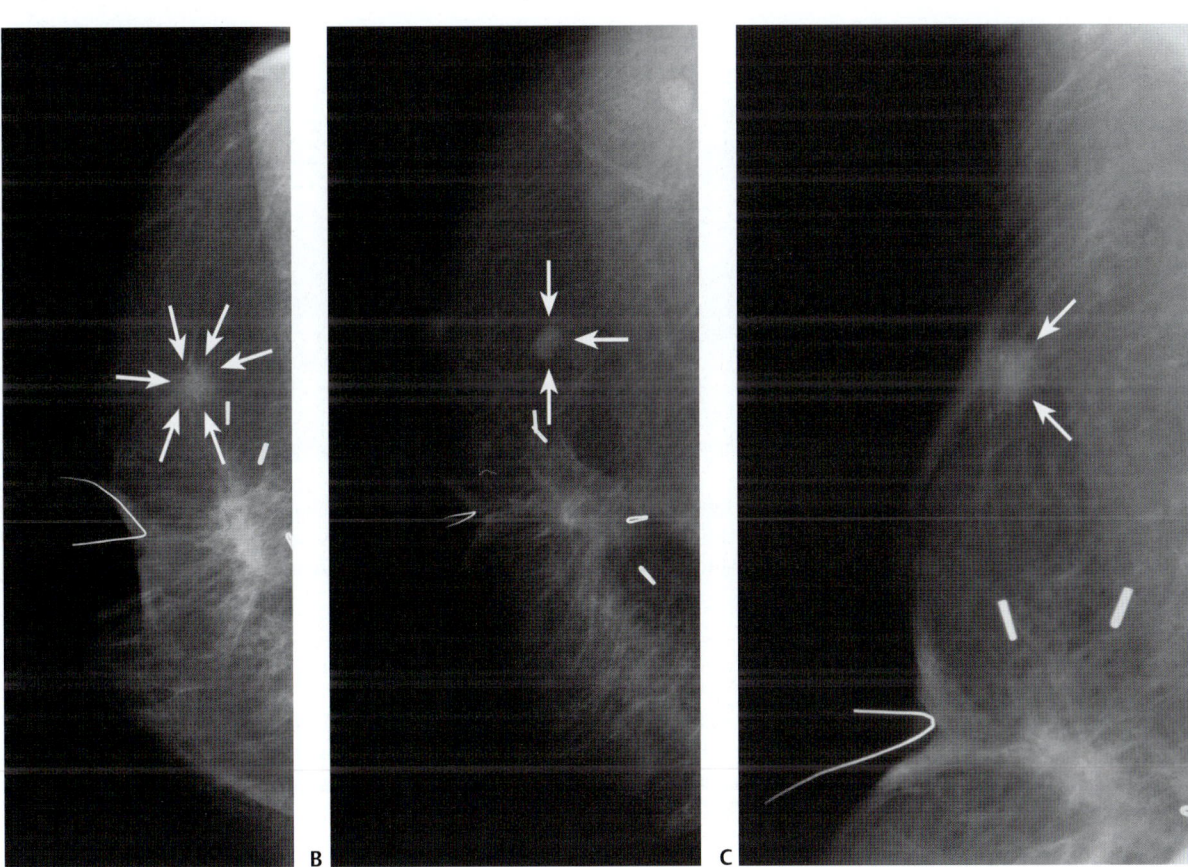

Fig. 7.21 There is a spiculated density deep to the right nipple. This density corresponds to the scar from the patient's lumpectomy. In the upper outer breast, there is a new spiculated mass (*arrows*) that is separate from the main scar. The new spiculated mass was described in Case 7.3. (**A**) Right LM mammogram. (**B**) Right CC mammogram. (**C**) Right mammogram tangential to spiculated mass (*arrows*).

152 Irregular Masses

Ultrasound

Frequency
- 10 MHz

Mass (Fig. 7.22)
- Margin: ill defined
- Echogenicity: hypoechoic
- Retrotumoral acoustic appearance: severe shadowing
- Shape: irregular

Pathology
- Fat necrosis (the new spiculated mass in the right upper outer quadrant)
- Scar (showed no evidence of recurrence and was not rebiopsied)

Management
- BI-RADS assessment category 4, suspicious; biopsy should be considered.

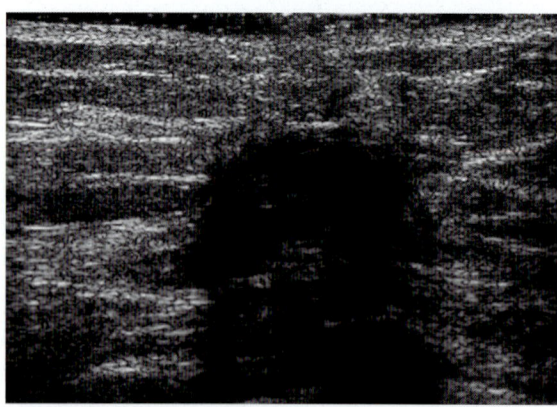 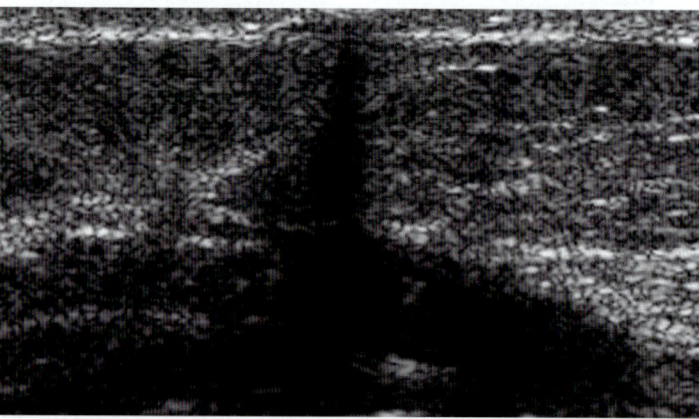

Fig. 7.22 The lumpectomy scar is distinguished from the adjacent spiculated mass by both its location and appearance. Although the scar is wide in the antiradial view (**A**), it is extremely narrow in the radial view (**B**). The adjacent spiculated mass depicted in **Fig. 7.23** is the same width in both views (see Case 7.3). (**A**) Right antiradial breast sonogram. (**B**) Right radial breast sonogram.

> **Pearls and Pitfalls**
>
> - Sonographically, scars are irregular spiculated masses. They can be distinguished from malignancy when the scar produces architectural distortion without a mass. This case illustrates the appearance of a benign scar. Although one view exhibits hypoechoic architectural distortion, the other view demonstrates no mass, only a thin line of tissue irregularity. However, if a scar develops a hypoechoic mass from fibrosis or fat necrosis, then malignancy cannot be excluded.

Suggested Reading

Sohn C, Blohmer J-U, Hamper UM. Sonography in the follow-up of breast cancer. In: Sohn C, Blohmer J-U, Hamper UM, eds. Breast Ultrasound. New York: Thieme; 1999:98–102

Tohno E, Cosgrove DO, Sloane JP. Postoperative scarring. In: Tohno D, Cosgrove DO, Sloane JP, eds. Ultrasound Diagnosis of Breast Diseases. New York: Churchill Livingstone; 1994:146–147

Benign Masses

Case 7.10: Myofibroblastoma

Case History
A 50-year-old woman presents with erythema and a new mass in the upper outer quadrant of the left breast. Physical exam and mammogram 6 months earlier were negative.

Physical Examination
- Left breast: palpable mass at the 3 o'clock position
- Right breast: normal exam

Mammogram

Mass (Fig. 7.23)
- Margin: spiculated
- Shape: irregular
- Density: high density

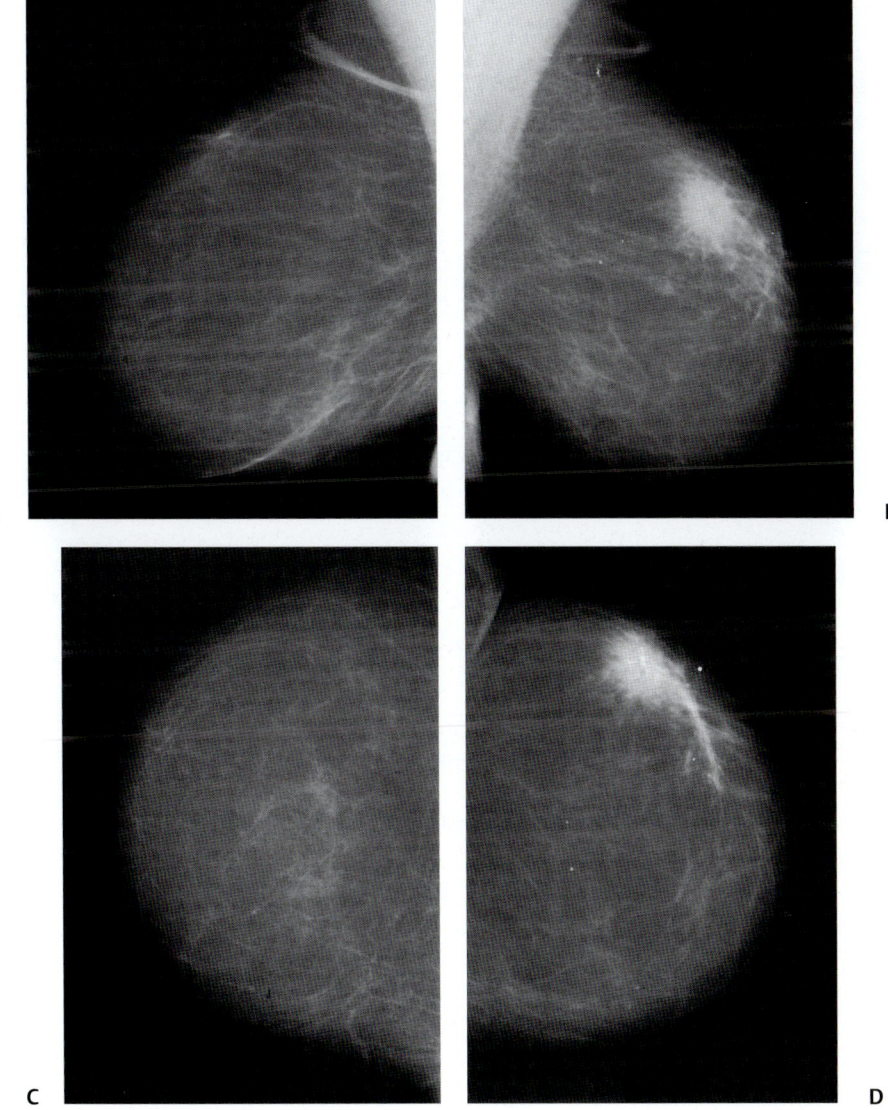

Fig. 7.23 There is an ill-defined mass with irregular margins in the upper outer left breast. (**A**) Right MLO mammogram. (**B**) Left MLO mammogram. (**C**) Right CC mammogram. (**D**) Left CC mammogram.

Ultrasound

Frequency
- 8 MHz

Mass (Fig. 7.24)
- Margin: ill defined
- Echogenicity: hypoechoic
- Retrotumoral acoustic appearance: bilateral edge shadowing
- Shape: irregular

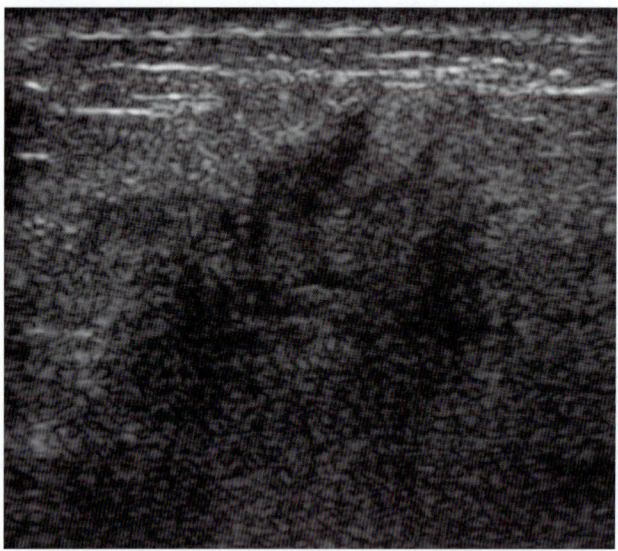

Fig. 7.24 Left radial breast sonogram. The mammographic mass (**Fig. 7.23**) corresponds to a palpable ill-defined, hypoechoic mass.

Pathology
- Myofibroblastoma

Management
- BI-RADS assessment category 4, suspicious; biopsy should be considered.

Pearls and Pitfalls

- Myofibroblastoma is a benign tumor composed of breast stromal fibroblasts and/or myofibroblasts. This lesion most commonly presents as a palpable mass in patients 50 to 70 years old. Men are affected more often than women.
- Mammographically, these lesions are most commonly noncalcified, oval, or lobulated masses with either well-defined or ill-defined margins.
- Sonographically, myofibroblastomas are generally oval or lobular well-defined hypoechoic masses with variable decreased acoustic transmission. This case has an unusual mammographic and sonographic appearance.

Suggested Reading

Greenberg JS, Kaplan SS, Grady C. Myofibroblastoma of the breast in women: imaging appearances. AJR Am J Roentgenol 1998;171:71–72

Pina L, Apesteguía L, Cojo R, et al. Myofibroblastoma of male breast: report of three cases and review of the literature. Eur Radiol 1997;7:931–934

8 Irregular Masses: Malignant Masses

Case 8.1: Infiltrating Ductal Carcinoma

Case History
A 64-year-old woman presents with back pain, abnormal bone scan, and a right breast lump.

Physical Examination
- Right breast: palpable lump in the outer breast
- Left breast: normal exam

Mammogram

Mass (Fig. 8.1)
- Margin: spiculated
- Shape: irregular
- Density: high density

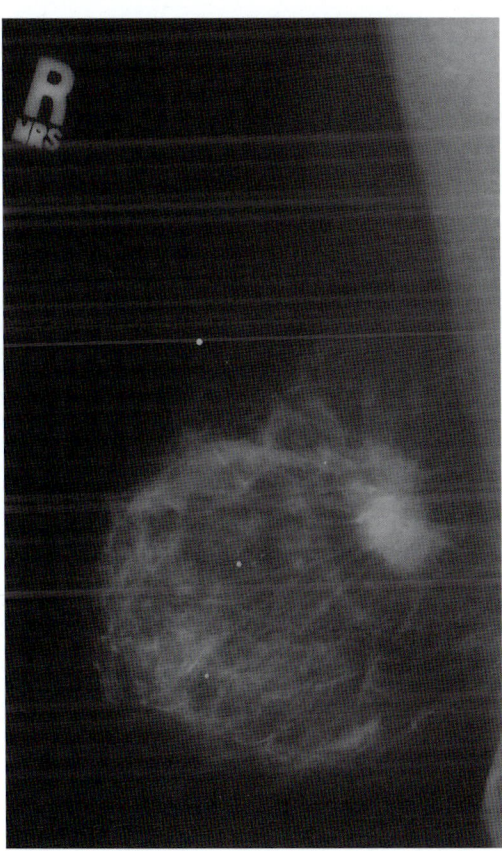
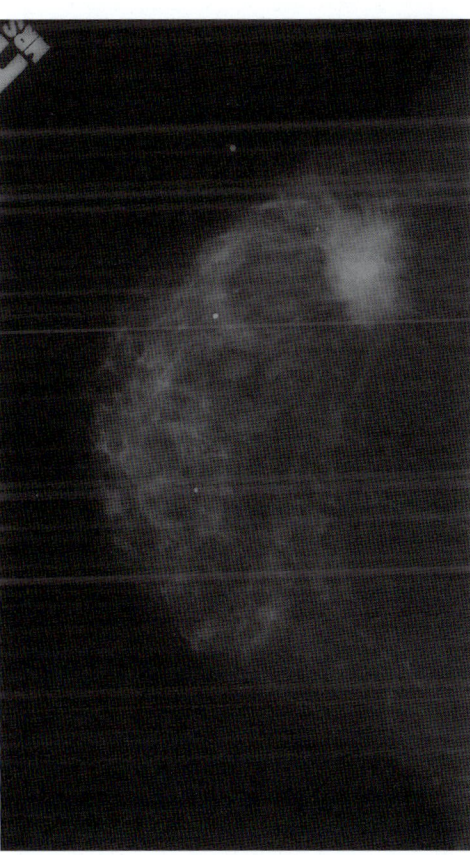

Fig. 8.1 In the upper outer quadrant, there is a spiculated mass that corresponds to the patient's palpable mass. (**A**) Right MLO mammogram. (**B**) Right CC mammogram.

Other Modalities: Bone Scan (Fig. 8.2)

Bone Scan Findings
The bone scan demonstrates that the patient's back pain is due to metastatic disease. Biopsies confirmed that these bone metastases originated from her breast cancer.

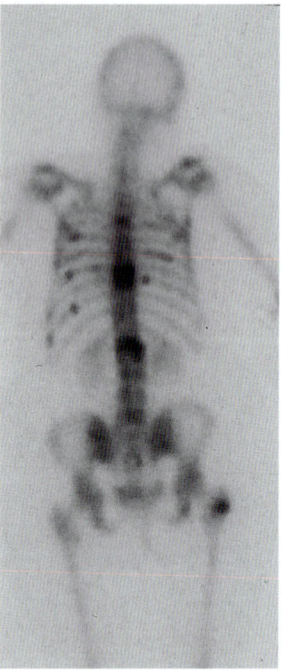

Fig. 8.2 Technetium-99m whole-body bone scan, posterior view. There are multiple areas of abnormal uptake in the ribs, spine, and right hip consistent with metastatic bony disease.

Pathology
- Infiltrating ductal carcinoma

Management
- BI-RADS assessment category 5, highly suggestive of malignancy

Pearls and Pitfalls

- Infiltrating ductal carcinoma is the most common breast cancer histology. This cell type represents between 47 and 79% of all invasive breast cancers. The lower percentage has been reported in Japan and the higher percentages in the United States and Scandinavia.
- Two thirds of invasive ductal carcinomas appear as irregular mammographic masses. The spiculations consist of a combination of fibrosis and infiltrating tumor. This case illustrates this classic presentation.
- In this case, since this mass is highly suggestive of malignancy, and the bone biopsy demonstrated metastatic disease, no biopsy was performed prior to excision. However, if the surgeon wishes to obtain a breast biopsy prior to excision, then one may perform a sonographically guided biopsy may be appropriate as these lesions are generally easily identified with this method.

Suggested Reading

Tabar L, Dean PB. Stellate/spiculated lesions. In: Tabar L, Dean PB. Teaching Atlas of Mammography. 3rd ed. New York: Thieme; 2001:93–147

Tavassoli FA. Infiltrating carcinoma: common and familiar special types. In: Tavassoli FA, Fattaneh A. Pathology of the Breast. 2nd ed. Stamford: Appleton and Lange; 1999:401–480

Case 8.2: Infiltrating Ductal Carcinoma

Case History
An 80-year-old woman presents with left nipple retraction.

Physical Examination
- Left breast: retracted nipple, associated with skin thickening; no definite mass identified
- Right breast: normal exam

Mammogram

Mass (Fig. 8.3)
- Margin: spiculated
- Shape: irregular
- Density: high density

Calcifications
- Type: dystrophic
- Distribution: grouped/clustered

Associated Findings
Architectural distortion, skin retraction, skin thickening, trabecular thickening, nipple retraction (**Fig. 8.3**)

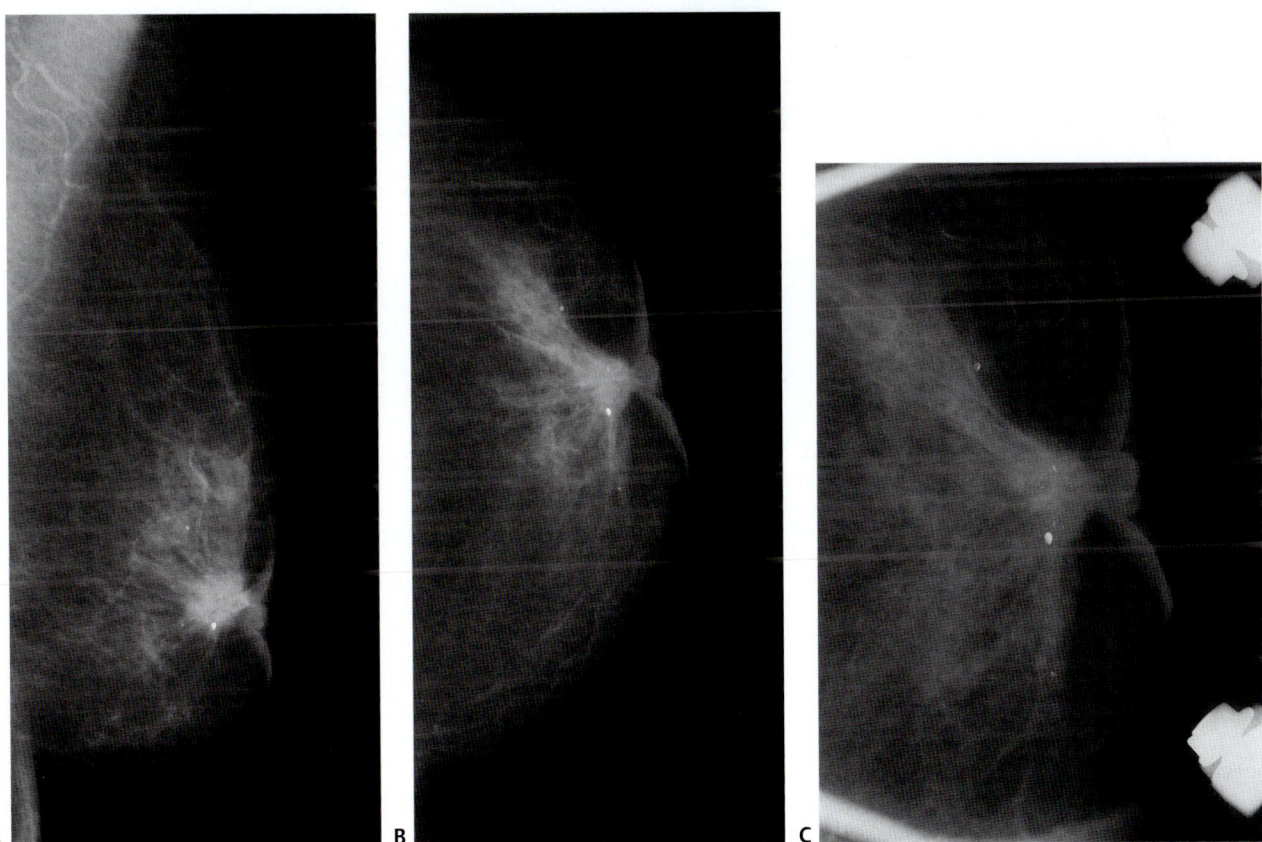

Fig. 8.3 There is a spiculated subareolar mass associated with calcifications, skin thickening, and nipple retraction. (**A**) Left MLO mammogram. (**B**) Left CC mammogram. (**C**) Left CC spot magnification mammogram.

Ultrasound

Frequency
- 8 MHz

Mass (Fig. 8.4)
- Margin: spiculation/architectural distortion
- Echogenicity: hypoechoic
- Retrotumoral acoustic appearance: bilateral edge shadowing
- Shape: irregular

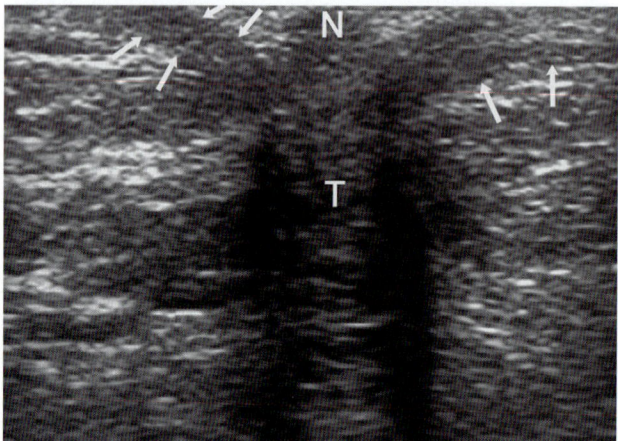

Fig. 8.4 Left transverse breast sonogram. The sonogram is centered over the nipple (N). Superficially, skin thickening is present (*arrows*). Deep to the nipple is a solid, irregular, ill-defined, hypoechoic tumor (T).

Pathology
- Invasive ductal carcinoma

Management
- BI-RADS assessment category 5, highly suggestive of malignancy

Pearls and Pitfalls
- Nipple inversion is due to many etiologies. Benign causes include congenital position, duct ectasia, subareolar abscess, granulomatous mastitis, and postoperative scarring. If the inversion is relatively recent, then carcinoma should be considered.
- The mass in this case is highly suggestive of malignancy, so sonography is not needed for characterization of the mass. Sonography was performed for biopsy guidance.

Suggested Reading
Evans AJ, Wilson ARM, Blamey RW, Robertson JFR, Ellis IO, Elston CW. Atlas of Breast Disease Management. Philadelphia: WB Saunders; 1998:32–34

Tavassoli FA, Fattaneh A. Pathology of the Breast, 2nd ed. Stamford: Appleton and Lange; 1999:792–793

Case 8.3: Infiltrating Ductal Carcinoma

Case History
A 54-year-old woman presents for screening mammogram.

Physical Examination
- Normal exam

Mammogram

Mass (Fig. 8.5)
- Margin: spiculated
- Shape: irregular
- Density: equal density

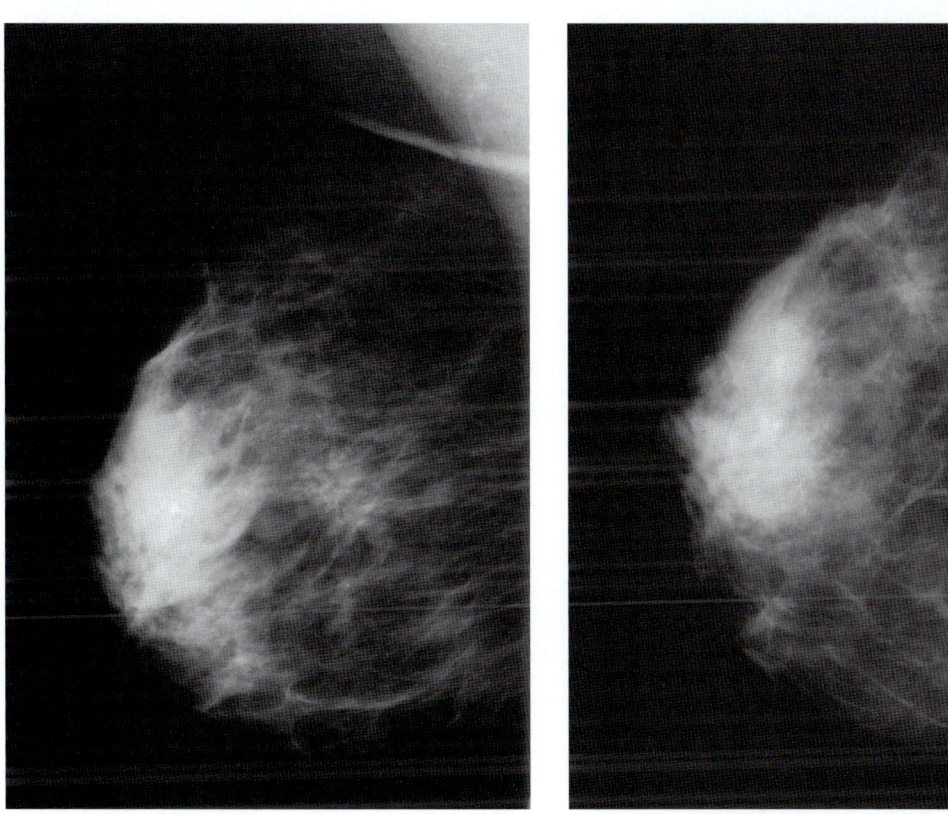

Fig. 8.5 A spiculated mass is in the right upper outer quadrant. (**A**) Right MLO mammogram. (**B**) Right CC mammogram.

Irregular Masses

Ultrasound

Frequency
- 11.5 MHz

Mass (Figs. 8.6 and 8.7)
- Margin: ill defined
- Echogenicity: hypoechoic
- Retrotumoral acoustic appearance: severe shadowing, mass completely obscured
- Shape: irregular

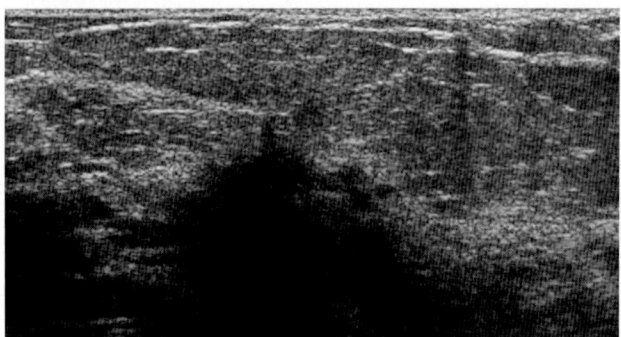

Fig. 8.6 Right radial breast sonogram. The spiculated mass identified in **Fig. 8.5** corresponds to an irregular hypoechoic mass with severe acoustic shadowing.

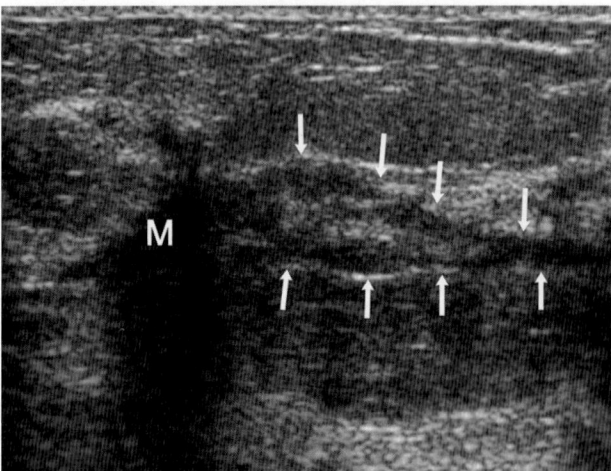

Fig. 8.7 Right radial breast sonogram. A few dilated ducts (*arrows*) extend from the main mass (M) (shown in **Fig. 8.6**) toward the nipple. The size of the main sonographic mass matches the mammographic size (approximately 2.5 cm). However, if one adds the length of the abnormal ducts, the total length of the abnormality is 5 cm. Only a small portion of the main mass is displayed in this image.

Pathology

Infiltrating ductal carcinoma. The main mass consisted of well-differentiated infiltrating ductal carcinoma. The sonographically dilated ducts histologically corresponded to dilated ducts with infiltrating carcinoma within the walls (**Fig. 8.8**).

Management

- BI-RADS assessment category 5, highly suggestive of malignancy

Fig. 8.8 Low-power microscopic image of the malignancy demonstrates direct infiltration of tumor cells creating spiculation (*arrows*).

Pearls and Pitfalls

- The breast sonogram suggests that the malignancy is larger than the mammographic density. To confirm this information, sonographically guided biopsies of both the mass and the abnormal ducts were performed. Both the biopsies and the excisional specimen confirmed that the tumor size matched the sonographic size.
- Sonographically, dilated ducts that extend from a tumor mass should be viewed as suspicious for additional carcinoma.

Suggested Reading

Tohno D, Cosgrove DO, Sloane JP, eds. Ultrasound Diagnosis of Breast Diseases. New York: Churchill Livingstone; 1994:165–166

Case 8.4: Infiltrating Ductal Carcinoma

Case History
A 65-year-old woman has right breast microcalcifications that have been stereotactically mammographically biopsied and are malignant. She now presents for needle localization of these microcalcifications before lumpectomy.

Physical Examination
- Normal exam

Mammogram

Mass (Fig. 8.9)
- Margin: indistinct
- Shape: irregular
- Density: equal density
- Calcifications
- Type: fine linear/branching
- Distribution: grouped/clustered

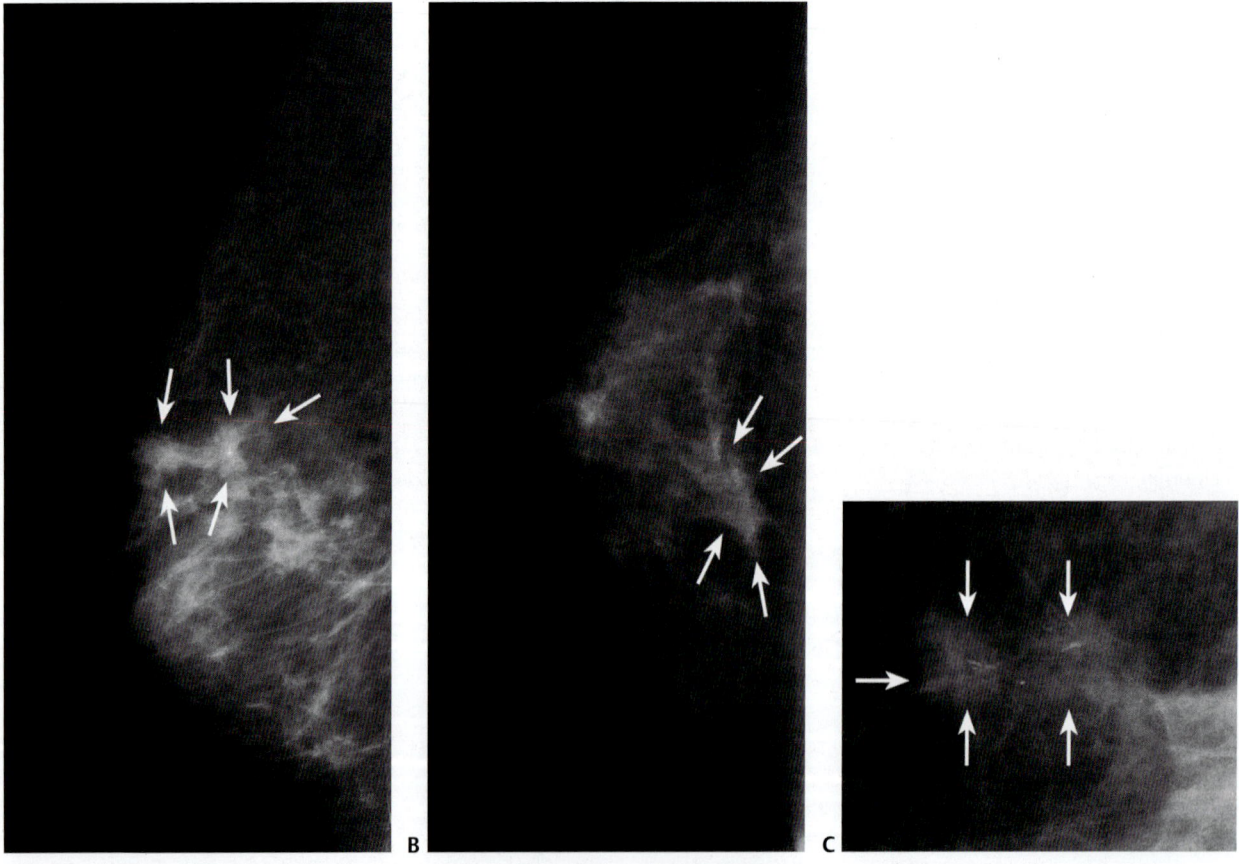

Fig. 8.9 In the upper inner quadrant, there is a cluster of fine linear calcifications. These calcifications are associated with a dumbbell-shaped ill-defined mass (*arrows*). The shape of this mass and the subtle multinodular pattern of the surrounding parenchyma suggest that the tumor may be multifocal. (**A**) Right ML mammogram. (**B**) Right CC mammogram. (**C**) Right MLO magnification mammogram.

Ultrasound

Frequency
- 10 MHz

Mass (Figs. 8.10, 8.11, and 8.12)
- Margin: ill defined
- Echogenicity: hypoechoic
- Retrotumoral acoustic appearance: posterior shadowing distal to mass
- Shape: irregular

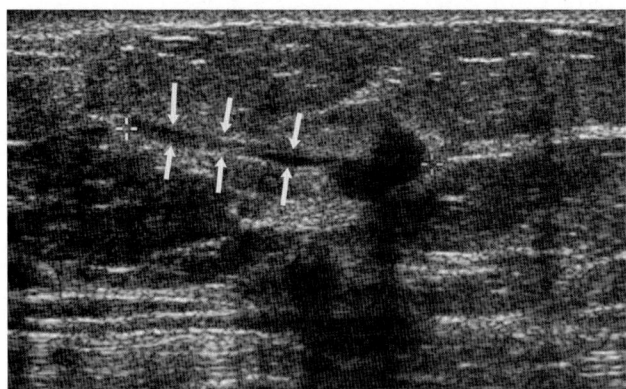

Fig. 8.10 Right radial breast sonogram. At the 2 o'clock position, a spiculated mass is associated with the stereotactic biopsy track (*arrows*). This mass corresponds to the mammographic mass containing the microcalcifications (**Fig. 8.9**).

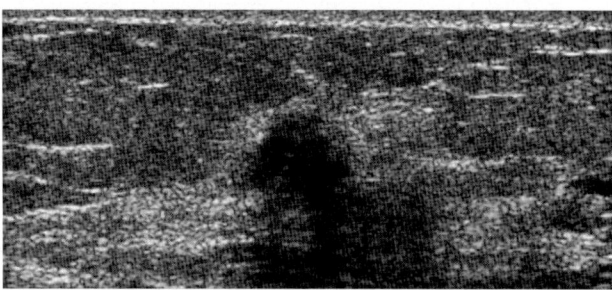

Fig. 8.11 Right radial breast sonogram. At the 12 o'clock position, a second spiculated solid, mass is present. This mass may be part of the dumbbell structure identified mammographically (**Fig. 8.9**).

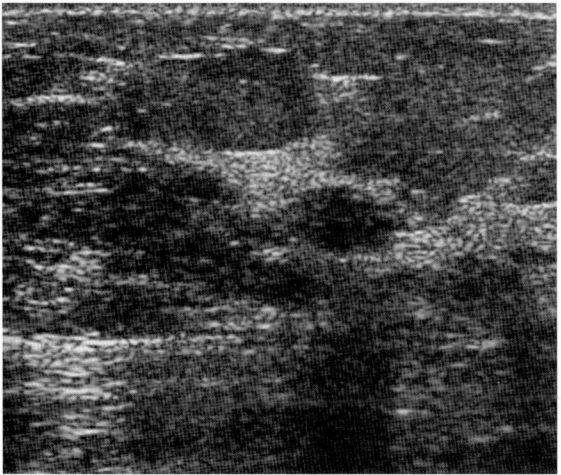

Fig. 8.12 Right radial breast sonogram. At the 9 o'clock position there is an oval, ill-defined, solid, shadowing mass. This mass is not mammographically identifiable. Sonographically guided biopsies of this mass and the one in **Fig. 8.11** confirmed that they were both malignant.

Pathology
Infiltrating ductal carcinoma. Mastectomy specimen: grossly, the tumor was 4 cm, but random sections outside this mass demonstrated small foci of infiltrating and in situ ductal carcinoma, so the overall size of the malignancy could not be defined. The tumor appeared to be an extensive multifocal malignancy.

Management
- BI-RADS assessment category 4, suspicious; biopsy should be considered.

Pearls and Pitfalls
- Although the terms *multifocal* and *multicentric* appear to be synonymous, they have distinct meanings when applied to malignancy. Multifocality refers to one tumor appearing with multiple closely spaced foci. Multicentricity refers to the simultaneous development of multiple different malignancies. Usually, a tumor is considered multifocal if the foci are either within the same quadrant of the breast or within 5 cm of each other.
- Mammographically, it is important to consider multifocality if there is a suggestion of multiple ill-defined masses closely related to a highly suspicious mass. Sometimes, with multiple oblique magnification views, one can identify spiculations extending from one mass to another. Sonography and an MRI are useful methods to clarify multifocality and guide for biopsy.

Suggested Reading
Berg WA, Gilbreath PL. Multicentric and multifocal cancer: whole-breast US in preoperative evaluation. Radiology 2000; 214:59–66

Johnson JE, Dutt PL, Page DL. Extent and multicentricity of in situ and invasive carcinoma. In: Bland KI, Copeland EM, eds. The Breast. Philadelphia: WB Saunders; 1998:296–306

Lagios MD. Multicentricity of breast carcinoma demonstrated by routine correlated serial subgross and radiographic examination. Cancer 1977;40:1726–1734

Case 8.5: Infiltrating Ductal Carcinoma

Case History
A 57-year-old woman presents with new right breast dimpling. Mammographically, two suspicious abnormalities are identified: lesion A in the medial inferior breast (which corresponds to the skin dimpling) and lesion B at the 12 o'clock position. Unfortunately, only the 12 o'clock position mass (B) is adequately localized for biopsy. The medial inferior abnormality (A) is not confidently identified during an attempt to perform mammographic stereotactic biopsy and is not localized on the initial breast sonogram. Lesion A is identified only sonographically after breast MRI demonstrates the mass.

Physical Examination
- Right breast: subtle skin dimpling in medial breast associated with vague firmness
- Left breast: normal exam

Mammogram

Mass (Fig. 8.13)
- Margin: indistinct
- Shape: irregular
- Density: equal density

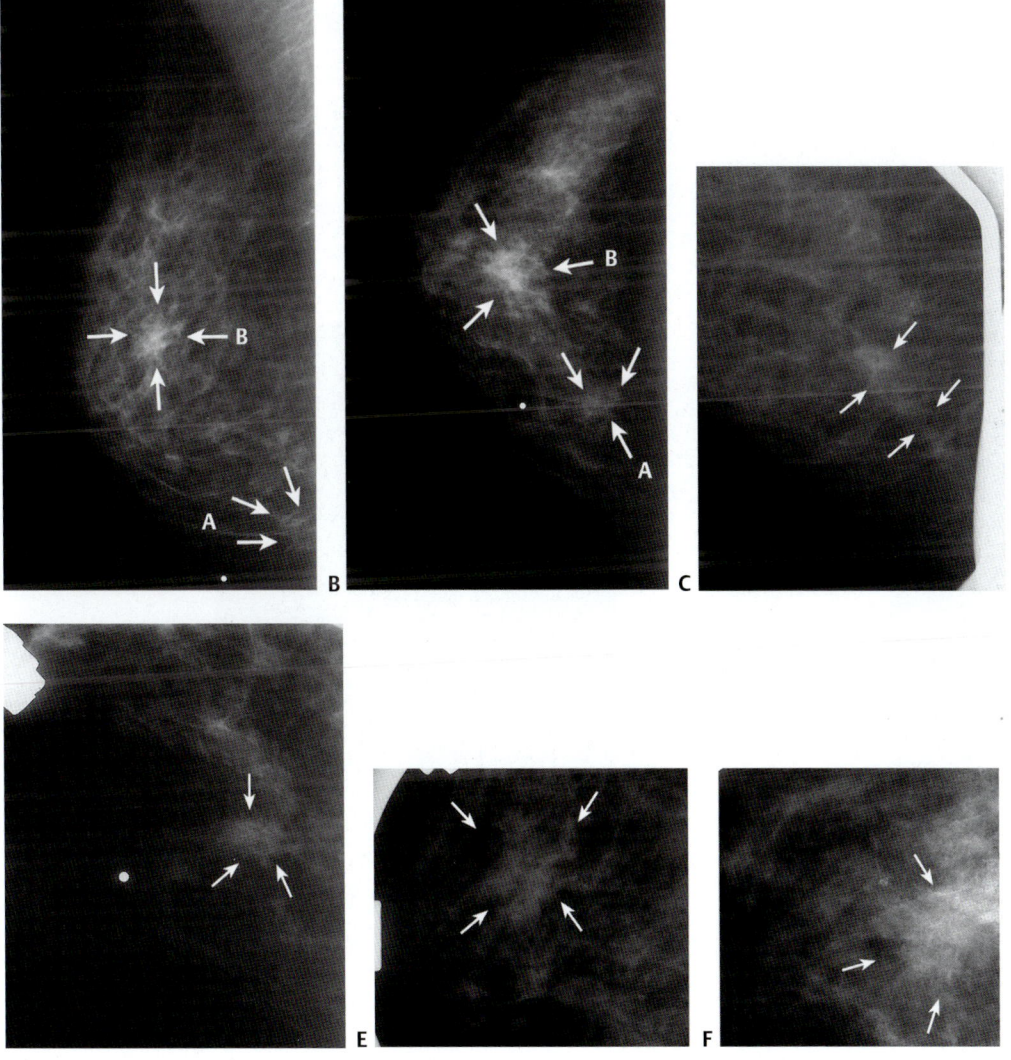

Fig. 8.13 The skin dimpling in the medial inferior quadrant (marked by a radiopaque dot) is associated with lesion A, an ill-defined mass, which is better identified on the CC spot compression (**D**). Lesion A appears as a subtle density associated with architectural distortion in part (**C**) and MLO spot compression (*arrows*). Lesion B is a second ill-defined mass at the 12 o'clock position. (**A**) Right MLO mammogram. (**B**) Right CC mammogram. (**C**) Right MLO spot compression of medial inferior area of skin dimpling (lesion A; *arrows*). (**D**) Right CC spot compression of medial inferior area of skin dimpling (lesion A; *arrows*). (**E**) Right MLO spot compression of the 12 o'clock position mass (lesion B; *arrows*). (**F**) Right CC spot compression of the 12 o'clock position mass (lesion B; *arrows*).

Ultrasound

Frequency
- 11.5 MHz

Mass (Figs. 8.14 and 8.15)
- Margin: ill defined
- Echogenicity: hypoechoic
- Retrotumoral acoustic appearance: posterior shadowing distal to mass
- Shape: irregular

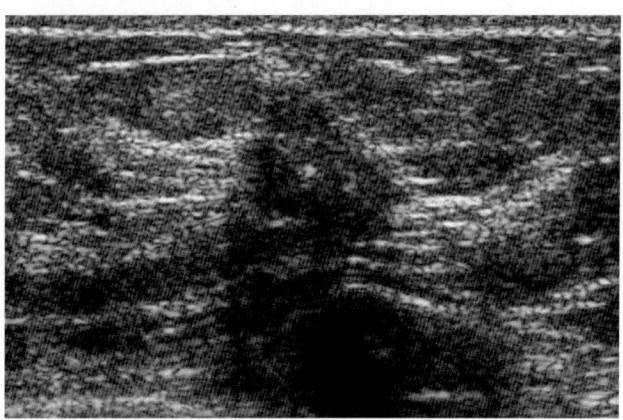

Fig. 8.14 Right radial breast sonogram. This ill-defined hypoechoic mass, which corresponds to **Fig. 8.13**, lesion A, was initially missed sonographically. After the right breast MRI (**Fig. 8.16**) demonstrated the mass, the patient was reexamined sonographically, and this mass was identified.

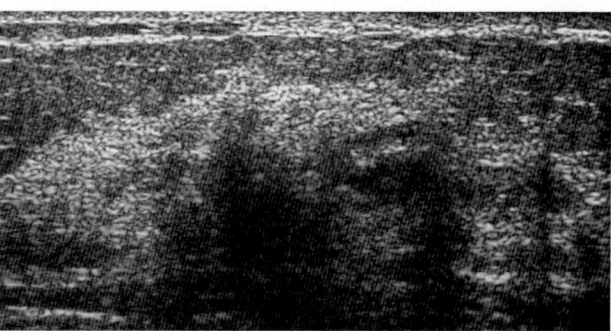

Fig. 8.15 Right radial breast sonogram. This irregular hypoechoic mass corresponds to the mammographic mass at the 12 o'clock position (which is **Fig. 8.13**, lesion B).

Other Modalities: MRI (Figs. 8.16 and 8.17)

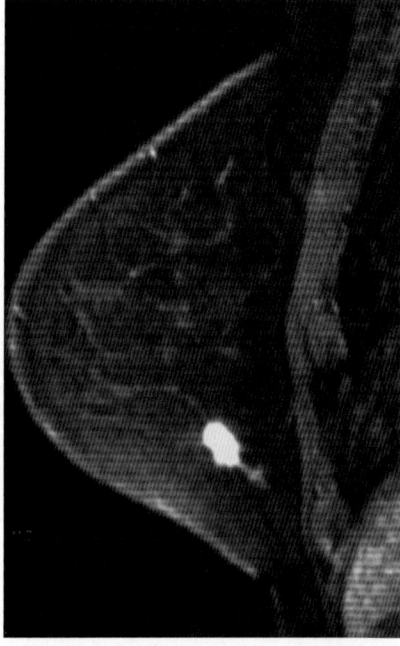

Fig. 8.16 Right sagittal dynamic bolus 3D volume gradient series breast MRI. In the inferior medial breast, a mass exhibits abnormal early enhancement. This mass corresponds to the area of skin dimpling (**Fig. 8.13**, lesion A).

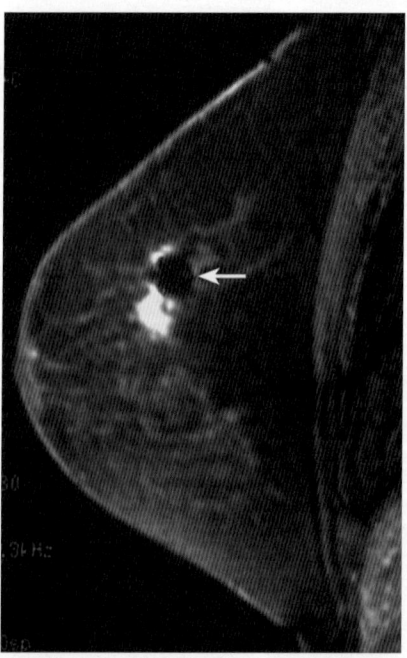

Fig. 8.17 Right sagittal dynamic bolus 3D volume gradient series breast MRI. **Fig. 8.13**, lesion B is in the upper breast at the 12 o'clock position. Lesion B exhibits low-intensity clip artifact from previous mammographic stereotactic core biopsy.

Pathology
- Infiltrating ductal carcinoma
- Mastectomy specimen showed three separate tumor masses. Two of the masses matched the MRI tumors. The third malignancy was identified pathologically in the inferior breast and could not be identified retrospectively by MRI.

Management
- BI-RADS assessment category 4, suspicious; biopsy should be considered.

Pearls and Pitfalls

- This case illustrates multicentric malignancies. Due to differences in pathologic examination and definition of multicentricity, studies have reported the prevalence of multicentricity as between 9 and 75%. The probable true prevalence is between 25 and 50% for all histologies. Invasive ductal carcinoma has a lower rate of multicentricity (19%) compared with other histologies.

Suggested Reading

Gump FE, Shikora S, Habif DV, Kister S, Logerfo P, Estabrook A. The extent and distribution of cancer in breasts with palpable primary tumors. Ann Surg 1986;204:384–390

Johnson JE, Dutt PL, Page DL. Extent and multicentricity of in situ and invasive carcinoma. In: Bland KI, Copeland EM, eds. The Breast. Philadelphia: WB Saunders; 1998:296–306

Tavassoli FA, Fattaneh A. Pathology of the Breast. 2nd ed. Stamford: Appleton and Lange; 1999:56–74

Case 8.6: Infiltrating Ductal Carcinoma

Case History
A 63-year-old woman presents with a palpable left breast lump. This is the same patient as in Case 35.1.

Physical Examination
- Firm lump in outer left breast near the 3 o'clock position

Mammogram

Mass (Fig. 8.18)
- Margin: ill defined
- Shape: oval
- Density: high density

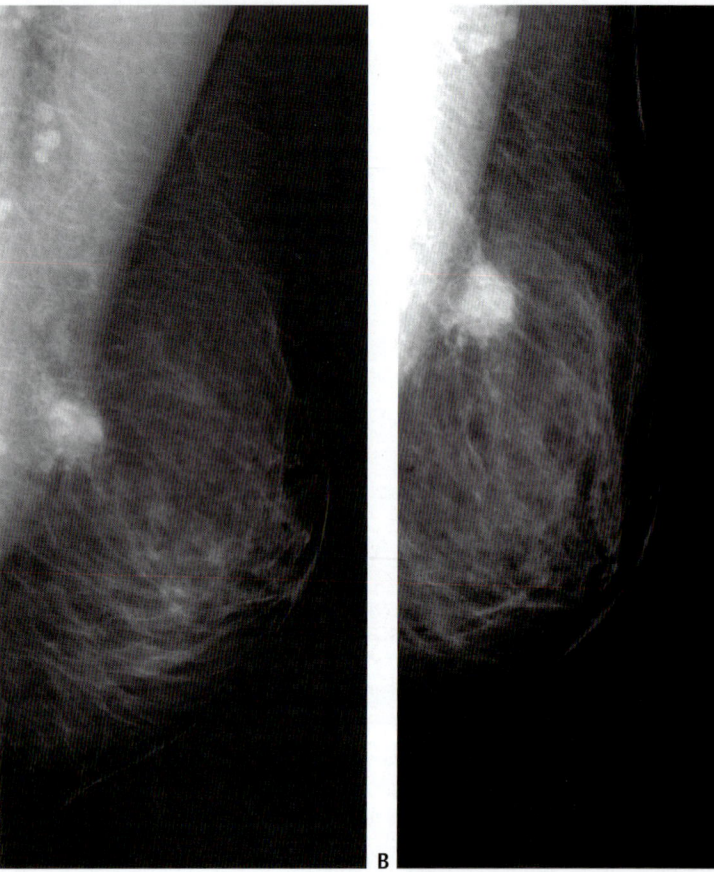

Fig. 8.18 In the outer quadrant, there is an ill-defined oval mass. (**A**) Left MLO mammogram. (**B**) Left exaggerated craniocaudal (XCCL) mammogram.

Ultrasound

Frequency
- 14 Mz

Mass (Fig. 8.19)
- Margins: irregular
- Echogenicity: hypoechoic
- Shape: irregular

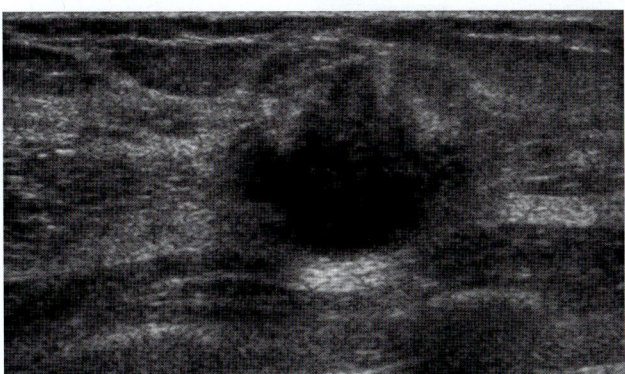

Fig. 8.19 Left breast antiradial sonogram. The mammographic mass and palpable lump correspond to an irregular hypoechoic solid mass near the 3 o'clock position that is associated with spiculations. The mass also distorts the Cooper's ligament and surrounding glandular architecture.

Other Modalities: MRI (Figs. 8.20, 8.21, and 8.22)

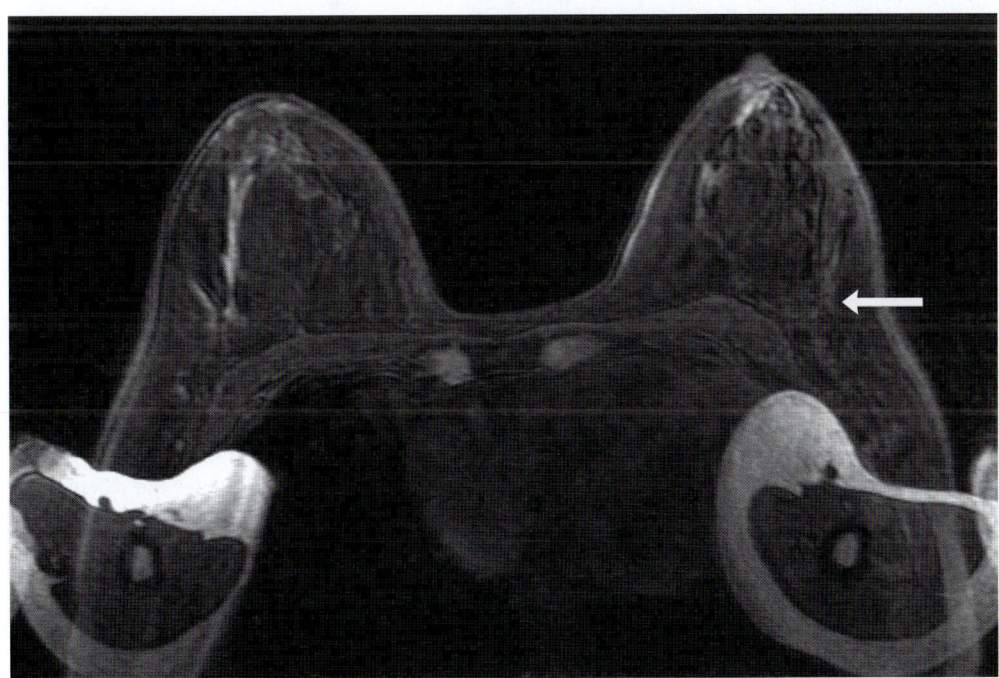

Fig. 8.20 Dynamic bolus T1-weighted, 2-minute axial bilateral breast MRI. This is the patient's first MRI. This image does not demonstrate the known primary malignancy (*arrow* points to area of known malignancy).

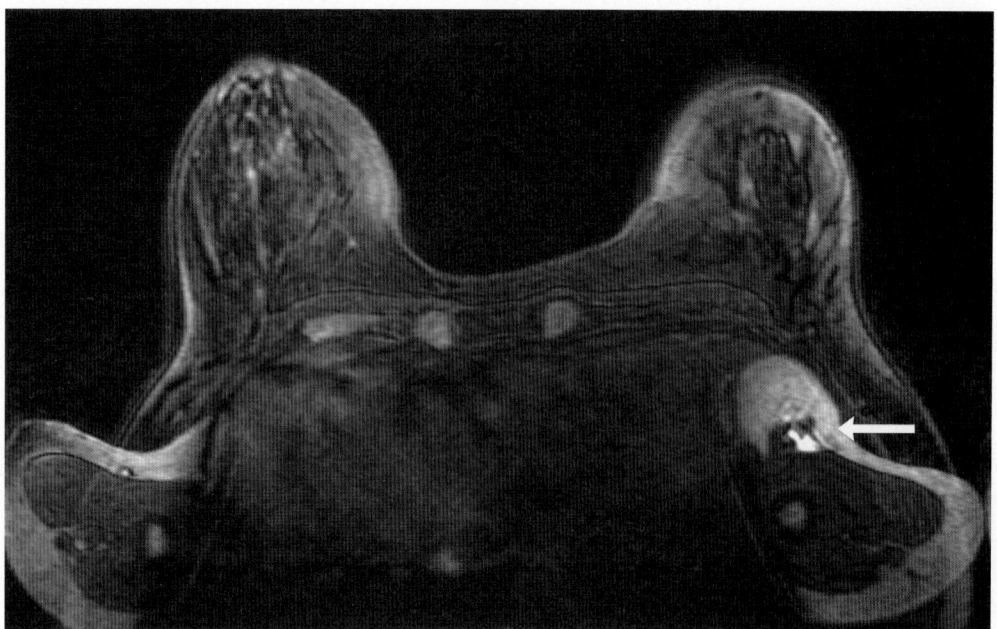

Fig. 8.21 Dynamic bolus T1-weighted, 5-minute axial bilateral breast MRI. Image from first MRI. This image from a series performed 3 minutes later than in **Fig. 8.20** shows intravenous contrast still within the left arm (*arrow*). The lack of visualization of the primary malignancy is due to a severely delayed bolus. In this case, the patient had a small amount of contrast extravasation in the arm but not enough to explain the poor imaging result.

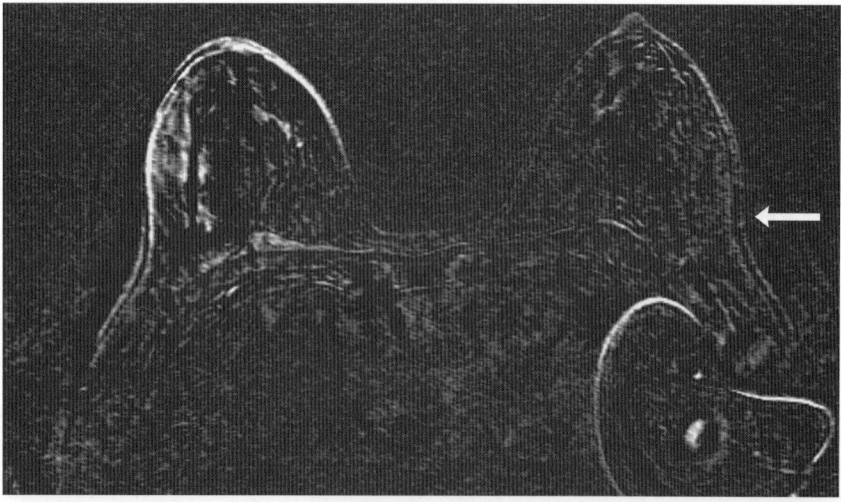

A

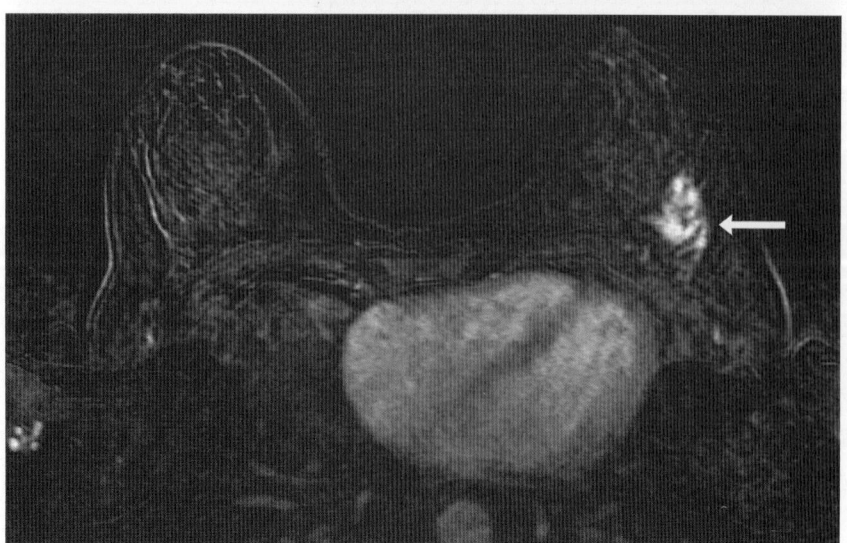

B

Fig. 8.22 During the first MRI, the bolus was severely delayed, so the early T1-weighted dynamic images are not diagnostic. The patient was informed of this problem, and she returned for a second MRI examination. This set of figures demonstrates the difference in appearance of the known malignancy (*arrow*) between (**A**) the first examination with inadequate IV contrast compared with (**B**) the second examination in which the IV contrast bolus is administered properly. (**A**) Dynamic bolus T1-weighted, 2-minute subtraction axial bilateral breast MRI with inadequate contrast bolus. (**B**) Dynamic bolus T1-weighted, 2-minute subtraction axial bilateral breast MRI with adequate contrast bolus.

Pathology
- Invasive ductal carcinoma

Management
- BI-RADS assessment category 4, suspicious; biopsy should be considered.

Pearls and Pitfalls
- The primary method to identify malignancies with MRI is to identify a rapidly enhancing mass. Therefore, if the intravenous (IV) contrast is not administered in a rapid bolus, the MRI diagnostic quality is severely compromised. In this case, it is not clear why the bolus was late. The patient did not appear to have signs of extravasation of contrast in her arm, and the IV connection appeared adequate. However, the lack of contrast within the vascular structures and heart, as well as the absence of liver enhancement, signals the lack of adequate circulating IV contrast.

Suggested Reading

Berg WA. Magnetic resonance imaging. In: Berg WA, Birdwell RL, Gombos EC, Wang S-C, Parkinson BT, Raza S, Green GE, Kennedy A, Kettler MD, eds. Diagnostic Imaging Breast. Altona, Manitoba: Friesens; 2006:II/0: 36–39

Mitchell DG, Cohen MS. Intravenous water-soluble contrast agents. In: Mitchell DG, Cohen MS, eds. MRI Principles. 2nd ed. Philadelphia: Elsevier, 2004:275–293

Ojeda-Fournier H, Choe KA, Mahoney MC. Recognizing and interpreting artifacts and pitfalls in MR imaging of the breast. Radiographics 2007;27(Suppl 1):S147–S164

Padhani AR. Contrast agent dynamics in breast MRI. In: Warren R, Coulthard A, eds. Breast MRI in Practice. London: Martin Dunitz; 2002:43–54

Rausch DR, Hendrick RE. How to optimize clinical breast MR imaging practices and techniques on your 1.5-T system. Radiographics 2006;26:1469–1484

Case 8.7: Invasive Lobular Carcinoma

Case History

A 73-year-old woman presents with a palpable left breast mass.

Physical Examination
- Left breast: palpable mass at the 5 o'clock position
- Right breast: normal exam

Mammogram

Mass (Fig. 8.23)
- Margin: indistinct
- Shape: irregular
- Density: equal density

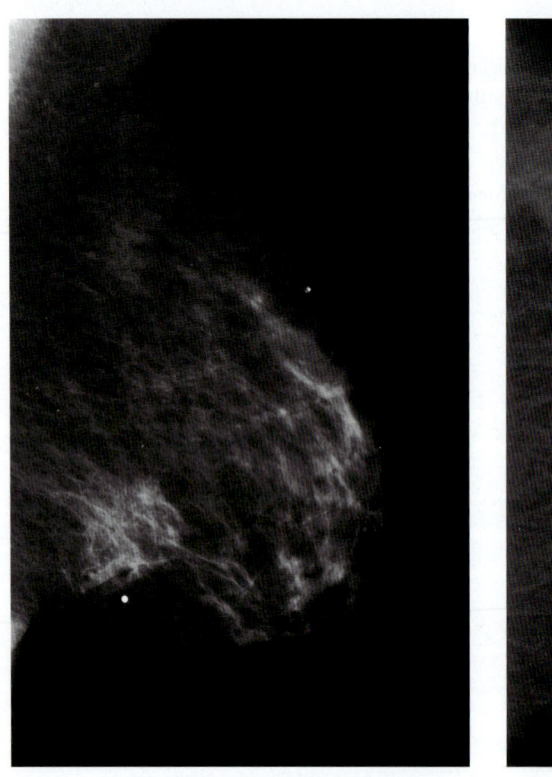
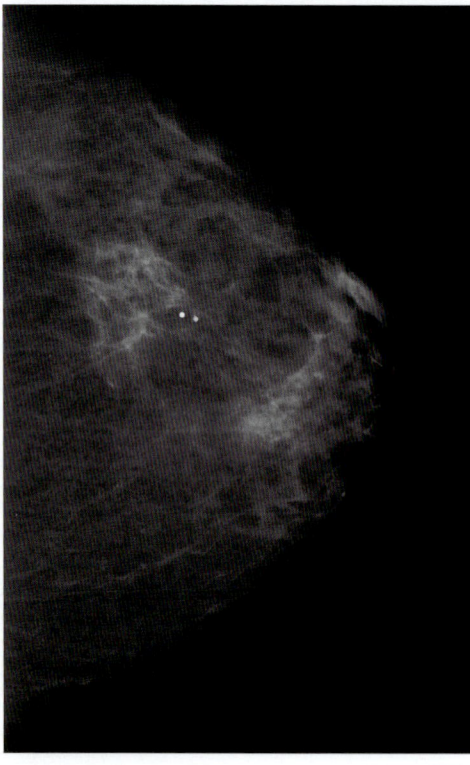

Fig. 8.23 An ill-defined mass is in the lower outer quadrant. This mass is associated with skin retraction and corresponds to the palpable lump. (**A**) Left MLO mammogram. (**B**) Left CC mammogram.

Ultrasound

Frequency
- 7 MHz

Mass (Fig. 8.24)
- Margin: spiculation/architectural distortion
- Echogenicity: heterogeneous (mixed)
- Retrotumoral acoustic appearance: severe shadowing, mass partially obscured
- Shape: irregular

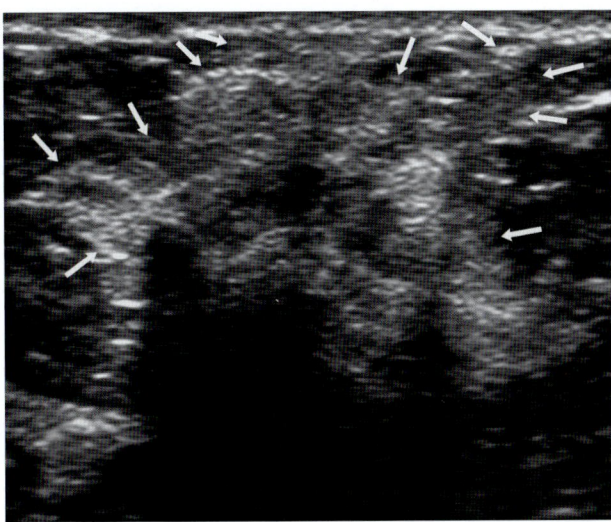

Fig. 8.24 Left radial breast sonogram. The palpable mass corresponds to an irregular mass (*arrows*) of heterogeneous echogenicity. Posterior acoustic shadowing partially obscures the mass.

Pathology
- Invasive lobular carcinoma (**Fig. 8.25**)

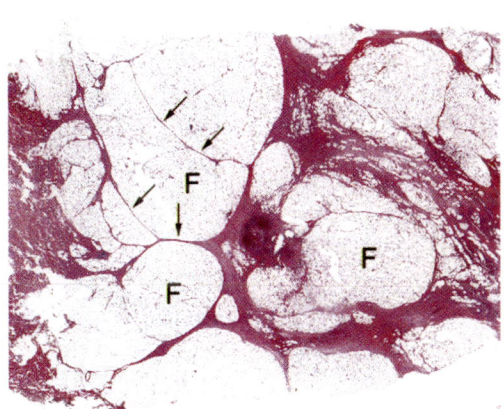
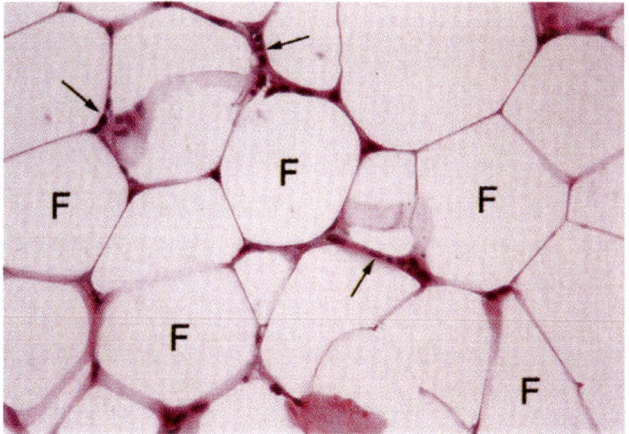

Fig. 8.25 Surgical specimen demonstrates that the malignant cells infiltrate the normal breast tissues without distorting the structure of the tissues. Normal fat cells (F) are distributed between thin columns (*arrows*) of malignant cells and produce the low-density mammographic mass. (**A**) Low-power microscopic view. (**B**) High-power microscopic view.

Management
- BI-RADS assessment category 4, suspicious abnormality; biopsy should be considered.

Pearls and Pitfalls

- Studies report that lobular carcinoma accounts for 1 to 15% of all breast malignancies. The median age of patients is between 45 and 57 years.
- Mammographically, this tumor may exhibit relatively low density because the malignancy extends into the breast stroma via small cords of cells or as isolated single cells. If the malignant cells are surrounded by fat (as in this case), the radiographic density is relatively low for a large mass.
- Sonographically, lobular carcinoma may be missed because it may present (particularly at lower frequencies) as a predominantly hyperechoic mass with shadowing. The mass may blend into the surrounding hyperechoic parenchyma. The main clue that helps to differentiate this mass from the surrounding parenchyma is focal shadowing from the mass.

Suggested Reading

Butler RS, Venta LA, Wiley EL, Ellis RL, Dempsey PJ, Rubin E. Sonographic evaluation of infiltrating lobular carcinoma. AJR Am J Roentgenol 1999;172:325–330

Rissanen T, Tikkakoski T, Autio AL, Apaja-Sarkkinen M. Ultrasonography of invasive lobular breast carcinoma. Acta Radiol 1998;39:285–291

Tavassoli FA. Infiltrating carcinoma: common and familiar special types. In: Tavassoli FA, Fattaneh A. Pathology of the Breast. 2nd ed. Stamford: Appleton and Lange; 1999:401–480

Case 8.8: Invasive Lobular Carcinoma

Case History
A 59-year-old woman presents with a new density identified by screening mammography.

Physical Examination
- Normal exam
- Mammogram

Mass (Fig. 8.26)
- Margin: indistinct
- Shape: irregular
- Density: equal density

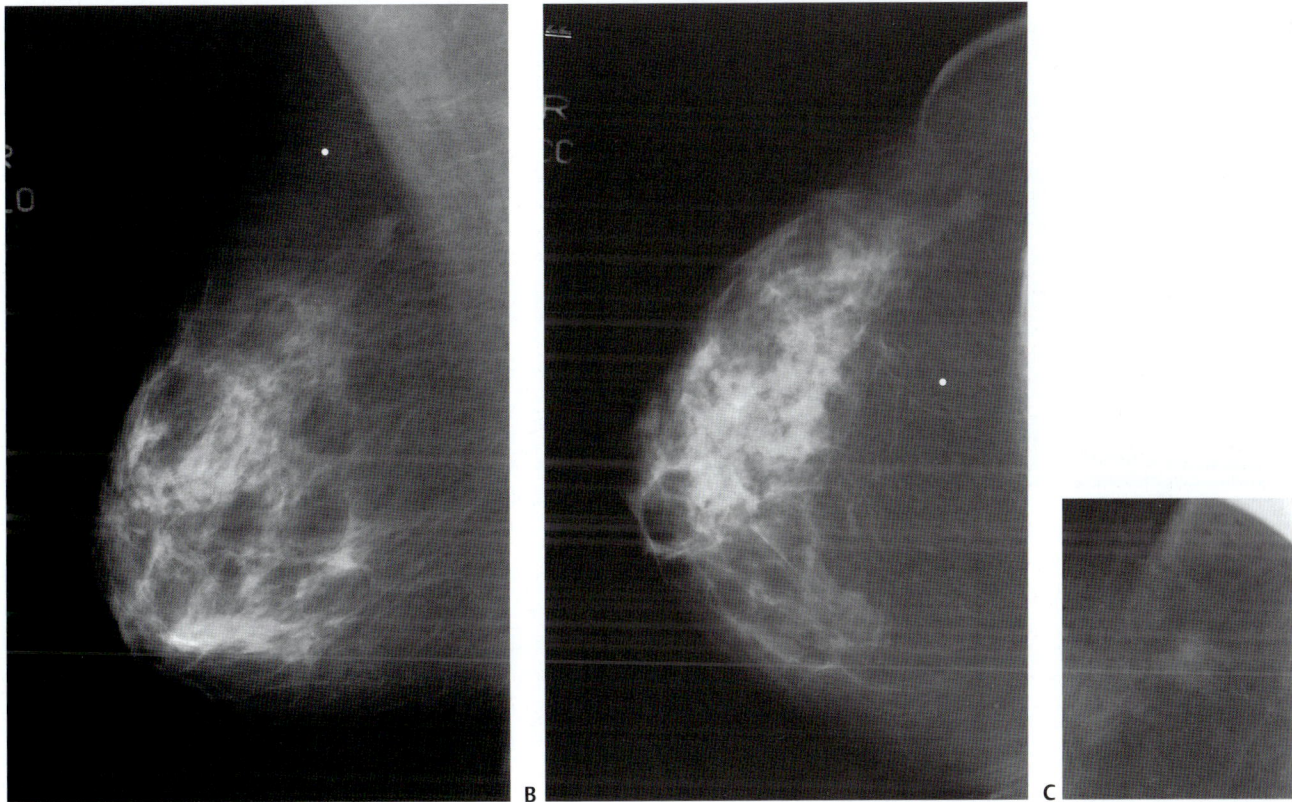

Fig. 8.26 There is a small irregular mass in the right upper outer breast. Radiopaque marker (*dot*) labels a skin mole. (**A**) Right MLO mammogram. (**B**) Right CC mammogram. (**C**) Right CC spot compression mammogram.

Ultrasound

Low Frequency

Frequency
- 7 MHz

Mass (Fig. 8.27)
- Margin: ill defined
- Echogenicity: heterogeneous (mixed)
- Retrotumoral acoustic appearance: posterior shadowing distal to mass
- Shape: irregular

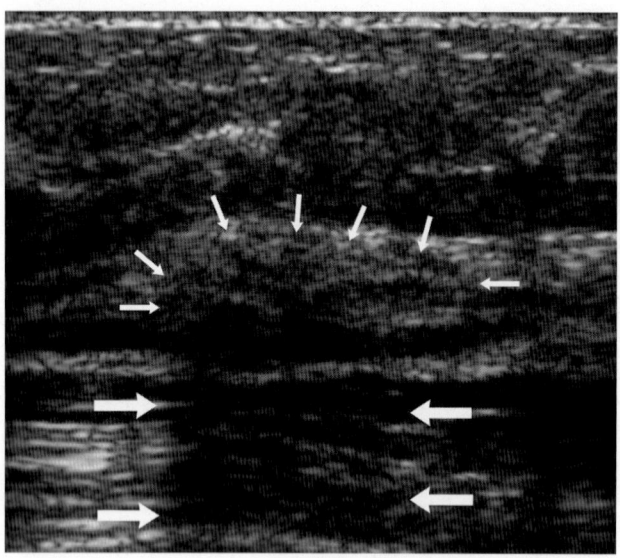

Fig. 8.27 Right radial breast sonogram. The mass identified in **Fig. 8.26** corresponds to minimal sonographic architectural distortion (*small arrows*) and posterior acoustic shadowing (*large arrows*).

Malignant Masses

High Frequency

Frequency
- 10 MHz

Associated Findings
The mass is much easier to identify on the higher-frequency examination (**Fig. 8.28**) compared with the lower frequency examination (**Fig. 8.27**) because the heterogeneous echogenicity of the mass is subtle on the lower-frequency study (**Fig. 8.28**).

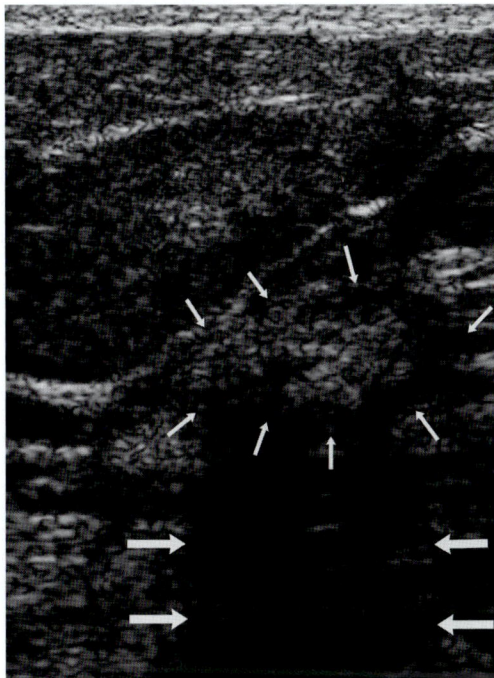

Fig. 8.28 Right radial breast sonogram. Higher frequency sonographic examination of same mass as in **Figs. 8.26** and **8.27** demonstrates a mass with heterogeneous echogenicity (*small arrows*) and acoustic shadowing (*large arrows*).

Pathology
- Invasive lobular carcinoma

Management
- BI-RADS assessment category 4, suspicious abnormality; biopsy should be considered.

Pearls and Pitfalls
- This case illustrates that higher-frequency sonographic technique greatly improves the detectability of breast masses.

Suggested Reading
Evans N, Lyons K. The use of ultrasound in the diagnosis of invasive lobular carcinoma of the breast less than 10 mm in size. Clin Radiol 2000;55:261–263

Skaane P, Skjørten F. Ultrasonographic evaluation of invasive lobular carcinoma. Acta Radiol 1999;40:369–375

Case 8.9: Lymphoma

Case History
A 70-year-old woman presents with non-Hodgkin lymphoma and a new right breast mammographic mass.

Physical Examination
- Breasts: no palpable masses
- Bilateral palpable cervical, axillary, and inguinal adenopathy

Mammogram

Mass (Fig. 8.29)
- Margin: indistinct
- Shape: irregular
- Density: equal density

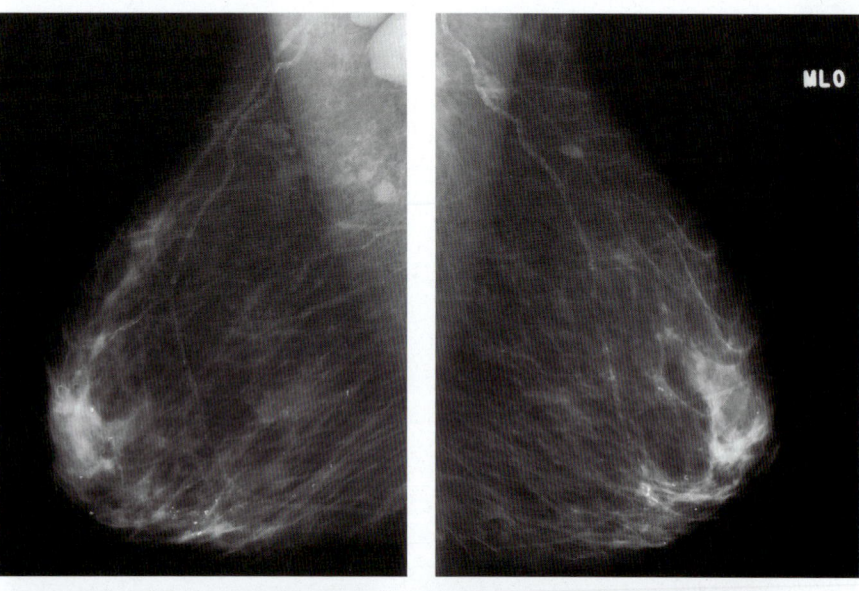

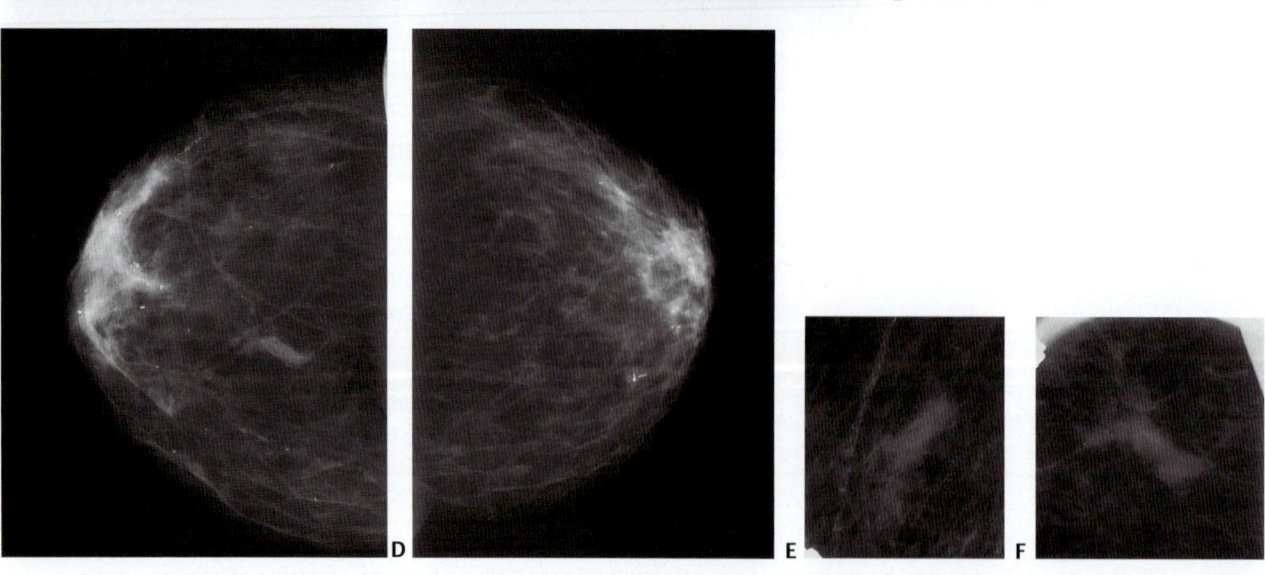

Fig. 8.29 In the 12 o'clock position of the right breast, there is an irregular, ill-defined mass. Large right axillary lymph nodes are also evident. (**A**) Right MLO mammogram. (**B**) Left MLO mammogram. (**C**) Right CC mammogram. (**D**) Left CC mammogram. (**E**) Right MLO spot compression mammogram. (**F**) Right CC spot compression mammogram.

Ultrasound

Frequency
- 13 MHz

Mass (Figs. 8.30 and 8.31)
- Margin: ill defined
- Echogenicity: hypoechoic
- Retrotumoral acoustic appearance: no shadowing
- Shape: irregular

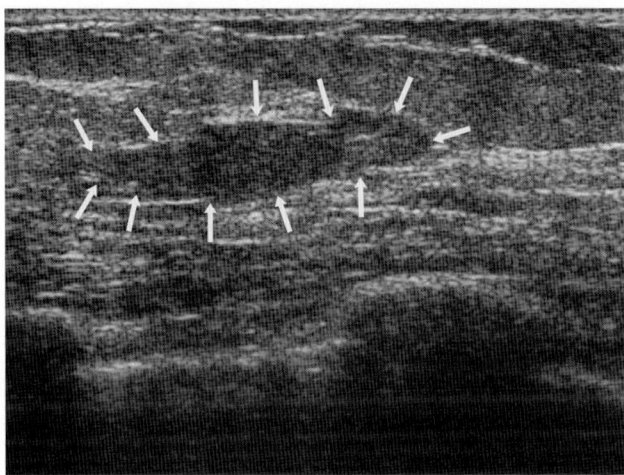

Fig. 8.30 Right radial breast sonogram. The mammographic mass (**Fig. 8.29**) corresponds to an ill-defined, hypoechoic mass (*arrows*).

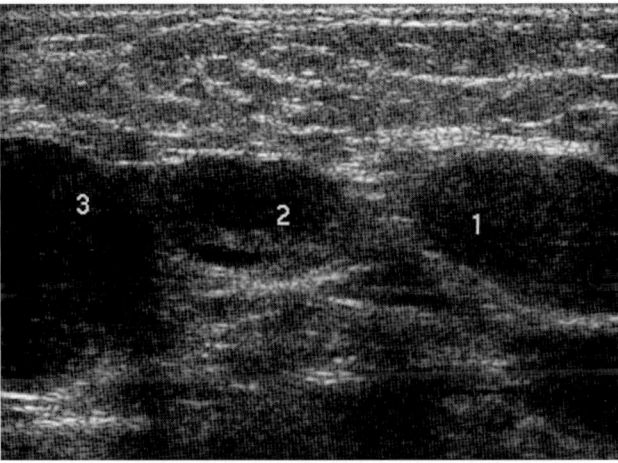

Fig. 8.31 Right radial breast sonogram. In the axilla, there are numerous enlarged lymph nodes (labeled 1, 2, 3).

Pathology
- Lymphoma
- Non-Hodgkin lymphoma, which matches the cell type of the patient's systemic lymphoma

Management
- BI-RADS assessment category 4, suspicious; biopsy should be considered.

Pearls and Pitfalls
- Lymphoma is one of the most common metastatic malignancies of the breast. Non-Hodgkin is more common than Hodgkin lymphoma. Generally, patients present with unilateral breast involvement.
- Mammographically, lymphoma presents as a circumscribed, irregular mass or as an ill-defined density associated with skin thickening.
- Sonographically, lymphoma generally is a circumscribed or irregular, hypoechoic mass. Sometimes the mass simulates a cyst by appearing anechoic with increased acoustic transmission.

Suggested Reading
Kiziltepe TT, Erden GA, Dingil G, Ince A. Breast metastasis from non-Hodgkin's lymphoma: evaluation with color Doppler sonography. AJR Am J Roentgenol 1996;167:1595–1596

Liberman L, Giess CS, Dershaw DD, Louie DC, Deutch BM. Non-Hodgkin lymphoma of the breast: imaging characteristics and correlation with histopathologic findings. Radiology 1994;192:157–160

McCrea ES, Johnston C, Haney PJ. Metastases to the breast. AJR Am J Roentgenol 1983;141:685–690

Meyer JE, Kopans DB, Long JC. Mammographic appearance of malignant lymphoma of the breast. Radiology 1980;135:623–626

Case 8.10: Tubular Carcinoma

Case History
A 75-year-old woman presents for screening mammogram.

Physical Examination
- Normal exam

Mammogram

Mass (Fig. 8.32)
- Margin: indistinct
- Shape: irregular
- Density: equal density

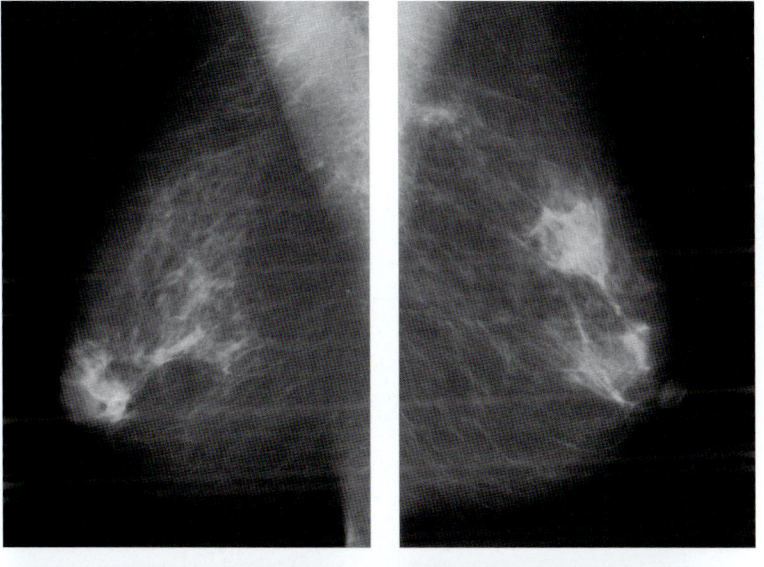
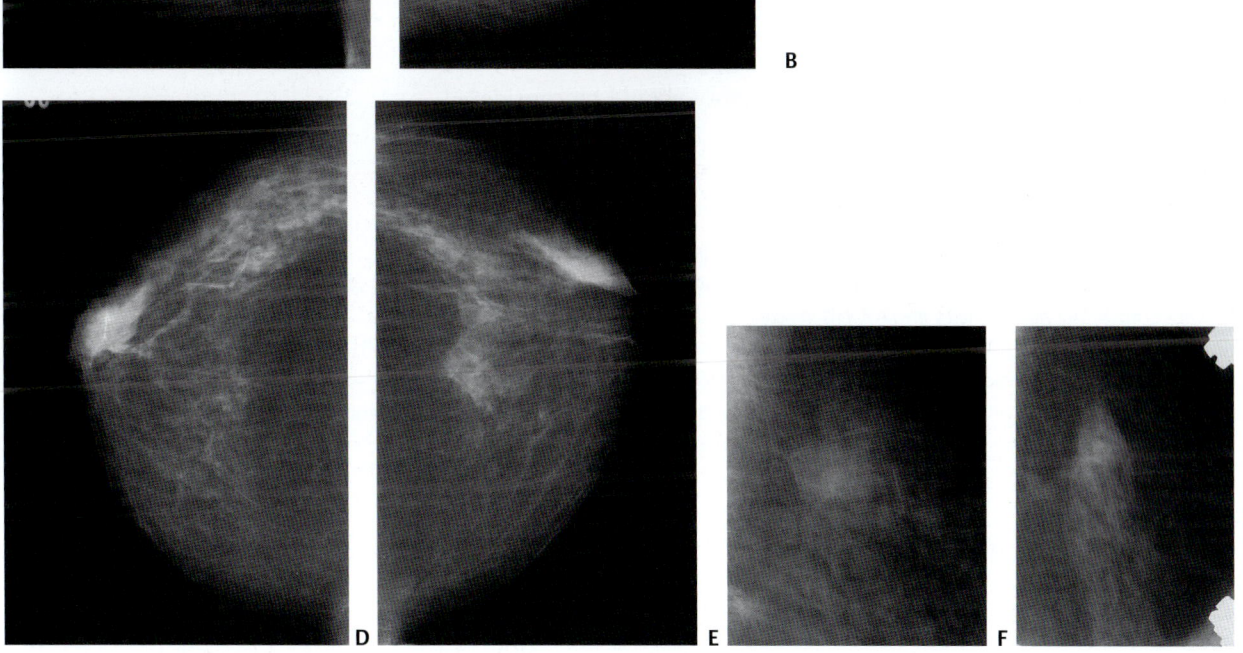

Fig. 8.32 In the left upper outer quadrant, there is an ill-defined mass. The mass is not visible on the routine CC view (**D**) but is identified on the exaggerated CC view (**F**). (**A**) Right MLO mammogram. (**B**) Left MLO mammogram. (**C**) Right CC mammogram. (**D**) Left CC mammogram. (**E**) Left MLO spot compression mammogram. (**F**) Left exaggerated CC spot compression mammogram.

Ultrasound

Frequency
- 7 MHz

Mass (Fig. 8.33)
- Margin: ill defined
- Echogenicity: hypoechoic
- Retrotumoral acoustic appearance: bilateral edge shadowing
- Shape: irregular

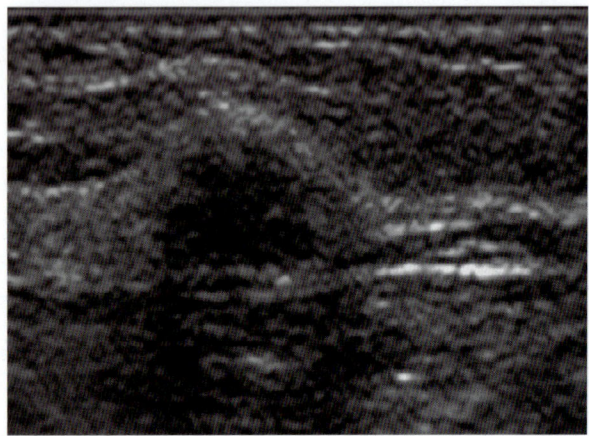

Fig. 8.33 Left radial breast sonogram. The mammographic mass corresponds to an irregular, hypoechoic mass.

Pathology
- Tubular carcinoma

Management
- BI-RADS assessment category 4, suspicious; biopsy should be considered

Pearls and Pitfalls

- Tubular carcinoma comprises 1 to 10% of all breast malignancies.
- Mammographically, tubular carcinomas are generally noncalcified, irregular masses with spiculated margins. They are commonly high density and < 1 cm in size.
- Sonographic findings of tubular carcinoma are similar to irregular masses produced by infiltrating ductal carcinoma. The mass is irregular, hypoechoic with posterior acoustic shadowing. High-frequency sonography may be necessary to detect very small masses. In this case, sonography was used to localize for percutaneous biopsy.

Suggested Reading

Elson BC, Helvie MA, Frank TS, Wilson TE, Adler DD. Tubular carcinoma of the breast: mode of presentation, mammographic appearance, and frequency of nodal metastases. AJR Am J Roentgenol 1993;161:1173–1176

Feig SA, Shaber GS, Patchefsky AS, Schwartz GF, Edeiken J, Nerlinger R. Tubular carcinoma of the breast: mammographic appearance and pathological correlation. Radiology 1978;129:311–314

Leibman AJ, Lewis M, Kruse B. Tubular carcinoma of the breast: mammographic appearance. AJR Am J Roentgenol 1993;160:263–265

Case 8.11: Tubular Carcinoma

Case History

A 55-year-old woman presents for screening mammogram.

Physical Examination
- Normal exam

Mammogram

Mass (Fig. 8.34)
- Margin: spiculated
- Shape: irregular
- Density: equal density

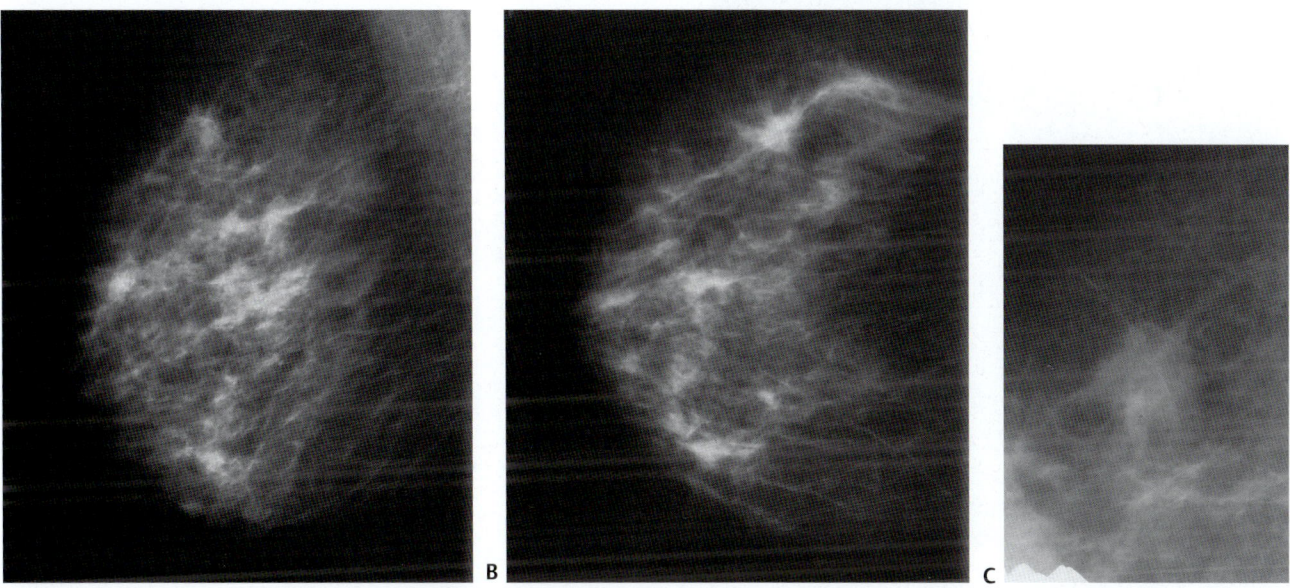

Fig. 8.34 There is a spiculated mass in the right upper outer quadrant. (**A**) Right MLO mammogram. (**B**) Right CC mammogram. (**C**) Right MLO spot magnification mammogram.

Irregular Masses

Ultrasound

Frequency
- 11.5 MHz

Mass (Fig. 8.35)
- Margin: ill defined
- Echogenicity: hypoechoic
- Retrotumoral acoustic appearance: severe shadowing, mass completely obscured
- Shape: irregular

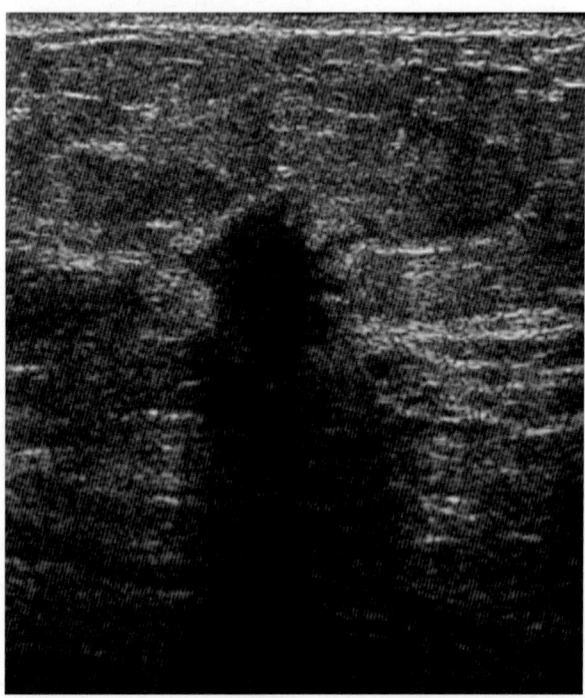

Fig. 8.35 Right radial breast sonogram. Sonographic examination of the mammographic spiculated mass (**Fig. 8.34**) demonstrates an irregular, hypoechoic mass with severe shadowing.

Pathology
- Tubular carcinoma (**Fig. 8.36**)

Management
- BI-RADS assessment category 4, suspicious; biopsy should be considered.

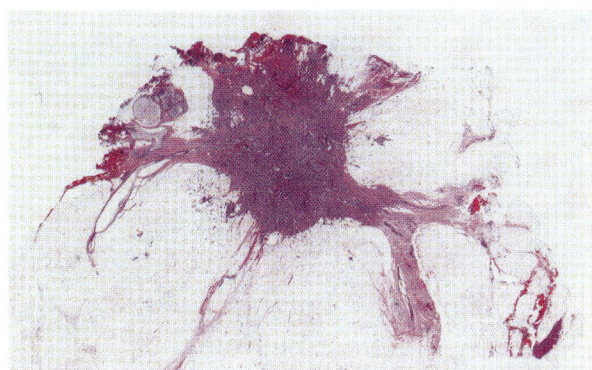

Fig. 8.36 Low-power microscopic image. The irregular shape of the pathologic specimen corresponds to the mammographic spiculated mass.

Pearls and Pitfalls

- Sonography detects between 88 and 100% of cases of tubular carcinomas. Sonography is useful when the tumor is mammographically occult or for guiding biopsy.
- Tubular carcinoma has been reported to be multicentric in 15 to 60% of patients and has been associated with another malignancy in the contralateral breast in 10 to 40% of patients. This patient also had abnormal calcifications in the left breast due to ductal carcinoma in situ.

Suggested Reading

Mitnick JS, Gianutsos R, Pollack AH, et al. Tubular carcinoma of the breast: sensitivity of diagnostic techniques and correlation with histopathology. AJR Am J Roentgenol 1999;172:319–323

Sheppard DG, Whitman GJ, Huynh PT, Sahin AA, Fornage BD, Stelling CB. Tubular carcinoma of the breast: mammographic and sonographic features. AJR Am J Roentgenol 2000;174:253–257

Case 8.12: Inflammatory Carcinoma

Case History

A 57-year-old woman presents with a new left breast lump.

Physical Examination
- Left breast: two palpable lumps at the 1 o'clock position; skin is thickened, red, and erythematous.
- Right breast: normal exam

Mammogram

Mass (Fig. 8.37)
- Margin: indistinct
- Shape: irregular
- Density: high density

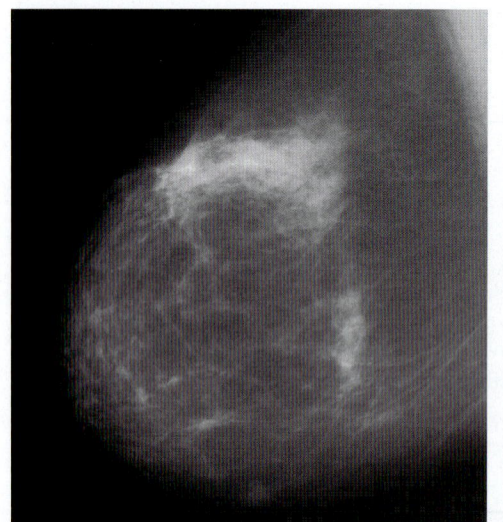
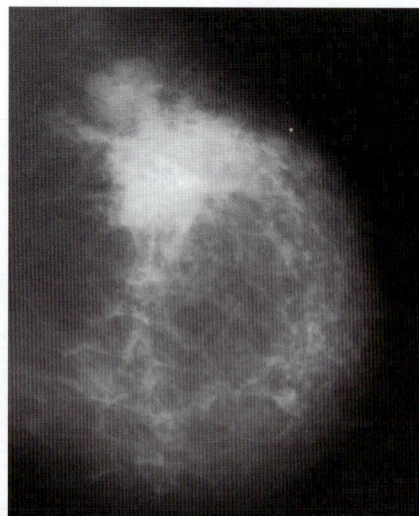
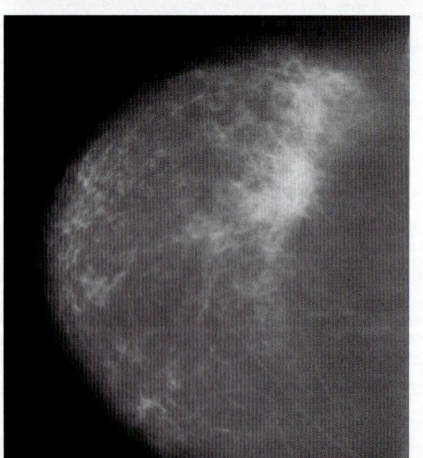
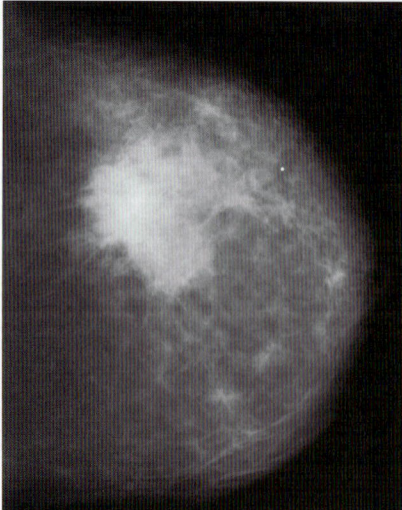
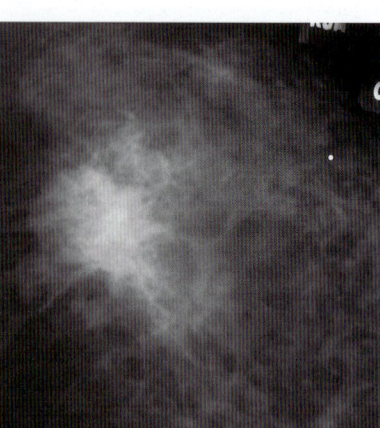

Fig. 8.37 In the left upper outer breast, there is an area of increased density associated with a dominant ill-defined, irregular mass. (**A**) Right MLO mammogram. (**B**) Left MLO mammogram. (**C**) Right CC mammogram. (**D**) Left CC mammogram. (**E**) Left CC spot compression mammogram.

Ultrasound

Frequency
- 10 MHz

Mass (Figs. 8.38 and 8.39)
- Margin: ill defined
- Echogenicity: hypoechoic
- Retrotumoral acoustic appearance: posterior shadowing distal to mass
- Shape: irregular

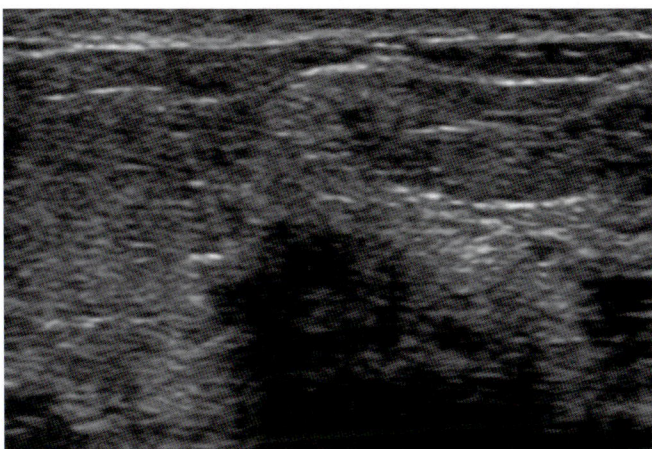

Fig. 8.38 Left radial breast sonogram. In the left upper outer quadrant, there are two palpable masses. The mass in this image corresponds to the dominant mammographically identified mass (**Fig. 8.37**).

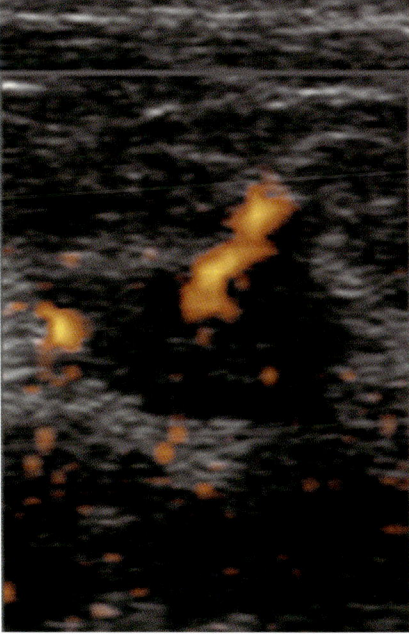

Fig. 8.39 Left radial color Doppler breast sonogram. A second palpable lump corresponds to this smaller, irregular, spiculated mass, which is a satellite lesion of the dominant mass in **Fig. 8.38**.

9 Calcifications: Large Linear

Case 9.1: Vascular

Case History
A 61-year-old woman presents for screening mammogram.

Physical Examination
- Normal exam

Mammogram

Calcifications (Fig. 9.1)
- Type: vascular
- Distribution: diffuse/scattered

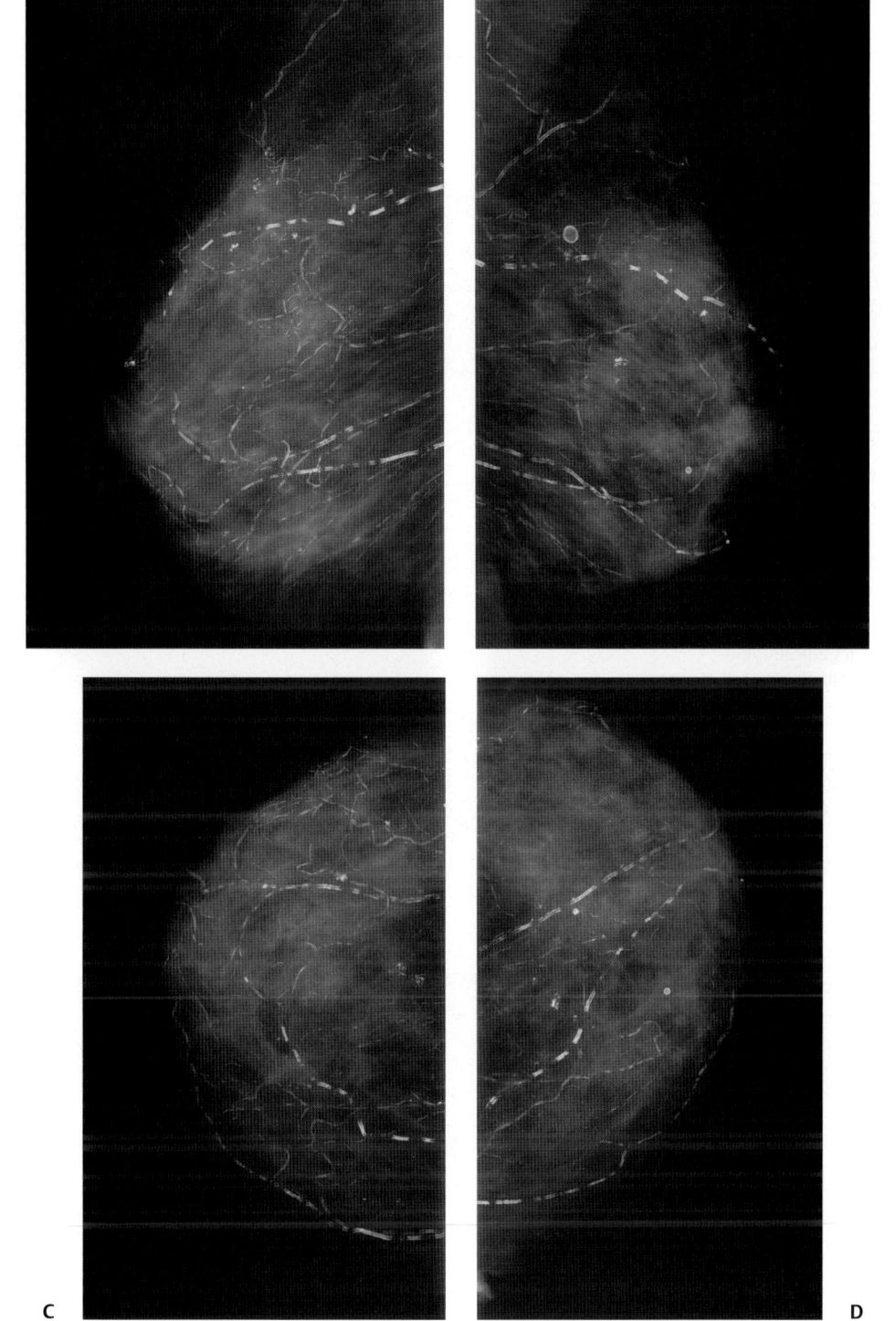

Fig. 9.1 Both breasts exhibit numerous linear vascular calcifications. (**A**) Right MLO mammogram. (**B**) Left MLO mammogram. (**C**) Right CC mammogram. (**D**) Left CC mammogram.

Pathology
- Atherosclerosis

Management
- BI-RADS assessment category 1, negative

Pearls and Pitfalls
- Atherosclerosis is the most common cause of vascular calcifications in the breast. These calcifications are linear and generally are easy to differentiate from malignant calcifications. Vascular calcifications may be increased in patients with renal failure. Occasionally, vessels that are poorly calcified may appear worrisome, but, generally, magnification views clarify the etiology of the calcification.

Suggested Reading

Cooper RA, Berman S. Extensive breast calcification in renal failure. J Thorac Imaging 1988;3:81–82

Kemmeren JM, Beijerinck D, van Noord PA, et al. Breast arterial calcifications: association with diabetes mellitus and cardiovascular mortality. Work in progress. Radiology 1996;201:75–78

Kragel PJ, Aquino MO, Fiorella R, Chapman J. Clinical, radiographic, and pathologic features of medial calcific sclerosis in the breast. South Med J 1997;90:518–521

Meybehm M, Pfeifer U. Vascular calcifications mimicking grouped microcalcifications on mammography. Breast Dis 1990;3:81–86

Sommer G, Kopsa H, Zazgornik J, Salomonowitz E. Breast calcifications in renal hyperparathyroidism. AJR Am J Roentgenol 1987;148:855–857

Case 9.2: Secretory Calcifications

Case History

A 76-year-old woman presents for routine mammogram.

Physical Examination

- Normal exam

Mammogram

Calcifications (Fig. 9.2)
- Type: large rodlike
- Distribution: diffuse/scattered

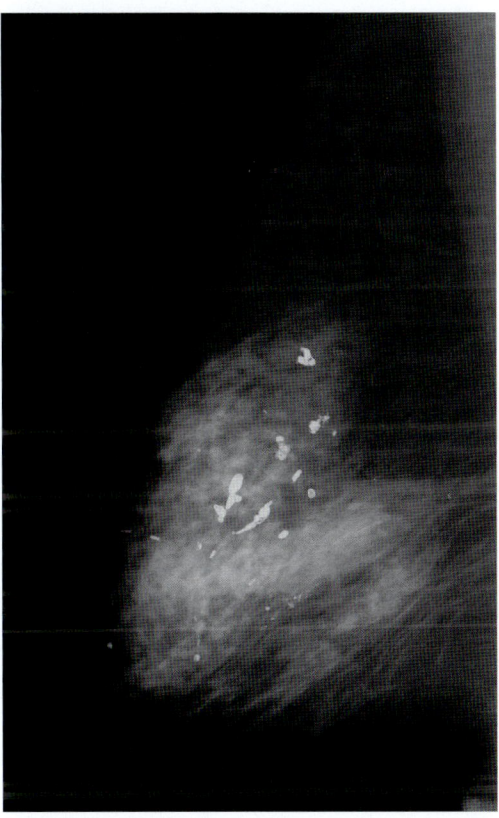
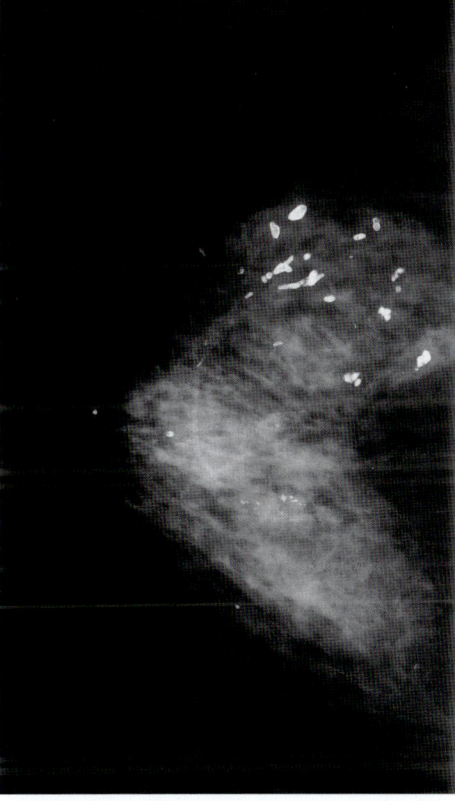

Fig. 9.2 There are diffuse, scattered, thick, linear, large oval and round calcifications in the upper half of the breast oriented toward the nipple. These calcifications are smooth bordered, and some have central lucencies. Most of the linear calcifications do not branch. (**A**) Right MLO mammogram. (**B**) Right CC mammogram.

Pathology
- Plasma cell mastitis

Management
- BI-RADS assessment category 2, benign finding

> **Pearls and Pitfalls**
>
> - Secretory calcifications result from ductal inflammation and are benign. This process is commonly bilateral. The large size, scattered distribution, and smooth borders distinguish these calcifications from malignant calcifications.
> - Secretory calcifications may present in one of two forms. They may be primarily linear, either with or without central lucency, or they may be spherical or globular in configuration with lucent centers. In this latter form, they are sometimes difficult to differentiate from multiple oil cysts. This case illustrates the spherical form.

Suggested Reading

De Paredes ES. Atlas of Film-Screen Mammography. 2nd ed. Baltimore: Urban & Schwarzenberg; 1988:191–276

Gershon-Cohen J, Ingleby H, Hermel MB. Calcification in secretory disease of the breast. Am J Roentgenol Radium Ther Nucl Med 1956;76:132–135

Case 9.3: Secretory Calcifications

Case History
A 79-year-old woman presents for a screening mammogram.

Physical Examination
- Normal exam

Mammogram

Calcifications (Fig. 9.3)
- Type: large rodlike
- Distribution: diffuse/scattered

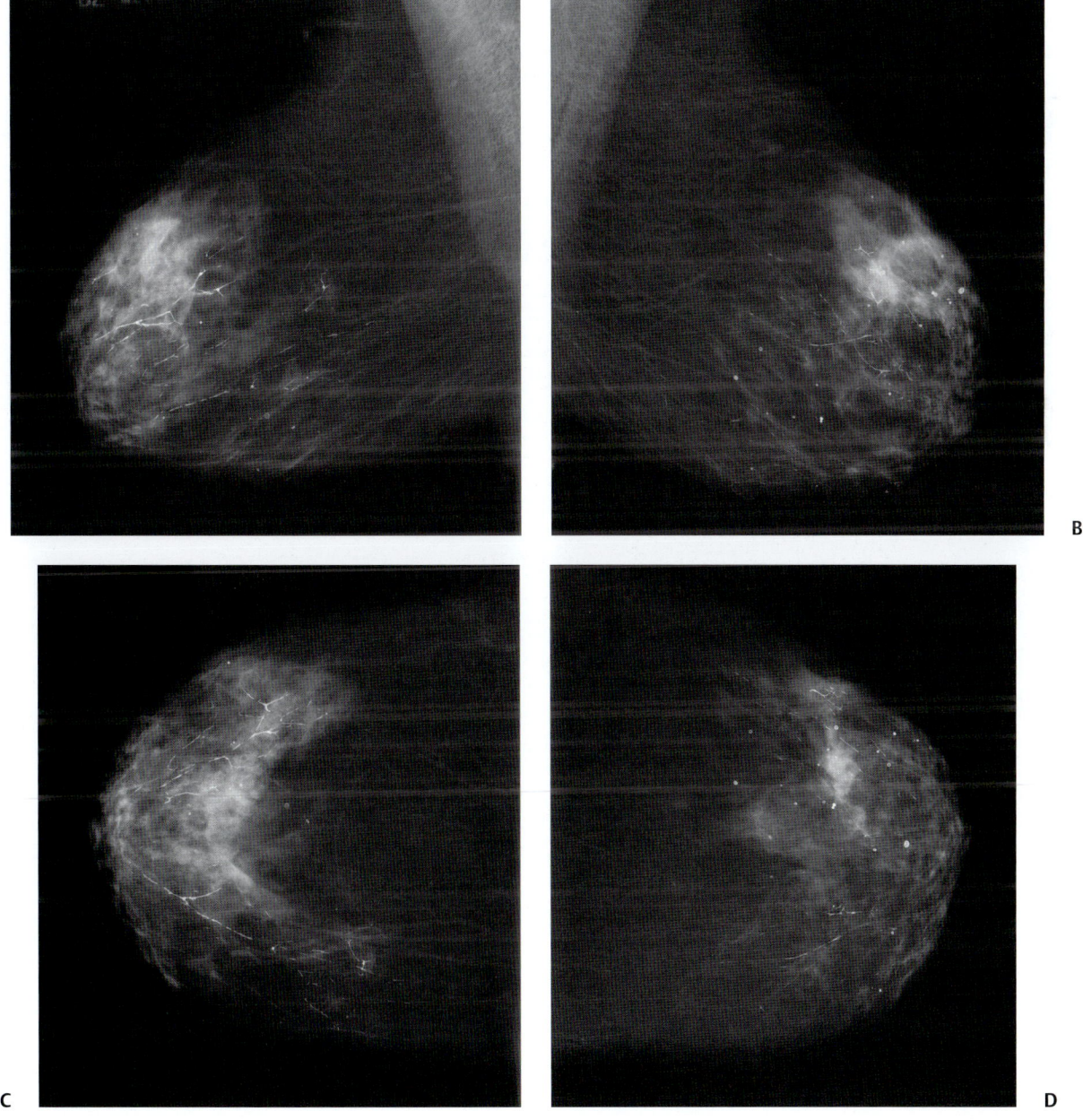

Fig. 9.3 There are numerous, large, smooth-bordered, solid, linear calcifications in both breasts. The calcifications are oriented toward the nipple, and some of the calcifications exhibit a branching pattern. (**A**) Right MLO mammogram. (**B**) Left MLO mammogram. (**C**) Right CC mammogram. (**D**) Left CC mammogram.

Pathology
- Plasma cell mastitis

Management
- BI-RADS assessment category 2, benign finding

> **Pearls and Pitfalls**
>
> - Secretory calcifications result from plasma cell mastitis, which is a periductal inflammatory condition. Because the calcifications may be within the ducts, in the walls of the ducts, or adjacent to the walls of the ducts, the calcification pattern parallels the ductal pattern. These large calcifications are oriented toward the nipple and may branch. This case illustrates the predominantly linear form of this condition.

Suggested Reading

Asch T, Frey C. Radiographic appearance of mammary duct ectasia with calcification. N Engl J Med 1962;266:86–87

Kopans DB. Pathologic, mammographic, and sonographic correlation. In: Kopans DB. Breast Imaging. 2nd ed. Philadelphia: Lippincott-Raven; 1998:511–516

Levitan LH, Witten DM, Harrison EG Jr. Calcification in breast disease: mammographic-pathologic correlation. Am J Roentgenol Radium Ther Nucl Med 1964;92:29–39

10 Calcifications: Milk of Calcium

Case 10.1: Milk of Calcium

Case History
A 50-year-old woman presents with right breast calcifications on her baseline mammogram.

Physical Examination
- Normal exam

Mammogram

Calcifications (Fig. 10.1)
- Type: milk of calcium
- Distribution: grouped/clustered

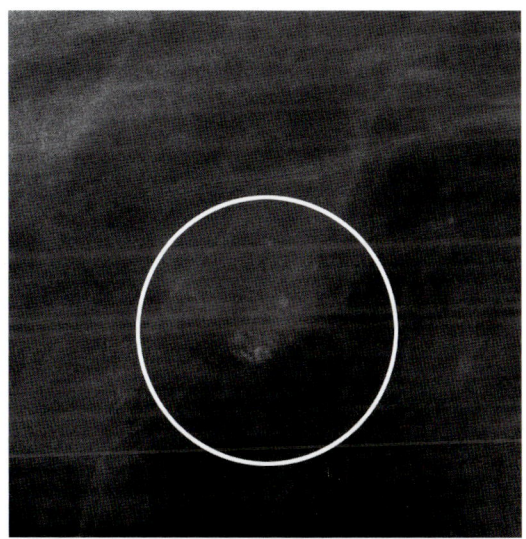
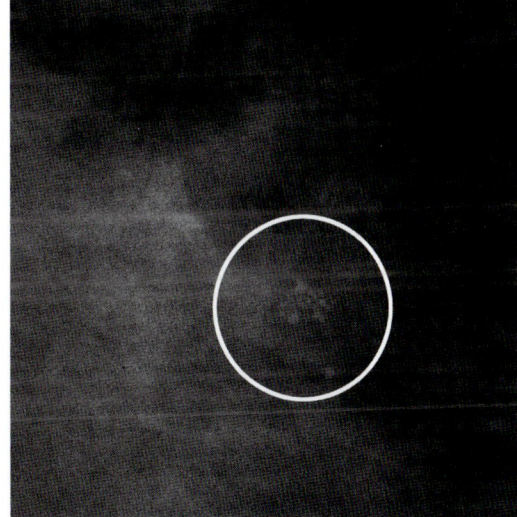

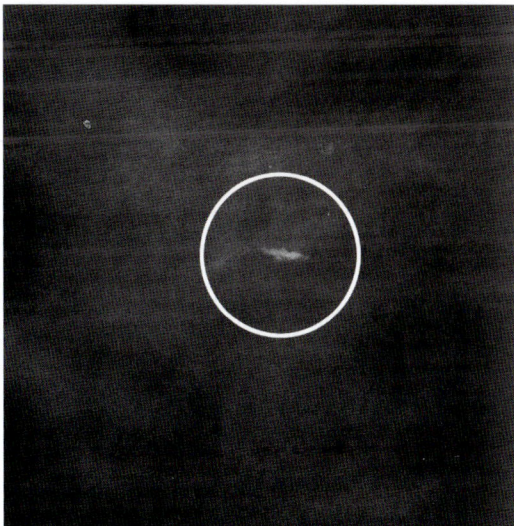

Fig. 10.1 A cluster of calcifications is present in the right inner inferior quadrant (*circle*). On both the right MLO magnification view (**A**) and the right CC magnification view (**B**), the calcifications are predominantly round or oval. (**C**) In the right ML magnification view, the calcifications produce a linear layer consistent with milk of calcium. (**A**) Right MLO magnification mammogram. (**B**) Right CC magnification mammogram. (**C**) Right ML magnification mammogram.

Ultrasound

Frequency
- 10 MHz (**Fig. 10.4**)

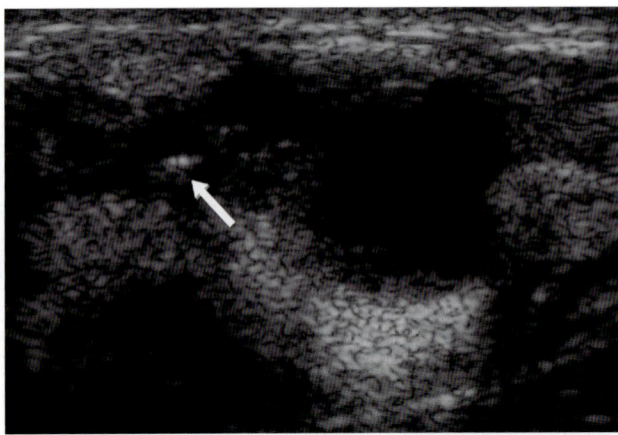

Fig. 10.4 Left longitudinal left breast sonogram. Sonographically, this breast has numerous cysts. In some of these cysts, hyperechoic layering material is present (*arrow*). This hyperechoic material corresponds to the mammographic milk of calcium calcifications.

Pathology
- Microcysts with milk of calcium

Management
- BI-RADS assessment category 2, benign finding

Pearls and Pitfalls

- In this case, macrocysts have sonographic evidence of milk of calcium. Sonographically, milk of calcium may appear as a hyperechoic material that layers in the dependent portion of the cyst. Milk of calcium may also appear as punctate high-intensity foci, which are "piled up" within a cyst.

Suggested Reading
Sickles EA, Abele JS. Milk of calcium within tiny benign breast cysts. Radiology 1981;141:655–658

11 Calcifications: Large Round

Case 11.1: Large Round

Case History
A 72-year-old woman presents for screening mammogram.

Physical Examination
- Normal exam

Mammogram

Calcifications (Fig. 11.1)
- Type: round
- Distribution: diffuse/scattered

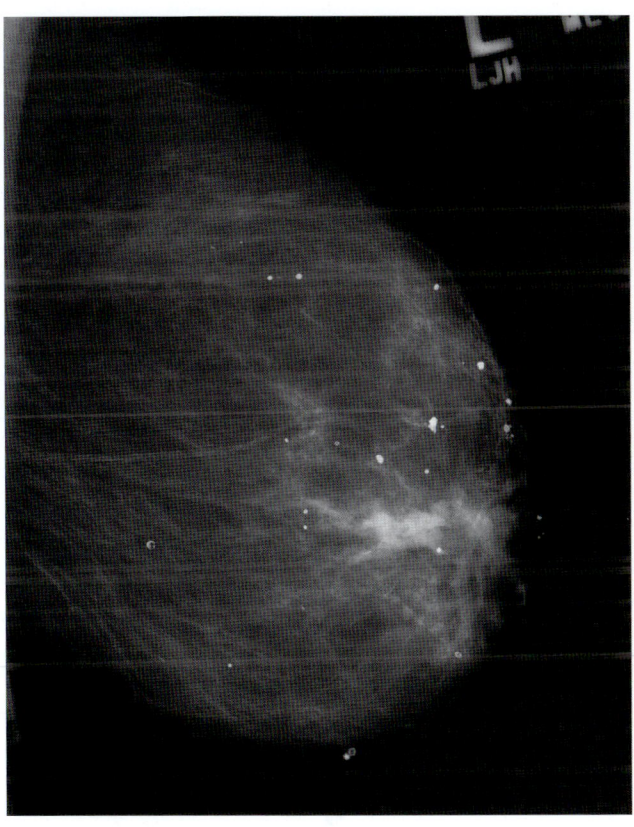 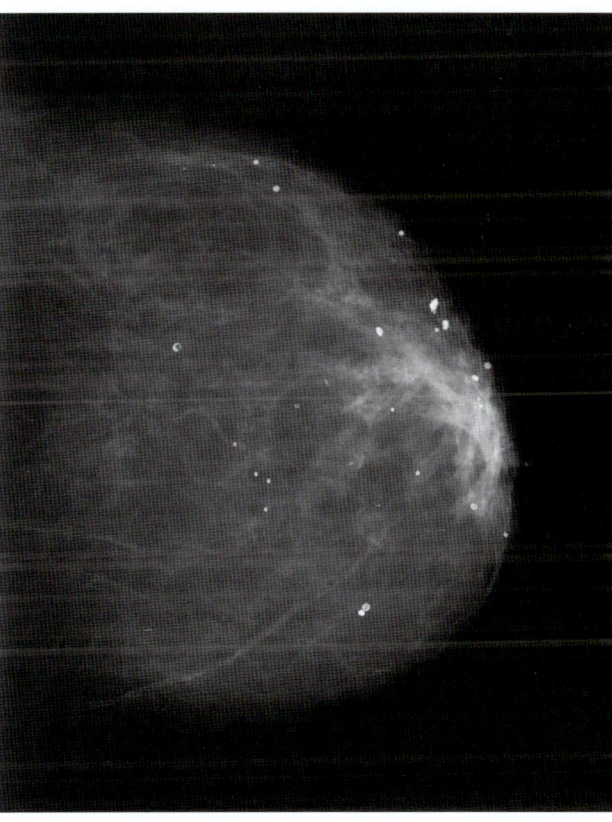

Fig. 11.1 In the left breast there are scattered round, oval calcifications. Some are solid, and others have lucent centers. (**A**) Left MLO mammogram. (**B**) Left CC mammogram.

Pathology
- Oil cyst

Management
- BI-RADS assessment category 2, benign finding

> **Pearls and Pitfalls**
>
> - When the walls of an oil cyst calcify, the calcification is round or oval and may have either a solid white or lucent center. Sometimes only part of the wall is calcified, so only a curvilinear calcification is evident.

Suggested Reading

Monsees BS. Evaluation of breast microcalcifications. Radiol Clin North Am 1995;33:1109–1121

12 Calcifications: Round Lucent Center

Case 12.1: Round Lucent Center

Case History

A 30-year-old woman presents with a small lump near her nipple.

Physical Examination
- Right breast: 5 mm palpable lump next to nipple
- Left breast: normal exam

Mammogram

Calcifications (Fig. 12.1)
- Type: lucent center
- Distribution: diffuse/scattered

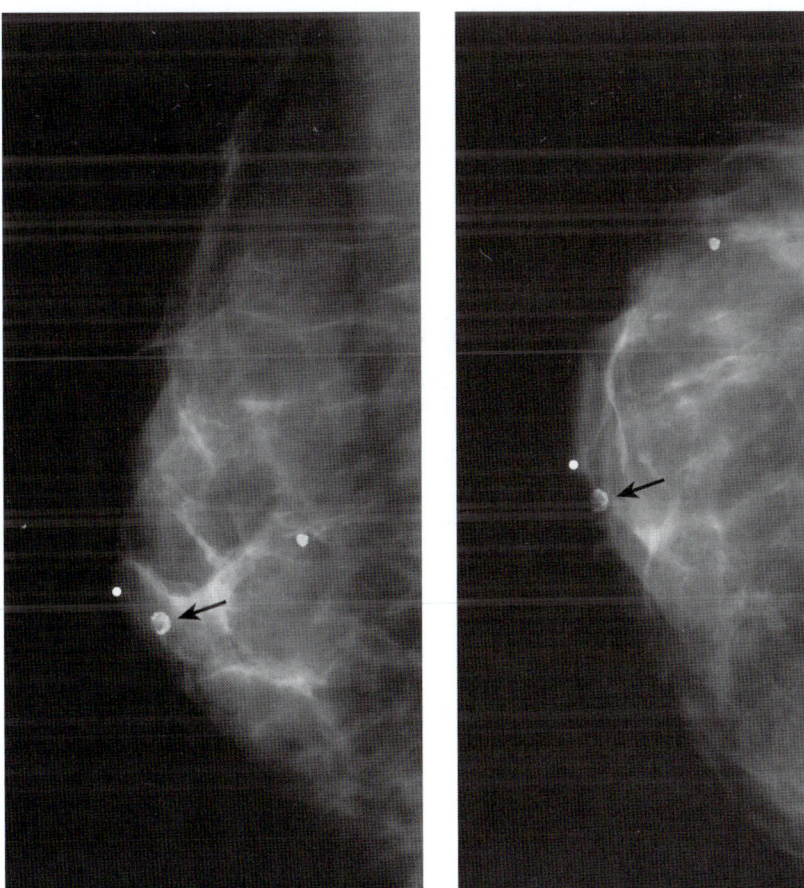
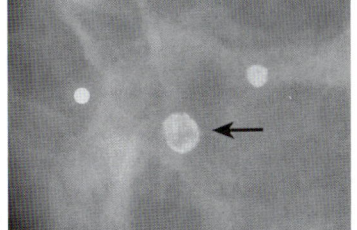

Fig. 12.1 There are two large round calcifications. A radiopaque marker is adjacent to the larger calcification (*arrow*) near the nipple. The round skin BB marker adjacent to the large calcification indicates that a palpable mass is present. (**A**) Right MLO mammogram. (**B**) Right CC mammogram. (**C**) Right MLO spot compression mammogram.

Ultrasound

Frequency
- 13 MHz (**Fig. 12.2**)

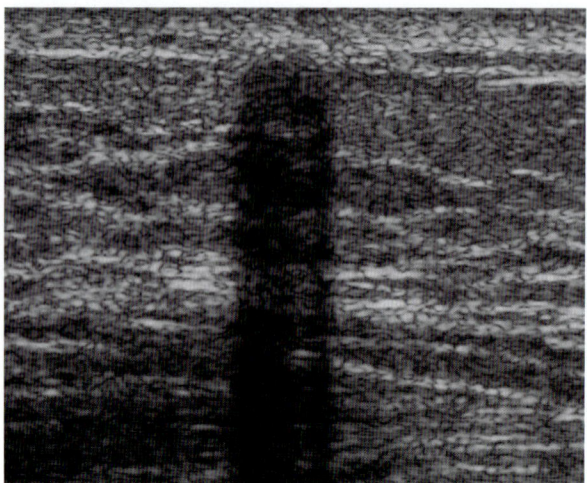

Fig. 12.2 Right antiradial breast sonogram. The palpable lump near the nipple corresponds to a well-defined hypoechoic nodule with posterior acoustic shadowing. This sonographic nodule corresponds to the mammographic oil cyst.

Pathology
- Oil cyst

Management
- BI-RADS assessment category 2, benign finding

Pearls and Pitfalls

- The sonographic appearances of oil cysts include a well-defined, heavily shadowing, oval or round mass (as in this case) or a nonshadowing, hypoechoic, well-defined cystic mass.
- The differential diagnosis of the sonographic mass in this case is either an oil cyst or a simple cyst surrounded by a fibrotic capsule.

Suggested Reading

Morgan CL, Trought WS, Peete W. Xeromammographic and ultrasonic diagnosis of a traumatic oil cyst. AJR Am J Roentgenol 1978;130:1189–1190

Case 12.2: Round Lucent Center

Case History
A 45-year-old woman presents for screening mammogram. She had a benign breast biopsy several years ago.

Physical Examination
- Right breast: faint scar at the 5 o'clock position near the areola
- Left breast: normal exam

Mammogram

Calcifications (Fig. 12.3)
- Type: lucent center
- Distribution: regional

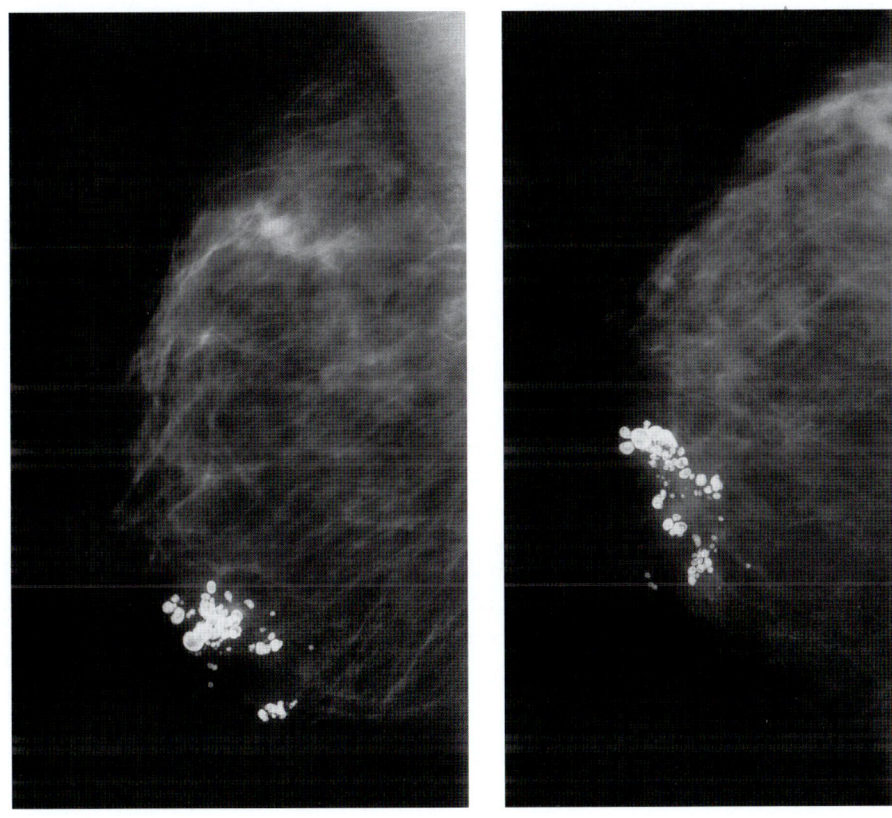

Fig. 12.3 In the inferior medial right breast, there are numerous round calcifications with lucent centers. (**A**) Right MLO mammogram. (**B**) Right CC mammogram.

Pathology
- Oil cyst

Management
- BI-RADS assessment category 2, benign finding

Pearls and Pitfalls
- Oil cysts result from fat necrosis. In this case, the fat necrosis was the consequence of a previous biopsy.
- Oil cysts may be solitary, scattered, or regional; this case is regional. They may appear as solid round, eggshell, lucent centered, or partial rim calcifications. The lucent center form is the most common presentation.

Suggested Reading
Bassett LW, Gold RH, Cove HC. Mammographic spectrum of traumatic fat necrosis: the fallibility of "pathognomonic" signs of carcinoma. AJR Am J Roentgenol 1978;130:119–122

Jackson VP, Jahan R, Fu YS. Benign breast lesions. In: Bassett LW, Jackson VP, Jahan R, Fu YS, Gold RH, eds. Diagnosis of Diseases of the Breast. Philadelphia: WB Saunders; 1997:357–443

13 Calcifications: Eggshell/Rim

Case 13.1: Eggshell/Rim

Case History

A 58-year-old woman arrives for screening mammogram.

Physical Examination

- Normal exam

Mammogram

Calcifications (Fig. 13.1)
- Type: eggshell/rim
- Distribution: single

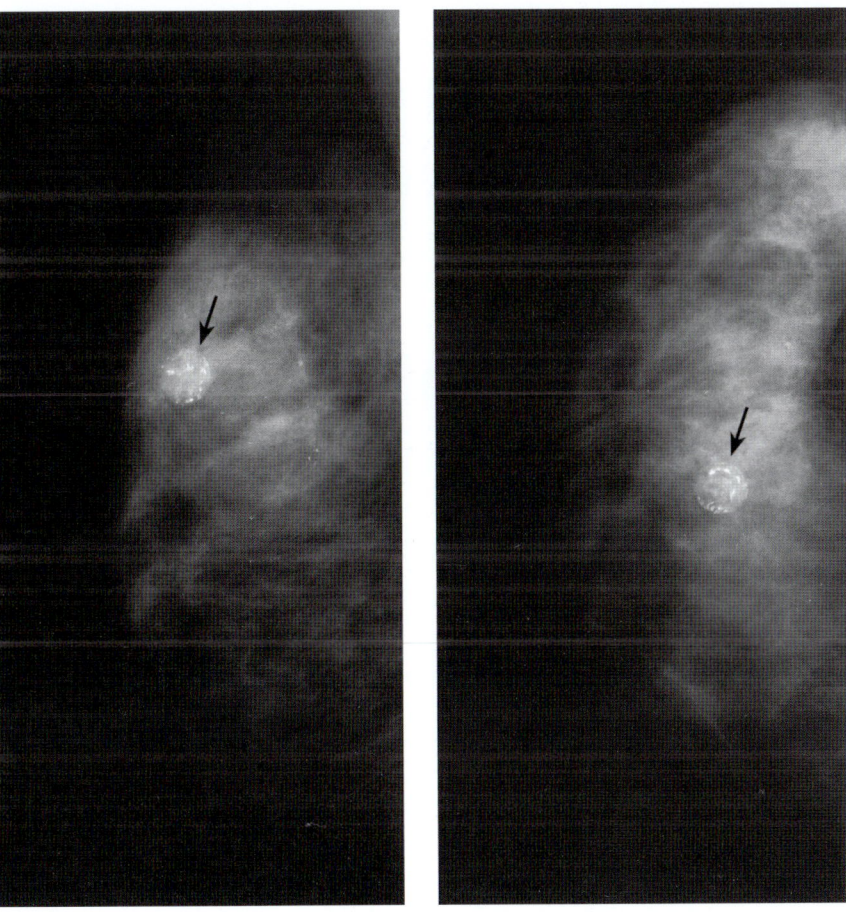

Fig. 13.1 In the 12 o'clock position of the right breast (*arrow*), there is a spherical calcification characteristic of a calcified cyst. (**A**) Right MLO mammogram. (**B**) Right CC mammogram.

Pathology
- Cyst

Management
- BI-RADS assessment category 2, benign finding

Pearls and Pitfalls

- Calcification of cyst walls appears as spherical or as a dense rim with a more lucent center (eggshell).

Suggested Reading

De Paredes ES. Atlas of Film Screen Mammography. 2nd ed. Baltimore: Williams & Wilkins; 1992:299–416

Jackson VP, Jahan R, Fu YS. Benign breast lesions. In: Bassett LW, Jackson VP, Jahan R, Fu YS, Gold RH, eds. Diagnosis of Diseases of the Breast. Philadelphia: WB Saunders, 1997:357–443

Case 13.2: Eggshell/Rim

Case History
An 84-year-old woman presents status post–left lumpectomy and radiation therapy 3 years ago.

Physical Examination
- Left breast: lumpectomy scar in the left upper outer quadrant
- Right breast: normal exam

Mammogram

Calcifications (Fig. 13.2)
- Type: eggshell/rim
- Distribution: single

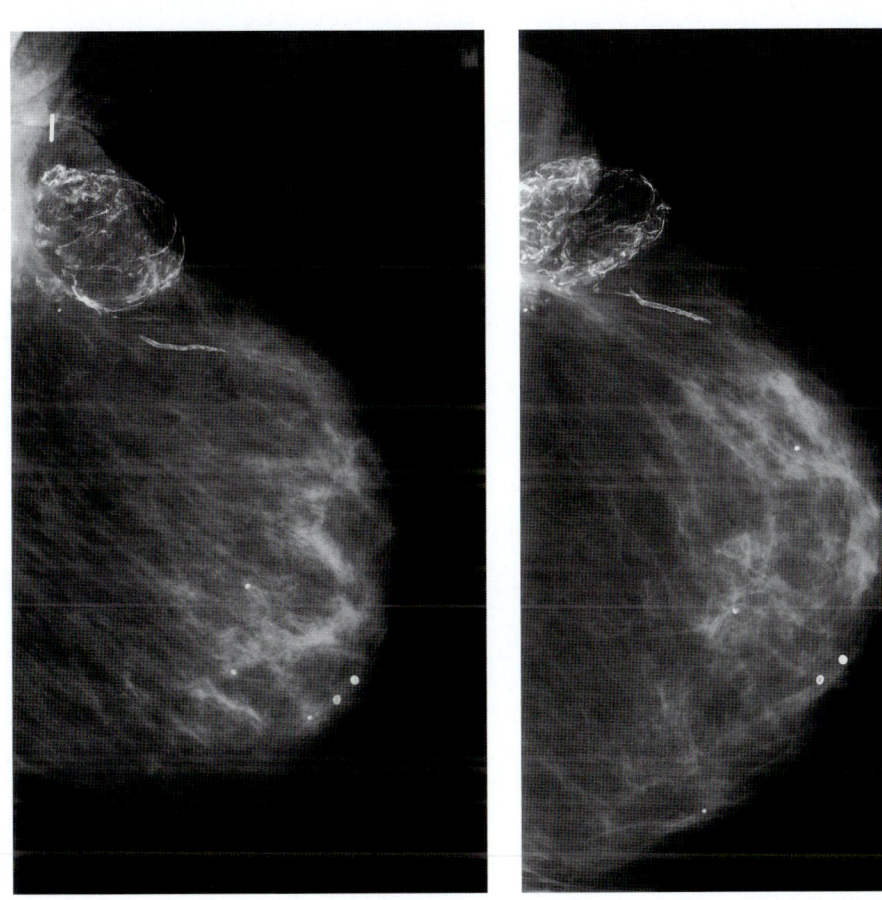

Fig. 13.2 In the left upper outer quadrant, there is a spherical rim calcification in the area of the patient's lumpectomy site. (**A**) Left MLO mammogram. (**B**) Left exaggerated CC mammogram.

Pathology
- Fat necrosis

Management
- BI-RADS assessment category 2, benign finding

Pearls and Pitfalls
- Calcifications from fat necrosis may appear as round lucent center, coarse irregular dystrophic, thin rim, or eggshell calcifications.

Suggested Reading
Bassett LW, Gold RH, Cove HC. Mammographic spectrum of traumatic fat necrosis: the fallibility of "pathognomonic" signs of carcinoma. AJR Am J Roentgenol 1978;130:119–122

Bassett LW, Gold RH, Mirra JM. Nonneoplastic breast calcifications in lipid cysts: development after excision and primary irradiation. AJR Am J Roentgenol 1982;138:335–338

14 Calcifications: Coarse/Popcorn–Fibroadenoma

Case 14.1: Coarse/Popcorn–Fibroadenoma

Case History
A 69-year-old woman presents for screening mammogram.

Physical Examination
- Normal exam

Mammogram

Calcifications (Figs. 14.1 and 14.2)
- Type: coarse/popcorn
- Distribution: single

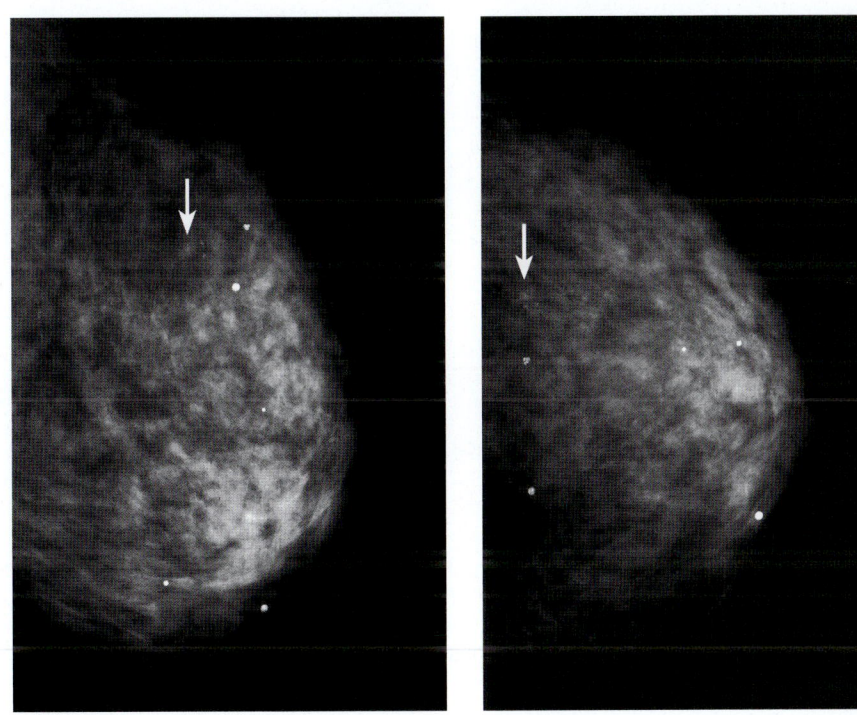

Fig. 14.1 Faint coarse calcifications are present in the upper outer breast (*arrow*). (**A**) Left MLO mammogram. (**B**) Left CC mammogram.

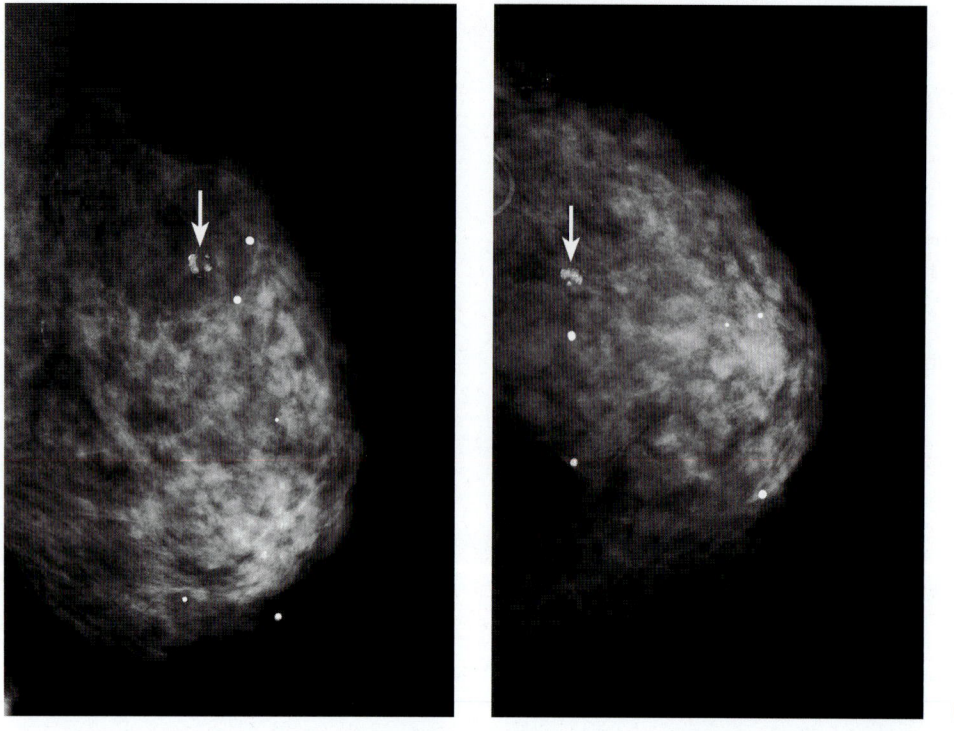

Fig. 14.2 Exam performed 3 years after **Fig. 14.1**. The calcifications (*arrow*) have enlarged and are now characteristic of an involuting fibroadenoma. (**A**) Left MLO mammogram. (**B**) Left CC mammogram.

Pathology
- Fibroadenoma

Management
- BI-RADS assessment category 2, benign finding

> **Pearls and Pitfalls**
>
> - Differential diagnosis of large, coarse calcifications includes fibroadenoma, fat necrosis, and calcium deposition from hypercalcemia (i.e., hyperparathyroidism, renal failure).

Suggested Reading
Gershon-Cohen J, Ingleby H. Roentgenography of fibroadenoma of the breast. Radiology 1952;59:77–87

Han SY, Witten DM. Diffuse calcification of the breast in chronic renal failure. AJR Am J Roentgenol 1977;129:341–342

Case 14.2: Coarse/Popcorn–Fibroadenoma

Case History
A 43-year-old woman presents status 2 years post–right lumpectomy for breast cancer, now with left breast lump.

Physical Examination
- Right breast: surgical scar in the inferior right breast
- Left breast: 1 cm lump near the left nipple

Mammogram

Calcifications (Fig. 14.3)
- Type: coarse/popcorn
- Distribution: single

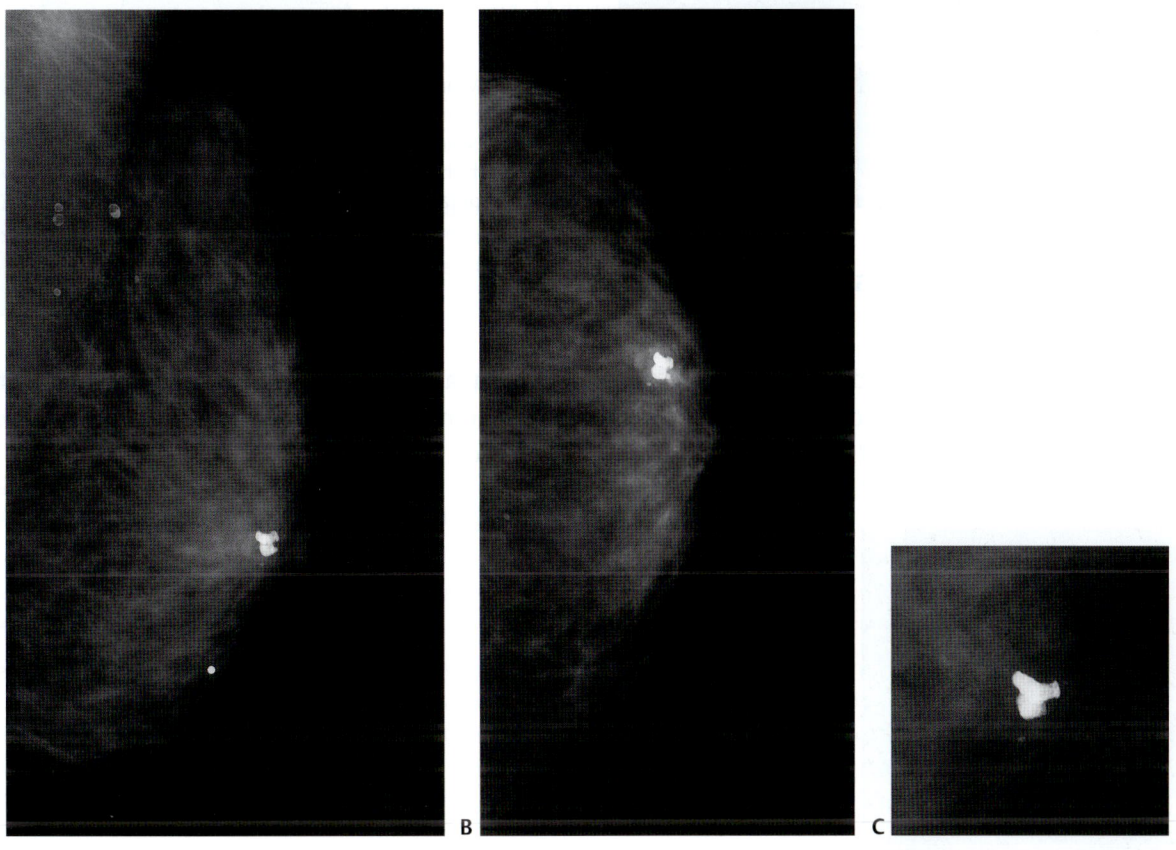

Fig. 14.3 In the subareolar region of the left breast, there is a large, coarse, lobulated calcification characteristic of a fibroadenoma. (**A**) Left MLO mammogram. (**B**) Left CC mammogram. (**C**) Left MLO spot magnification mammogram.

Ultrasound

Frequency
- 13 MHz

15 Calcifications: Dystrophic

Case 15.1: Fat Necrosis

Case History

An 84-year-old woman presents for screening mammogram.

Physical Examination

- Scars in both breasts from previous reduction mammoplasties

Mammogram

Calcifications (Fig. 15.1)
- Type: dystrophic
- Distribution: diffuse/scattered

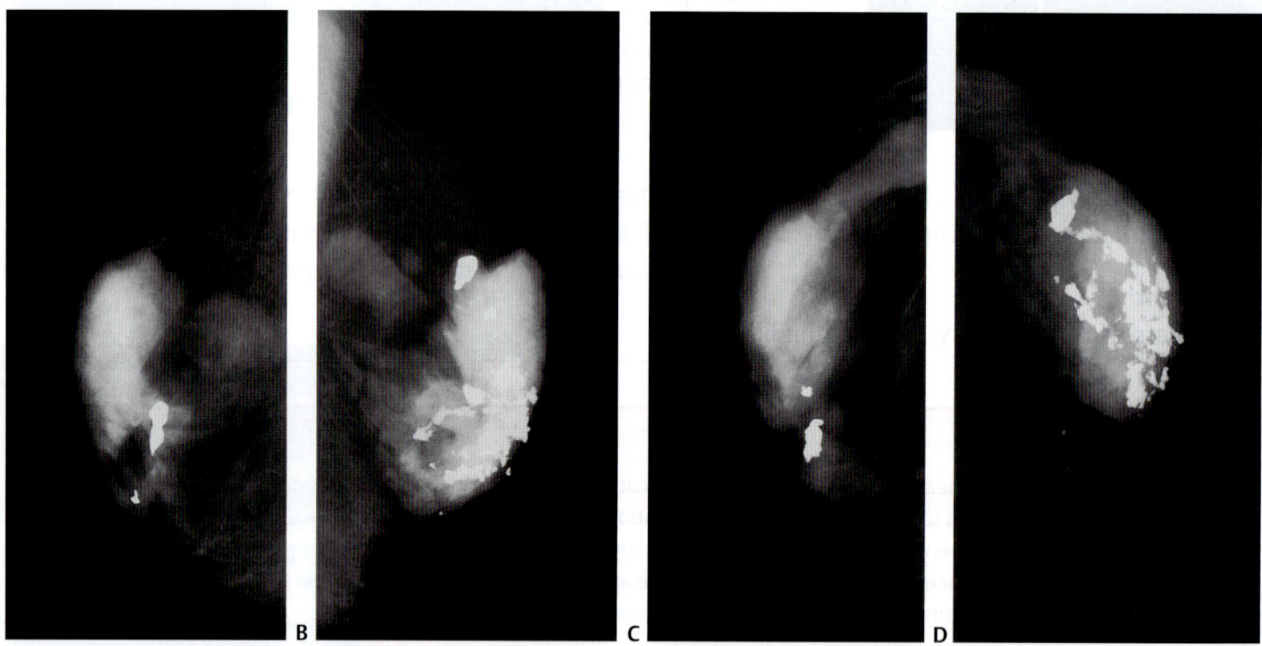

Fig. 15.1 In both breasts there are large, coarse, dystrophic calcifications that have resulted from this patient's bilateral reduction mammoplasties. (**A**) Right MLO mammogram. (**B**) Left MLO mammogram. (**C**) Right CC mammogram. (**D**) Left CC mammogram.

Pathology
- Fat necrosis

Management
- BI-RADS assessment category 2, benign finding

Pearls and Pitfalls
- Fat necrosis may be associated with round (oil cyst), eggshell/rim, or large, irregular calcifications. This case is an example of the last type of calcification.

Suggested Reading
Sickles EA. Breast calcifications: mammographic evaluation. Radiology 1986;160:289–293

Case 15.2: Fat Necrosis

Case History
A 79-year-old woman presents with right breast calcifications.

Physical Examination
- Normal exam

Mammogram

Calcifications (Figs. 15.2 and 15.3)
- Type: dystrophic
- Distribution: grouped/clustered

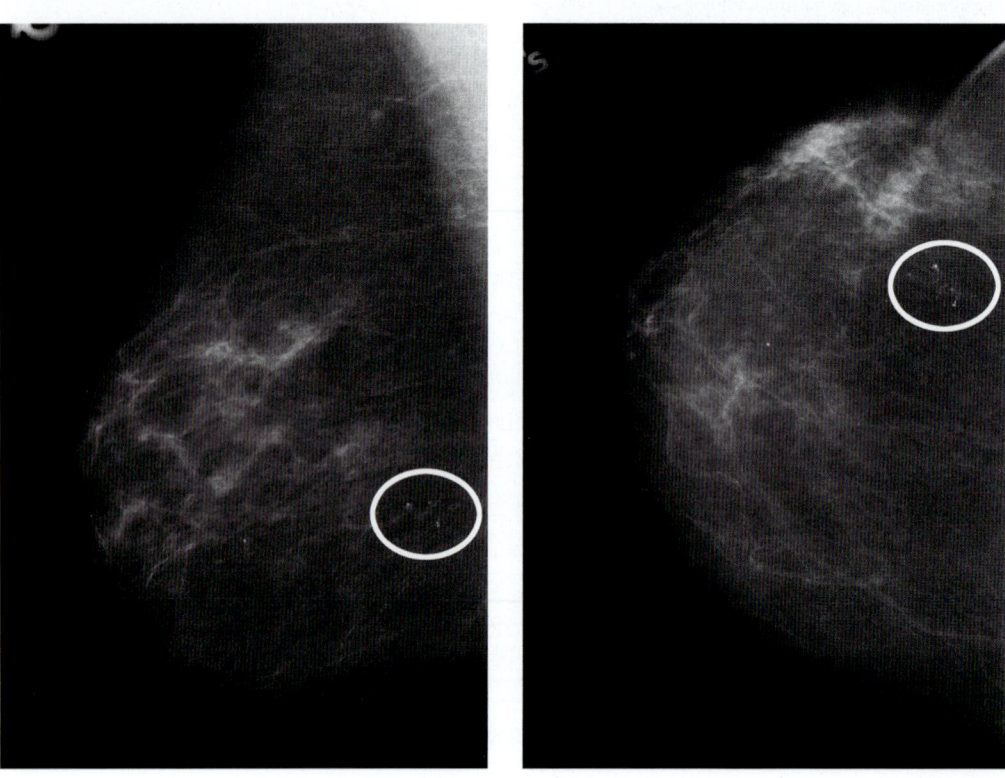

Fig. 15.2 In the right outer breast, there is a cluster of calcifications (*circle*) that was biopsied after this examination. (**A**) Right MLO mammogram. (**B**) Right CC mammogram.

Dystrophic **219**

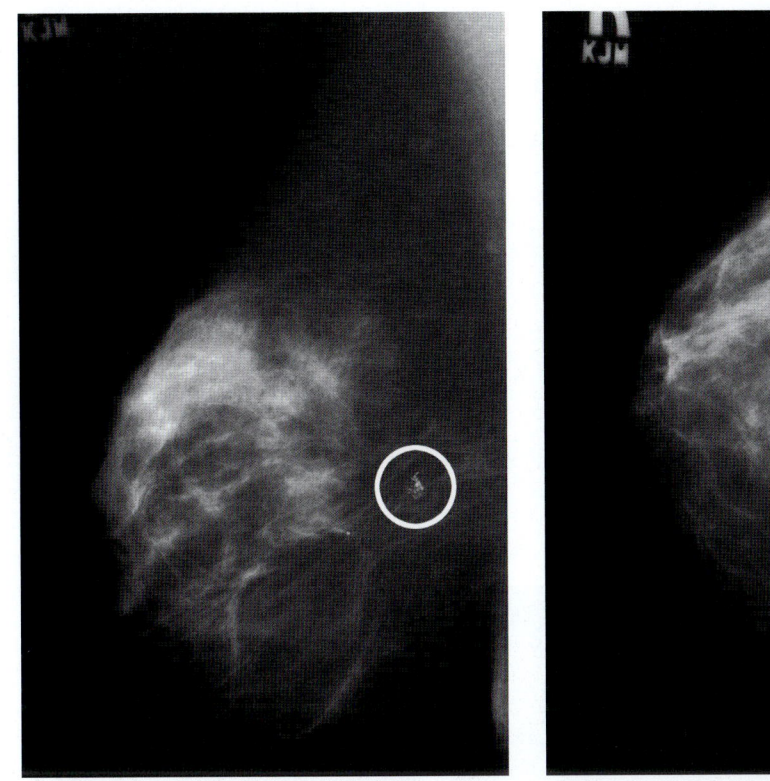

Fig. 15.3 Five years after the mammographic examination shown in **Fig. 15.2**, the calcifications (*circle*) have become large and coarse. (**A**) Right MLO mammogram. (**B**) Right CC mammogram.

Pathology
- Scar

Management
- BI-RADS assessment category 2, benign finding

Pearls and Pitfalls

- Early dystrophic scar calcifications may be difficult to differentiate from ductal carcinoma in situ or invasive malignancy. However, when the calcifications are large and coarse, they can confidently be considered benign.

Suggested Reading
Bassett LW. Mammographic analysis of calcifications. Radiol Clin North Am 1992;30:93–105

De Paredes ES. Atlas of Film Screen Mammography. 2nd ed. Baltimore: Williams & Wilkins; 1992:299–416

Case 15.3: Fat Necrosis

Case History
A 70-year-old woman, who is 9 years status post–right lumpectomy and radiation therapy, presents with increasing calcifications in the lumpectomy site.

Physical Examination
- Right breast: well-healed right upper breast scar; no new masses
- Left breast: normal exam

Mammogram

Calcifications (Fig. 15.4)
- Type: dystrophic
- Distribution: grouped/clustered

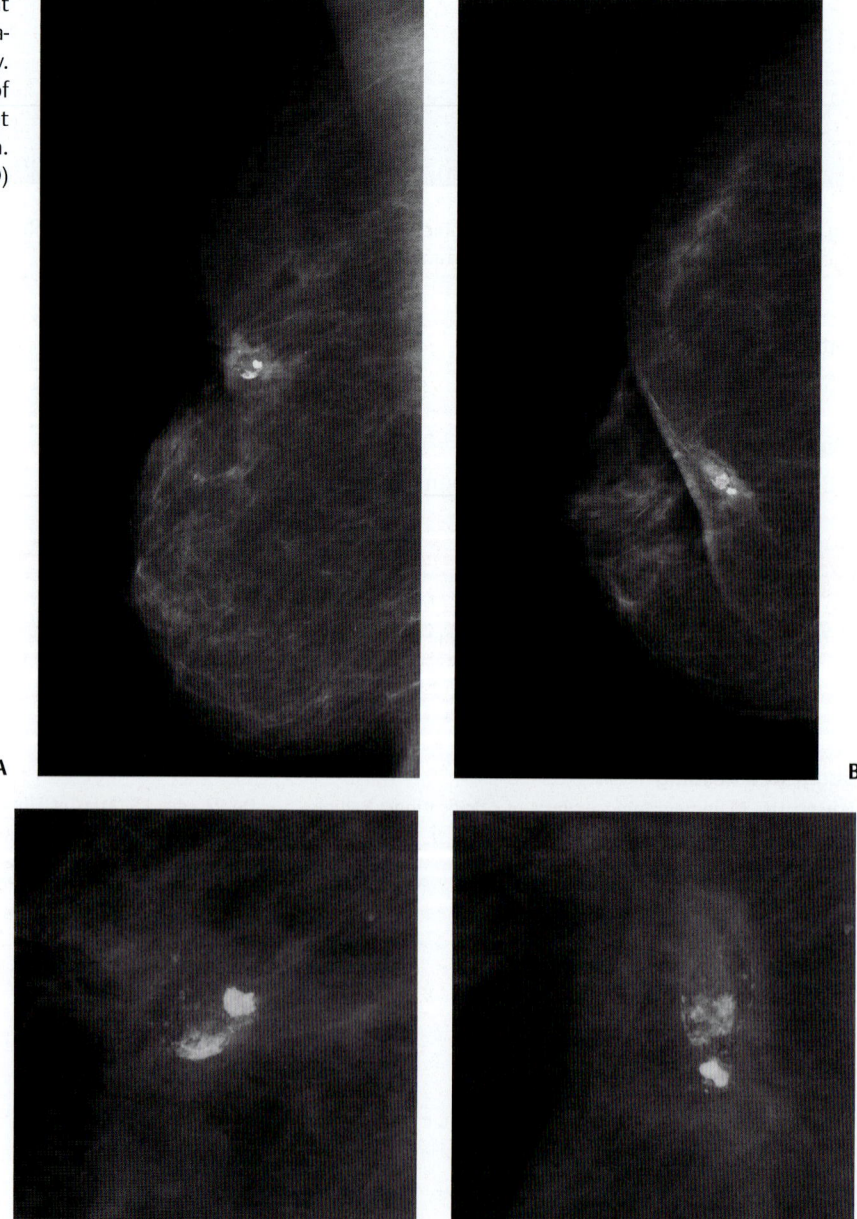

Fig. 15.4 In the 12 o'clock position of the right breast, there is a scar associated with calcifications from the patient's previous lumpectomy. There has been an increase in the number of calcifications since the previous year. (**A**) Right MLO mammogram. (**B**) Right CC mammogram. (**C**) Right MLO magnification mammogram. (**D**) Right CC magnification mammogram.

Ultrasound

Frequency
- 10 MHz

Mass (Fig. 15.5)
- Margin: ill defined
- Echogenicity: hypoechoic
- Retrotumoral acoustic appearance: severe shadowing, mass completely obscured
- Shape: irregular

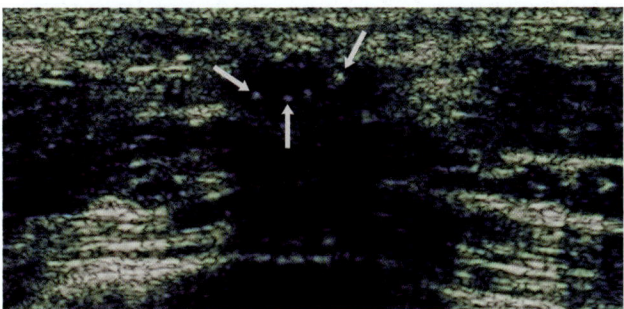

Fig. 15.5 Right antiradial breast sonogram. In the area of the lumpectomy scar, the sonographic findings include architectural distortion of the superficial tissue lines, calcifications (*arrows*), and an irregular, hypoechoic mass with posterior acoustic shadowing.

Pathology
- Scar

Management
- BI-RADS assessment category 2, benign finding

Pearls and Pitfalls

- In this case, the sonographic findings are confusing, which complicates management. Because there is a faint density associated with the scar on the mammogram, the sonogram will most likely demonstrate a mass; furthermore, it may be difficult to differentiate fibrosis from recurrent neoplasm. Therefore, if there is any concern about the increasing calcifications, then management should be determined by the mammographic appearance of the calcifications.

Suggested Reading

Dershaw DD. Evaluation of the breast undergoing lumpectomy and radiation therapy. Radiol Clin North Am 1995;33:1147–1160

Dershaw DD, Shank B, Reisinger S. Mammographic findings after breast cancer treatment with local excision and definitive irradiation. Radiology 1987;164:455–461

Case 15.4: Foreign Body

Case History

A 43-year-old woman, for aplastic anemia, presents for screening mammogram.

Physical Examination
- Normal exam

Mammogram

Mass
- Margin: circumscribed
- Shape: square
- Density: high

Calcifications (Fig. 15.6)
- Type: dystrophic
- Distribution: single

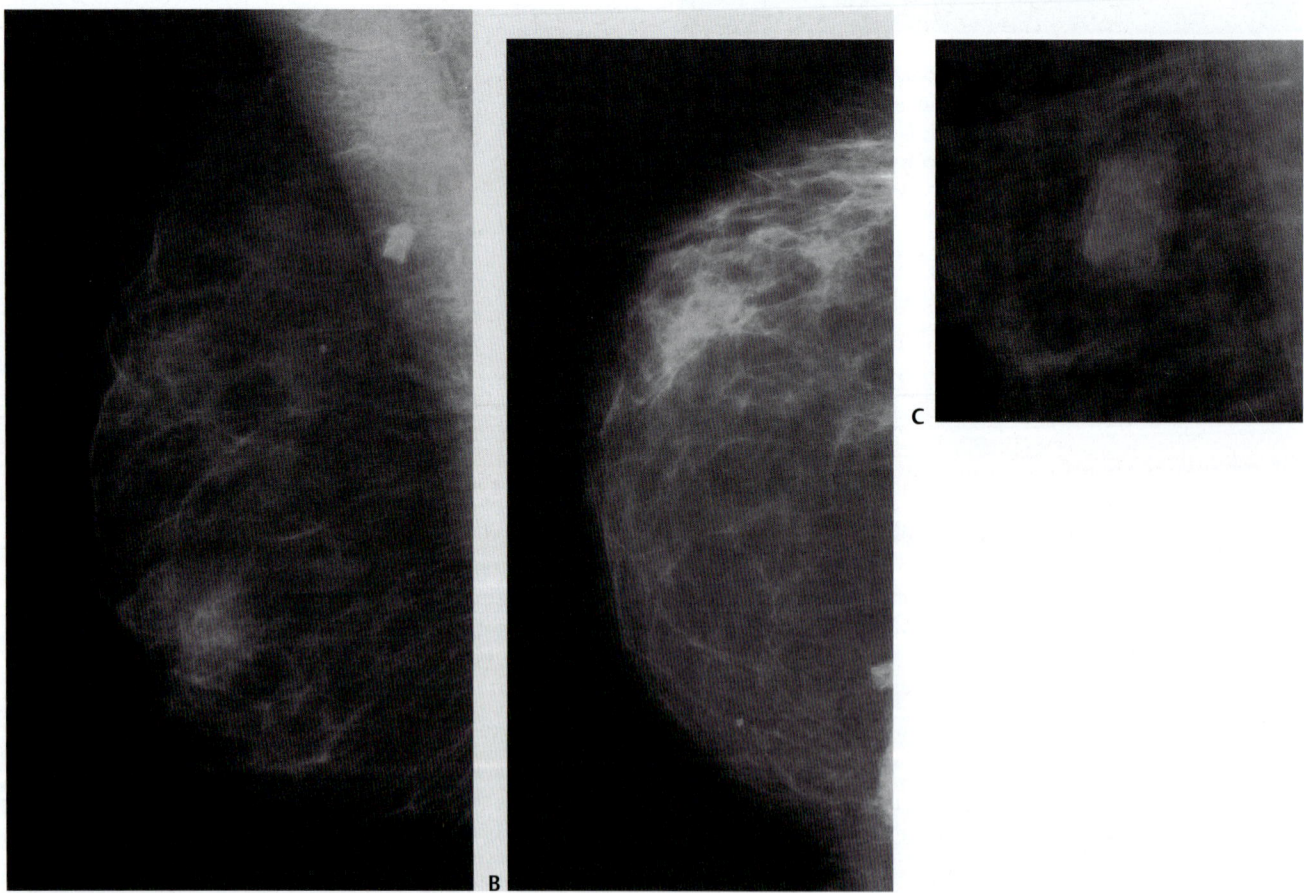

Fig. 15.6 In the upper medial breast there is a well-defined square density with associated coarse, dystrophic calcifications. (**A**) Right MLO mammogram. (**B**) Right exaggerated medial CC mammogram. (**C**) Right MLO magnification mammogram.

Pathology
- Foreign body reaction

Management
- BI-RADS assessment category 2, benign finding

Pearls and Pitfalls

- This is an example of a foreign body causing breast calcification. The density identified in **Fig. 15.6** is a Hickman catheter hub. The patient had been treated with IV chemotherapy through a Hickman catheter for aplastic anemia. The hub was inadvertently retained in the chest after the Hickman catheter was removed. Other foreign bodies such as sutures will produce irregular breast calcifications.

Suggested Reading

Beyer GA, Thorsen MK, Shaffer KA, Walker AP. Mammographic appearance of the retained Dacron cuff of a Hickman catheter. AJR Am J Roentgenol 1990;155:1203–1204

Davis SP, Stomper PC, Weidner N, Meyer JE. Suture calcification mimicking recurrence in the irradiated breast: a potential pitfall in mammographic evaluation. Radiology 1989;172:247–248

Jackson VP, Jahan R, Fu YS. Benign breast lesions. In: Bassett LW, Jackson VP, Jahan R, Fu YS, Gold RH, eds. Diagnosis of Diseases of the Breast. Philadelphia: WB Saunders; 1997:357–443

16 Calcifications: Small Round/Punctate

Case 16.1: Skin

Case History

A 41-year-old woman presents for screening mammogram.

Physical Examination

- Normal exam

Mammogram

Calcifications (Fig. 16.1)
- Type: skin calcifications
- Distribution: scattered, diffuse

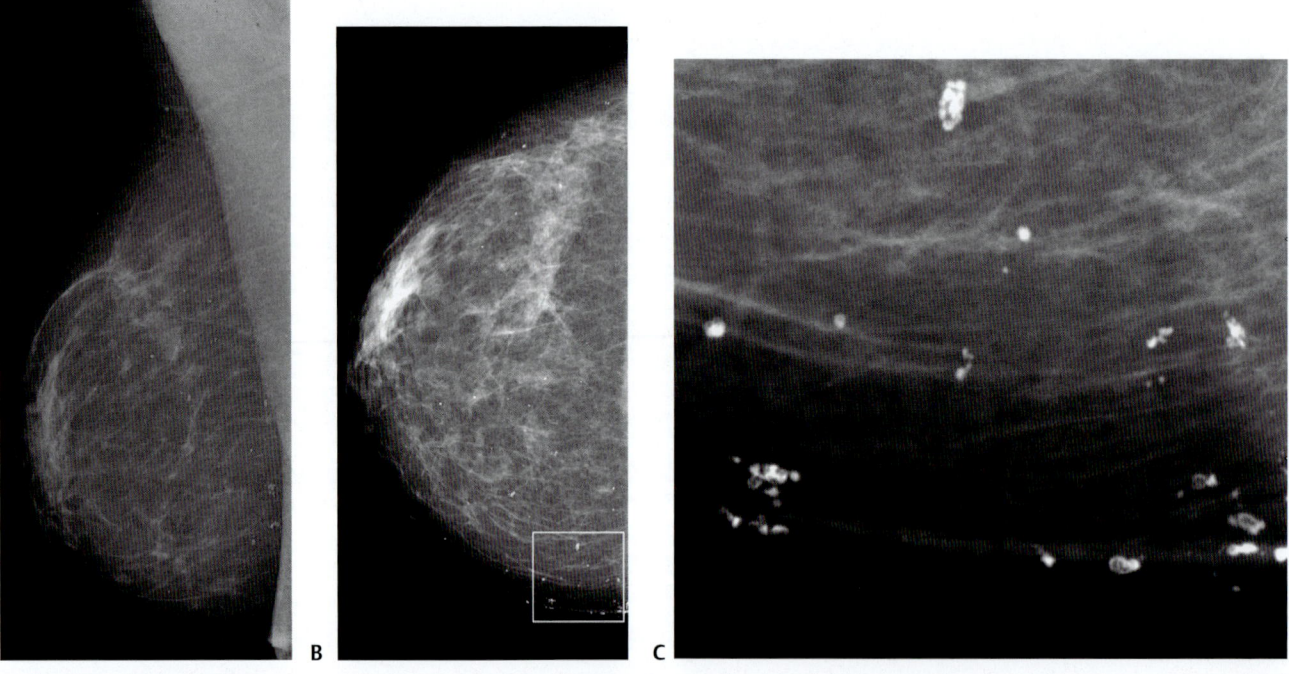

Fig. 16.1 There are multiple scattered round and polygonal skin calcifications, many with lucent centers. (**A**) Right MLO mammogram. (**B**) Right CC mammogram. (**C**) Enlargement of medial CC mammogram, which is marked by a square on **B**.

Management
- BI-RADS assessment category 2, benign finding

Pearls and Pitfalls

- Skin calcifications are commonly in the medial side of the breast. They are well defined, round or polygonal in shape, with lucent centers. If they are superimposed upon the breast parenchyma, they may be mistaken for intraparenchymal calcifications. Tangential views will distinguish skin calcifications from intraparenchymal ones. This case illustrates that digital mammography is superior to film screen technique in displaying these calcifications, because the skin and subcutaneous tissues are better visualized with the digital technique.
- These calcifications are within the sebaceous glands and may be the result of chronic folliculitis.

Suggested Reading
Kopans DB, Meyer JE, Homer MJ, Grabbe J. Dermal deposits mistaken for breast calcifications. Radiology 1983;149:592–594

Case 16.2: Fibrocystic Change

Case History
A 49-year-old woman presents with new left subareolar calcifications on her screening mammogram.

Physical Examination
- Normal exam

Mammogram

Calcifications (Figs. 16.2 and 16.3)
- Type: punctate
- Distribution: regional

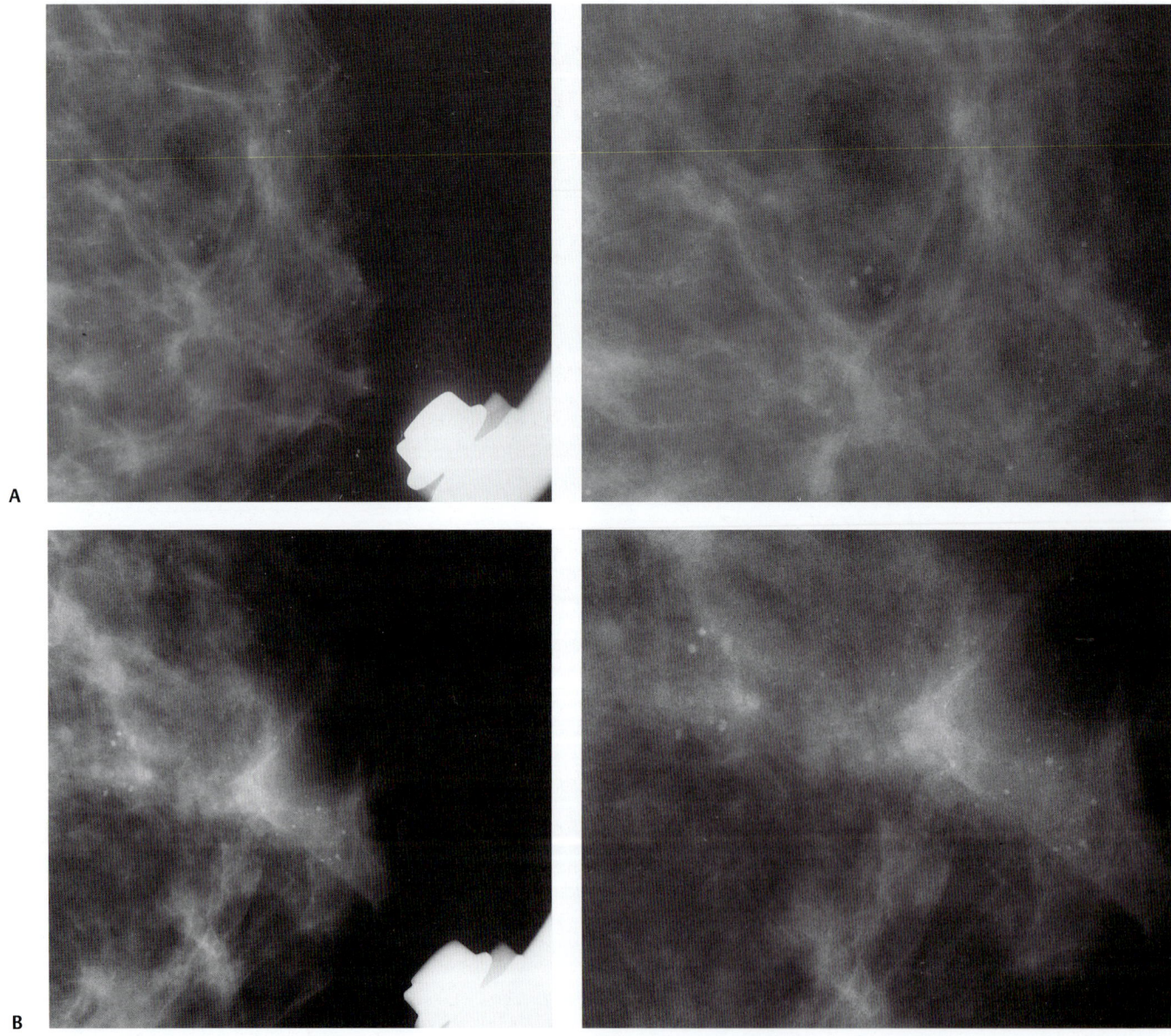

Fig. 16.2 Numerous round, punctate calcifications are present in the subareolar region. (**A**) Left MLO magnification mammogram. (**B**) Enlargement of calcifications in (**A**). (**C**) Left CC magnification mammogram. (**D**) Enlargement of calcifications in (**C**).

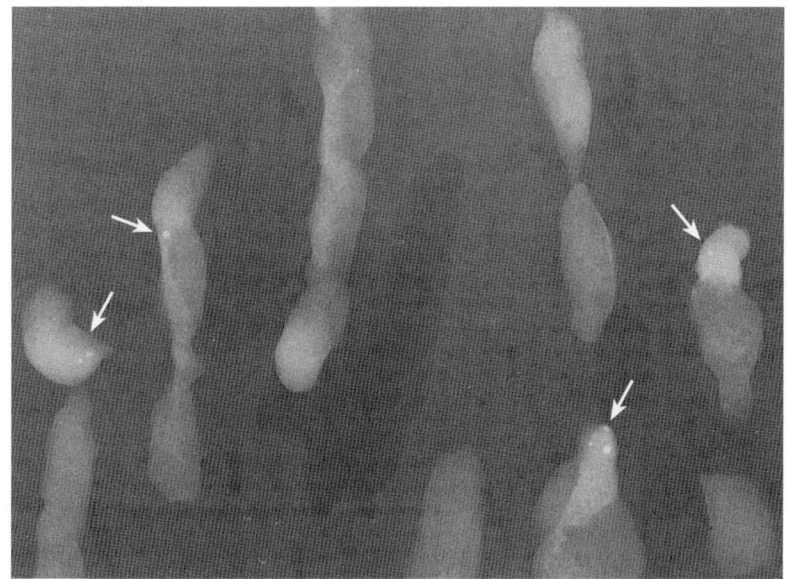

Fig. 16.3 Specimen needle core biopsy radiograph. The round, punctate calcifications (*arrows*) are easily identified within this biopsy specimen.

Ultrasound

Frequency
- 10 to 13 MHz (**Figs. 16.4** and **16.5**)

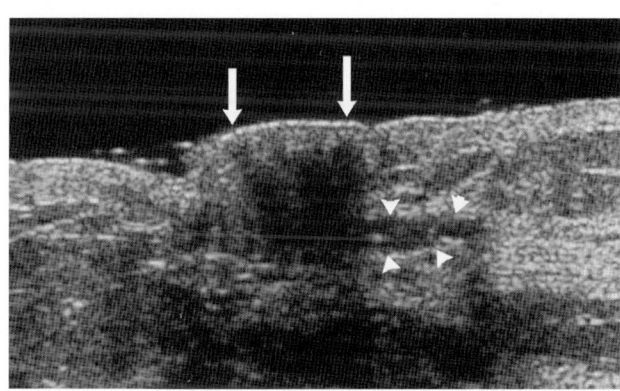

Fig. 16.4 Left radial breast sonogram. Under the nipple (*large arrows*), there were several main ducts (*arrowheads*).

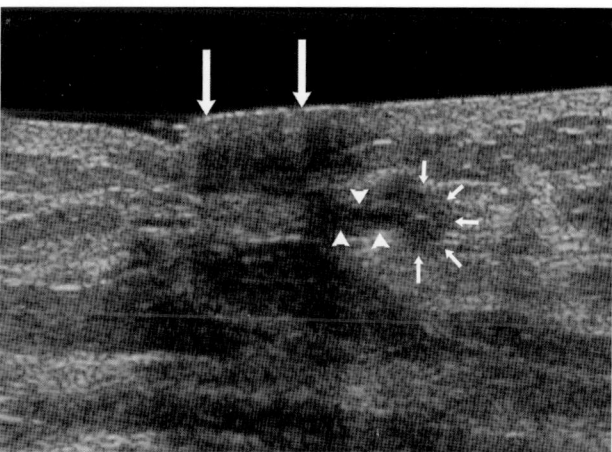

Fig. 16.5 Left radial breast sonogram. The main ducts (*arrowheads*) led to lobulated structures (*small arrows*), consistent with lobular hyperplasia. Nipple (*large arrows*).

Pathology
- Cysts; besides calcifications within microcysts, atypical lobular hyperplasia was present.

Management
- BI-RADS assessment category 3, probably benign; short-interval follow-up

Pearls and Pitfalls
- The calcifications in this case are round because they are within microcysts. This atypical lobular hyperplasia was inadvertently adjacent to these microcysts.
- High-frequency sonography is able to delineate ductal and lobular details that were not visible with lower-resolution equipment.

Suggested Reading
Gershon-Cohen J, Berger SM, Curcio BM. Breast cancer with microcalcifications: diagnostic difficulties. Radiology 1966;87:613–622

Teboul M, Halliwell M. Atlas of Ultrasound and Ductal Echography of the Breast. 2nd ed. Cambridge: Blackwell Science; 1996:154–201

Case 16.3: Fibrocystic Change

Case History
A 45-year-old woman presents with right breast calcifications that have increased in number since her prior screening mammogram performed 2 years ago.

Physical Examination
- Normal exam

Mammogram

Calcifications (Figs. 16.6 and 16.7)
- Type: punctate
- Distribution: diffuse/scattered

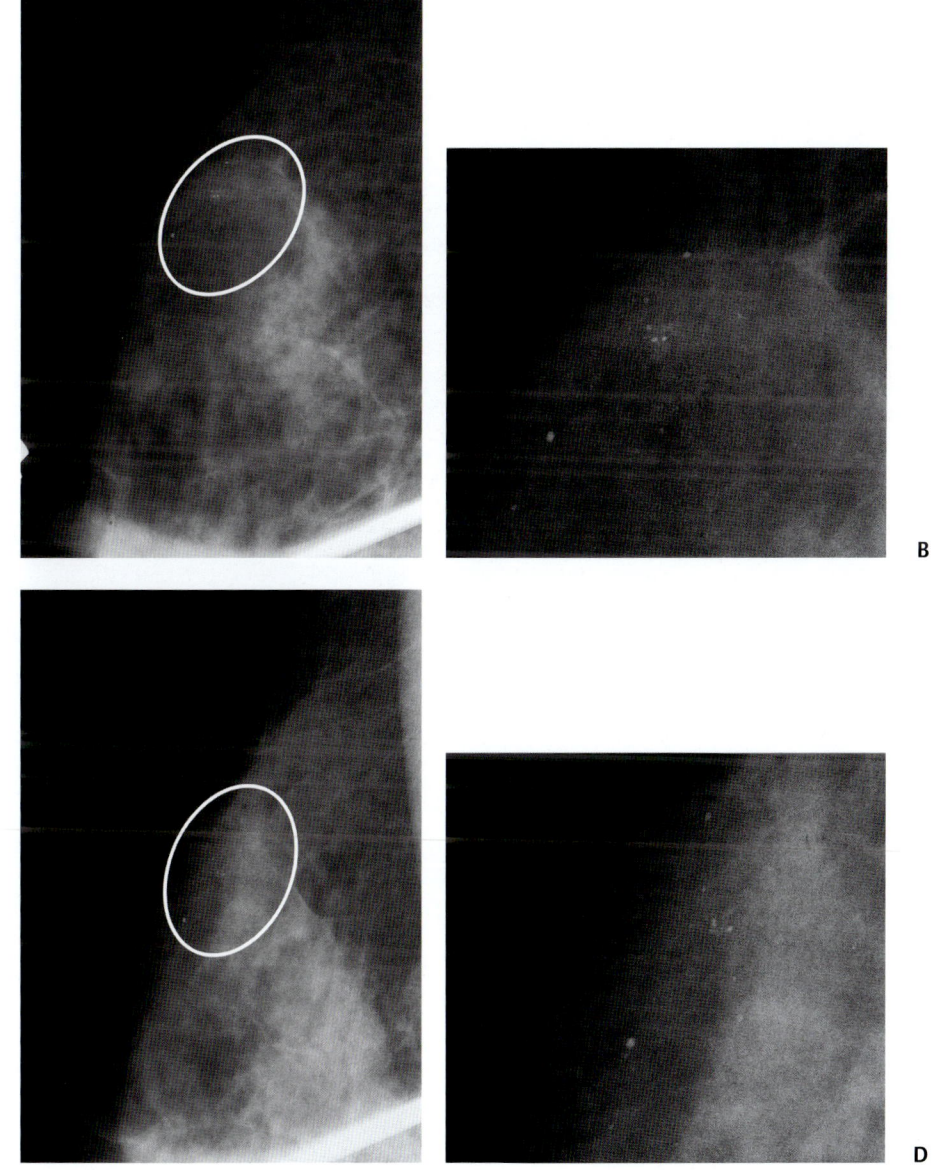

Fig. 16.6 In the upper outer quadrant, there are scattered round, punctate calcifications (*circle*). (**A**) Right MLO magnification view. (**B**) Enlargement of calcifications in **A**. (**C**) Right accentuated CC magnification view.

230 Calcifications

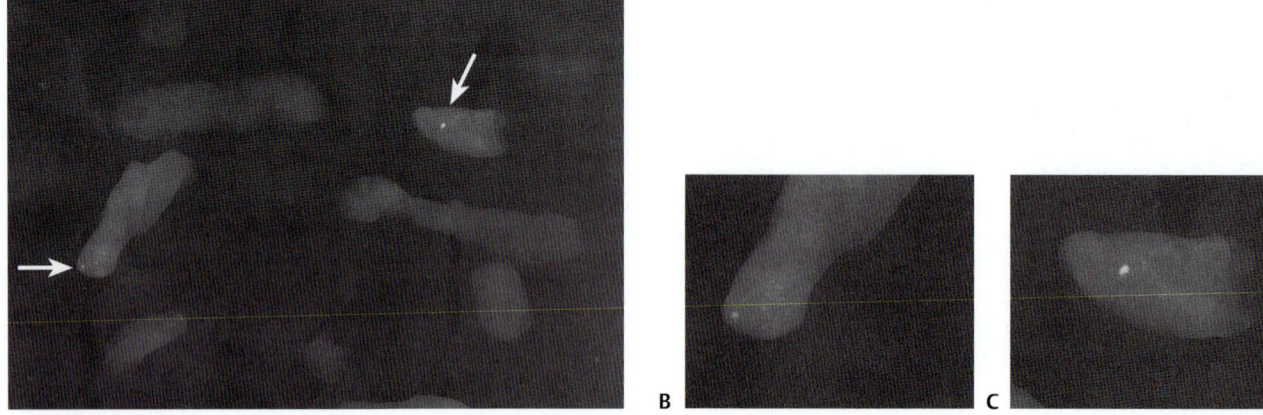

Fig. 16.7 (**A**) Specimen radiograph of breast tissue cores from percutaneous biopsy. The punctate calcifications in the specimen (*arrows*) mirror the appearance of the punctate calcifications in **Fig. 16.6**. (**B**) and (**C**) Enlargements of calcifications in (**A**).

Pathology
- Cysts; benign fibrous and cystic changes with calcifications in cysts

Management
- BI-RADS assessment category 2, benign finding

Pearls and Pitfalls

- Scattered punctate or round microcalcifications are produced by a variety of benign conditions, including cystic hyperplasia, papillomatosis, sclerosing adenosis, adenosis, and atypical lobular hyperplasia.

Suggested Reading
Gershon-Cohen J, Berger SM, Curcio BM. Breast cancer with microcalcifications: diagnostic difficulties. Radiology 1966;87:613–622

Case 16.4: Fibrocystic Change

Case History
A 57-year-old woman presents with increasing right breast calcifications.

Physical Examination
- Normal exam

Mammogram

Calcifications (Fig. 16.8)
- Type: punctate
- Distribution: grouped/clustered

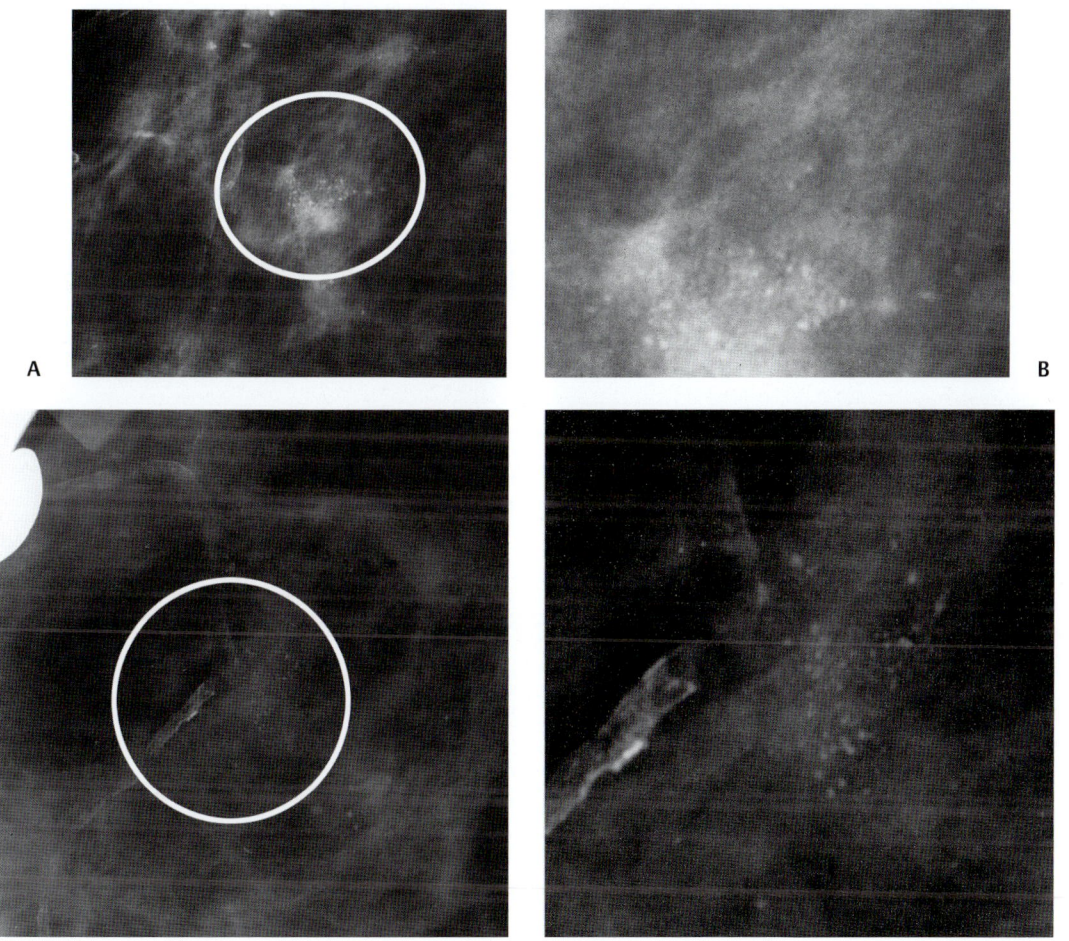

Fig. 16.8 In the upper outer quadrant of the right breast, there is a cluster of punctate calcifications (*circle*). (**A**) Right MLO magnification mammogram. (**B**) Enlargement of calcifications in **A**. (**C**) Right CC magnification mammogram. (**D**) Enlargement of calcifications in **C**.

Pathology
- Fibrocystic changes
- Calcifications in adenosis

Management
- BI-RADS assessment category 4, suspicious abnormality; biopsy should be considered.

Pearls and Pitfalls

- One of the common problems faced by mammographers is to assign assessment categories to small round, punctate, and amorphous clusters of calcifications. If the calcifications are uniform in density and size and are clearly round in shape with smooth borders, then the cluster may be assigned a category 3 (or category 2 if they have been stable for 2 to 3 years). However, if the calcifications are increasing in number or ill defined (amorphous) to identify the shape or borders, then a category 4 is appropriate.
- Punctate calcifications are produced by fibrocystic changes, lobular hyperplasia, atypical lobular hyperplasia, or ductal carcinoma in situ.

Suggested Reading
MacErlean DP, Nathan BE. Calcification in sclerosing adenosis simulating malignant breast calcification. Br J Radiol 1972;45:944–945

Case 16.5: Fibrocystic Change

Case History
A 54-year-old woman presents with new calcifications on her screening mammogram.

Physical Examination
- Normal exam

Mammogram

Calcifications (Fig. 16.9)
- Type: punctate
- Distribution: linear

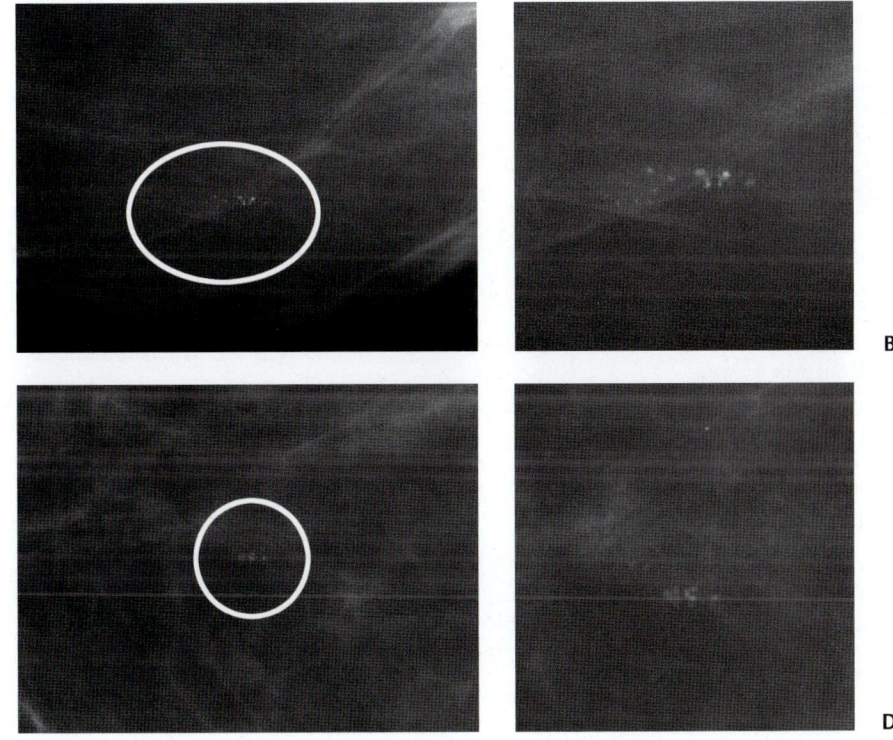

Fig. 16.9 A linear cluster of round, punctate calcifications is present in the inner inferior quadrant of the left breast (*circle*). (**A**) Left LM magnification mammogram. (**B**) Enlargement of calcification in A. (**C**) Left CC magnification mammogram. (**D**) Enlargement of calcifications.

Ultrasound

Frequency
- 7 MHz (**Fig. 16.10**)

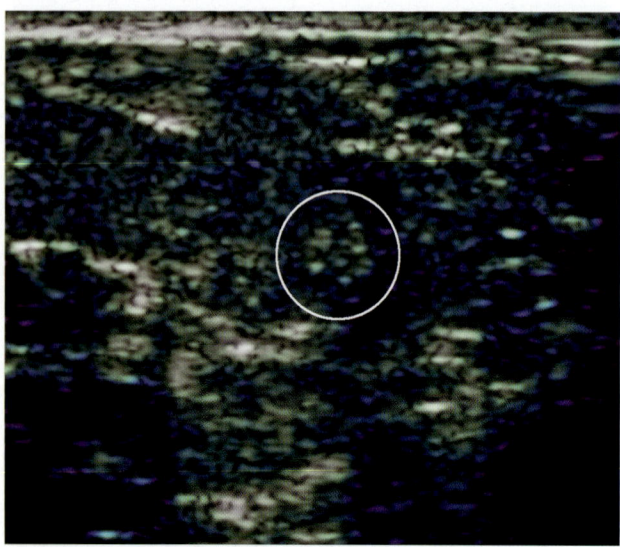

Fig. 16.10 Left antiradial breast sonogram. The mammographic calcifications identified in **Fig. 16.9** correspond to a group of high acoustic intensity foci (*circle*). Sonographically, these calcifications were grouped in a cylindrical pattern that matched the linear pattern of the mammogram. No associated abnormal ducts or masses were present.

Pathology
- Fibroadenoma (not otherwise specified)

Management
- BI-RADS assessment category 4, suspicious abnormality; biopsy should be considered.

Pearls and Pitfalls

- The punctate shape of the calcifications tends to suggest a benign etiology. However, the linear arrangement may be produced by ductal carcinoma in situ. The calcifications in this case are separate from the adjacent calcified vessel, so vascular calcifications are unlikely. As there is no sonographic abnormality other than the calcifications, the sonographic findings are nonspecific, so the management is based on the mammographic features of the calcifications.

Suggested Reading

Bassett LW. Mammographic analysis of calcifications. Radiol Clin North Am 1992;30:93–105

De Paredes E. Calcifications. In: De Paredes E, ed. Atlas of Film-Screen Mammography. Baltimore: Williams & Wilkins; 1992:299–416

Gershon-Cohen J, Ingleby H. Roentgenography of fibroadenoma of the breast. Radiology 1952;59:77–87

Case 16.6: Ductal Carcinoma in Situ

Case History

A 41-year-old woman presents with new calcifications on her screening mammogram.

Physical Examination
- Normal exam

Mammogram

Calcifications (Figs. 16.11 and 16.12)
- Type: punctate
- Distribution: grouped/clustered

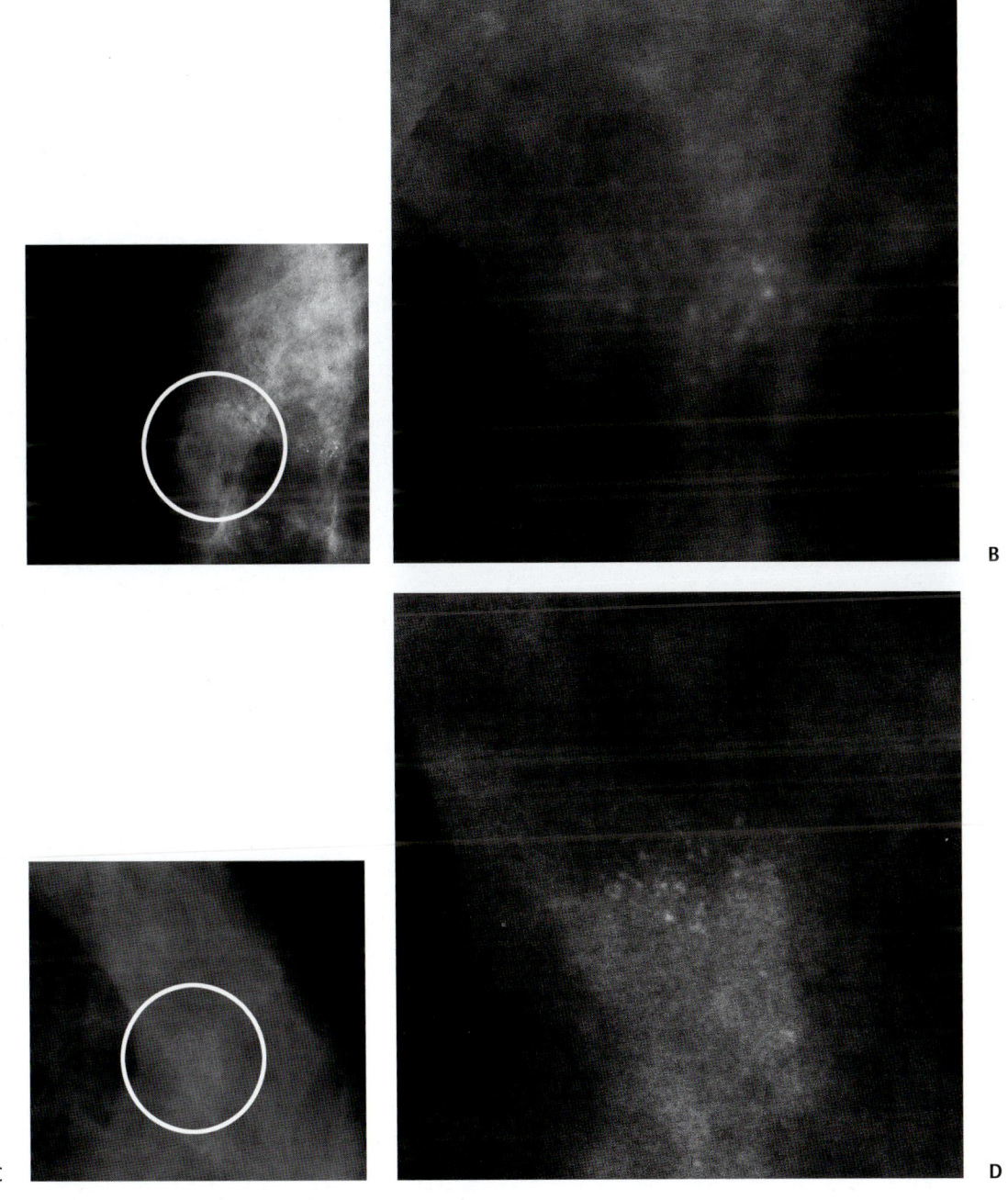

Fig. 16.11 In the left upper outer breast, there is a cluster of punctate calcifications (*circle*). (**A**) Left MLO magnification mammogram. (**B**) Enlargement of calcifications in **A**. (**C**) Left CC magnification mammogram. (**D**) Enlargement of calcifications in **C**.

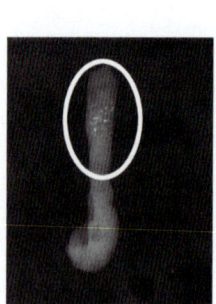 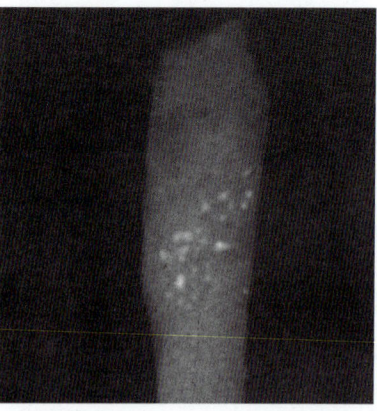

A   B

Fig. 16.12 (**A**) Specimen radiograph of percutaneous needle core biopsy of calcifications identified in **Fig. 16.11**. Most of the calcifications are in one core (*circle*). Predominant punctate shapes match the prebiopsy mammographic appearance of the calcifications. (**B**) Enlargement of circled calcifications in **A**.

Pathology
- Ductal carcinoma in situ

Management
- BI-RADS assessment category 4, suspicious abnormality; biopsy should be considered.

Pearls and Pitfalls
- A punctate shape generally suggests a benign etiology. However, in this case, the clustered distribution, variation in the density and size of the calcifications, and increasing number support classifying them in a suspicious category leading to biopsy.

Suggested Reading

Egan RL, McSweeney MB, Sewell CW. Intramammary calcifications without an associated mass in benign and malignant diseases. Radiology 1980;137(1 pt 1):1–77

Feig SA, Shaber GS, Patchefsky A, et al. Analysis of clinically occult and mammographically occult breast tumors. AJR Am J Roentgenol 1977;128:403–408

Millis RR, Davis R, Stacey AJ. The detection and significance of calcifications in the breast: a radiological and pathological study. Br J Radiol 1976;49:12–26

Case 16.7: Ductal Carcinoma in Situ

Case History
A 72-year-old woman developed a cluster of calcifications that increased in number when followed at 6-month intervals for 1 year.

Physical Examination
- Normal exam

Mammogram

Calcifications (Figs. 16.13 and 16.14)
- Type: punctate
- Distribution: grouped/clustered

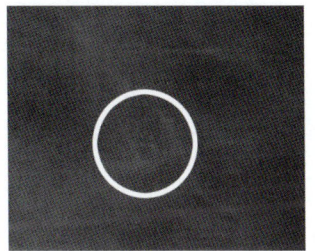

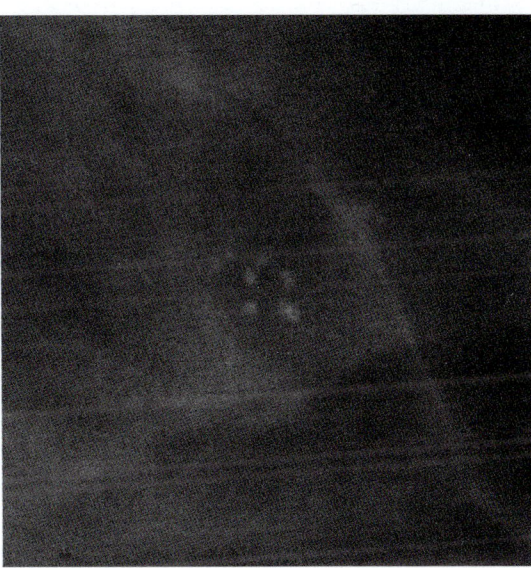

Fig. 16.13 (**A**) Left MLO magnification mammogram. A cluster of fairly uniform punctate calcifications is present inferior to the nipple (*circle*). No associated mass is appreciated on the mammogram. (**B**) Enlargement of circled calcifications in **A**.

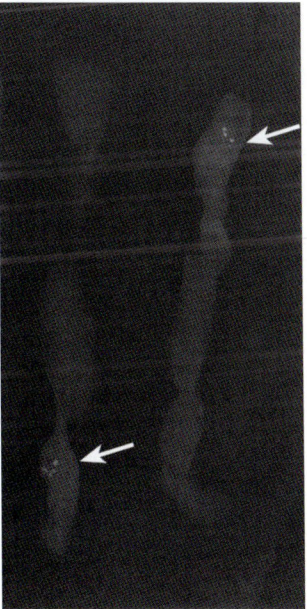

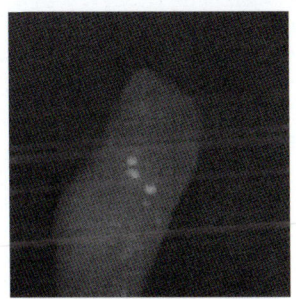

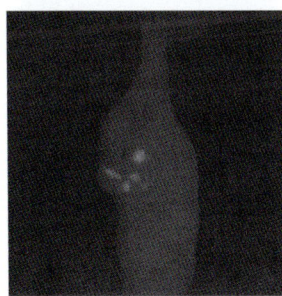

Fig. 16.14 (A) Specimen radiograph of 11-gauge core biopsy samples of the calcifications identified in **Fig. 16.13**. In addition to the smooth, fairly round calcifications, there are numerous, smaller, fainter, punctate microcalcifications (*arrows*). These small calcifications cannot be appreciated on the prebiopsy magnification view (**Fig. 16.13**). (**B**) and (**C**) are enlargements of circled calcifications in **A**.

Ultrasound

Low Frequency (Fig. 16.15)

Frequency
- 7 MHz

Mass
- Margin: ill defined
- Echogenicity: hypoechoic
- Retrotumoral acoustic appearance: single edge shadowing
- Shape: oval

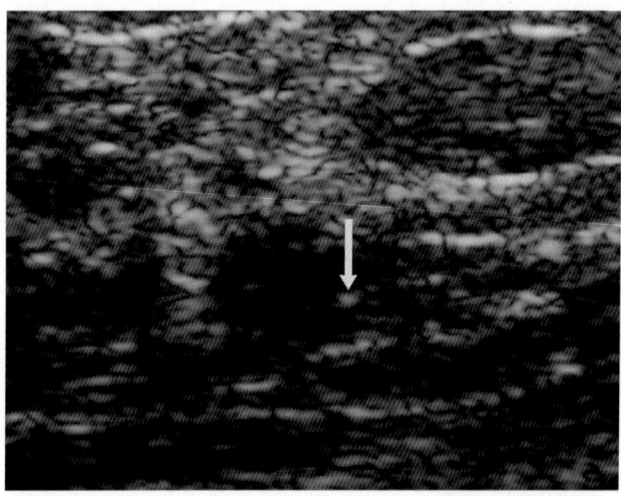

Fig. 16.15 Left breast radial, low-frequency sonogram. The calcifications (*arrow*) shown in **Fig. 16.13** were located within a 5 mm, oval, ill-defined, hypoechoic solid mass. The mass is not well characterized sonographically because this sonographic frequency exhibits inadequate resolution due to the small size of this mass.

High Frequency (Fig. 16.16)

Frequency
- 13 MHz

High Frequency Findings
The high-frequency sonographic study demonstrates an irregular, ill-defined, hypoechoic mass associated with the mammographic calcifications. The sonographic malignant features of the mass are better characterized by the high-frequency examination compared with the lower-frequency study. Although the calcifications are also more conspicuous with higher-frequency sonography, their sonographic appearance is still nonspecific.

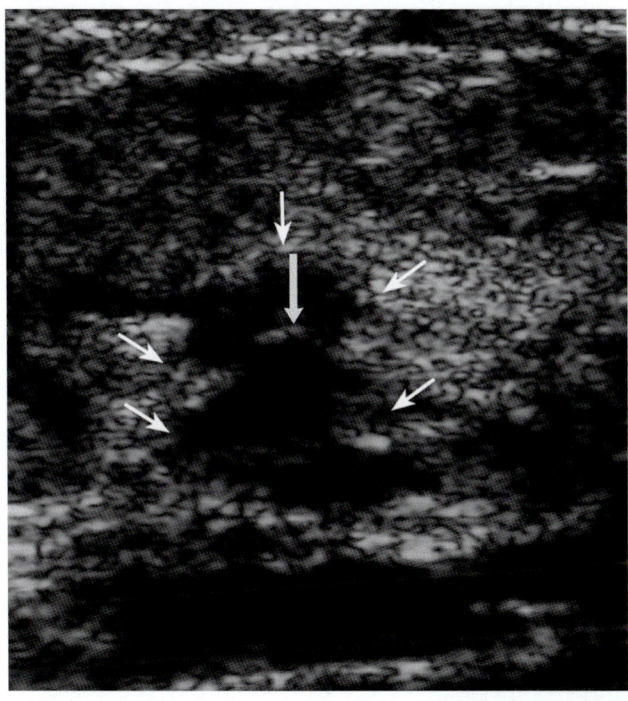

Fig. 16.16 Right breast radial high-frequency sonogram of the same mass as in **Fig. 16.15**. The borders of the mass are irregular and associated with spiculations. The calcifications (*large arrow*) are easily identified.

Pathology
- Invasive ductal carcinoma with a predominant intraductal component. At excision, a 3 mm area of invasive and intraductal carcinoma was evident.

Management
- BI-RADS assessment category 4, suspicious abnormality; biopsy should be considered.

Pearls and Pitfalls

- Although sonographic examination would not normally be performed, this case illustrates that high-frequency sonography may identify masses in association with calcifications, even when a mass is not apparent mammographically. With high-frequency sonography, 50 to 60% of mammographic malignant calcifications without density or mass are associated with a sonographic mass.

Suggested Reading

Cox BA, Kelly KM, Ko P, Hertzog L, Stain SC. Ultrasound characteristics of breast carcinoma. Am Surg 1998;64:934–938

Huang CS, Wu CY, Chu JS, Lin JH, Hsu SM, Chang KJ. Microcalcifications of non-palpable breast lesions detected by ultrasonography: correlation with mammography and histopathology. Ultrasound Obstet Gynecol 1999;13:431–436

Case 16.8: Ductal Carcinoma in Situ

Case History
A 53-year-old woman presents with new calcifications on her screening mammogram.

Physical Examination
- Normal exam

Mammogram

Calcifications (Fig. 16.17)
- Type: punctate
- Distribution: grouped/clustered

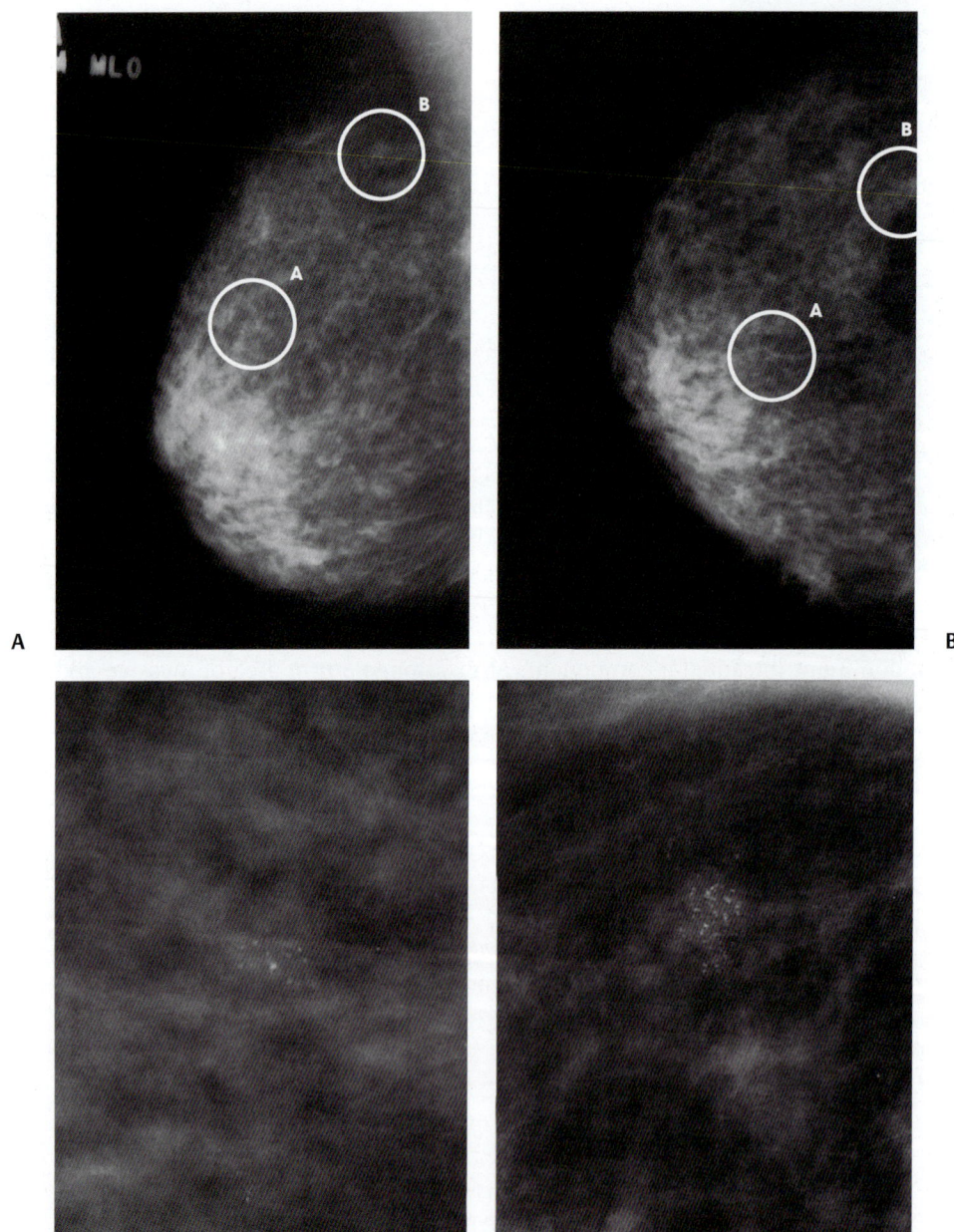

Fig. 16.17 Two clusters of calcifications are present in the right breast. Cluster A (*circle*) is a cluster of punctate calcifications at the 12 o'clock position. Cluster B (*circle*) is a cluster of heterogeneous calcifications in the upper outer breast. (**A**) Right MLO mammogram. (**B**) Right XCCL mammogram. (**C**) Right MLO magnification mammogram of cluster A. (**D**) Right CC magnification mammogram of cluster B.

Pathology
- Ductal carcinoma in situ
- Cluster A: ductal carcinoma in situ, low nuclear grade
- Cluster B: invasive and in situ ductal carcinoma

Management
- BI-RADS assessment category 4, suspicious; biopsy should be considered.

Pearls and Pitfalls
- The cluster of punctate calcifications is commonly due to benign etiologies. However, because the patient has a second highly suspicious area of heterogeneous calcifications, the punctate cluster should also be biopsied. Ductal carcinoma in situ is multifocal in about one third of women. The risk of multifocal ductal carcinoma in situ increases with increasing tumor size. Only 12 to 17% of patients with lesions ≤ 25 mm have multifocal disease compared with 47% with tumors > 25 mm.

Suggested Reading

Anastassiades O, Iakovou E, Stavridou N, Gogas J, Karameris A. Multicentricity in breast cancer: a study of 366 cases. Am J Clin Pathol 1993;99:238–243

Dershaw DD, Abramson A, Kinne DW. Ductal carcinoma in situ: mammographic findings and clinical implications. Radiology 1989;170:411–415

Lagios MD. Multicentricity of breast carcinoma demonstrated by routine correlated serial subgross and radiographic examination. Cancer 1977;40:1726–1734

Lagios MD, Westdahl PR, Margolin FR, Rose MR. Duct carcinoma in situ: relationship of extent of noninvasive disease to the frequency of occult invasion, multicentricity, lymph node metastases, and short-term treatment failures. Cancer 1982;50:1309–1314

Swain SM. Ductal carcinoma in situ. Cancer Invest 1992;10:443–454

Zavotsky J, Gardner B. Postexcisional recurrence of carcinoma of the breast. J Am Coll Surg 1996;182:71–77

Case 16.9: Invasive Ductal Carcinoma

Case History

A 56-year-old woman presents with increasing right breast calcifications.

Physical Examination

- Normal exam

Mammogram

Calcifications (Fig. 16.18)
- Type: punctate
- Distribution: linear

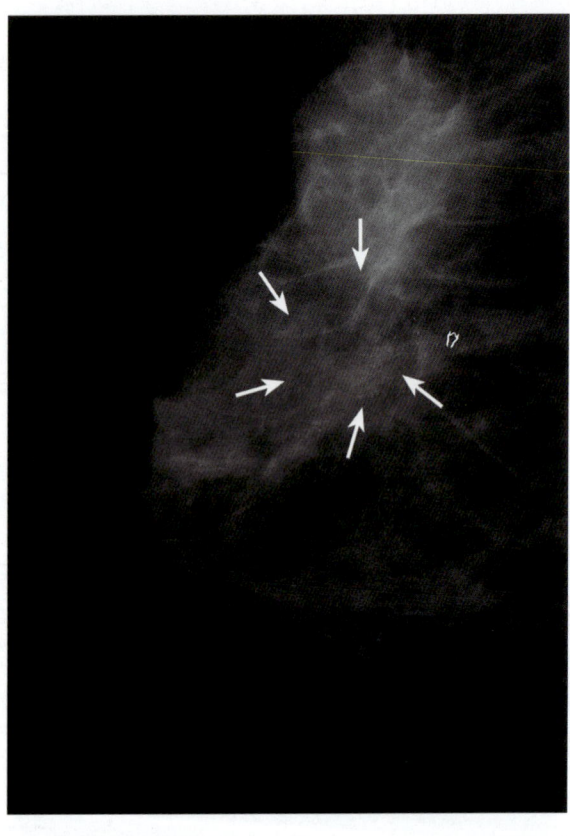
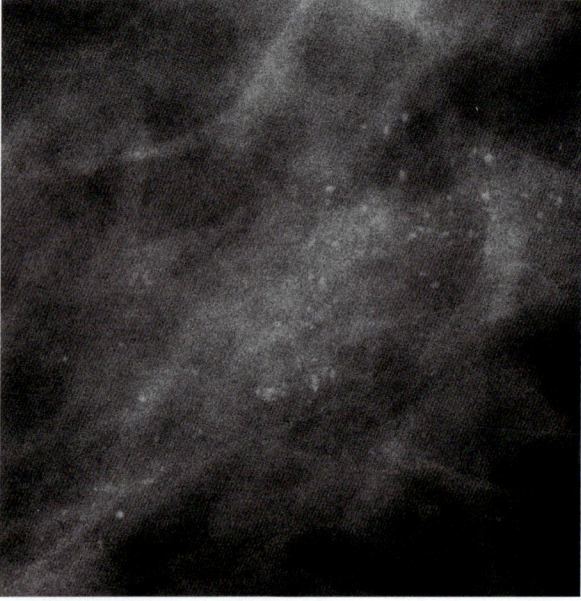

Fig. 16.18 (**A**) Right LM magnification mammogram. Numerous punctate calcifications are segmentally localized in the upper breast (*arrows*). A clip was placed after the patient's percutaneous biopsy. (**B**) Enlargement of calcifications in **A**.

Pathology
- Invasive ductal carcinoma with a predominantly intraductal component
- Greater than 20 mm area of ductal carcinoma in situ with a 3 mm area of invasive ductal carcinoma
- Extensive involvement of lobules with ductal carcinoma in situ

Management
- BI-RADS assessment category 4, suspicious abnormality; biopsy should be considered.

Pearls and Pitfalls
- Punctate calcifications are a less common presentation of malignancy. They sometimes result from extension of the neoplasm into the lobules.

Suggested Reading

Homer MJ, Safaii H. Cancerization of the lobule: implication regarding analysis of microcalcification shape. Breast Dis 1990;3:131–133

Lagios MD, Page DL. In situ carcinomas of the breast: ductal carcinoma in situ, Paget's disease, lobular carcinoma in situ. In: Bland KI, ed. The Breast: Comprehensive Management of Benign and Malignant Diseases. Philadelphia: WB Saunders;1998:261–283

17 Calcifications: Amorphous/Indistinct Microcalcifications

Case 17.1: Skin Powder/Deodorant

Case History
A 48-year-old woman presents with new densities on her right mammogram.

Physical Examination
- Normal exam

Mammogram

Calcifications (Figs. 17.1 and 17.2)
- Type: amorphous/indistinct
- Distribution: grouped/clustered

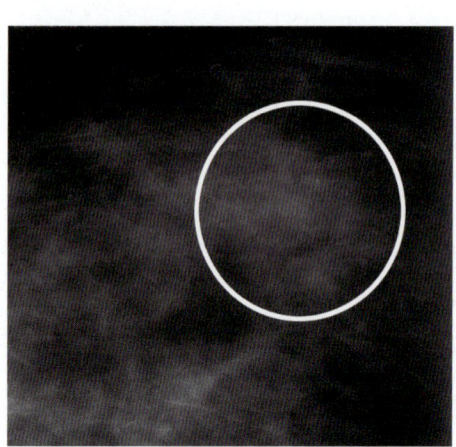

Fig. 17.1 (A) Right CC mammogram. In the outer breast, multiple amorphous densities were present (*circle*). These densities could only be identified on this view. (B) Enlargement of circled densities in **A**.

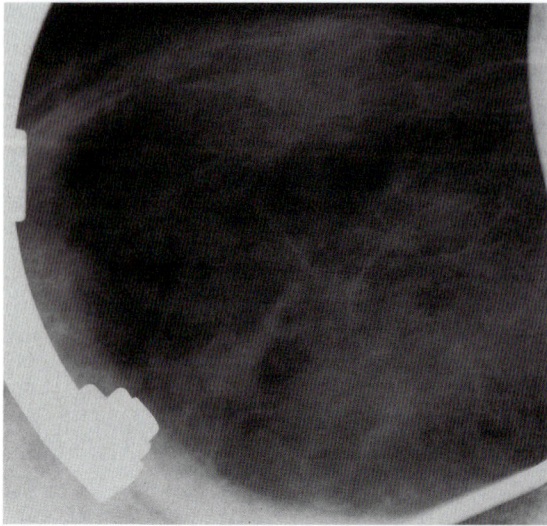

Fig. 17.2 Right CC spot magnification mammogram. The patient returned 5 days later, and the densities are no longer present.

Pathology
- Deodorant material on skin

Management
- BI-RADS assessment category 2, benign finding

Pearls and Pitfalls
- This case is an example of the appearance of skin powder. Various creams, powders, tattoos, and aluminum deodorants can produce densities that may appear to represent intraparenchymal calcifications. When the densities are extremely small and visible on only one view, this etiology should be considered.

Suggested Reading
Bartton JW III, Kornguth PJ. Mammographic deodorant and powder artifact: is there confusion with malignant microcalcifications? Breast Dis 1990;3:121–126

Pamilo M, Soiva M, Suramo I. New artifacts simulating malignant microcalcifications in mammography. Breast Dis 1989;1:321–327

Case 17.2: Fibrocystic Change

Case History
A 64-year-old woman presents with new calcifications on her screening mammogram.

Physical Examination
- Normal exam

Mammogram

Calcifications (Fig. 17.3)
- Type: amorphous/indistinct
- Distribution: grouped/clustered

246 Calcifications

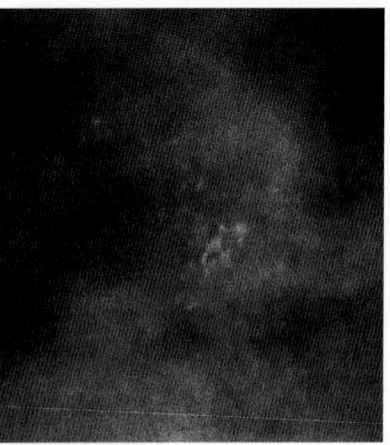
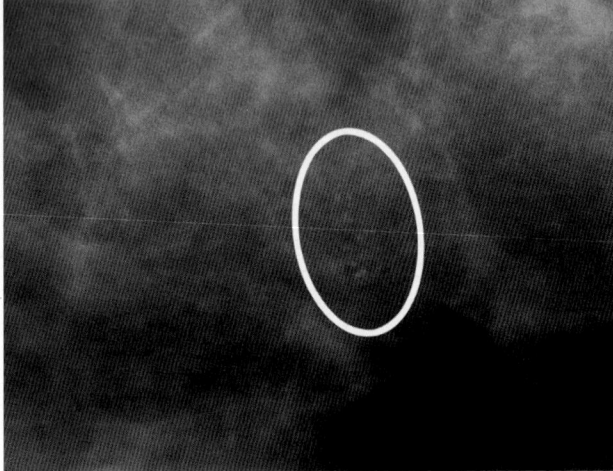

Fig. 17.3 In the upper outer quadrant of the right breast, there is a cluster of indistinct amorphous calcifications (*circle*). (**A**) Right MLO magnification mammogram. (**B**) Enlargement of circled calcifications in **A**. (**C**) Right CC magnification mammogram.

Ultrasound

Low Frequency

Frequency
- 7 MHz (**Fig. 17.4**)

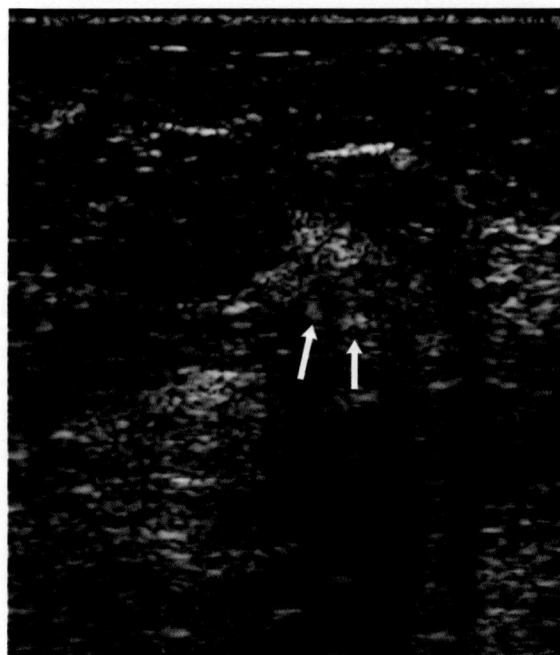

Fig. 17.4 Right radial low-frequency breast sonogram. The calcifications (*arrows*) identified in **Fig. 17.3** were localized sonographically. Lower-frequency sonography is generally more helpful when the breast tissue is extremely attenuating. In this case of fibroadenomatous hyperplasia, the lower frequency demonstrates that there is no mass in the area of the calcifications. Only benign-appearing hyperechoic tissue is present.

High Frequency (Fig. 17.5)

Frequency
- 10 MHz

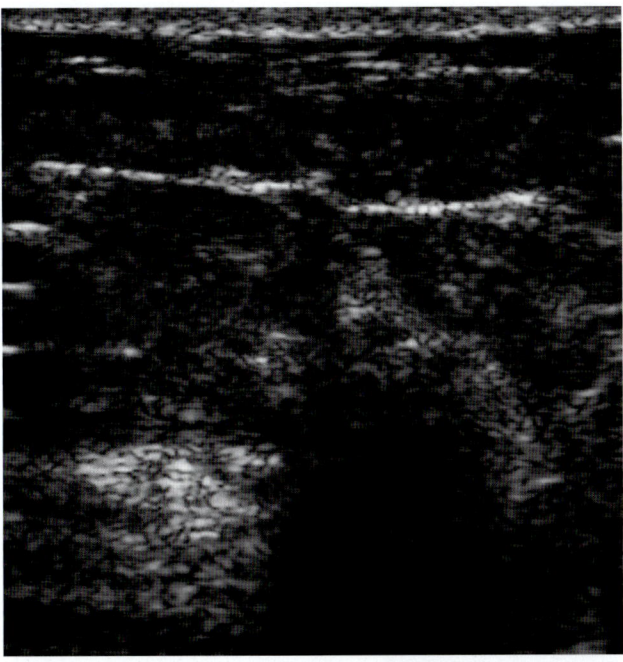

Fig. 17.5 Right radial high-frequency breast sonogram. When using the higher frequency, the area of calcification heavily shadows due to the highly attenuating fibrous tissue. The shadowing prevents one from differentiating attenuating benign tissue from malignant tissue.

Pathology
- Fibroadenomatoid hyperplasia

Management
- BI-RADS assessment category 4, suspicious abnormality; biopsy should be considered.

Pearls and Pitfalls

- These amorphous calcifications are moderately suspicious. Conditions that may produce these calcifications include fibrocystic changes, fibroadenomas, fat necrosis, and intraductal carcinoma.
- Fibrosis highly attenuates sound and commonly produces focal shadowing. To differentiate diffuse fibrosis from a focal malignant mass, one should utilize a lower frequency. A lower frequency may penetrate the tissue and demonstrate either the presence of a mass or the presence of benign tissue.

Suggested Reading
Kamal M, Evans AJ, Denley H, Pinder SE, Ellis IO. Fibroadenomatoid hyperplasia: a cause of suspicious microcalcification on mammographic screening. AJR Am J Roentgenol 1998;171:1331–1334

Case 17.3: Fibrocystic Change

Case History
A 49-year-old woman presents with left breast calcifications that are new since her previous screening mammogram 4 years ago.

Physical Examination
- Normal exam

Mammogram

Calcifications (Figs. 17.6 and 17.7)
- Type: amorphous/indistinct
- Distribution: segmental

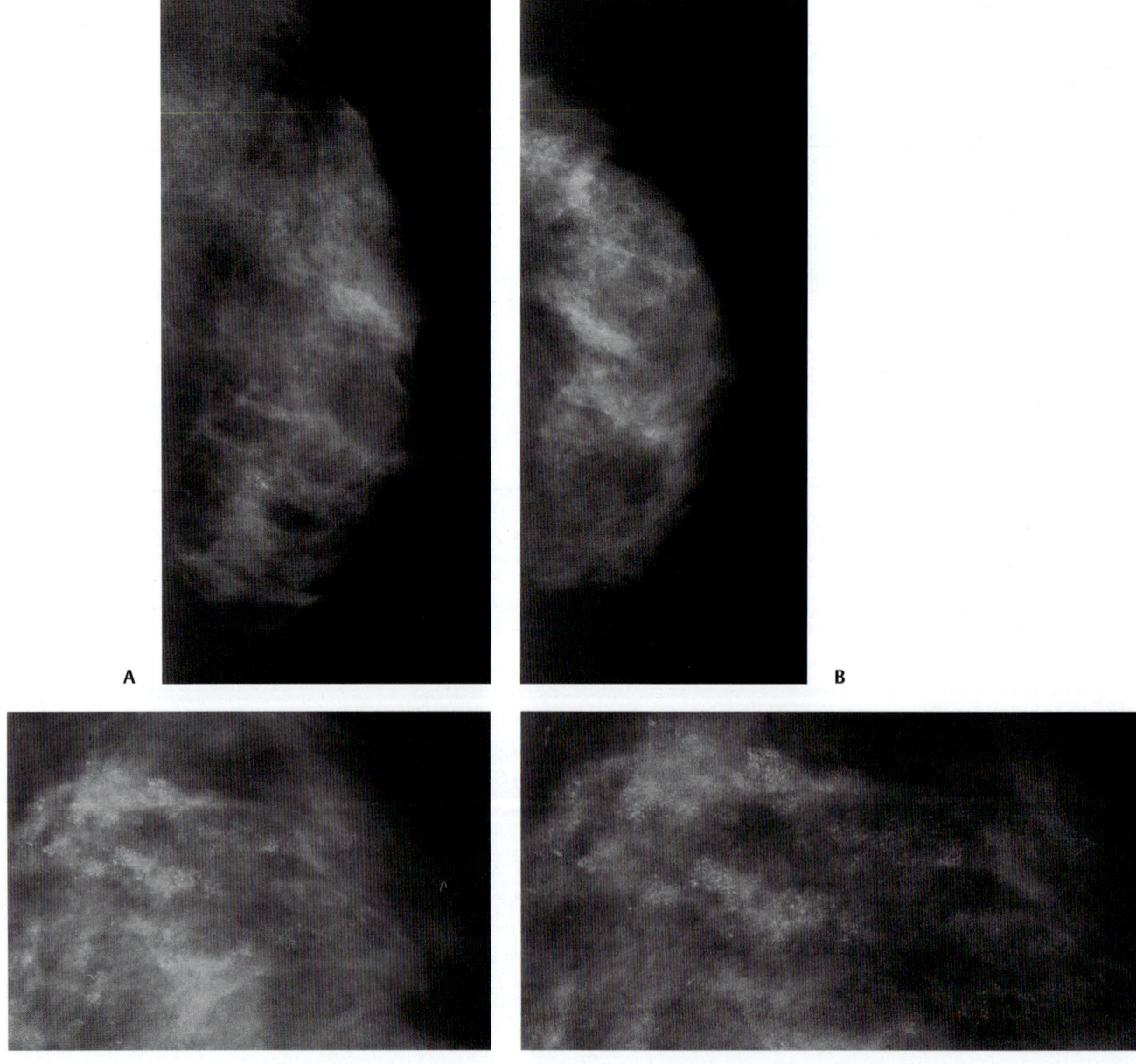

Fig. 17.6 Amorphous calcifications are present throughout the entire left upper outer quadrant. (**A**) Left MLO mammogram. (**B**) Left CC mammogram. (**C**) Left LM magnification mammogram. (**D**) Enlargement of calcifications in **C**.

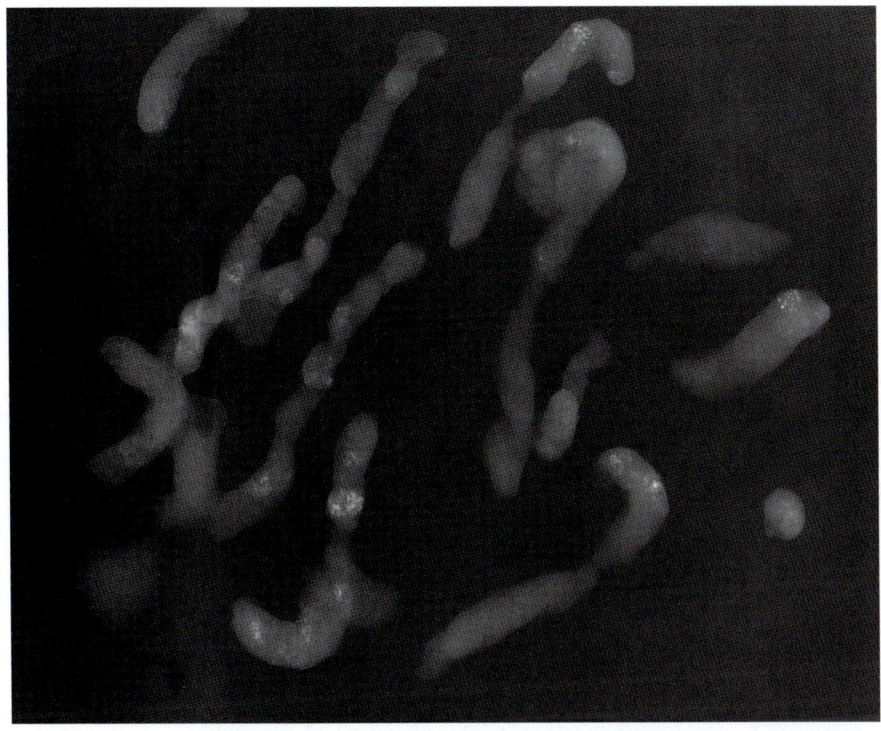

Fig. 17.7 Specimen radiograph from percutaneous mammographically guided stereotactic core biopsy. Most of the cores exhibit amorphous calcifications.

Pathology

Atypical ductal hyperplasia; both the percutaneous core biopsy and the partial mastectomy specimens demonstrated atypical duct epithelial hyperplasia without evidence of in situ or invasive carcinoma.

Management

- BI-RADS assessment category 4, suspicious; biopsy should be considered.

Pearls and Pitfalls

- Atypical ductal hyperplasia (ADH) is commonly associated with biopsied calcifications. If the sampled tissue only demonstrates ADH, reexcision of the tissue is recommended. About 50% of percutaneous biopsies showing only ADH are associated with malignancy after subsequent surgical excision. Larger tissue core sampling devices appear to reduce the chance of inadequate sampling to 10 to 20%.

Suggested Reading

Brem RF, Behrndt VS, Sanow L, Gatewood OM. Atypical ductal hyperplasia: histologic underestimation of carcinoma in tissue harvested from impalpable breast lesions using 11-gauge stereotactically guided directional vacuum-assisted biopsy. AJR Am J Roentgenol 1999;172:1405–1407

Burbank F. Stereotactic breast biopsy of atypical ductal hyperplasia and ductal carcinoma in situ lesions: improved accuracy with directional, vacuum-assisted biopsy. Radiology 1997;202:843–847

Jackman RJ, Burbank F, Parker SH, et al. Atypical ductal hyperplasia diagnosed at stereotactic breast biopsy: improved reliability with 14-gauge, directional, vacuum-assisted biopsy. Radiology 1997;204:485–488

Liberman L, Dershaw DD, Glassman JR, et al. Analysis of cancers not diagnosed at stereotactic core breast biopsy. Radiology 1997;203:151–157

Liberman L, Smolkin JH, Dershaw DD, Morris EA, Abramson AF, Rosen PP. Calcification retrieval at stereotactic, 11-gauge, directional, vacuum-assisted breast biopsy. Radiology 1998;208:251–260

Case 17.4: Lobular Calcifications

Case History
A 40-year-old woman presents for her baseline mammogram.

Physical Examination
- Normal exam

Mammogram

Calcifications (Figs. 17.8 and 17.9)
- Type: amorphous/indistinct
- Distribution: regional

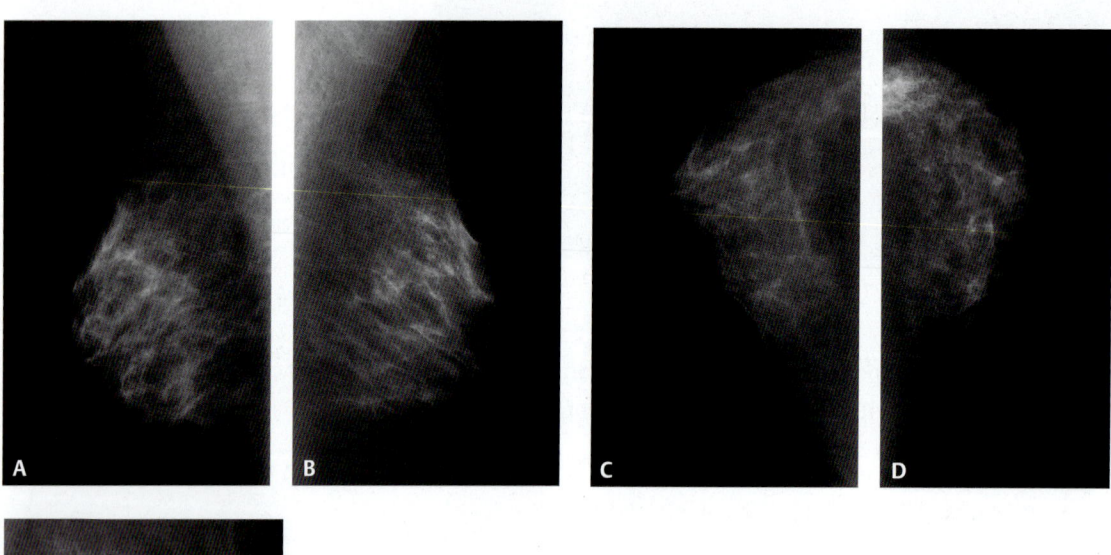

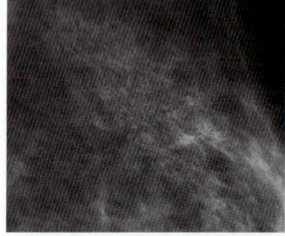

Fig. 17.8 Amorphous calcifications are distributed throughout the upper outer quadrant of the left breast. (**A**) Right MLO mammogram. (**B**) Left MLO mammogram. (**C**) Right CC mammogram. (**D**) Left CC mammogram. (**E**) Left MLO spot magnification mammogram.

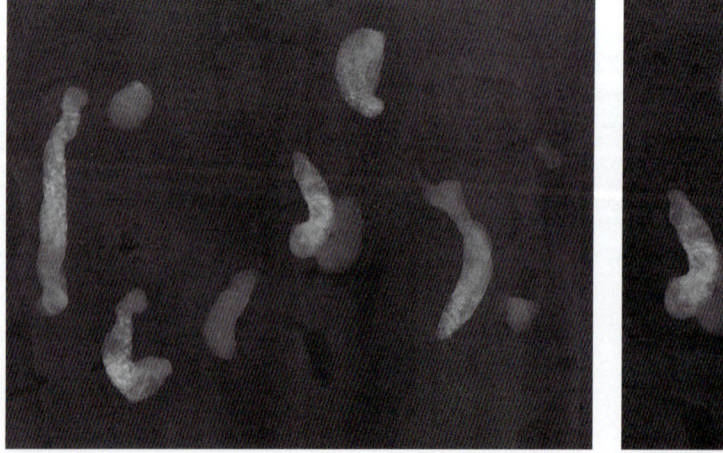
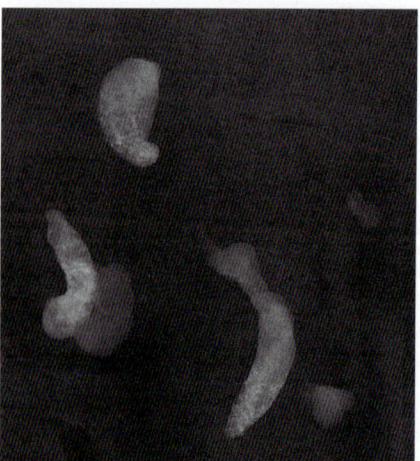

Fig. 17.9 (**A**) Specimen radiograph of percutaneous mammographically guided stereotactic core breast biopsy. The amorphous appearance of the calcifications is evident in all of the tissue cores. (**B**) Enlargement of calcifications in **A**.

Pathology
Lobular hyperplasia. Microscopically, the calcifications are within lobules.

Management
- BI-RADS assessment category 4, suspicious abnormality; biopsy should be considered.

Pearls and Pitfalls
- Microcalcifications within lobules may be either punctate or amorphous in appearance.

Suggested Reading
De Paredes ES. Atlas of Film Screen Mammography. 2nd ed. Baltimore: Williams & Wilkins; 1992:299–416

Pope TL Jr, Fechner RE, Wilhelm MC, Wanebo HJ, de Paredes ES. Lobular carcinoma in situ of the breast: mammographic features. Radiology 1988;168:63–66

Snyder RE. Mammography and lobular carcinoma in situ. Surg Gynecol Obstet 1966;122:255–260

Case 17.6: Ductal Carcinoma in Situ

Case History
A 64-year-old woman presents with new right breast calcifications.

Physical Examination
- Normal exam

Mammogram

Calcifications (Figs. 17.12 and 17.13)
- Type: amorphous/indistinct
- Distribution: grouped/clustered

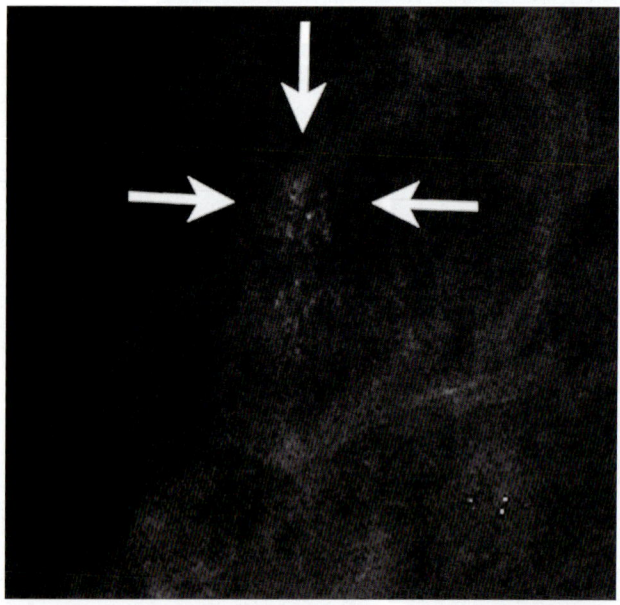

Fig. 17.12 Right MLO magnification mammogram. Faint amorphous calcifications (*arrows*) are present in the upper breast.

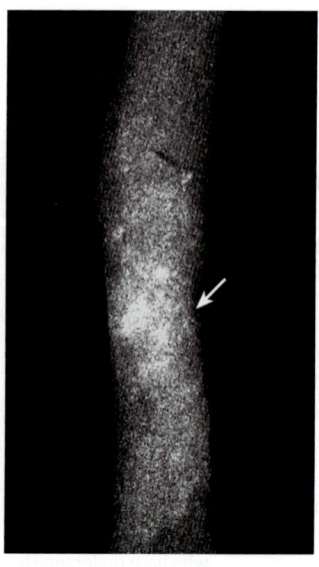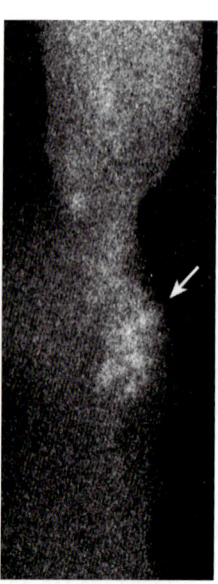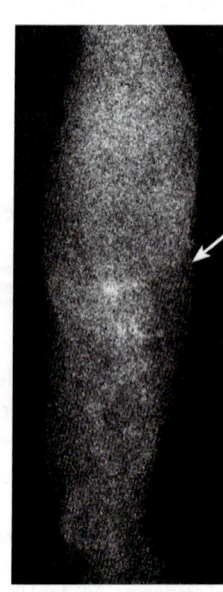

Fig. 17.13 Specimen radiograph of percutaneous core right breast biopsy. Cores from the biopsy of the calcifications identified in **Fig. 17.12** confirm the amorphous appearance of the calcifications (*arrows*).

Pathology
- Ductal carcinoma in situ, low nuclear grade, solid and cribriform type (**Figs. 17.14** and **17.15**)

Management
- BI-RADS assessment category 4, suspicious abnormality; biopsy should be considered.

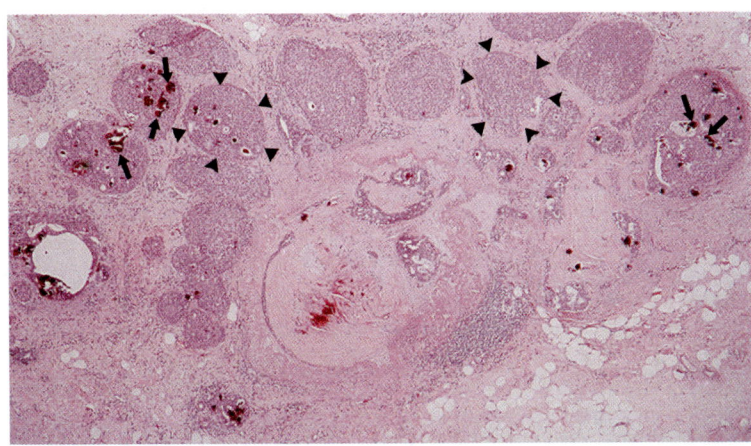

Fig. 17.14 The lobules (*arrowheads*) are filled with malignant cells and calcifications (*arrows*). This type of malignant calcification results in a nonlinear pattern that is more typical of low-grade ductal carcinoma in situ.

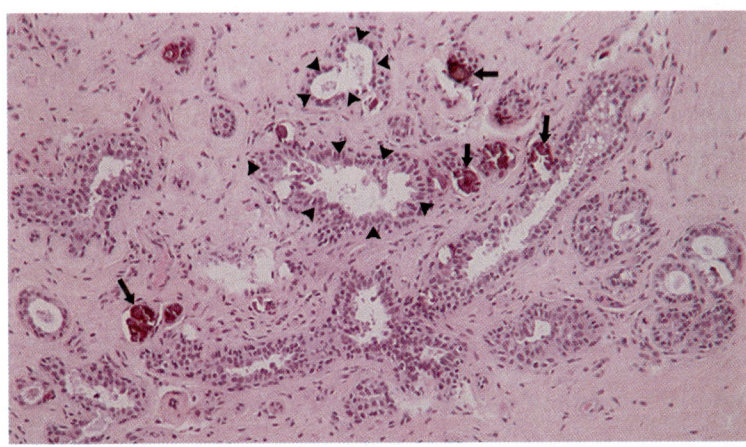

Fig. 17.15 This is a different patient with calcifications (*arrows*) within normal lobules (*arrowheads*). Unless the calcifications are well defined, round, and have smooth borders, this type of nonlinear cluster of calcifications may be difficult to differentiate from the malignant cluster in **Fig. 17.14**.

Pearls and Pitfalls

- Ductal carcinoma in situ (DCIS) may present as either clustered or fine linear/branching calcifications. When DCIS is not associated with comedo necrosis, the tumor tends to form dystrophic calcifications within ductal debris or between cribriform spaces. This pattern produces a nonlinear cluster pattern, as illustrated in this case. This type of malignancy calcifies less than the necrotic type, so the size of the tumor may be larger than the area of the mammographic calcifications.

Suggested Reading

Evans A, Pinder S, Wilson R, et al. Ductal carcinoma in situ of the breast: correlation between mammographic and pathologic findings. AJR Am J Roentgenol 1994;162:1307–1311

Holland R, Hendriks JHCL, Vebeek AL, Mravunac M, Schuurmans Stekhoven JH. Extent, distribution, and mammographic/histological correlations of breast ductal carcinoma in situ. Lancet 1990;335:519–522

Case 17.7: Lymph Node Calcifications

Case History
A 46-year-old woman presents for her baseline mammogram.

Physical Examination
- Normal exam

Mammogram

Calcifications (Fig. 17.16)
- Type: amorphous/indistinct
- Distribution: grouped/clustered

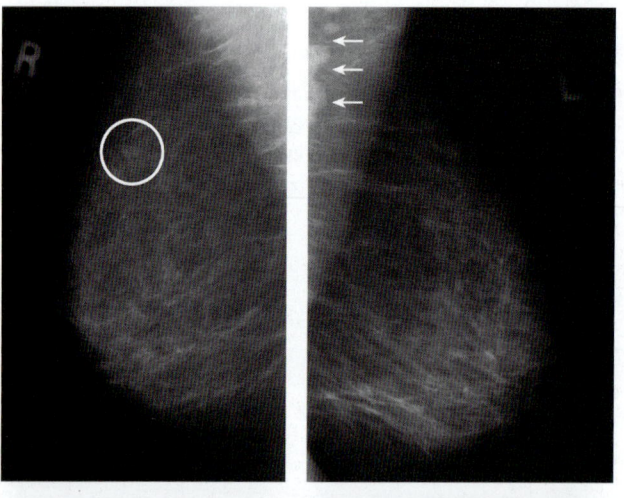

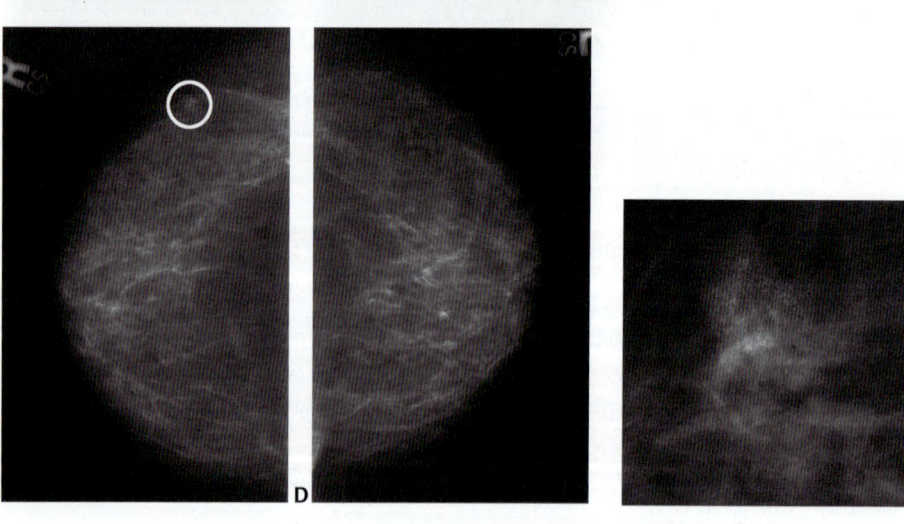

Fig. 17.16 In the right upper outer breast, there is a 9 mm nodular density containing numerous amorphous microcalcifications (*circle*). In the left breast, there are multiple axillary nodes (*arrows*), which exhibit amorphous microcalcifications that are identical to the right breast nodule. (**A**) Right MLO mammogram. (**B**) Left MLO mammogram. (**C**) Right CC mammogram. (**D**) Left CC mammogram. (**E**) Right MLO magnification mammogram.

Pathology
Dermatopathic lymphangitis. The lymph node exhibits normal internal architecture, but there are many sinusoidal macrophages that contain melanin. The calcifications are associated with a giant foreign body reaction.

Management
- BI-RADS assessment category 4, suspicious; biopsy should be considered.

Pearls and Pitfalls

- Lymph nodes may be associated with amorphous or coarse calcifications in metastatic disease and granulomatous diseases such as histoplasmosis, tuberculosis, and sarcoidosis. In patients with rheumatoid arthritis, gold therapy may cause metallic deposition in the nodes, which simulate calcifications.

Suggested Reading

Aqel NM, Peters EE. Kikuchi's disease in axillary lymph nodes draining breast carcinoma. Histopathology 2000;36:280–281

Bassett LW, Jackson VP, Jahan R, Fu YS, Gold RH. Diagnosis of Diseases of the Breast. Philadelphia: WB Saunders; 1997:363–365

Bruwer A, Nelson GW, Spark RP. Punctate intranodal gold deposits simulating microcalcifications on mammograms. Radiology 1987;163:87–88

Chen SW, Bennett G, Price J. Axillary lymph node calcification due to metastatic papillary carcinoma. Australas Radiol 1998;42:241–243

Eisenkraft BL, Som PM. The spectrum of benign and malignant etiologies of cervical node calcification. AJR Am J Roentgenol 1999;172:1433–1437

Hooley R, Lee C, Tocino I, Horowitz N, Carter D. Calcifications in axillary lymph nodes caused by fat necrosis. AJR Am J Roentgenol 1996;167:627–628

Yang WT, Suen M, Metreweli C. Mammographic, sonographic and histopathological correlation of benign axillary masses. Clin Radiol 1997;52:130–135

Case 17.8: Invasive Ductal Carcinoma

Case History
A 43-year-old woman initially presented at an outside institution with a pea-sized palpable mass near the right nipple and calcifications on her mammogram. The mass was biopsied at the outside institution.

Physical Examination
- Right breast: biopsy ecchymosis near right nipple; original nodule no longer detectable
- Left breast: normal exam

Mammogram

Calcifications (Fig. 17.17)
- Type: amorphous/indistinct
- Distribution: grouped/clustered

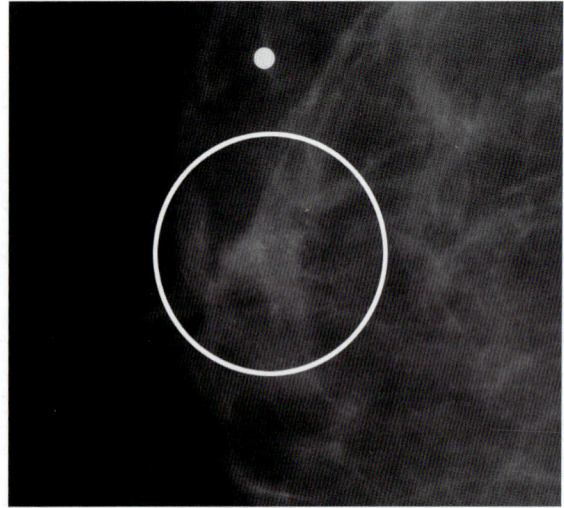 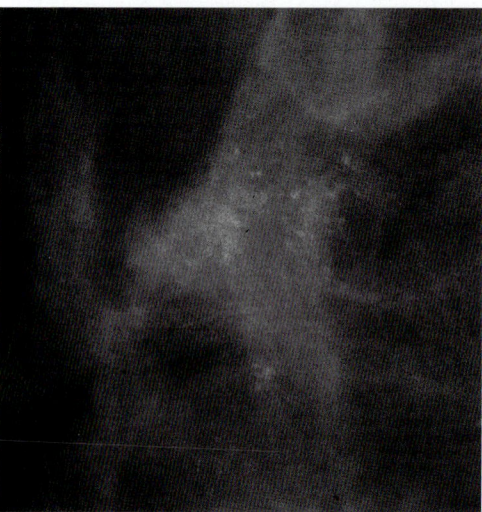

Fig. 17.17 (**A**) Right ML magnification mammogram. In the subareolar region there is a palpable lump marked by a radiopaque marker. The lump is associated with a cluster of amorphous calcifications (*circle*). (**B**) Enlargement of circled calcifications in **A**.

Ultrasound

Frequency
- 13 MHz

Mass (Fig. 17.18)
- Margin: ill defined
- Echogenicity: hypoechoic
- Retrotumoral acoustic appearance: severe shadowing, mass completely obscured
- Shape: irregular

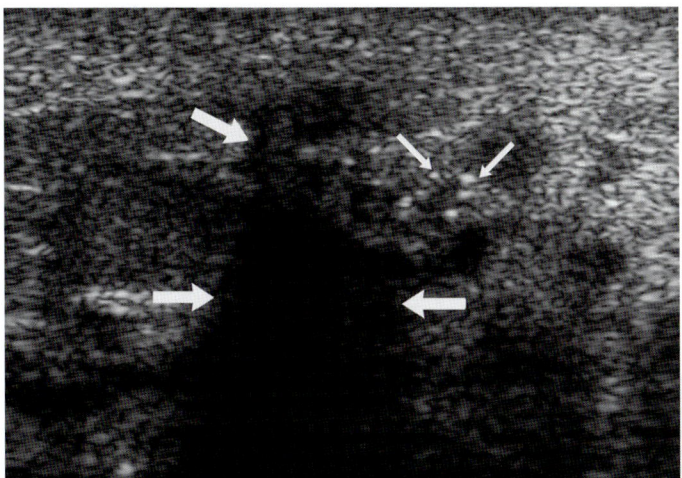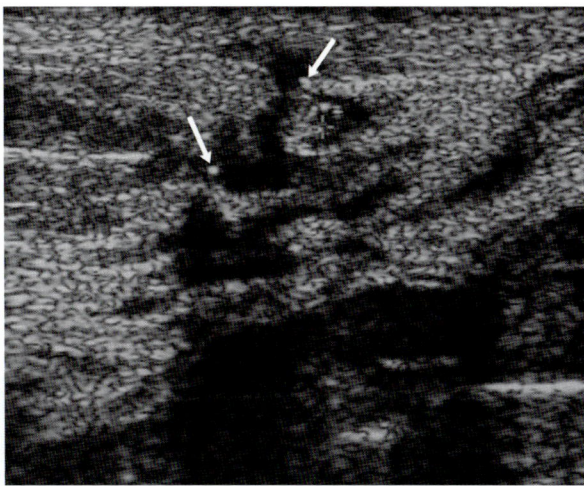

Fig. 17.18 (A) Right longitudinal breast sonogram. Associated with the subareolar calcifications (identified in **Fig. 17.16**) is a hypoechoic mass (*thick arrows*) with severe shadowing. Some calcifications (*thin arrows*) are associated with the mass. (**B**) Right transverse breast sonogram. Adjacent to the subareolar mass are abnormally dilated ducts with calcifications (*arrows*). (**B**) Right transverse breast sonogram.

Pathology
Final excisional specimen demonstrated 1 cm invasive ductal carcinoma with extensive intraductal component.

Management
- BI-RADS assessment category 4, suspicious abnormality; biopsy should be considered.

Pearls and Pitfalls

- The assessment of this case is based on the suspicious appearance of the mammographic calcifications alone. If one included the malignant-appearing sonographic mass, then the assessment would be category 5, highly suggestive of malignancy.
- Because the site of the mass and the calcifications were readily identifiable sonographically, the location of the lesion was marked on the skin sonographically. This site was reconfirmed intraoperatively, and the surgeon made a direct incision into the lesion without preoperative wire localization.

Suggested Reading

Leucht D, Madjar H. Microcalcification in sonography. In: Leucht D, ed. Teaching Atlas of Breast Ultrasound. New York: Thieme; 1996:189–204

Rickard MT. Ultrasound of malignant breast microcalcifications: role in evaluation and guided procedures. Australas Radiol 1996;40:26–31

Yang WT, Suen M, Ahuja A, Metreweli C. In vivo demonstration of microcalcification in breast cancer using high resolution ultrasound. Br J Radiol 1997;70:685–690

Case 18.2: Fibrocystic Changes

Case History
A 68-year-old woman presents with increasing number of calcifications on her right breast screening mammogram.

Physical Examination
- Normal exam

Mammogram

Calcifications (Fig. 18.3)
- Type: pleomorphic/heterogeneous
- Distribution: grouped/clustered

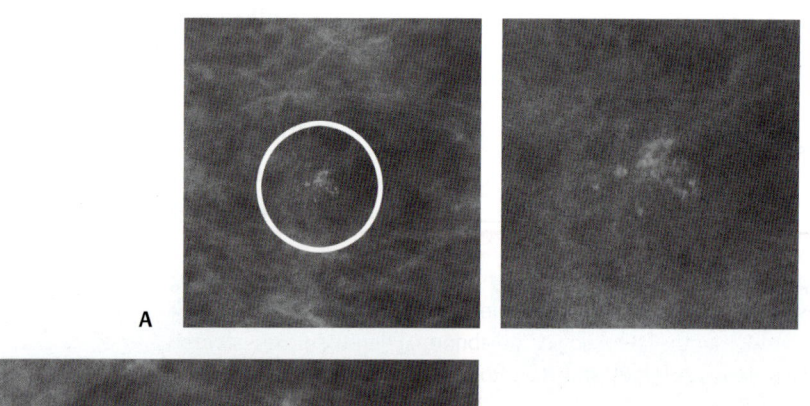
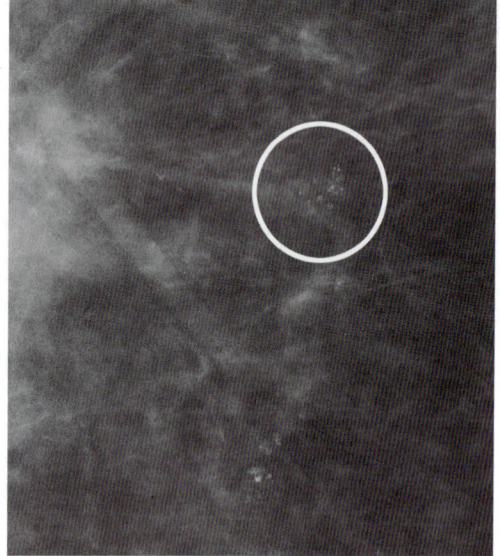
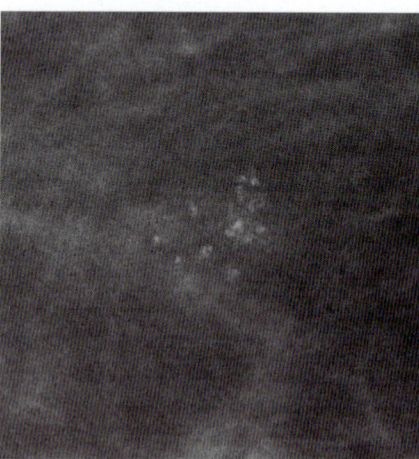

Fig. 18.3 In the right upper outer breast, there is a cluster of pleomorphic calcifications (*circle*). (**A**) Right ML magnification mammogram. (**B**) Enlargement of circled calcifications in **A**. (**C**) Right CC magnification mammogram. (**D**) Enlargement of circled calcifications in **C**.

Ultrasound

Frequency
- 11.5 MHz (**Fig. 18.4**)

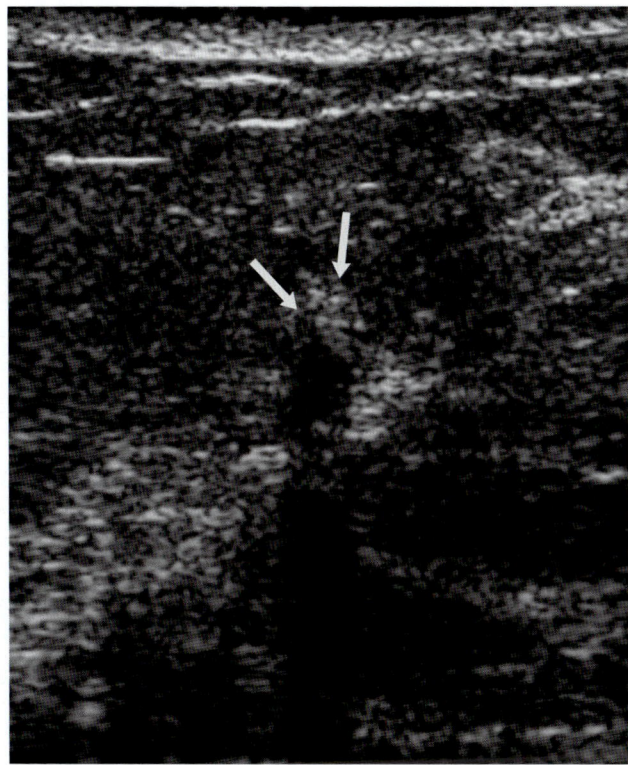

Fig. 18.4 Right transverse breast sonogram. The mammographic calcifications correspond to multiple high-intensity foci (*arrows*) associated with posterior acoustic shadowing. No sonographic mass is present.

Pathology
- Fibrocystic changes
- Predominantly fatty tissue with benign calcifications in small area of stromal fibrosis and epithelial hyperplasia

Management
- BI-RADS assessment category 4, suspicious abnormality; biopsy should be considered.

Pearls and Pitfalls

- Clustered heterogeneous calcifications are due to both benign and malignant etiologies. Benign etiologies include early calcification of fibroadenomas or fat necrosis. Papillomas and fibrocystic changes may also produce these types of calcifications. Malignant causes include ductal carcinoma in situ and invasive ductal carcinoma.

Suggested Reading
Bird RE. Critical pathways in analyzing breast calcifications. Radiographics 1995;15(4):928–934

Case 18.3: Fibroadenoma

Case History
A 69-year-old woman presents with new left breast calcifications.

Physical Examination
- Normal exam

Mammogram

Calcifications (Fig. 18.5)
- Type: pleomorphic/heterogeneous
- Distribution: grouped/clustered

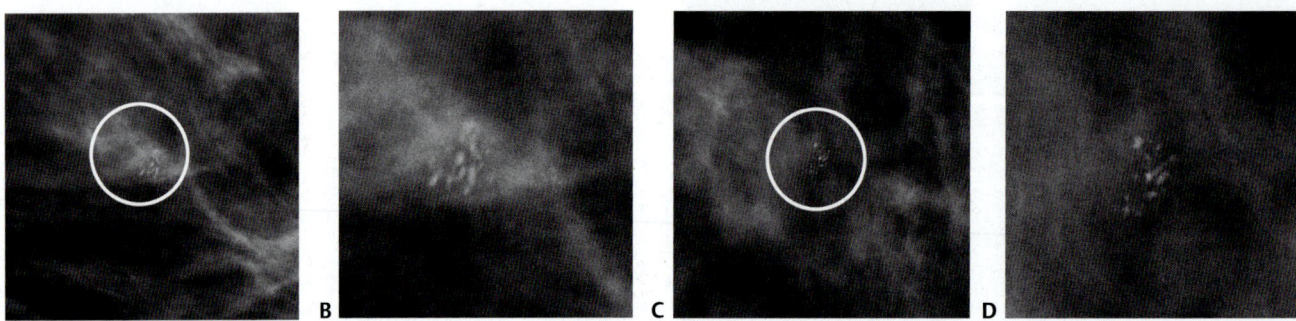

Fig. 18.5 A cluster of pleomorphic calcifications (*circle*) is in the left outer inferior breast. (**A**) Left ML magnification view. (**B**) Enlargement of circled calcifications in **A**. (**C**) Left CC magnification view. (**D**) Enlargement of circled calcifications in **C**.

Pathology
- Fibroadenomatoid hyperplasia

Management
- BI-RADS assessment category 4, suspicious abnormality; biopsy should be considered.

Pearls and Pitfalls
- Fibroadenomatous hyperplasia is an early stage of fibroadenoma formation. Calcifications formed during this process may be indistinguishable from malignant calcifications.

Suggested Reading
Kamal M, Evans AJ, Denley H, Pinder SE, Ellis IO. Fibroadenomatoid hyperplasia: a cause of suspicious microcalcification on mammographic screening. AJR Am J Roentgenol 1998;171(5):1331–1334

Tavassoli FA, Fattaneh A. Pathology of the Breast. 2nd ed. Stamford: Appleton & Lange; 1999:590–597

Case 18.4: Fibroadenoma

Case History

An 80-year-old woman presents with new calcifications on her screening mammogram.

Physical Examination
- Normal exam

Mammogram

Calcifications (Fig. 18.6)
- Type: pleomorphic/heterogeneous
- Distribution: grouped/clustered

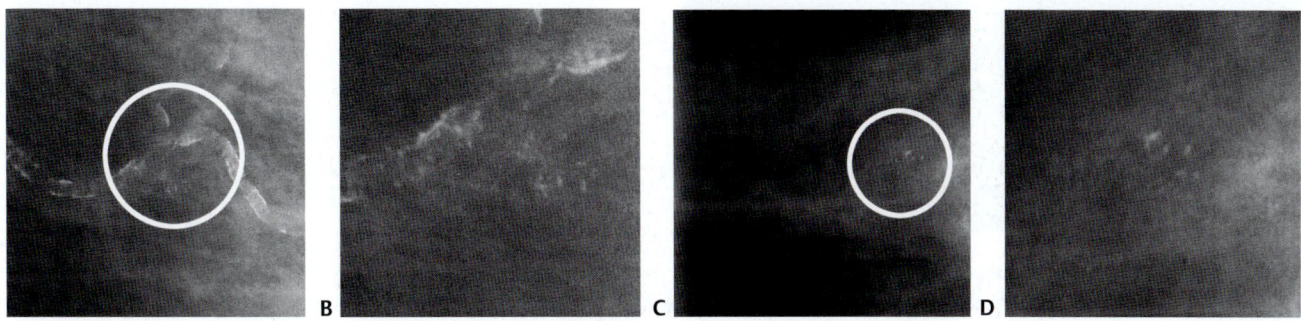

Fig. 18.6 In the left upper outer quadrant, there is a cluster of calcifications (*circle*). (**A**) Left LM magnification mammogram. (**B**) Enlargement of circled calcifications in **A**. (**C**) Left CC magnification mammogram. (**D**) Enlargement of circled calcifications in **C**.

Ultrasound

Low Frequency

Frequency
- 7 MHz (**Fig. 18.7**)

Mass
- Margin: well defined, oval/round
- Echogenicity: hypoechoic
- Retrotumoral acoustic appearance: no shadowing
- Shape: ellipsoid

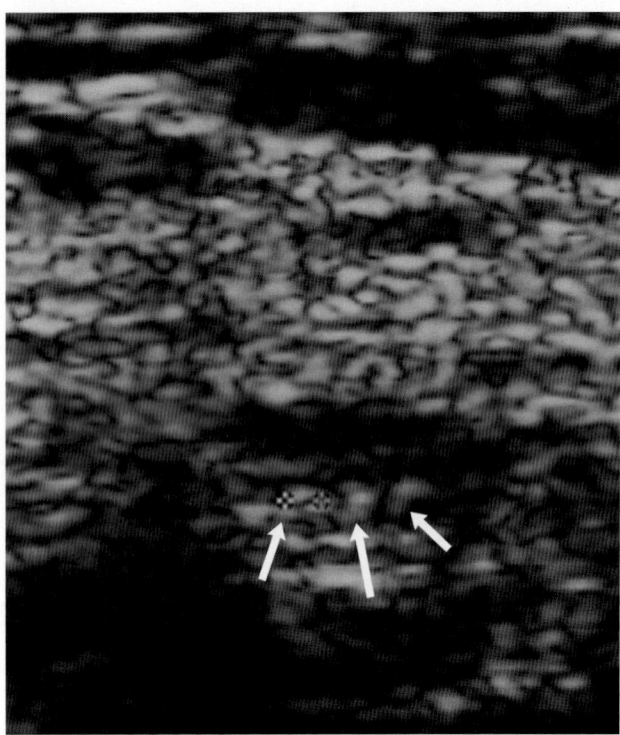

Fig. 18.7 Left radial low-frequency breast sonogram. The calcifications (*arrow*) identified in **Fig. 18.6** are associated with a hypoechoic mass. With this lower frequency, the hypoechoic mass is not well identified.

High Frequency (Fig. 18.8)

Frequency
- 11.5 MHz

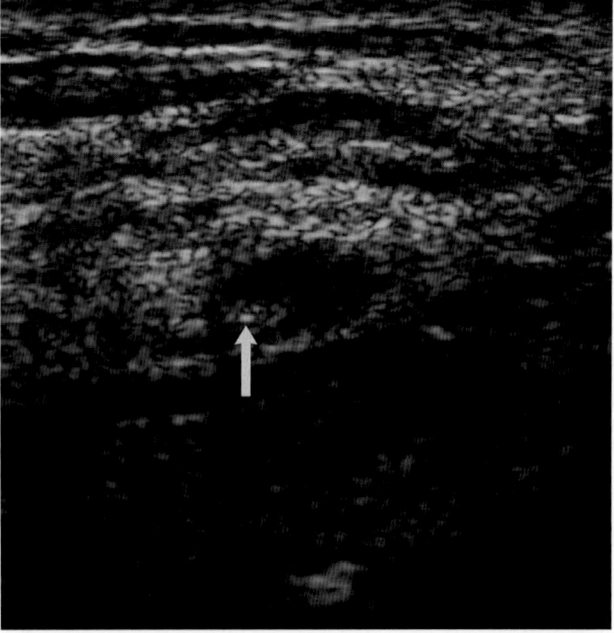

Fig. 18.8 Left radial high-frequency breast sonogram. The calcifications (*arrow*) are within a well-defined, oval, hypoechoic mass. The mass is more clearly identified with this high-frequency technique compared with the low-frequency exam.

Pathology
- Fibroadenoma (not otherwise specified)

Management
- BI-RADS assessment category 4, suspicious abnormality; biopsy should be considered.

Pearls and Pitfalls
- Although the mass has a more benign appearance on the higher-frequency sonographic exam, the small size prevents confident definition of the margins. This limitation and the presence of suspicious mammographic calcifications result in a suspicious, category 4 assessment.

Suggested Reading
Bassett LW. Mammographic analysis of calcifications. Radiol Clin North Am 1992;30(1):93–105

Gershon-Cohen J, Ingleby H. Roentgenography of fibroadenoma of the breast. Radiology 1952;59(1):77–87

Kopans DB. Breast Imaging. 2nd ed. Philadelphia: Lippincott-Raven; 1998:511–615

Case 18.5: Fat Necrosis

Case History
A 64-year-old woman, 6 months after right breast lumpectomy and radiation therapy, has new calcifications adjacent to her lumpectomy site.

Physical Examination
- Right breast: scar in upper outer quadrant of right breast from previous lumpectomy; no new masses
- Left breast: normal exam

Mammogram

Calcifications (Fig. 18.9)
- Type: pleomorphic/heterogeneous
- Distribution: grouped/clustered

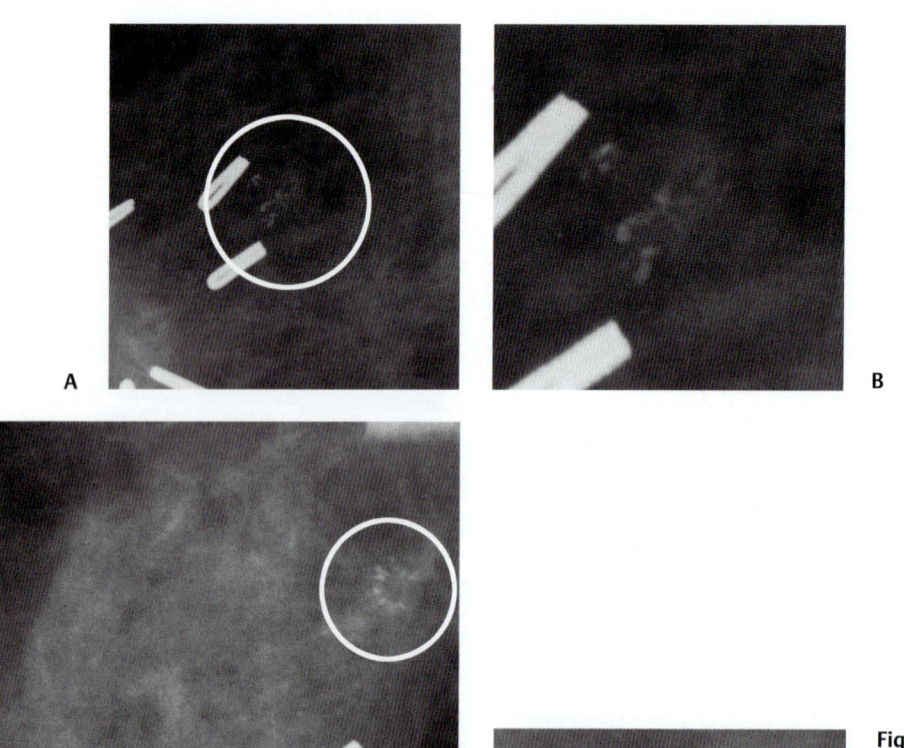

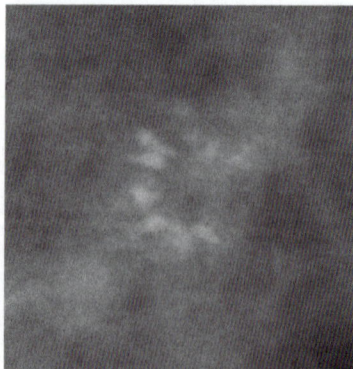

Fig. 18.9 In the right upper outer quadrant, there are clips associated with architectural distortion from a previous lumpectomy. Adjacent to the clips is a group of new heterogeneous calcifications (*circle*). (**A**) Right MLO magnification mammogram. (**B**) Enlargement of circled calcifications in **A**. (**C**) Right CC magnification mammogram. (**D**) Enlargement of circled calcifications in **C**.

Ultrasound

Frequency
- 5 MHz

Mass (18.10)
- Margin: spiculation/architectural distortion
- Echogenicity: hypoechoic
- Retrotumoral acoustic appearance: severe shadowing, mass completely obscured
- Shape: irregular

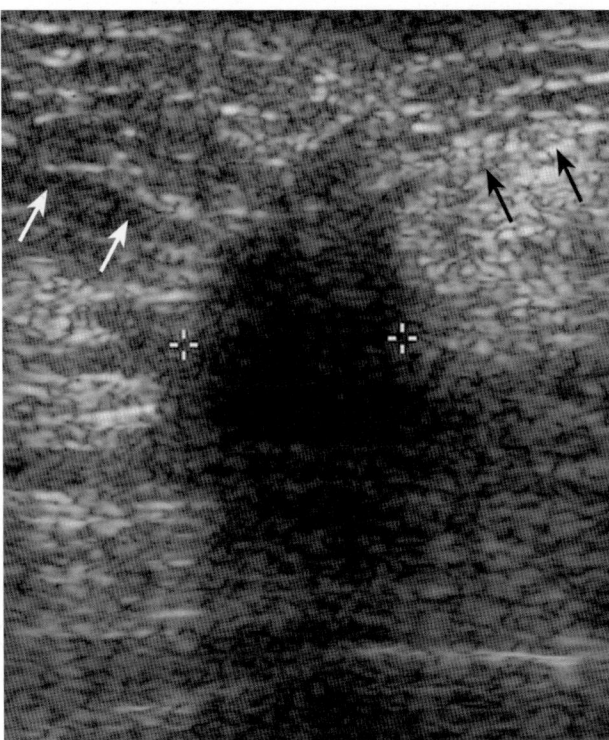

Fig. 18.10 Right longitudinal breast sonogram. The patient's lumpectomy scar is an irregular, hypoechoic, spiculated abnormality with severe posterior acoustic shadowing. The superficial tissue lines (*white and black arrows*) exhibit architectural distortion.

Pathology
- Scar

Management
- BI-RADS assessment category 4, suspicious abnormality; biopsy should be considered.

Pearls and Pitfalls
- Differential diagnosis for etiology of these calcifications is either fat necrosis from lumpectomy or malignancy.
- Sonographically, scars are hypoechoic areas with severe acoustic shadowing that are commonly associated with architectural distortion and spiculation.

Suggested Reading

Dershaw DD, Giess CS, McCormick B, et al. Patterns of mammographically detected calcifications after breast-conserving therapy associated with tumor recurrence. Cancer 1997;79(7):1355–1361

Liberman L, Van Zee KJ, Dershaw DD, Morris EA, Abramson AF, Samli B. Mammographic features of local recurrence in women who have undergone breast-conserving therapy for ductal carcinoma in situ. AJR Am J Roentgenol 1997;168(2): 489–493

Rissanen TJ, Mäkäräinen HP, Mattila SI, Lindholm EL, Heikkinen MI, Kiviniemi HO. Breast cancer recurrence after mastectomy: diagnosis with mammography and US. Radiology 1993;188(2):463–467

Vora SA, Wazer DE, Homer MJ. Management of microcalcifications that develop at the lumpectomy site after breast-conserving therapy. Radiology 1997;203(3):667–671

Case 18.6: Papilloma

Case History
A 79-year-old woman presents with new left breast calcifications.

Physical Examination
- Normal exam

Mammogram

Calcifications (Fig. 18.11)
- Type: pleomorphic/heterogeneous
- Distribution: grouped/clustered

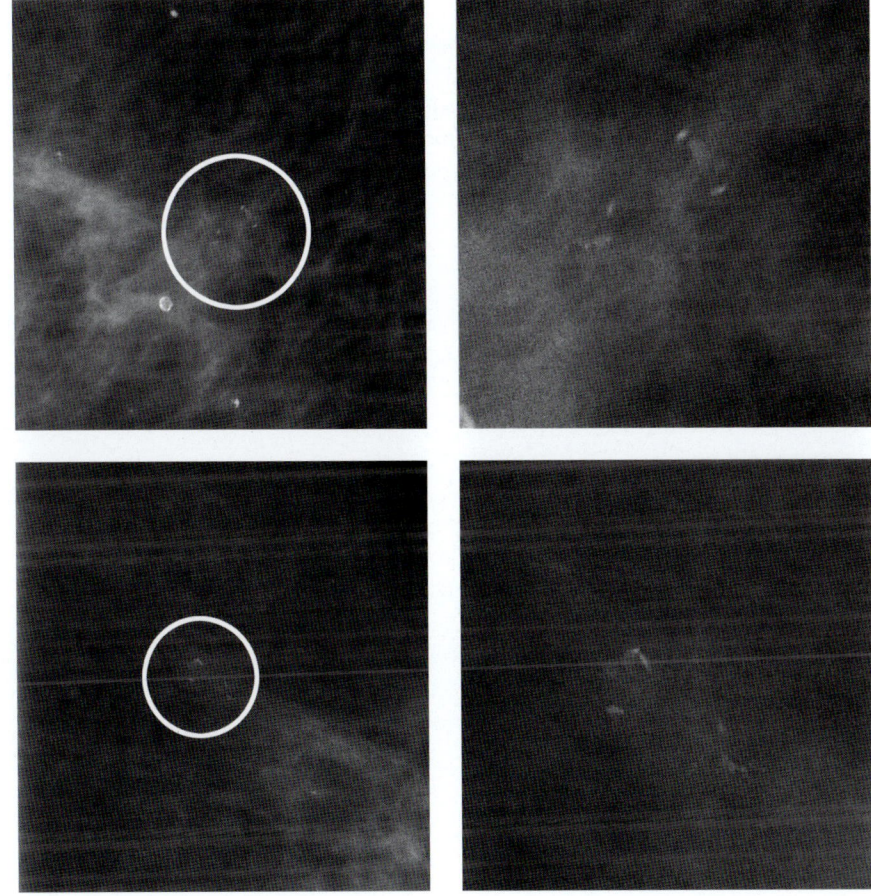

Fig. 18.11 In the left upper outer breast, there is a cluster of heterogeneous calcifications (*circle*). (**A**) Left LM magnification mammogram. (**B**) Left CC magnification mammogram.

Pathology
- Papilloma

Management
- BI-RADS assessment category 4, suspicious abnormality; biopsy should be considered.

> **Pearls and Pitfalls**
>
> - There are three types of papillomas: solitary central papilloma, multiple papillomas, and juvenile papillomatosis.
> - This case is an example of a solitary papilloma. Although this papilloma is peripheral, these masses are usually within a major duct in the subareolar region. Mammographically, they present as circumscribed masses or a cluster of calcifications.

Suggested Reading

De Paredes ES. Atlas of Film Screen Mammography. 2nd ed. Baltimore: Williams & Wilkins; 1992:299–416

Jackson VP, Jahan R, Fu YS. Benign breast lesions. In: Bassett LW, Jackson VP, Jahan R, Fu YS, Gold RH, eds. Diagnosis of Diseases of the Breast. Philadelphia: WB Saunders; 1997:357–443

Tabar L, Dean PB. Teaching Atlas of Mammography. 3rd ed. New York: Thieme; 2001:220–221

Case 18.7: Ductal Carcinoma in Situ

Case History

A 42-year-old woman presents with increasing calcifications.

Physical Examination

- Normal exam

Mammogram

Calcifications (Fig. 18.12)
- Type: pleomorphic/heterogeneous
- Distribution: segmental

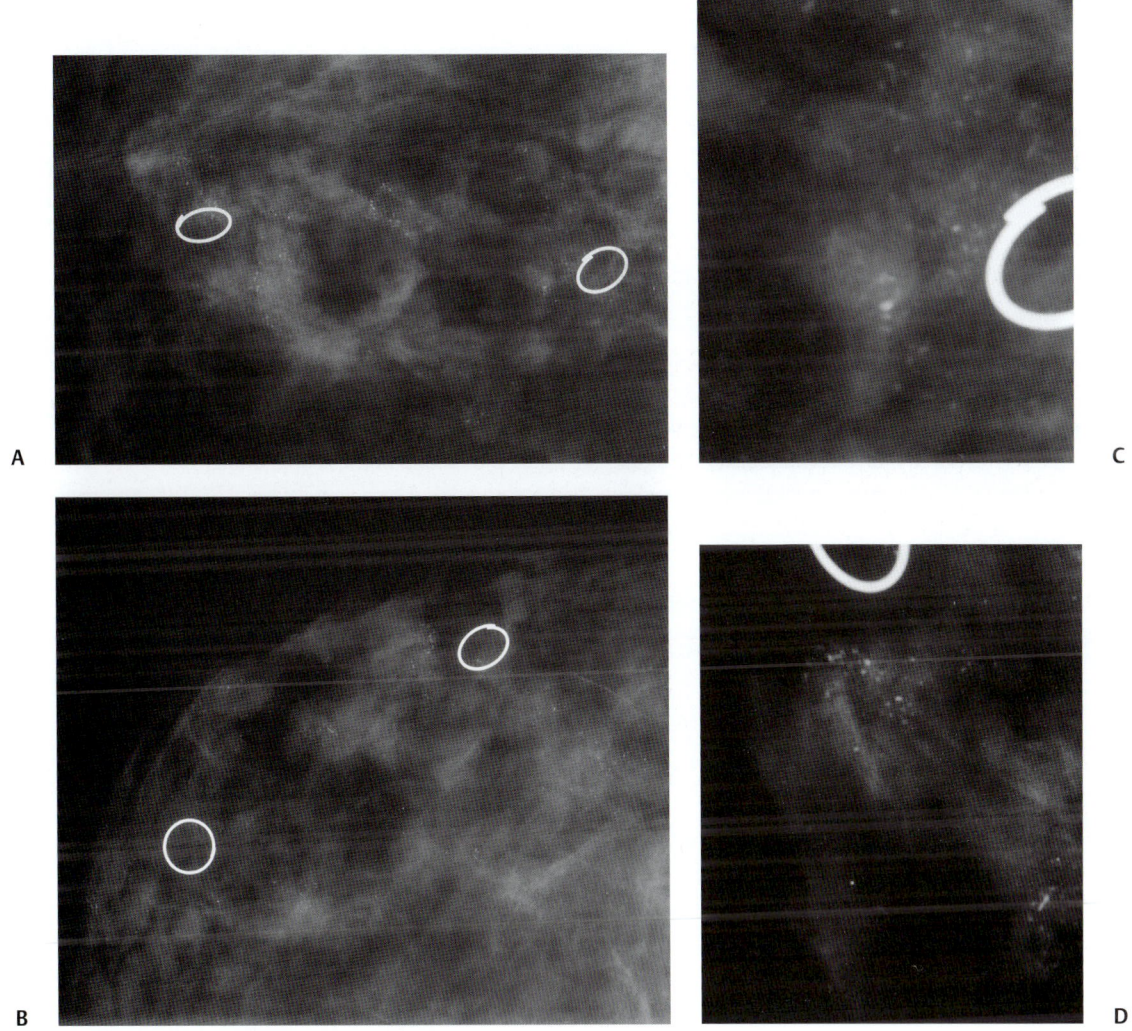

Fig. 18.12 In the inner breast, there are numerous clusters of pleomorphic calcifications. (**A**) Right ML magnification (mammogram). (**B**) Right CC magnification mammogram. (**C**) and (**D**) are an enlargement of the calcifications shown in **A** and **B**.

Calcifications

Ultrasound

Frequency
- 13 MHz (**Fig. 18.13**)

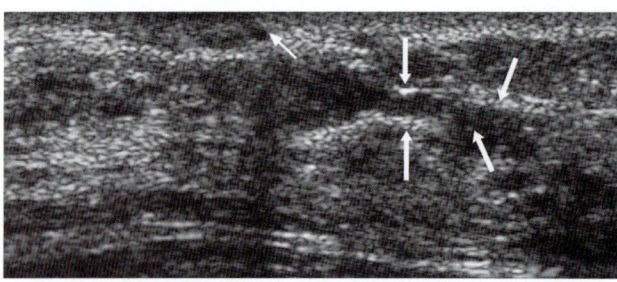

Fig. 18.13 Right radial breast sonogram. Abnormally dilated duct (*thicker arrows*) filled with punctate echogenic foci are present in the area associated with mammographic calcifications. Nipple (*thin arrow*).

Pathology
- Ductal carcinoma in situ

Management
- BI-RADS assessment category 4, suspicious abnormality; biopsy should be considered

Pearls and Pitfalls
- Sonographically, DCIS may appear as isolated calcifications, dilated ducts containing calcifications, an irregular solid mass, or a diffuse area of hypoechogenicity. This case illustrates the second of these appearances.

Suggested Reading
Tohno E, Cosgrove DO. Malignant diseases-primary carcinomas. In: Tohno D, Cosgrove DO, Sloane JP, eds. Ultrasound Diagnosis of Breast Diseases. New York: Churchill Livingstone; 1994:158–180

Case 18.8: Ductal Carcinoma In Situ

Case History
A 60-year-old woman presents for screening mammograms.

Physical Examination
- Normal exam

Mammogram

Calcifications (Fig. 18.14)
- Type: pleomorphic/heterogeneous
- Distribution: clustered and linear

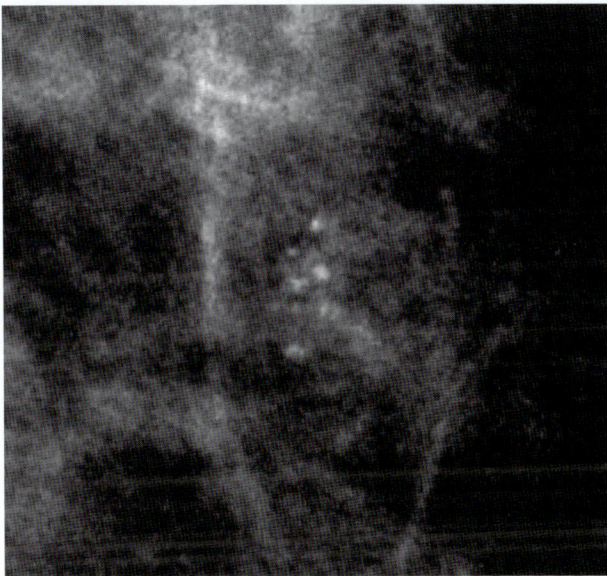

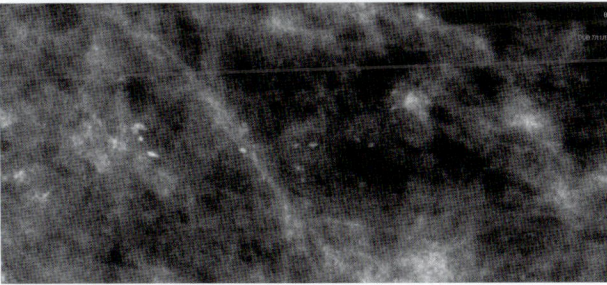

Fig. 18.14 There are multiple clusters of pleomorphic calcifications in the left lower outer quadrant. Some of the calcifications are clustered (**A**), and some are distributed in a linear pattern (**B**). (**A**) Left ML magnification mammogram. (**B**) Left CC magnification mammogram.

Other Modalities: MRI (Figs. 18.15 and 18.16)

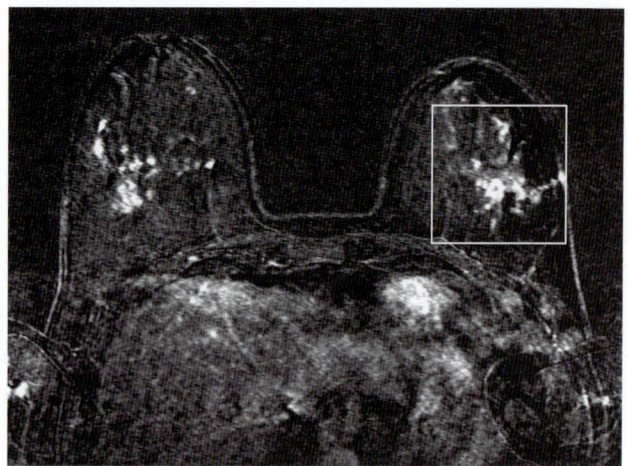

Fig. 18.15 Dynamic bolus T1-weighted 5-minute subtraction axial bilateral breast MRI. In the left lower outer breast, there is non-mass segmental heterogeneous clumped enhancement (*square*). This clumped enhancement corresponded to the left mammographic calcifications. Non-mass segmental enhancement in the right lower outer quadrant is also present.

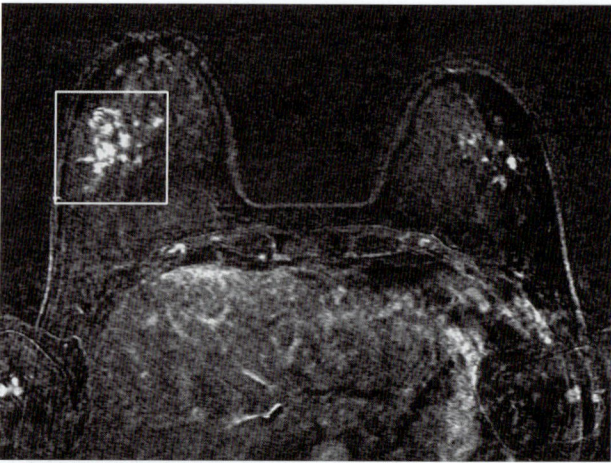

Fig. 18.16 Dynamic bolus T1-weighted 5-minute subtraction axial bilateral breast MRI. In the right lower outer breast, there is non-mass segmental heterogeneous clumped enhancement (*square*). This area was biopsied with MRI guidance because there were no mammographic calcifications in this area.

Pathology
- Left: ductal carcinoma in situ
- Right: ductal carcinoma in situ

Management
- BI-RADS assessment category 5, highly suggestive of malignancy

Pearls and Pitfalls
- Clumped enhancement has been described as appearing as a string of pearls, bunch of grapes, or cobblestone-like. The differential diagnosis of clumped enhancement is ductal carcinoma in situ (DCIS), invasive ductal or lobular carcinoma, lobular carcinoma in situ, fibrocystic change, atypical ductal hyperplasia, multiple papillomas, ruptured duct, chronic inflammation, and hemangiomas. Clumped enhancement is the most common pattern for DCIS.
- Rapid initial uptake with washout is most commonly present when DCIS presents as a mammographic mass as opposed to calcifications. When correlating MRI kinetics to mammographic findings of pure DCIS, Jansen and colleagues[1] found that this highly suspicious kinetic curve is associated with 90% of mammographic masses, 45% of pleomorphic, fine linear, or linear/branching calcifications, and only 22% amorphous calcifications.

Reference
1. Jansen SA, Newstead GM, Abe H, Shimauchi A, Schmidt RA, Karczmar GS. Pure ductal carcinoma in situ: kinetic and morphologic MR characteristics compared with mammographic appearance and nuclear grade. Radiology 2007;245(3):684–691

Suggested Reading
Raza S. Clumped. In: Berg WA, Birdwell RL, Gombos EC, Wang S-C, Parkinson BT, Raza S, Green GE, Kennedy A, Kettler MD, eds. Diagnostic Imaging Breast. Altona, Manitoba: Friesens, 2006, IV-1-166-167

Case 18.9: Infiltrating Ductal Carcinoma

Case History
A 44-year-old woman presents for screening mammography.

Physical Examination
- Normal exam

Mammogram

Calcifications (Fig. 18.17)
- Type: pleomorphic/heterogeneous
- Distribution: clustered

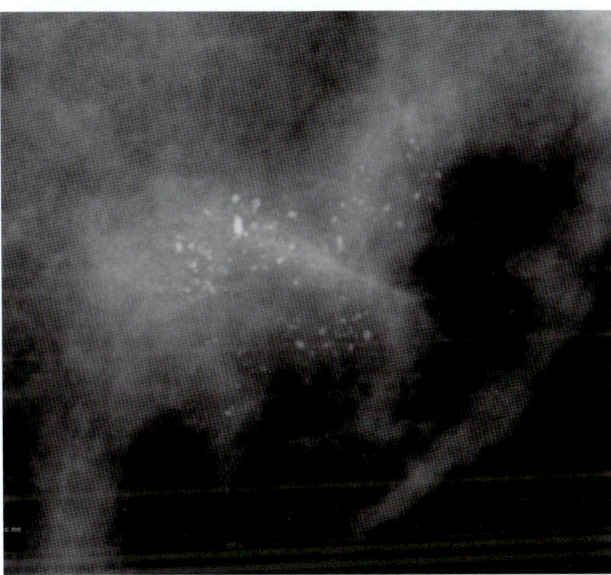

Fig. 18.17 Left CC spot magnification mammogram. In the left 9 o'clock position, there is a cluster of pleomorphic calcifications.

Ultrasound

Frequency (Fig. 18.18)
- 14 MHz

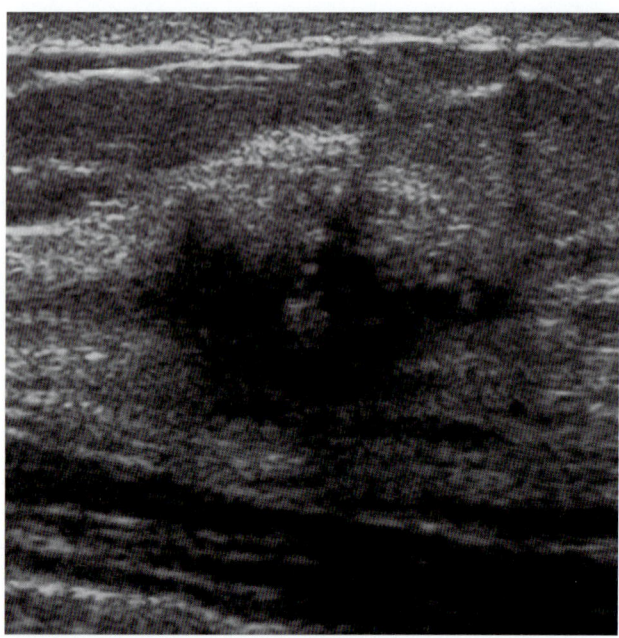

Fig. 18.18 Left radial breast sonogram. The mammographic cluster of calcifications corresponds to an irregular, hypoechoic solid mass with calcifications.

Other Modalities: MRI (Figs. 18.19 and 18.20)

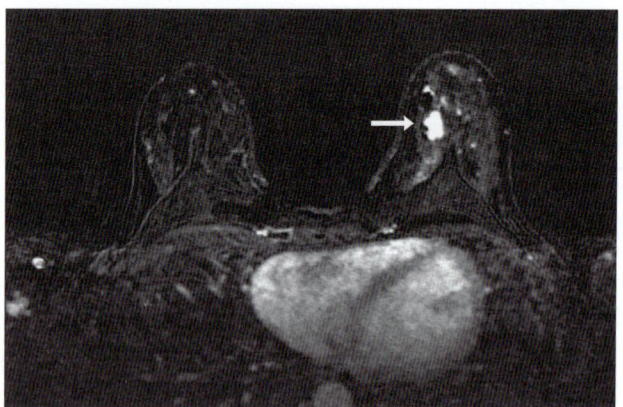

Fig. 18.19 Dynamic bolus T1-weighted 2-minute subtraction axial bilateral breast MRI. At the 9 o'clock position of the left breast, there is an irregular mass (*arrow*) with initial rapid enhancement corresponding to the mammographic mass.

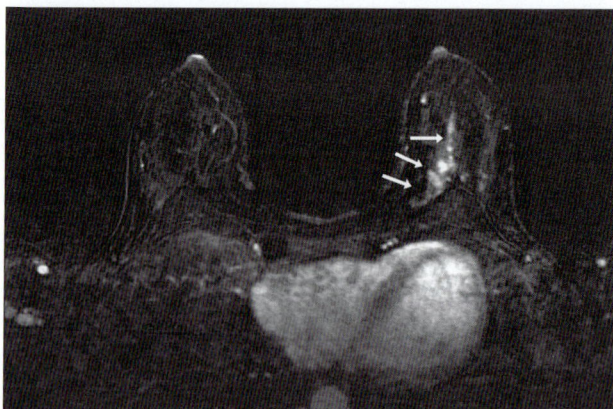

Fig. 18.20 Dynamic bolus T1-weighted 2-minute subtraction axial bilateral breast MRI. Inferior to the mass in **Fig. 18.17**, there is segmental non-mass heterogeneous, clumped enhancement (*arrows*) in the inner inferior quadrant.

Pathology
- Left mass with calcifications at the 9 o'clock position: invasive ductal carcinoma
- Left inner inferior non-mass enhancement: invasive ductal and ductal carcinoma in situ

Management
- Left mammographic calcifications at the 9 o'clock position: BI-RADS assessment category 5, highly suggestive of malignancy
- Left inner inferior non-mass MRI enhancement: BI-RADS assessment category 4, suspicious; biopsy should be considered.

Pearls and Pitfalls

- MRI is less sensitive at identifying ductal carcinoma in situ compared with invasive cancer. MRI sensitivities generally range from 90 to 100% for invasive cancer versus 77 to 96% for ductal carcinoma in situ.
- With MRI, ductal carcinoma in situ most commonly appears as a non-mass enhancement (65%) rather than as an enhancing mass (35%). The most common non-mass appearances are clumped internal enhancement with ductal or segmental distribution.

Suggested Reading

Menell JH. Ductal carcinoma in situ. In: Morris EA, Liberman L, eds. Breast MRI. New York: Springer; 2005:164-172

Raza S, Vallejo M, Chikarmane SA, Birdwell RL. Pure ductal carcinoma in situ: a range of MRI features. AJR Am J Roentgenol 2008;191(3):689–699

Case 18.10: Infiltrating Ductal Carcinoma

Case History
A 39-year-old woman presents with a right breast palpable lump. She is 6-months postpartum and is still breast-feeding. She was initially studied with the lower-frequency sonography. Her sonogram was interpreted as BI-RADS category 3 (probably benign lesion, short-term follow-up recommended). After 1 month, because symptoms persisted, she was examined with the high-frequency sonography. As a result of her high-frequency sonogram, the mammograms were then performed.

Physical Examination
- Right breast: palpable lump at the 6 o'clock position
- Left breast: normal exam

Mammogram

Calcifications (Fig. 18.21)
- Type: pleomorphic/heterogeneous
- Distribution: grouped/clustered

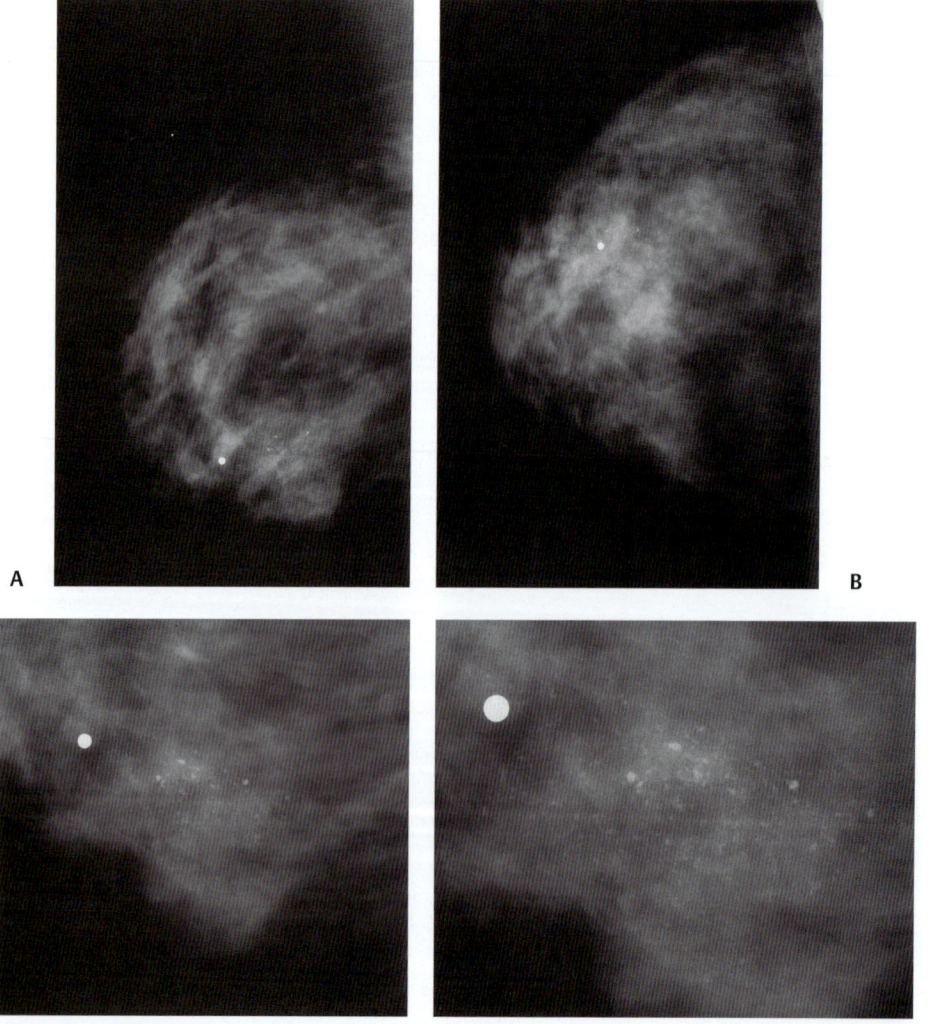

Fig. 18.21 Near the right 6 o'clock position, there is a cluster of pleomorphic calcifications that correspond to a palpable lump, which is marked with a radiopaque marker. (**A**) Right MLO mammogram. (**B**) Right CC mammogram. (**C**) Right MLO magnification mammogram. (**D**) Right CC magnification mammogram.

Ultrasound

Low Frequency (18.22)

Frequency
- 7 MHz

Mass
- Margin: well defined, lobulated
- Echogenicity: hypoechoic
- Retrotumoral acoustic appearance: bilateral edge shadowing
- Shape: lobulated

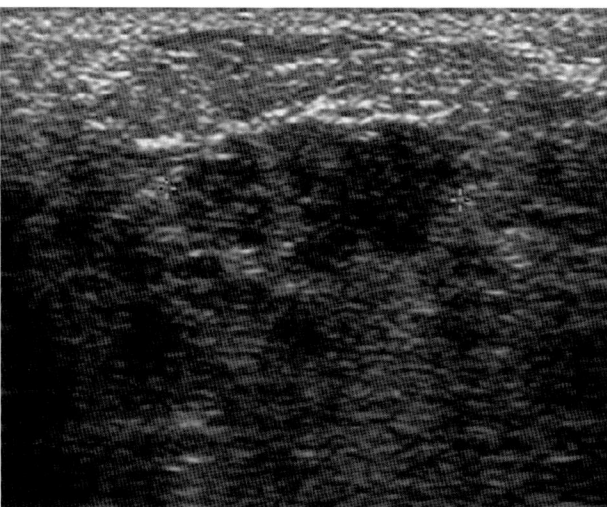

Fig. 18.22 Right radial low-frequency breast sonogram. A palpable lump corresponded to a lobulated hypoechoic mass.

High Frequency (Fig. 18.23)

Frequency
- 13 MHz

High Frequency Findings
High frequency better displays the irregularity of the margins of the mass. Furthermore, the high-frequency examination demonstrates calcifications that were not visible on the lower-frequency study. Mammography subsequently confirmed the presence of malignant calcifications (**Fig. 18.20**).

Case 18.11: Infiltrating Ductal Carcinoma

Case History

A 58-year-old woman presents for screening mammograms.

Physical Examination

- Normal exam

Mammogram

Calcifications (Fig. 18.25)
- Type: heterogeneous/pleomorphic
- Distribution: clustered

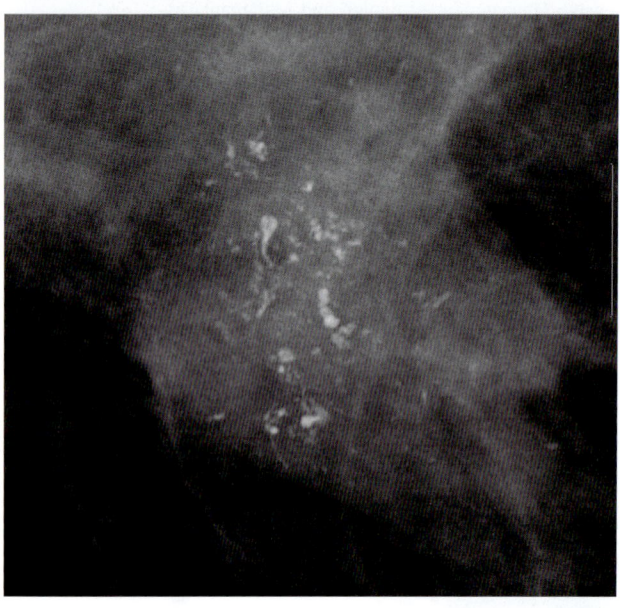

Fig. 18.25 Right CC magnification mammogram. Near the 1 o'clock position of the right breast there is a cluster of pleomorphic calcifications associated with an irregular mass.

Ultrasound

Frequency (Figs. 18.26 and 18.27)
- 14 MHz

Mass
- Margin: ill defined
- Echogenicity: hypoechoic
- Shape: irregular

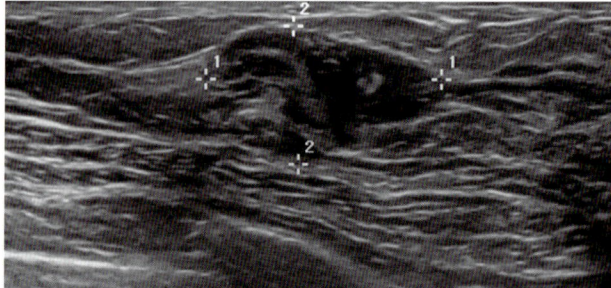

Fig. 18.26 Right radial breast sonogram. The mammographic pleomorphic calcifications sonographically correspond to an irregular solid mass that is subsequently sonographically biopsied and found to be malignant. Mass is outlined by electronic calipers.

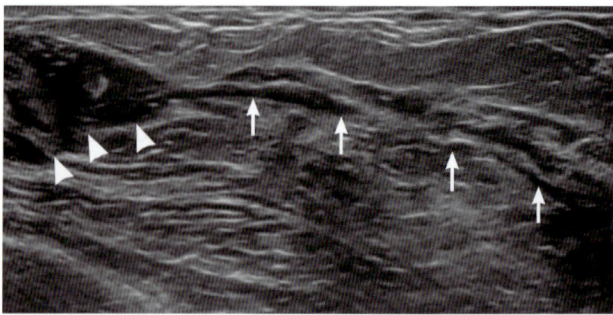

Fig. 18.27 Right radial breast sonogram. At one edge of the mass (*arrowheads*), there are dilated ducts (*arrows*) consistent with ductal extension of tumor.

Other Modalities: MRI and Second Look Sonography (Figs. 18.28, 18.29, and 18.30)

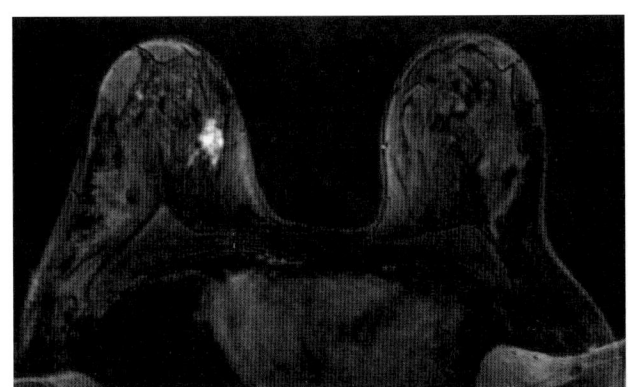
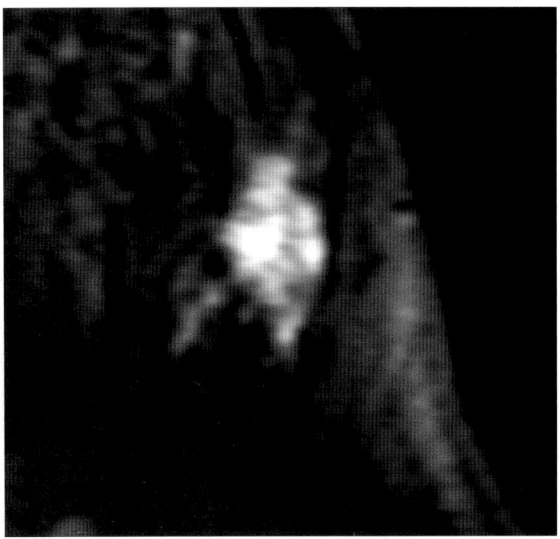

Fig. 18.28 With breast MRI, the known right breast cancer appears as an irregular enhancing mass with dark nonenhancing lines. These internal nonenhancing lines should not be confused with benign nonenhancing septations. This mass has been recently sonographically biopsied, and these lines are probably due to the postbiopsy effect. The overall morphology of the mass is obviously malignant. (**A**) Bilateral contrast-enhanced axial breast high-resolution MRI. (**B**) Enlargement of right breast cancer.

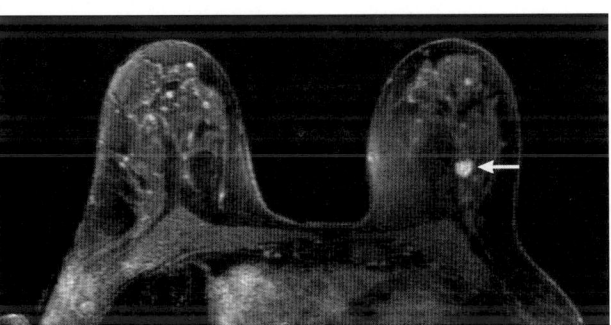
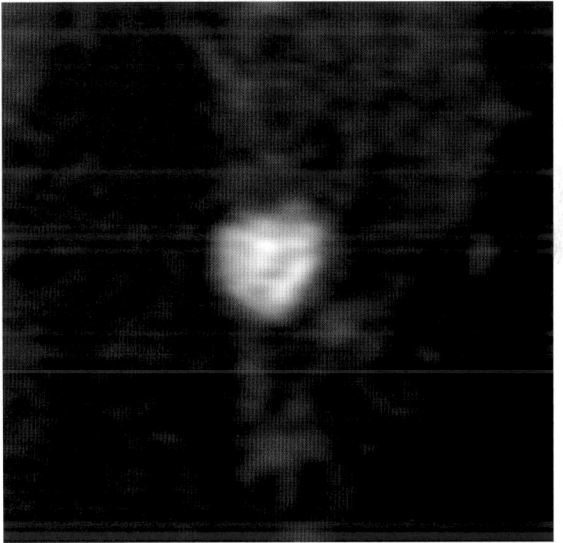

Fig. 18.29 The breast MRI demonstrates a second mass. There is a circumscribed oval enhancing mass (arrow) with a central nonenhancing septation near the left 3 o'clock position. (**A**) Bilateral contrast-enhanced axial breast high-resolution MRI. (**B**) Enlargement of an oval mass at the left 3 o'clock position.

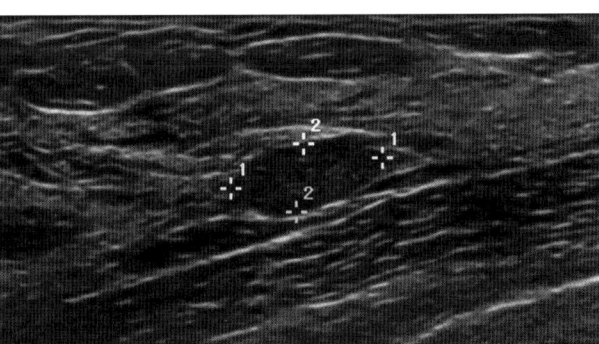

Fig. 18.30 Left radial breast sonogram. This sonogram is performed to identify the left MRI mass. The MRI mass corresponds to a circumscribed solid hypoechoic mass. Although this mass appears to be benign by MRI and sonography, it is subsequently sonographically biopsied as part of the patient's staging protocol.

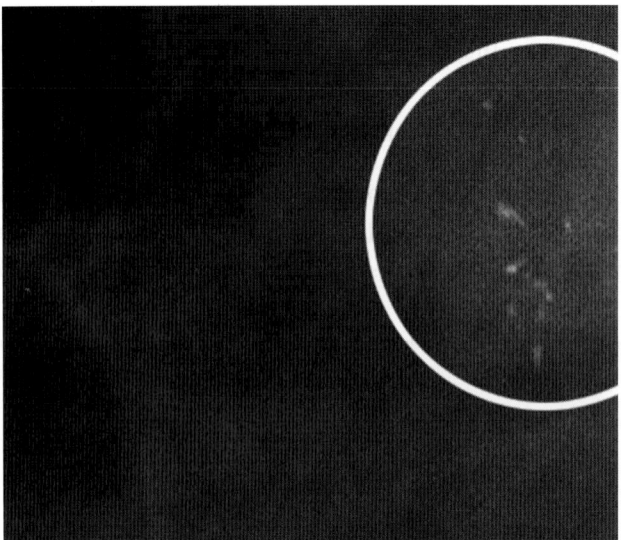

Fig. 18.32 Right MLO magnification mammogram. The cluster of calcifications (*circle*) identified in **Fig. 18.30** consists of numerous punctate and linear heterogeneous calcifications.

Ultrasound

Frequency
- 11.5 MHz

Mass (Fig. 18.33)
- Margin: ill defined
- Echogenicity: hypoechoic
- Retrotumoral acoustic appearance: posterior shadowing distal to mass
- Shape: irregular

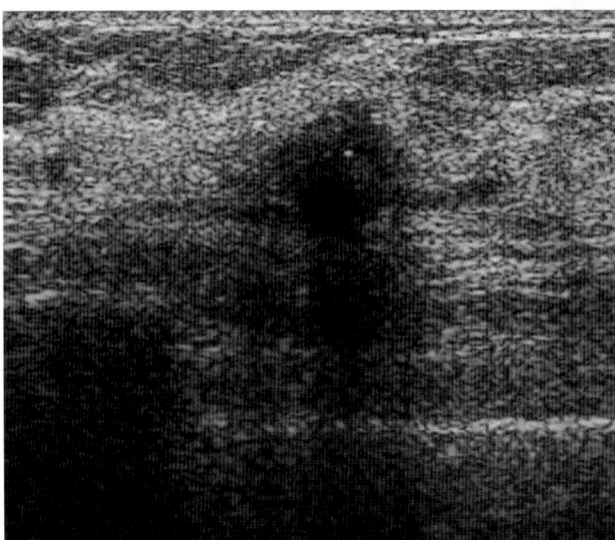

Fig. 18.33 Right breast radial sonogram. The calcifications identified in **Figs. 18.30** and **18.31** correspond to an ill-defined hypoechoic mass with posterior acoustic shadowing. Calcification is present within the mass.

Pathology
- Apocrine carcinoma

Management
- BI-RADS assessment category 4, suspicious abnormality; biopsy should be considered.

Pearls and Pitfalls

- Apocrine carcinoma is a variant of ductal carcinoma that represents < 1% of ductal malignancies. Because this tumor is rare, imaging information is limited. These malignancies have been reported to present as mammographic masses, usually with ill-defined margins. However, sometimes these masses are well defined. Calcifications have also been associated with these masses. The sonographic features would be expected to be similar to other ductal malignancies. Like this case, these masses would be solid, hypoechoic, with varying degrees of shadowing. Clinically, these tumors behave in a manner similar to ductal carcinoma.

Suggested Reading
Gilles R, Lesnik A, Guinebretière JM, et al. Apocrine carcinoma: clinical and mammographic features. Radiology 1994;190(2):495–497

19 Calcifications: Fine Linear/Branching Microcalcifications

Case 19.1: Adenoymyoepithelioma

Case History

A 68-year-old woman has increasing calcifications on her screening mammogram. She has a past history of lung cancer and bladder cancer. Stereotactic core needle biopsy of the calcifications was not conclusive, so a needle localization and excisional biopsy were performed. The patient was unable to maintain an upright position for the needle localization, so sonographic guidance of the wire localization was performed.

Physical Examination
- Normal exam

Mammogram

Calcifications (Figs. 19.1 and 19.2)
- Type: fine linear/branching
- Distribution: linear

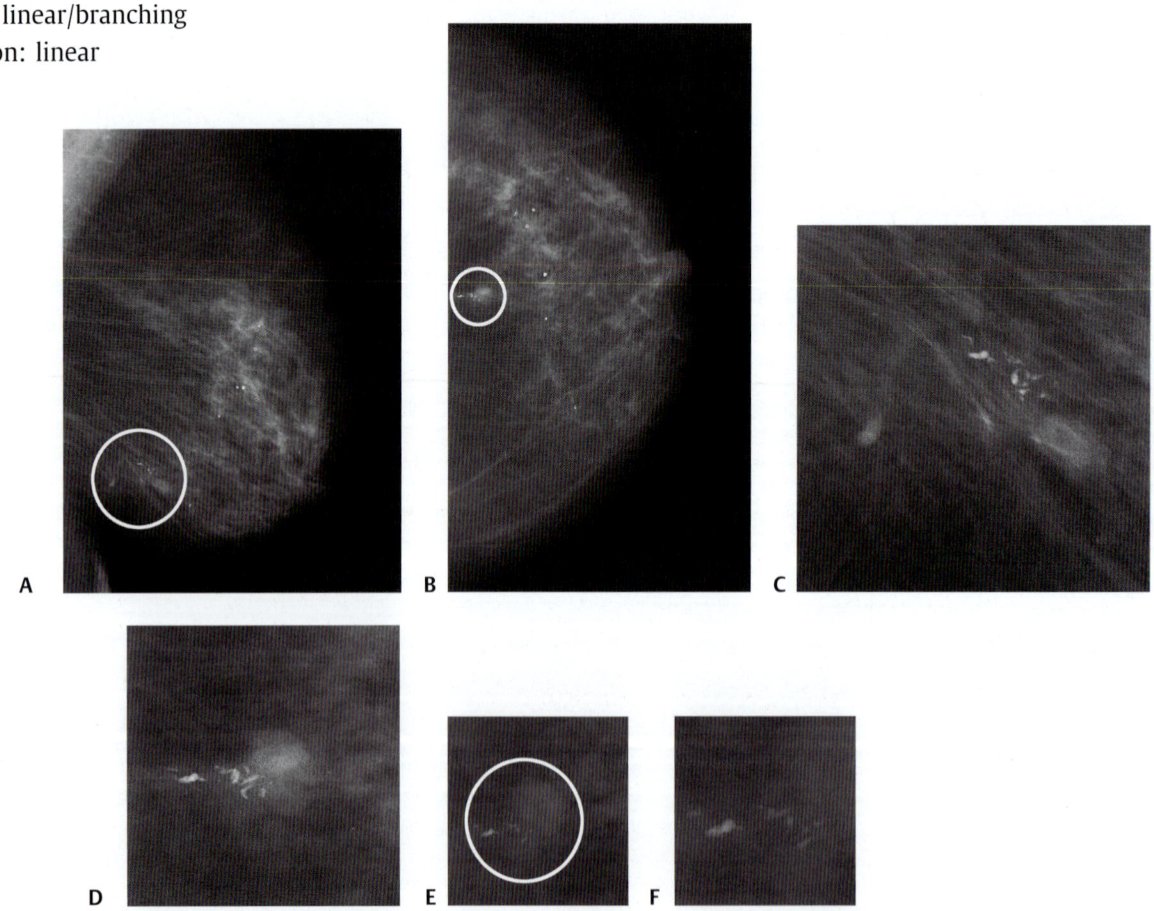

Fig. 19.1 In the 6 o'clock position of the left breast, there is a nodular density associated with linear calcifications (*circle*). (**A**) Left MLO mammogram. (**B**) Left CC mammogram. (**C**) Enlargement of circled calcifiations in **A**. (**D**) Enlargement of circled calcifications in **B**.

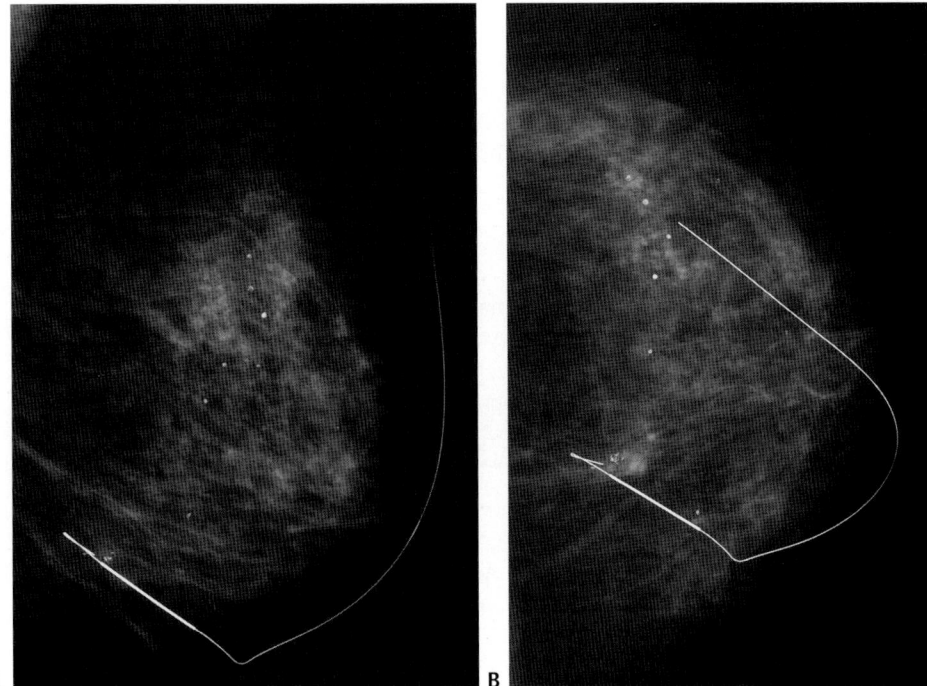

Fig. 19.2 Mammograms performed after sonographic guidance of needle localization demonstrate that the wire is in excellent position with respect to the calcifications. (**A**) Left ML mammogram after needle localization. (**B**) Left CC mammogram after needle localization.

Ultrasound

Frequency
- 13 MHz

Mass (Fig. 19.3)
- Margin: ill defined
- Echogenicity: hypoechoic
- Retrotumoral acoustic appearance: bilateral edge shadowing
- Shape: ellipsoid

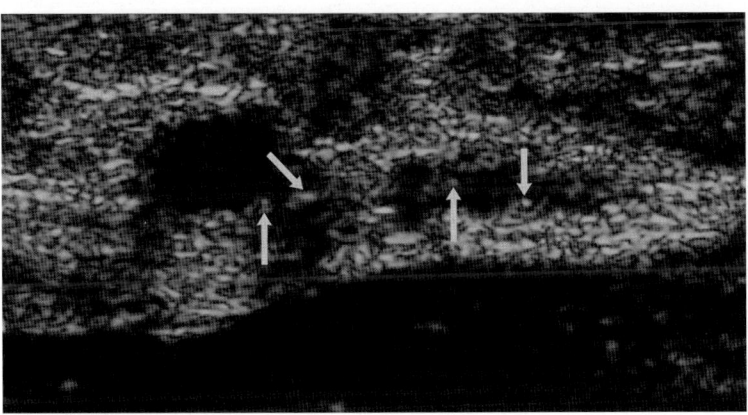

Fig. 19.3 Left radial breast sonogram. The calcifications identified in **Fig. 19.1** corresponded to a focally dilated tubular structure associated with a solid nodule. Both the tubular structure and the nodule contained multiple calcifications (*arrows*). Sonographic needle localization was performed using this image. After localization, mammographic images were taken to confirm the wire position (**Fig. 19.2**).

Pathology
- Adenomyoepithelioma

Management
- BI-RADS assessment category 4, suspicious abnormality; biopsy should be considered.

> **Pearls and Pitfalls**
> - Adenomyoepithelioma is an unusual breast tumor that is generally benign but may recur after local excision. Occasionally, carcinoma or malignant myoepithelioma will arise within an adenomyoepithelioma.
> - Sonographic guidance for needle localization of calcifications is rarely necessary. To perform this procedure, it is critical that one be confident in locating the calcifications. High-frequency sonography is generally a necessity in this situation.

Suggested Reading

Leucht D, Madjar H. Microcalcification in sonography. In: Leucht D, ed. Teaching Atlas of Breast Ultrasound. New York: Thieme, 1996:189–204

Tavassoli FA, Fattaneh A. Pathology of the Breast, 2nd ed. Stamford: Appleton & Lange; 1999:763–791

Case 19.2: Ductal Carcinoma in Situ

Case History
A 70-year-old woman presents with new right breast calcifications on her screening mammogram.

Physical Examination
- Normal exam

Mammogram

Calcifications (Fig. 19.4)
- Type: fine linear/branching
- Distribution: grouped/clustered

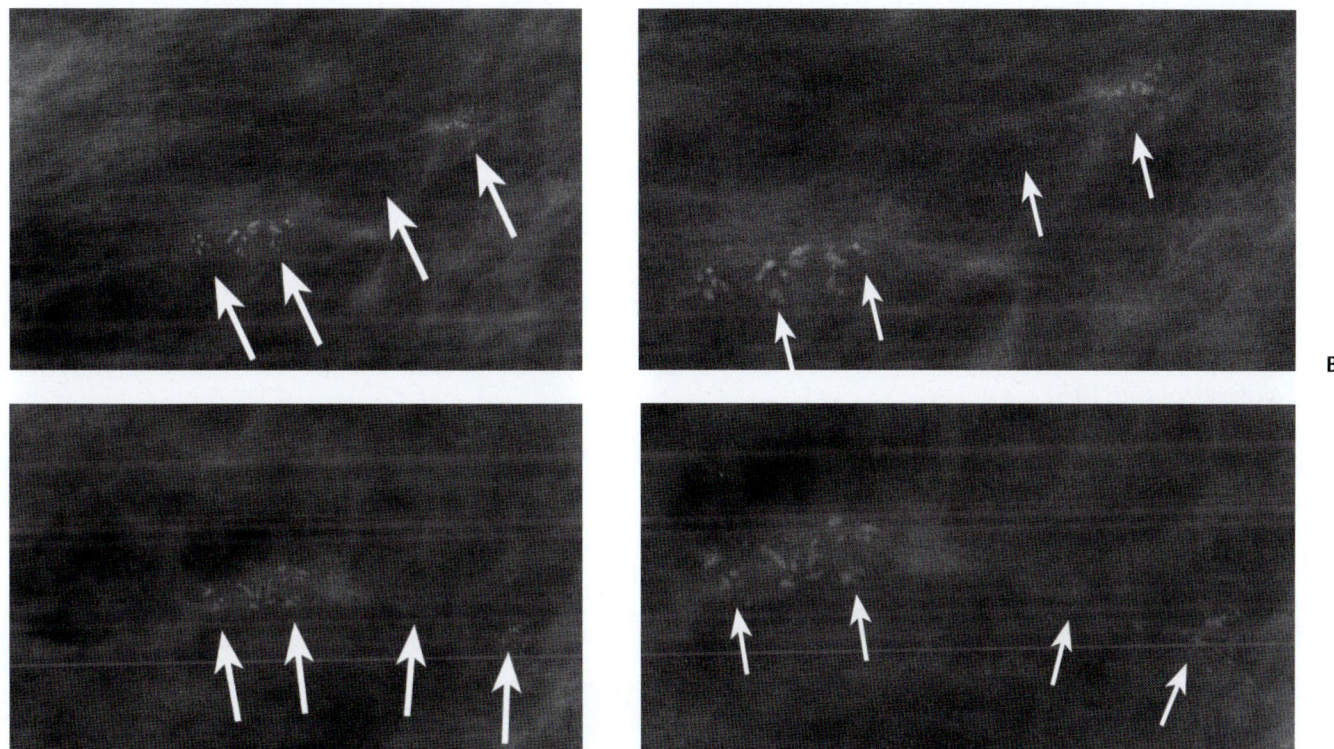

Fig. 19.4 In the inferior outer breast, there is a cluster of heterogeneous calcifications that are arranged in a linear pattern (*arrows*). (**A**) Right MLO magnification mammogram. (**B**) Right exaggerated CC magnification mammogram.

Pathology
- Ductal carcinoma in situ
- Solid type with high nuclear grade and high mitotic rate and with comedo necrosis and dystrophic calcifications

Management
- BI-RADS assessment category 4, suspicious abnormality; biopsy should be considered.

Pearls and Pitfalls

- Calcification in DCIS with comedo necrosis usually occurs in the center of the necrotic tumor debris within the ducts. As a result, the mammographic calcification pattern of this histology is commonly fine linear or branching. However, there is considerable mammographic overlap between the different DCIS subtypes, so histologic subtype cannot be mammographically predicted with great accuracy.

Suggested Reading

Hermann G, Keller RJ, Drossman S, et al. Mammographic pattern of microcalcifications in the preoperative diagnosis of comedo ductal carcinoma in situ: histopathologic correlation. Can Assoc Radiol J 1999;50:235–240

Stomper PC, Connolly JL. Ductal carcinoma in situ of the breast: correlation between mammographic calcification and tumor subtype. AJR Am J Roentgenol 1992;159:483–485

Case 19.3: Ductal Carcinoma in Situ

Case History
A 45-year-old woman presents for screening mammogram.

Physical Examination
- Normal exam

Mammogram

Calcifications (Fig. 19.5)
- Type: linear and branching pleomorphic/heterogeneous
- Distribution: segmental

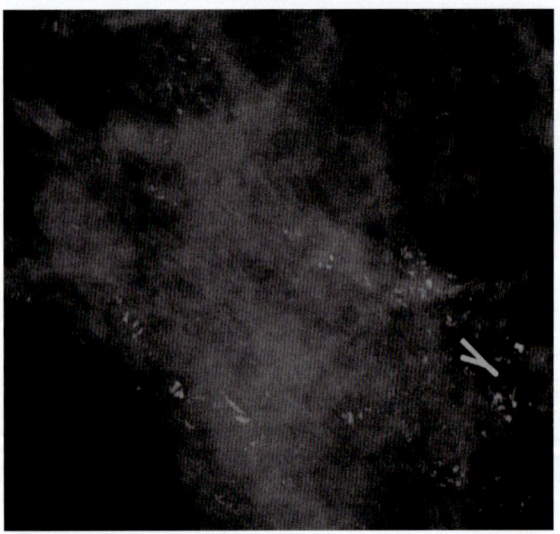
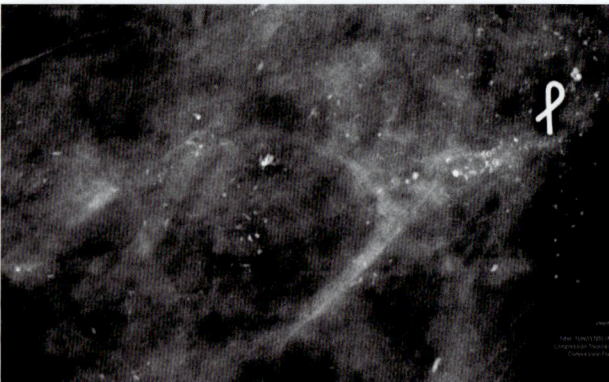

Fig. 19.5 In the left upper outer quadrant, there is segmental distribution of linear and branching pleomorphic calcifications. (**A**) Left ML magnification mammogram. (**B**) Left CC magnification mammogram.

Fine Linear/Branching Microcalcifications 295

Ultrasound

Frequency (Fig. 19.6)
- 14 MHz

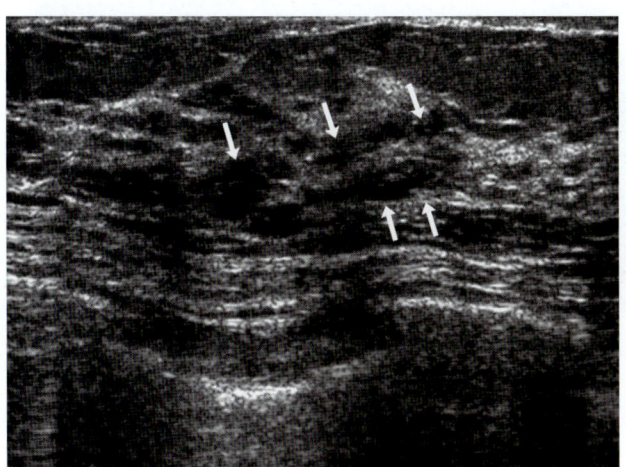
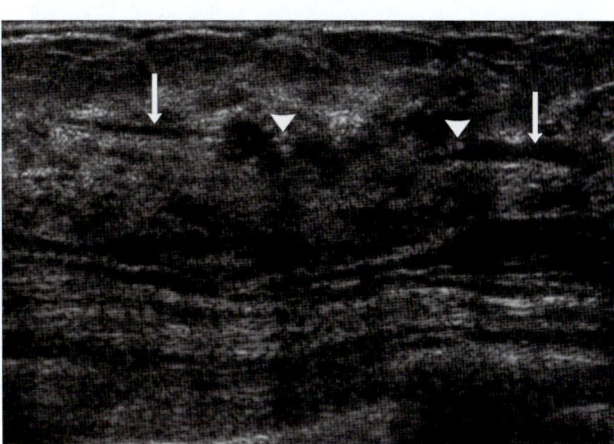
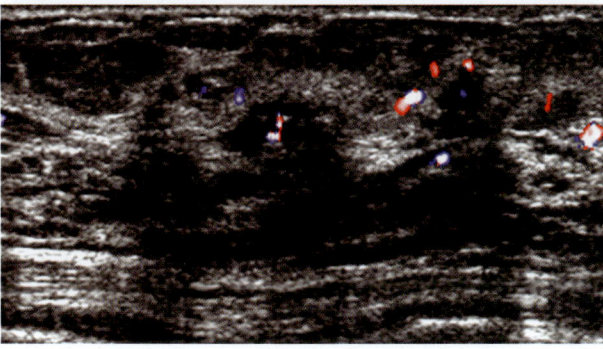

Fig. 19.6 Sonographic examination of the left upper outer quadrant demonstrates numerous diffusely dilated ducts (*arrows*) with focal dilatation containing punctate calcifications (*arrowheads*), which do not shadow. Color flow Doppler of this area is increased compared with other areas of the breast. (**A**) Left breast antiradial sonogram. (**B**) Left radial sonogram. (**C**) Left breast radial sonogram with color flow Doppler.

Other Modalities: MRI (Fig. 19.7)

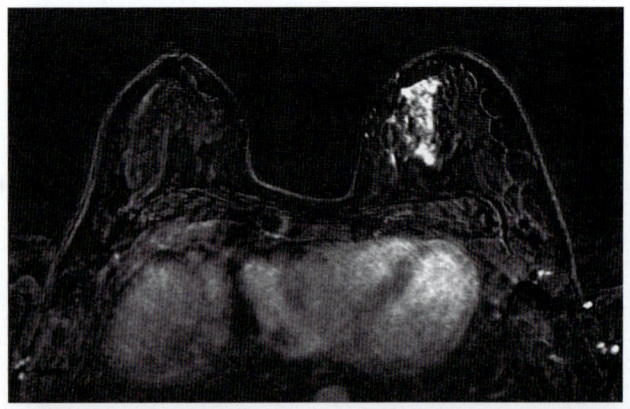
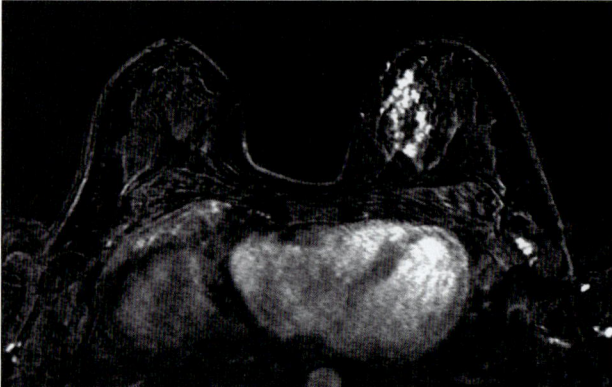
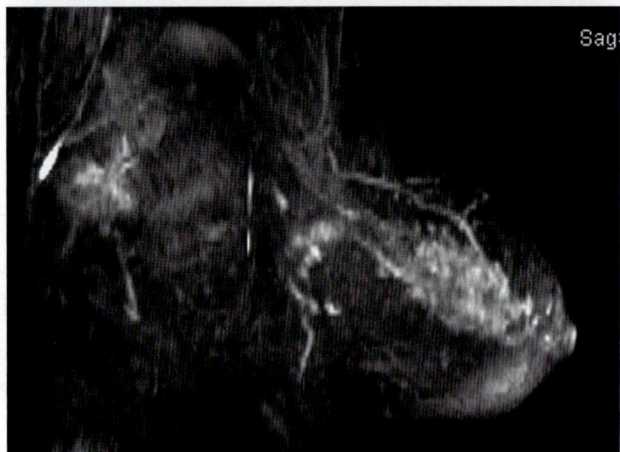

Fig. 19.7 Breast MRI shows segmental rapid enhancement of the upper outer quadrant. In most of the segment, the enhancement is homogeneous (**A**), but some of the enhancement has a clumped pattern (**B**). (**A**) Dynamic bolus T1-weighted 2-minute subtraction axial bilateral breast MRI. (**B**) Dynamic bolus T1-weighted 2-minute subtraction axial bilateral breast MRI 5 mm inferior to **A**. (**C**) Contrast-enhanced right breast MRI maximum projection intensity (MIP) image.

Pathology
- Mastectomy: invasive ductal carcinoma, grade 3, with extensive ductal carcinoma in situ

Management
- BI-RADS assessment category 5, highly suggestive of malignancy

Pearls and Pitfalls
- This is an example of a common sonographic presentation of ductal carcinoma in situ (DCIS). Unlike invasive malignancy, DCIS routinely does not appear as a sonographic mass. Instead, DCIS may appear as abnormal ducts. Abnormal ductal findings include intraductal mass, debris, calcifications, thickened wall, and focal or diffuse ectasia. Color Doppler is also commonly increased in areas of ductal carcinoma in situ compared with surrounding normal breast tissue. When cross-correlating sonography with MRI lesions, review the MRI to anticipate the sonographic findings. When the MRI lesion presents as non-mass enhancement, search for sonographic features of ductal carcinoma in situ.

Suggested Reading
Hashimoto BE. Sonographic assessment of breast calcifications. Curr Probl Diagn Radiol 2006;35:213–218

Hashimoto BE. Sonography of ductal carcinoma in situ. Ultrasound Clin 2007;1:631–643

Stavros TA. Malignant solid breast nodules: specific types. In: Stavros TA. Breast Ultrasound. Philadelphia: Lippincott Williams & Wilkins; 2004:597–688

Case 19.4: Ductal Carcinoma in Situ

Case History
A 42-year-old woman presents with left breast calcifications identified on screening mammogram.

Physical Examination
- Normal exam

Mammogram

Calcifications (Figs. 19.8 and 19.9)
- Type: fine linear/branching
- Distribution: segmental

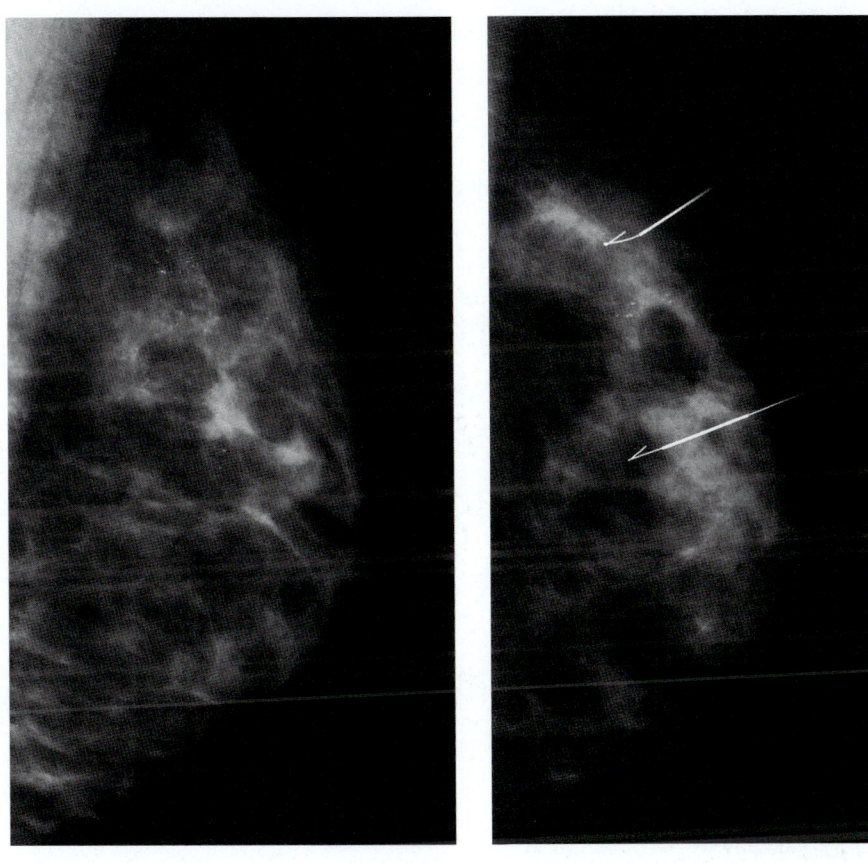

Fig. 19.8 In the upper outer left breast there are fine linear/branching calcifications. (**A**) Left ML mammogram. (**B**) Left CC mammogram.

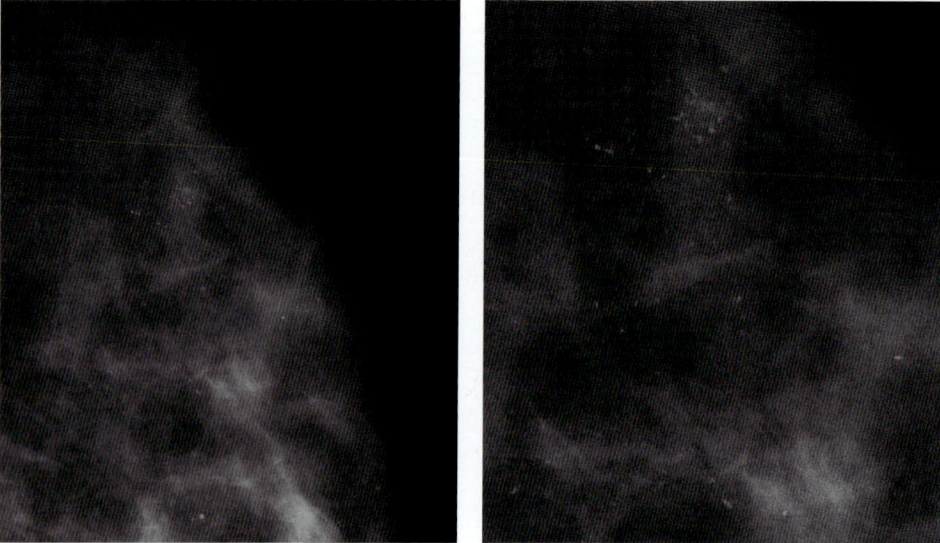

Fig. 19.9 Left ML magnification view mammogram. The calcifications form a linear/branching pattern.

Pathology
- Ductal carcinoma in situ
- High nuclear grade, solid to focal cribriform growth, with comedo-type necrosis and microcalcifications (**Fig. 19.10**)

Management
- BI-RADS assessment category 5, highly suggestive of malignancy

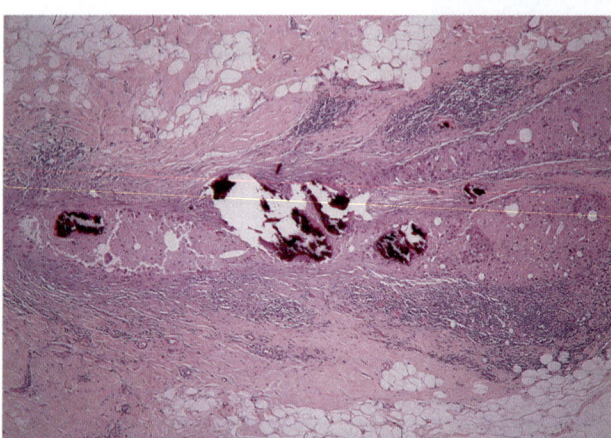

Fig. 19.10 This malignancy is associated with extensive intraductal calcifications. The intraductal location of these calcifications results in the mammographically visible linear pattern.

Pearls and Pitfalls

- About 75% of cases of DCIS appear as isolated mammographic calcifications. In 10%, both calcifications and a soft tissue mass are mammographically demonstrated, and in another 10% only a soft tissue mass is evident. In 5%, the DCIS is incidentally discovered adjacent to a benign mammographic lesion.

Suggested Reading

Stomper PC, Connolly JL, Meyer JE, Harris JR. Clinically occult ductal carcinoma in situ detected with mammography: analysis of 100 cases with radiologic-pathologic correlation. Radiology 1989;172:235–241

Stomper PC, Margolin FR. Ductal carcinoma in situ: the mammographer's perspective. AJR Am J Roentgenol 1994;162:585–591

Case 19.5: Invasive Ductal Carcinoma

Case History
A 43-year-old woman presents with left breast calcifications identified on screening mammogram.

Physical Examination
- Normal exam

Mammogram

Calcifications (Fig. 19.11)
- Type: fine linear/branching
- Distribution: segmental

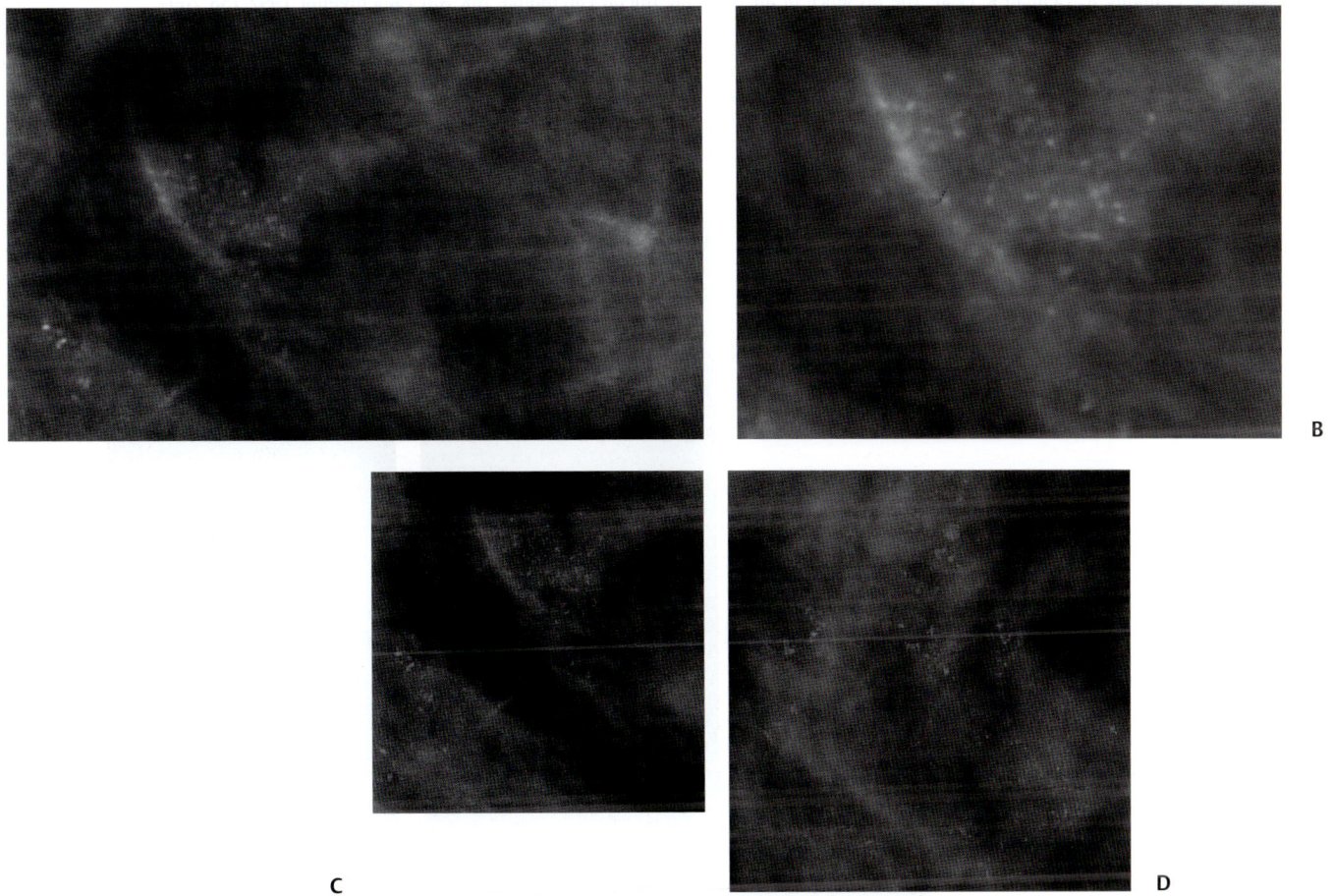

Fig. 19.11 In the left outer inferior breast, there are numerous clusters of heterogeneous linear-shaped calcifications. (**A**) Left MLO magnification view. (**C**) Left exaggerated CC magnification view. (**B**) and (**D**) are enlargements of calcifications in **A** and **C**.

Pathology
- Invasive ductal carcinoma with a predominant intraductal component

Management
- BI-RADS assessment category 5, highly suggestive of malignancy

Ultrasound

Frequency
- 7.5 MHz

Mass (Figs. 19.13 and 19.14)
- Margin: ill defined
- Echogenicity: hypoechoic
- Retrotumoral acoustic appearance: increased acoustic transmission
- Shape: irregular

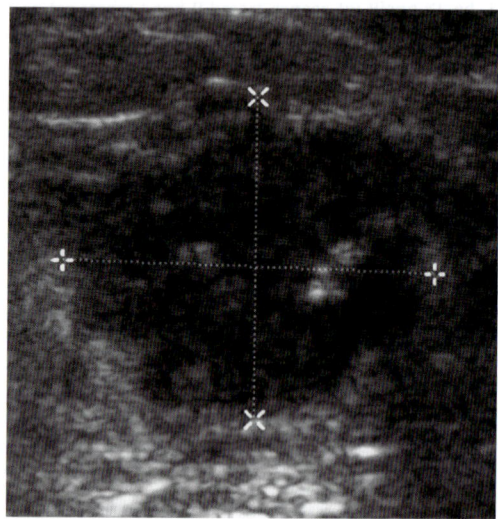

Fig. 19.13 Right radial breast sonogram. The palpable lump located within the segment of abnormal calcifications identified in **Fig. 19.9** corresponds to an ill-defined, hypoechoic solid mass with calcifications.

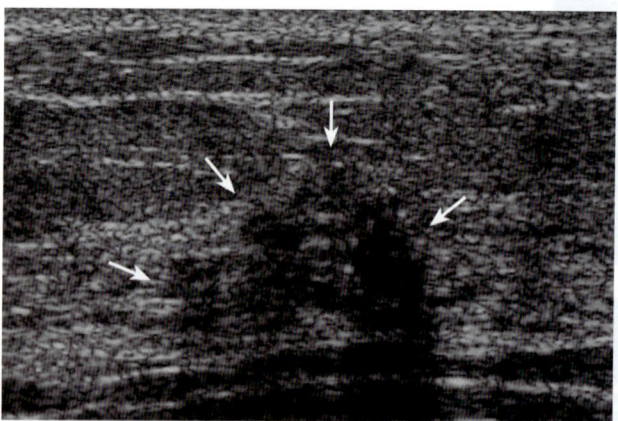

Fig. 19.14 Right radial breast sonogram. After chemotherapy, the hypoechoic mass (*arrows*) shrank from 18 to 12 mm and was no longer palpable.

Other Modalities: Breast Sestamibi Scans (Figs. 19.15 and 19.16)

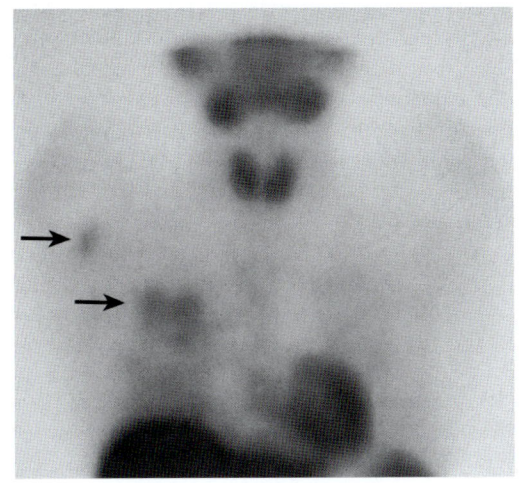

Fig. 19.15 Breast sestamibi scan prior to preoperative chemotherapy demonstrates abnormal activity consistent with a primary right breast malignancy associated with metastatic adenopathy (*arrows*). (**A**) Breast sestamibi scan. Right anteroposterior position. (**B**) Breast sestamibi scan. Right lateral position.

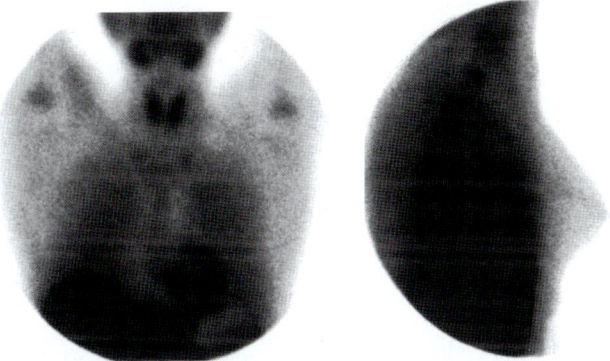

Fig. 19.16 Breast sestamibi scan performed after preoperative chemotherapy shows that the abnormal activity in the right breast and axilla has resolved. (**A**) Breast sestamibi scan. Anteroposterior position. (**B**) Breast sestamibi scan. Right lateral position.

Pathology
Invasive ductal carcinoma with a predominant intraductal component. Mastectomy specimen obtained after chemotherapy demonstrated extensive fibrosis with residual ductal carcinoma in situ measuring 3 × 2.5 cm with 1 mm focus of infiltrating ductal carcinoma. Four axillary nodes were negative.

Management
- BI-RADS assessment category 5, highly suggestive of malignancy

Pearls and Pitfalls

- In patients undergoing preoperative chemotherapy, clinical and mammographic information is in agreement in 79% of cases. In this case they were discordant, but the mammographic information reflected the pathologic findings more accurately.
- Technetium-labeled sestamibi imaging is useful in following these patients. This technique has a sensitivity of 92%, specificity of 89%, positive predictive value of 81%, and negative predictive value of 96%. However, false-negative findings increase with malignancies < 1 cm. Metastatic lymph nodes can be detected with a sensitivity of 84% and specificity of 91%.
- Some studies have shown that the sonographic tumor size correlates closer to the pathologic size and that sonography correlates better with tumor shrinkage than mammography.

Suggested Reading

Fornage BD, Toubas O, Morel M. Clinical, mammographic, and sonographic determination of preoperative breast cancer size. Cancer 1987;60:765–771

Khalkhali I, Cutrone JA, Mena IG, et al. Scintimammography: the complementary role of Tc-99m sestamibi prone breast imaging for the diagnosis of breast carcinoma. Radiology 1995;196:421–426

Moskovic EC, Mansi JL, King DM, Murch CR, Smith IE. Mammography in the assessment of response to medical treatment of large primary breast cancer. Clin Radiol 1993;47:339–344

Powles TJ, Hickish TF, Makris A, et al. Randomized trial of chemoendocrine therapy started before or after surgery for treatment of primary breast cancer. J Clin Oncol 1995;13:547–552

Taillefer R, Robidoux A, Lambert R, Turpin S, Laperrière J. Technetium-99m-sestamibi prone scintimammography to detect primary breast cancer and axillary lymph node involvement. J Nucl Med 1995;36:1758–1765

Asymmetry

This is a schematic diagram of the diagnostic approach to mammographic increased density. For further discussion, see Chapter 1.

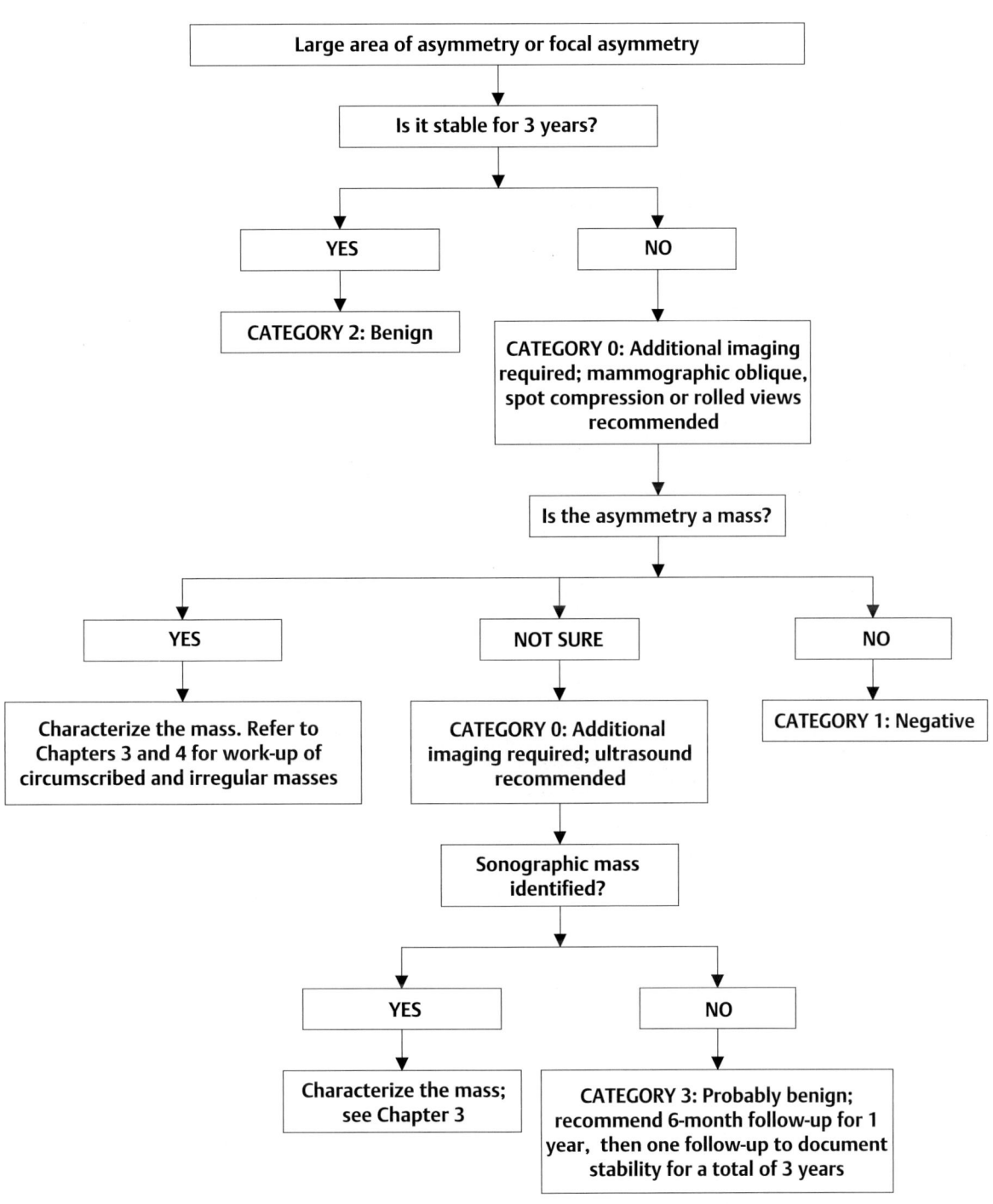

20 Global Asymmetry

Case 20.1: Lymphedema

Case History

An 84-year-old woman presents 2 years after left axillary dissection for left arm melanoma and right lumpectomy for breast cancer.

Physical Examination
- Right breast: well-healed scar in the upper outer breast
- Left breast: diffuse swelling without redness

Mammogram
- Global asymmetry (**Fig. 20.1**)

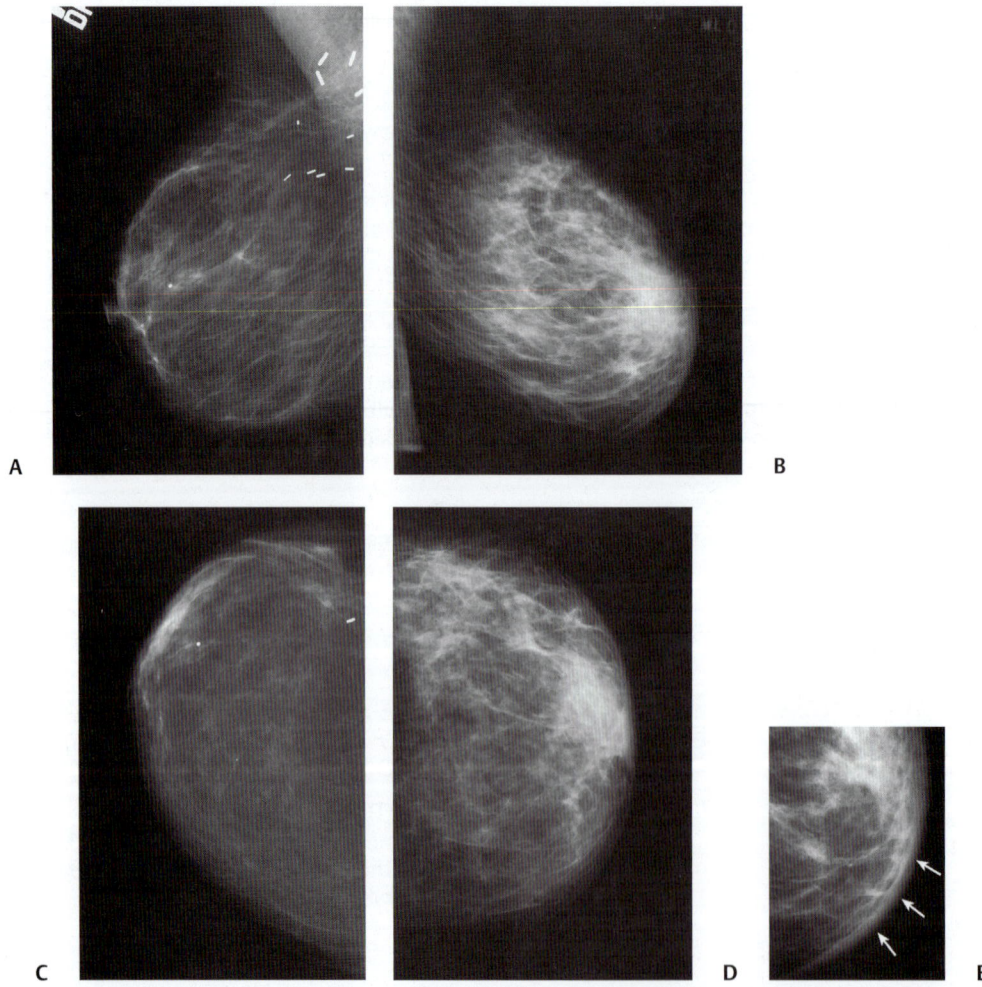

Fig. 20.1 The left breast exhibits diffuse increased density with skin thickening (skin thickening highlighted by *arrows* in (**E**)). Clips in the right upper outer quadrant are from a previous lumpectomy. (**A**) Right MLO mammogram. (**B**) Left MLO mammogram. (**C**) Right CC mammogram. (**D**) Left CC mammogram. (**E**) Left MLO mammogram (close-up).

Pathology
- Lymphedema

Management
- BI-RADS assessment category 2, benign finding

Pearls and Pitfalls

- Lymphedema is due to five main etiologies: (1) obstruction of axillary nodes (due to either malignant involvement or surgical removal of nodes), (2) general lymphatic obstruction from contralateral breast cancer, (3) inflammation, (4) postradiation effect, and (5) systemic fluid overload (e.g., from congestive heart failure or renal failure). In this case, the patient's lymphedema resulted from an axillary dissection performed for melanoma staging.

Suggested Reading
Tabar L, Dean PB. Thickened skin syndrome of the breast. In: Tabar L, Dean PB. Teaching Atlas of Mammography. 3rd ed. New York: Thieme; 2001:239–247

Asymmetry

Case 20.2: Mastitis

Case History
Two weeks after a normal vaginal delivery, this 34-year-old woman develops severe left breast pain and erythema. Clinically, she appears to have mastitis and is started on antibiotics.

Physical Examination
- Left breast: diffusely tender and erythematous
- Right breast: normal exam

Mammogram
- Global asymmetry (**Figs. 20.2** and **20.3**)

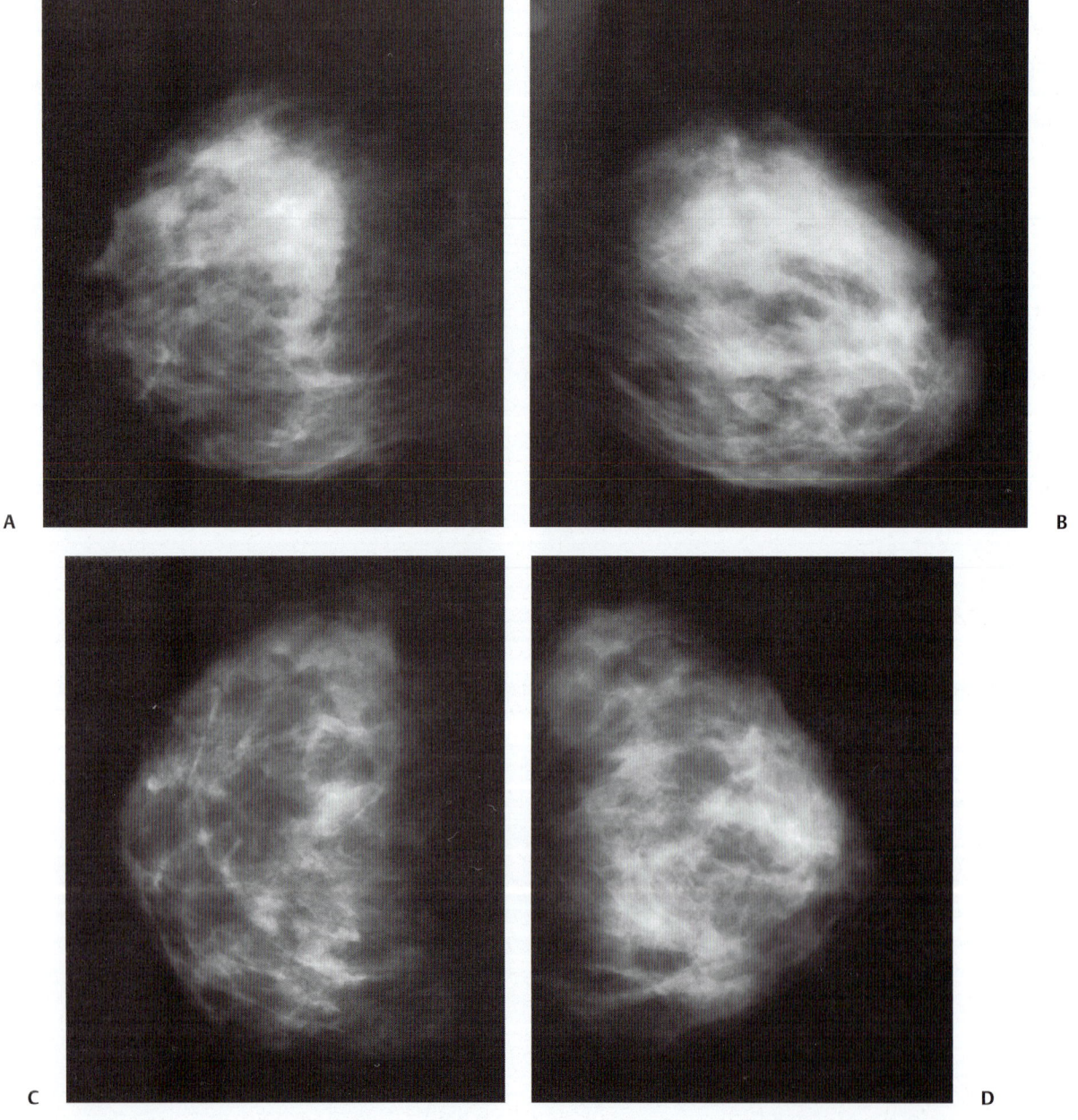

Fig. 20.2 Although both breasts exhibit diffuse increased density, the left breast is slightly more dense than the right breast. (**A**) Right MLO mammogram. (**B**) Left MLO mammogram. (**C**) Right CC mammogram. (**D**) Left CC mammogram.

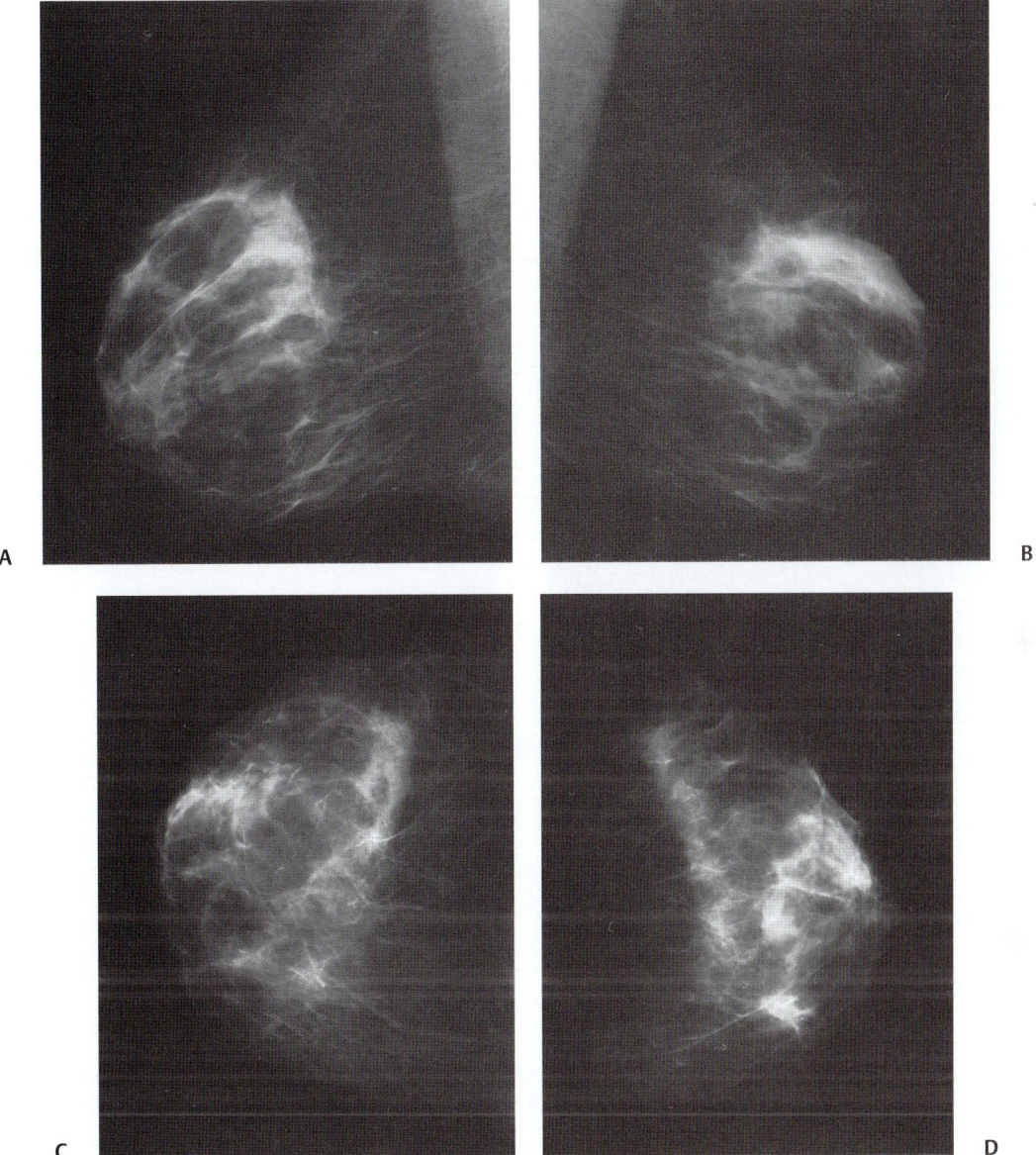

Fig. 20.3 Nine months after the examination in Fig. 20.2, bilateral mammograms demonstrate a reduction in the overall density. (A) Right MLO mammogram. (B) Left MLO mammogram. (C) Right CC mammogram. (D) Left CC mammogram.

Ultrasound

Frequency
- 7.5 MHz (**Fig. 20.4**)

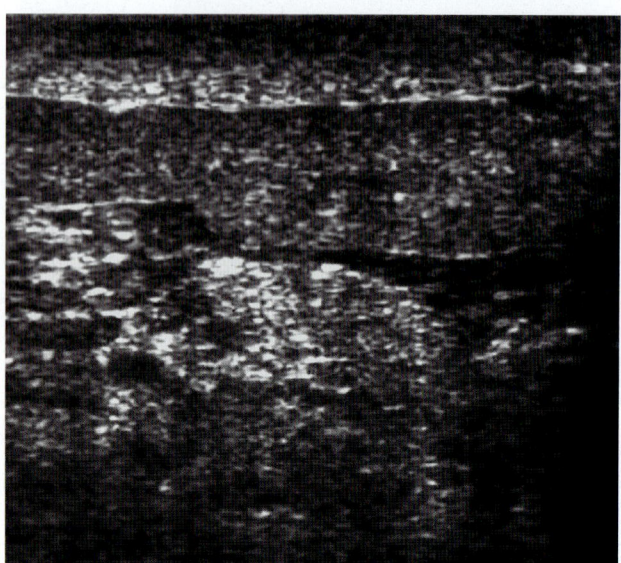

Fig. 20.4 Left radial breast sonogram. Sonography is performed at the same time as the mammograms in **Fig. 20.2** to identify a possible abscess. No abscess is identified. There is skin thickening and multiple linear fluid collections throughout the parenchyma.

Pathology
- Mastitis

Management
- BI-RADS assessment category 3, probably benign; short-interval follow-up

Pearls and Pitfalls

- This case illustrates bilateral global asymmetry due to prominent postpartum glandular tissue. The slight left global asymmetry is due to mastitis.
- Sonographically, mastitis produces thickening of the skin, subcutaneous fat, and glandular tissue. The interface between the fat and glandular tissue is indistinct. Numerous thin, linear fluid collections are present. With progression of inflammation, an abscess may form. Abscesses are generally hypoechoic round or oval masses. The margins may be either smooth or irregular. Commonly, abscesses contain solid material, septations, or movable internal echoes. Sonography is useful to identify and drain abscesses.

Suggested Reading

Heywang-Kobrunner SH, Schreer I, Dershaw DD. Diagnostic Breast Imaging. New York: Thieme; 1997:194–201

Tohno D, Cosgrove DO, Sloane JP, eds. Ultrasound Diagnosis of Breast Diseases. New York: Churchill Livingstone; 1994:136–138

Case 20.3: Inflammatory Carcinoma

Case History
A 63-year-old woman presents with right breast swelling.

Physical Examination
- Right breast: mild diffuse erythema and peau d'orange; no focal palpable mass
- Left breast: normal exam

Mammogram
- Global asymmetry (**Fig. 20.5**)

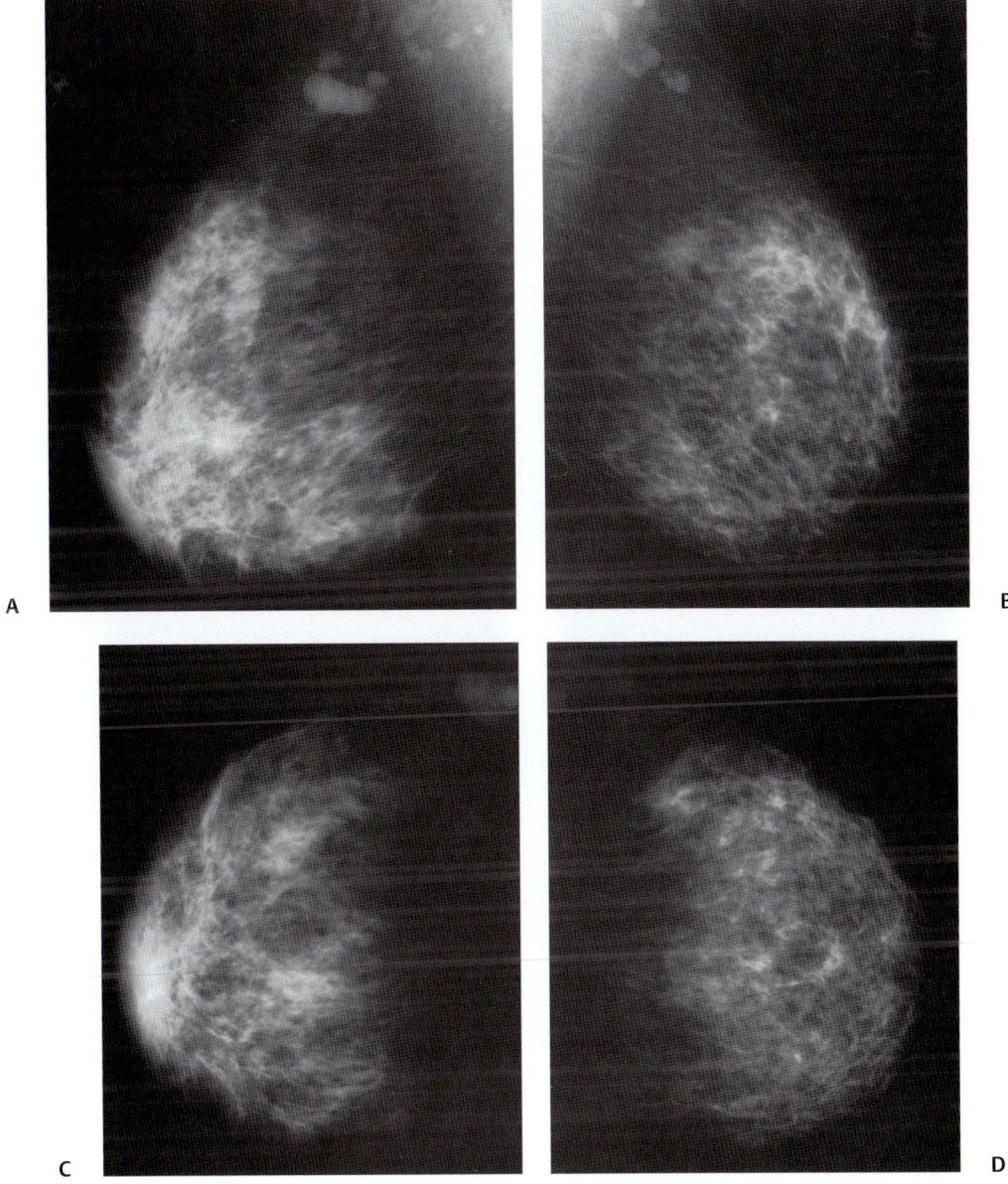

Fig. 20.5 The right breast exhibits global asymmetry, trabecular thickening, and periareolar skin thickening. Multiple enlarged right axillary nodes are present. (**A**) Right MLO mammogram. (**B**) Left MLO mammogram. (**C**) Right CC mammogram. (**D**) Left CC mammogram.

Pathology
- Infiltrating ductal carcinoma. The patient was treated with chemotherapy prior to mastectomy. Residual tumor was 1.5 cm. No dermal lymphatic invasion was present, but lack of involvement may be due to tumor response to chemotherapy. Six of 14 axillary nodes had metastatic disease.

Management
- BI-RADS assessment category 5, highly suggestive of malignancy

Pearls and Pitfalls
- The definition of inflammatory carcinoma is mildly controversial. Some have defined this entity clinically (i.e., skin erythema, edema, and warmth), and others insist on microscopic confirmation of metastatic involvement of the dermal lymphatics. Some patients do not fit these criteria. Only 80% of women with skin changes have dermal lymphatic involvement, and 4% with dermal lymphatic tumor do not have skin abnormalities.

Suggested Reading
Cardenosa G. Breast Imaging Companion. Philadelphia: Lippincott-Raven; 1997:166–167

Case 20.4: Estrogen Effect

Case History
A 74-year-old woman presents for screening mammogram.

Physical Examination
- Normal exam

Mammogram
- Global asymmetry (**Figs. 20.6** and **20.7**)

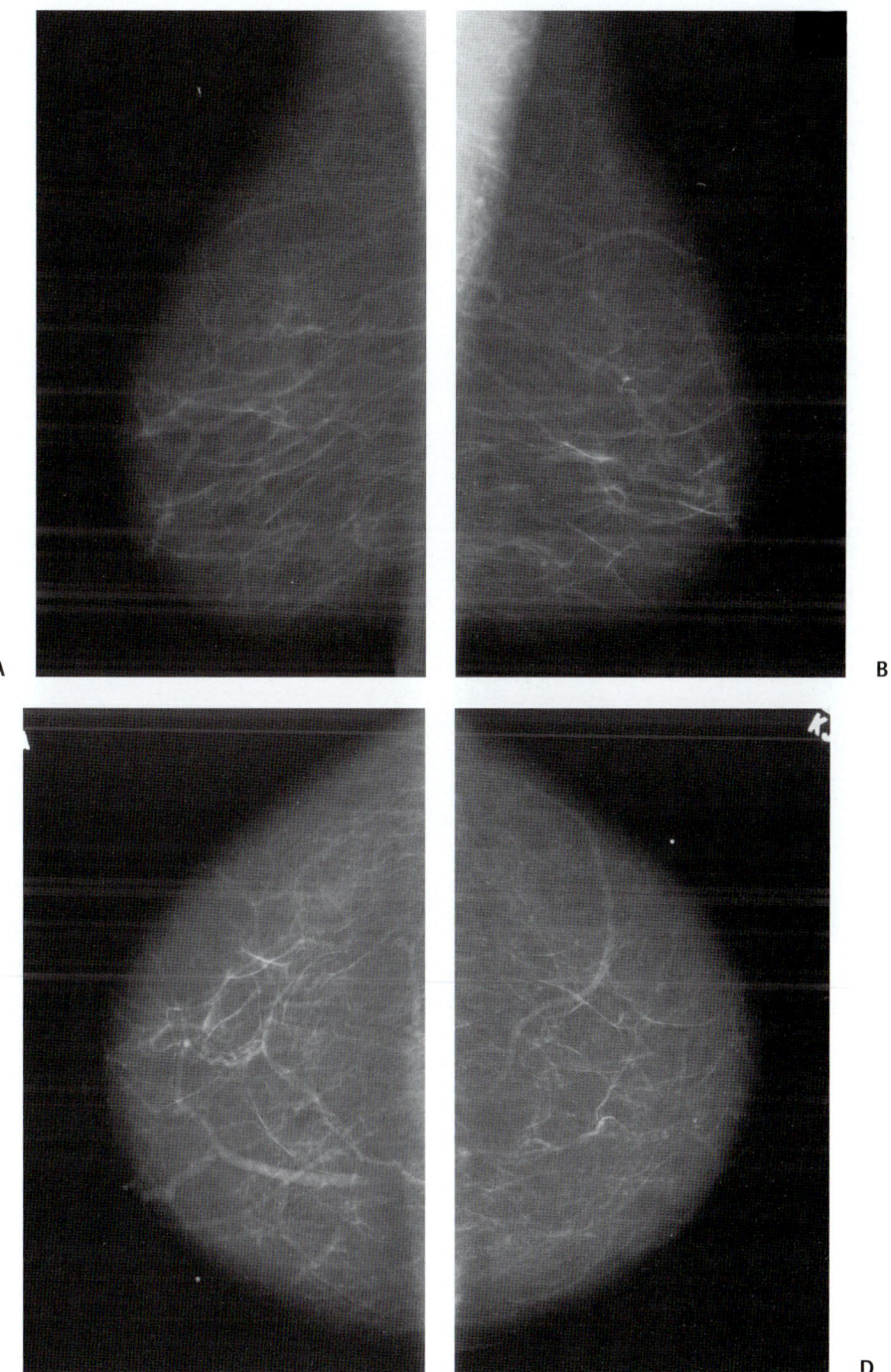

Fig. 20.6 Normal fatty breast pattern. (**A**) Right MLO mammogram. (**B**) Left MLO mammogram. (**C**) Right CC mammogram. (**D**) Left CC mammogram.

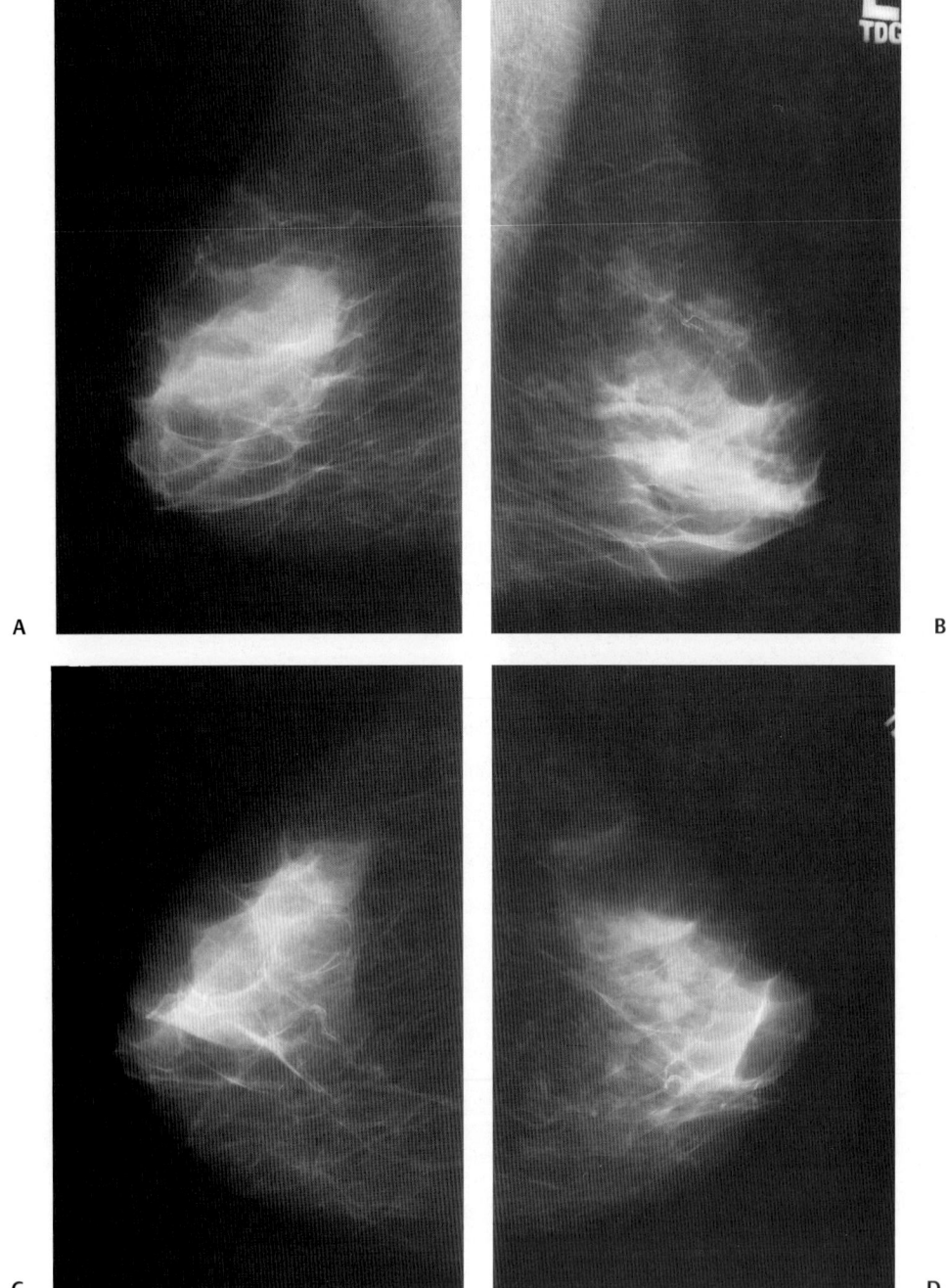

Fig. 20.7 This bilateral mammographic examination was performed 2 years later on the same patient as in **Fig. 20.6**. (**A**) Right MLO mammogram. (**B**) Left MLO mammogram. (**C**) Right CC mammogram. (**D**) Left CC mammogram.

Pathology
- Normal breast tissue

Management
- BI-RADS assessment category 1, negative

Pearls and Pitfalls

- The patient started hormone replacement therapy (HRT) just after the earlier mammographic examination (**Fig. 20.6**). Studies have shown that approximately 24% of women develop increased mammographic density after starting HRT. Estrogen stimulates growth of ductal epithelium and periductal connective tissue. Although progesterone is an antagonist to these proliferative effects, progesterone enhances the effect of estrogen by encouraging distal ductal development.
- Besides causing diffuse increased density, HRT causes asymmetric densities and cystic formation.

Suggested Reading

Cyrlak D, Wong CH. Mammographic changes in postmenopausal women undergoing hormonal replacement therapy. AJR Am J Roentgenol 1993;161:1177–1183

Laya MB, Gallagher JC, Schreiman JS, Larson EB, Watson P, Weinstein L. Effect of postmenopausal hormonal replacement therapy on mammographic density and parenchymal pattern. Radiology 1995;196:433–437

McNicholas MMJ, Heneghan JP, Milner MH, Tunney T, Hourihane JB, MacErlaine DP. Pain and increased mammographic density in women receiving hormone replacement therapy: a prospective study. AJR Am J Roentgenol 1994;163:311–315

Stomper PC, Van Voorhis BJ, Ravnikar VA, Meyer JE. Mammographic changes associated with postmenopausal hormone replacement therapy: a longitudinal study. Radiology 1990;174:487–490

Case 20.5: Fat Necrosis

Case History
A 70-year-old woman, who sustained severe right breast injury during a fall 1 year ago, presents with a right breast lump in the area of the previous trauma.

Physical Examination
- Right breast: palpable lump in the upper outer quadrant
- Left breast: normal exam

Mammogram
- Global asymmetry (**Figs. 20.8** and **20.9**)

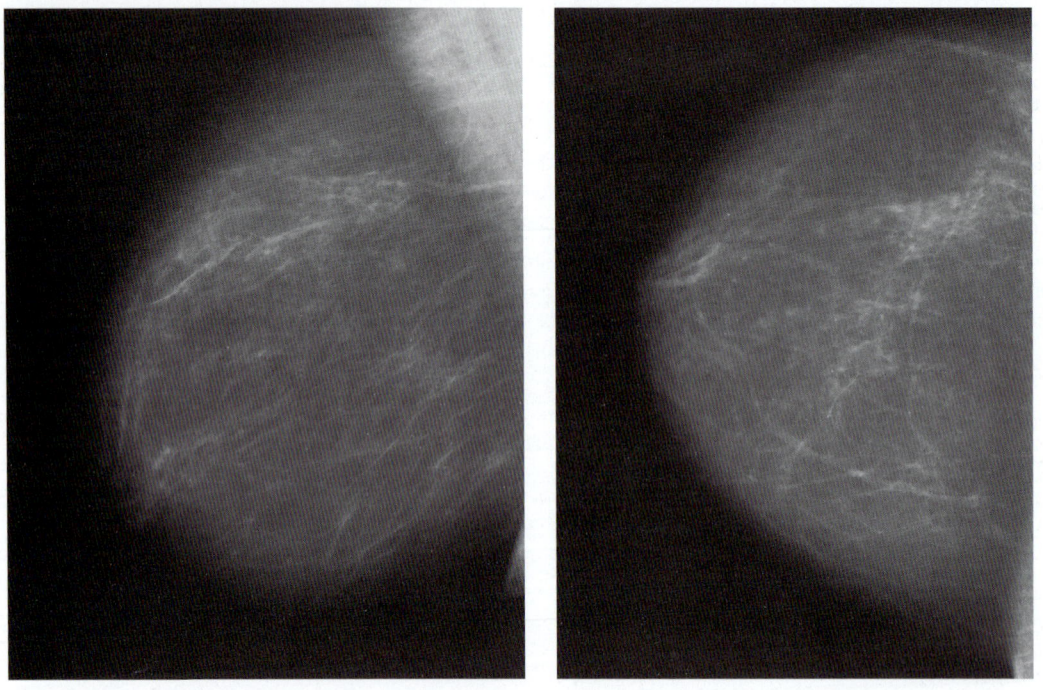

Fig. 20.8 Prior to the injury, the patient's right breast mammogram was normal. (**A**) Right MLO mammogram. (**B**) Right CC mammogram.

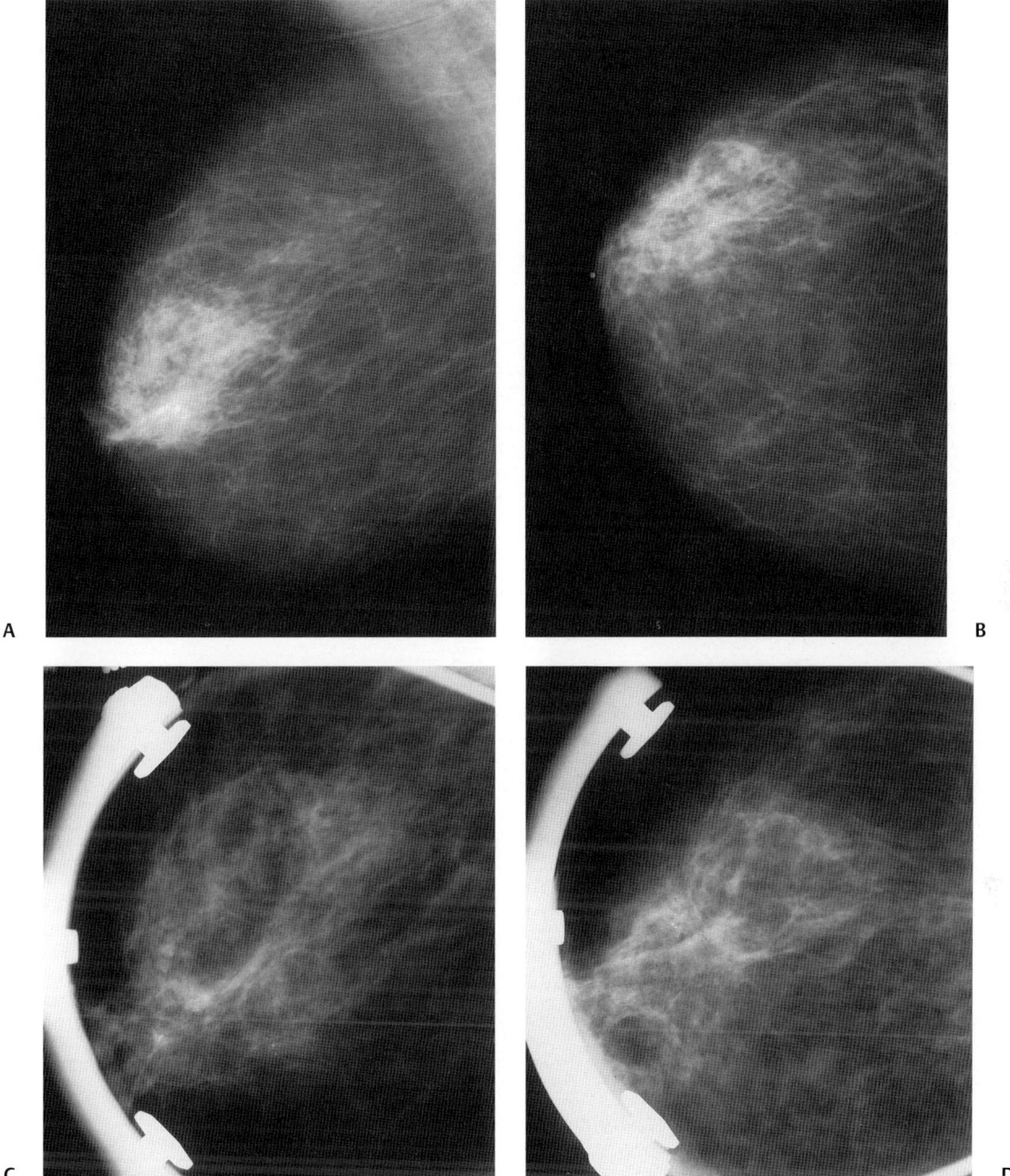

Fig. 20.9 One year after the injury, there is a new global asymmetry which is most pronounced in the right upper outer quadrant. (**A**) Right MLO mammogram. (**B**) Right CC mammogram. (**C**) Right MLO spot compression. (**D**) Right CC spot compression.

Ultrasound

Frequency
- 8 MHz

Mass (Fig. 20.10)
- Margin: ill defined
- Echogenicity: hypoechoic
- Retrotumoral acoustic appearance: posterior shadowing distal to mass
- Shape: irregular

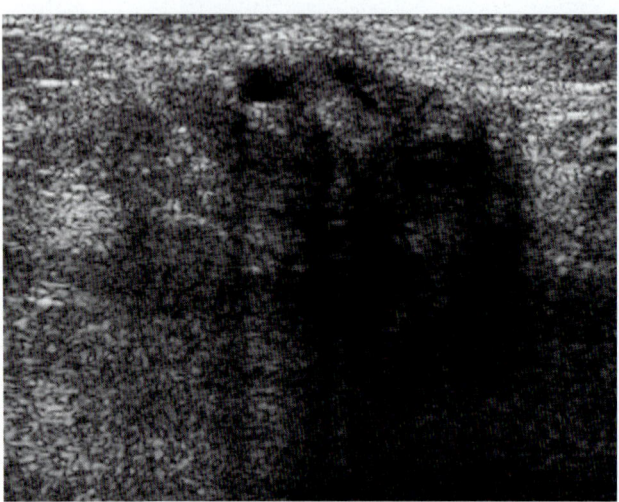

Fig. 20.10 Right radial breast sonogram. In the right upper outer quadrant, the palpable mass corresponds to an irregular hypoechoic mass. This mass corresponds to the mammographic global asymmetry.

Pathology
- Fat necrosis

Management
- BI-RADS assessment category 4, suspicious; biopsy should be considered.

Pearls and Pitfalls

- Trauma (such as this case), infection or inflammation, HRT, and malignancy produce large areas of increased mammographic density.
- In cases of infection or trauma, sonographic examination is useful to identify abscess or hematoma.
- If the asymmetric density is stable for longer than 3 years, recommend routine mammographic screening. For densities that have been stable for 1 to 3 years, proceed with short-term follow-up. For new asymmetries or those increasing in size or density, biopsy is recommended.

Suggested Reading

Heywang-Kobrunner SH, Schreer I, Dershaw DD. Diagnostic Breast Imaging. New York: Thieme, 1997:353–357

Case 20.6: Malignant Disease

Case History
A 65-year-old woman presents with a left breast lump. This is her first mammographic examination.

Physical Examination
- Left breast: 10 cm hard mass in the superior breast
- Right breast: normal exam

Mammogram
- Global asymmetry (**Fig. 20.11**)

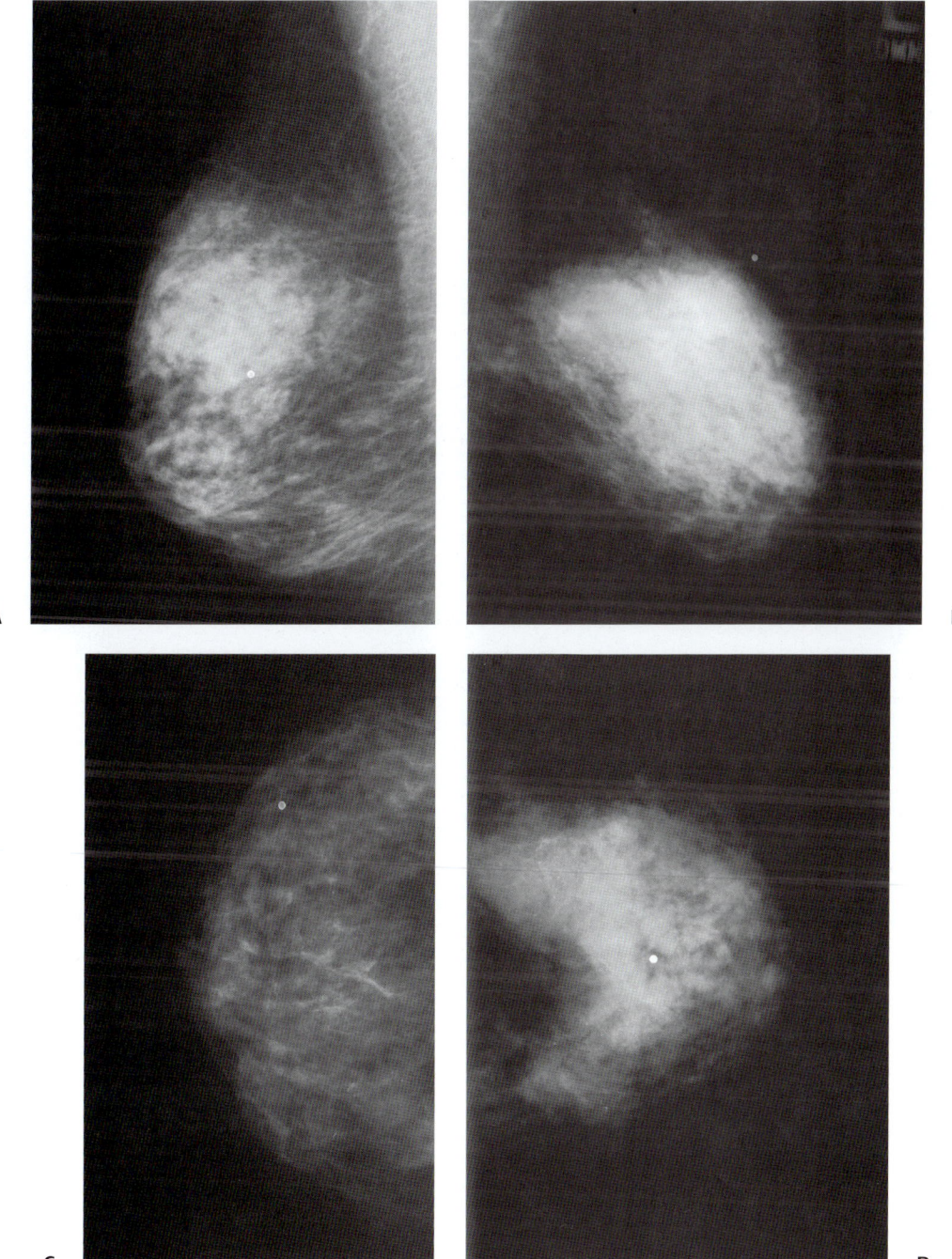

Fig. 20.11 There is global asymmetry in the left upper breast, which is associated with a palpable mass (palpable mass marked with a radiopaque marker). (**A**) Right MLO mammogram. (**B**) Left MLO mammogram. (**C**) Right CC mammogram. (**D**) Left CC mammogram.

Pathology
- Ductal carcinoma in situ with small area of invasion. The left mastectomy specimen demonstrated a 9 cm mass that predominantly consisted of ductal carcinoma in situ of low to intermediate grade. Only 0.1 cm of infiltrating ductal carcinoma was identified within the mass.

Management
- BI-RADS assessment category 5, highly suggestive of malignancy

Pearls and Pitfalls
- This case differs from inflammatory carcinoma because the patient did not have any skin changes. Any large malignancy may produce an increase in mammographic density. Besides ductal carcinoma in situ or infiltrating ductal carcinoma, invasive lobular carcinoma may also cause generalized increased breast density.

Suggested Reading
Harvey JA, Fechner RE, Moore MM. Apparent ipsilateral decrease in breast size at mammography: a sign of infiltrating lobular carcinoma. Radiology 2000;214:883–889

Case 20.7: Malignant Disease

Case History
A 36-year-old woman felt two left breast lumps. Histology from biopsy of both lumps was infiltrating ductal carcinoma. The patient's mammograms were interpreted as normal, and the surgeon recommended a lumpectomy. The patient was seen at our institution for a second opinion.

Physical Examination
- Left breast: two healing biopsy incisions at the 1:30 position on the clock, approximately 5 cm apart; no other palpable masses
- Right breast: normal exam

Mammogram
- Global asymmetry (**Fig. 20.12**)

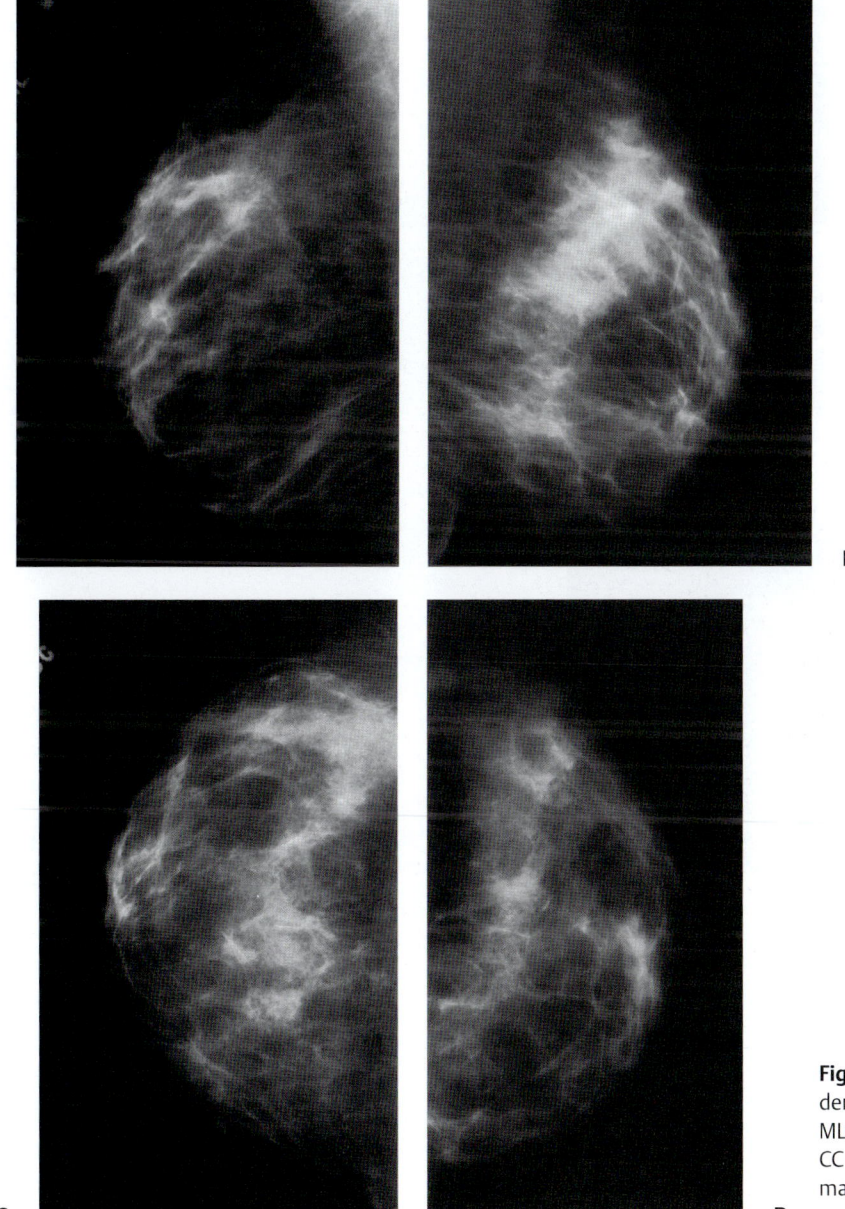

Fig. 20.12 There is a band of asymmetric increased density in the posterior third of the left breast on the MLO view. This asymmetry is not evident on the left CC view. (**A**) Right MLO mammogram. (**B**) Left MLO mammogram. (**C**) Right CC mammogram. (**D**) Left CC mammogram.

Ultrasound

Frequency
- 10 MHz

Mass (Figs. 20.13 and 20.14)
- Margin: ill defined
- Echogenicity: hypoechoic
- Retrotumoral acoustic appearance: bilateral edge shadowing
- Shape: irregular

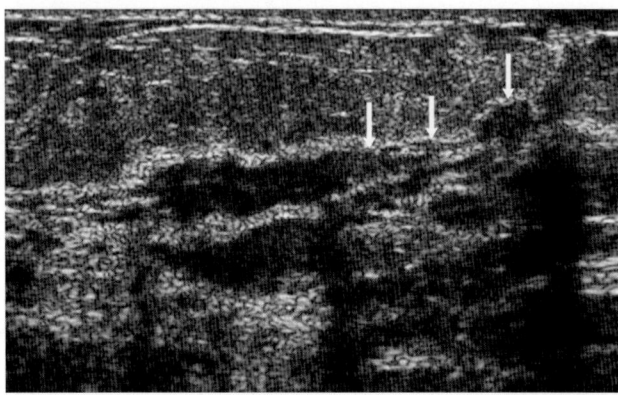

Fig. 20.13 Left radial breast sonogram at the 1:30 clock position. Sonographically, the patient had numerous (too many to count) masses between the 12 o'clock and 5 o'clock positions of the left breast. These masses had a variety of appearances. At the 1:30 position (area of original palpable lumps), there is a large hypoechoic mass that was responsible for both lumps. The mass exhibited ductal extension toward the nipple (*arrows*).

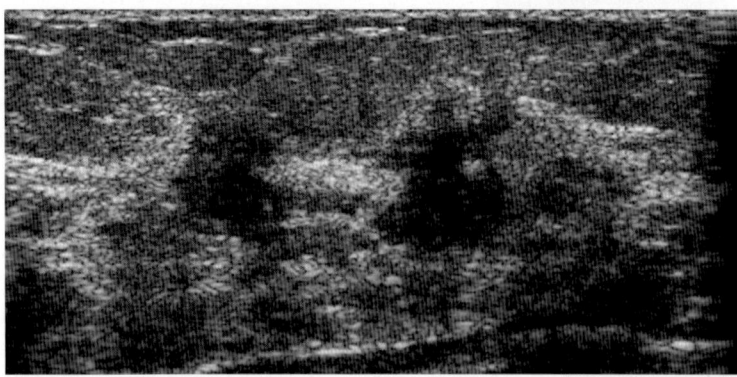

Fig. 20.14 Left radial breast sonogram at the 3 o'clock position. In this area, there is a series of spiculated masses that follow the ductal system.

Other Modalities: MRI (Fig. 20.15)

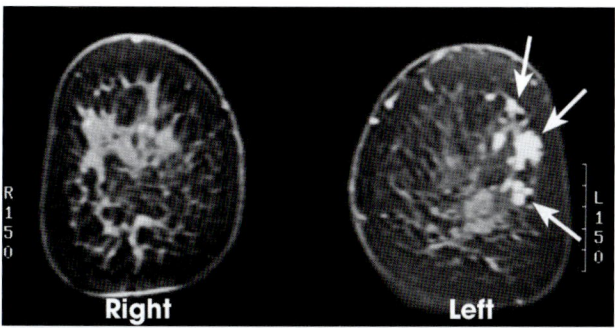

Fig. 20.15 Bilateral coronal dynamic bolus three-dimensional volume gradient breast MRI. There is abnormal contrast enhancement in the left breast (*arrows*), indicating extensive neoplastic involvement.

Pathology
- Invasive ductal carcinoma with a predominant intraductal component. The mastectomy specimen demonstrated multifocal infiltrating ductal carcinoma with 40% in situ carcinoma. Over 10 nodules were identified during gross inspection.

Management
- BI-RADS assessment category 5, highly suggestive of malignancy

Pearls and Pitfalls
- In cases where multicentric neoplasm is suspected and there are no discrete mammographic masses or abnormal calcifications, sonography and MRI are useful methods to identify multiple malignant foci. Therefore, the mammographic assessment in this case would be category 0. The final assessment of imaging for this case (category 5) is based on the sonographic and MRI findings. Findings from either of these modalities and the clinical information should lead to the conclusion that the patient has multicentric disease. Although most cases of multicentric disease are treated with mastectomy, in certain cases a partial mastectomy may be preferred. MRI provides a better global image for surgical planning. However, sonography is useful for biopsy and needle localization guidance.

Suggested Reading

Berg WA, Gilbreath PL. Multicentric and multifocal cancer: whole-breast US in preoperative evaluation. Radiology 2000;214:59–66

Heywang-Kobrunner SH, Schreer I, Dershaw DD. Diagnostic Breast Imaging. New York: Thieme; 1997:224–225

Rosenblatt R, Fineberg SA, Sparano JA, Kaleya RN. Stereotactic core needle biopsy of multiple sites in the breast: efficacy and effect on patient care. Radiology 1996;201:67–70

Case 21.2: Lobular Carcinoma

Case History
A 51-year-old woman presents for screening mammogram.

Physical Examination
- Left breast: ill-defined, firm area in left upper outer breast
- Right breast: normal exam

Mammogram
- Focal asymmetry (**Figs. 21.3** and **21.4**)

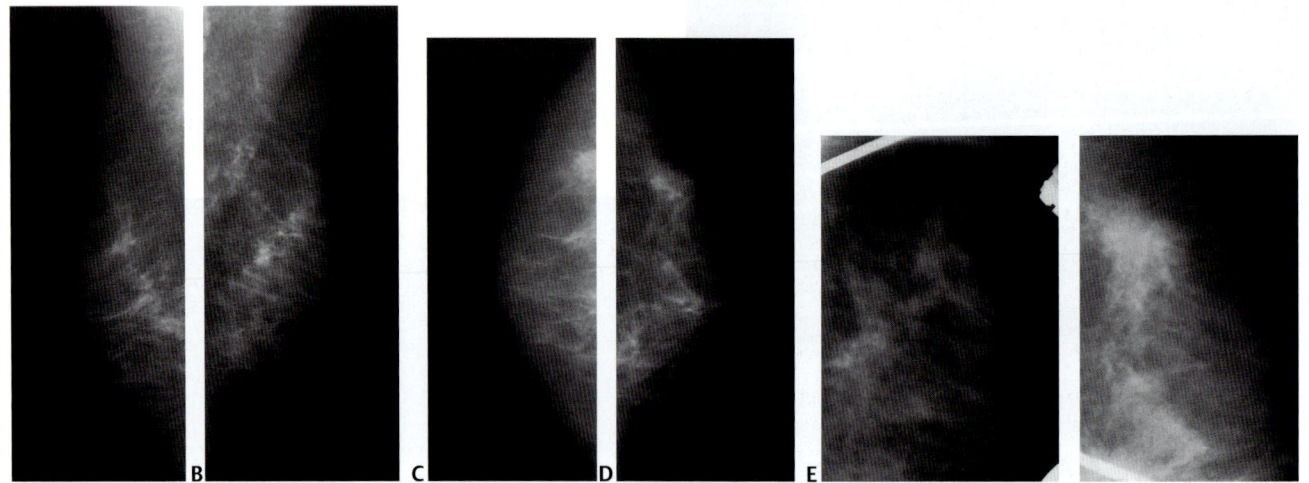

Fig. 21.3 There is a focal asymmetric density in the left outer breast visible only on the CC views. (**A**) Right MLO mammogram. (**B**) Left MLO mammogram. (**C**) Right CC mammogram. (**D**) Left CC mammogram. (**E**) Left MLO spot compression mammogram. (**F**) Left CC spot compression mammogram.

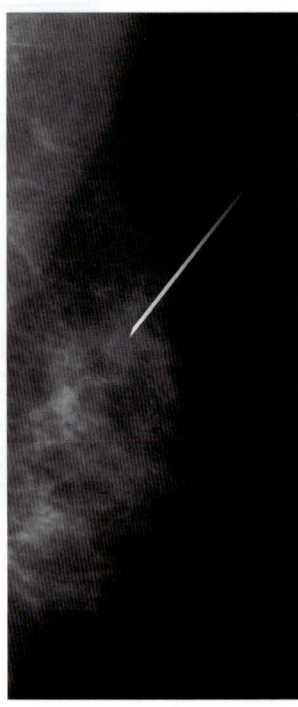

Fig. 21.4 Left MLO after sonographically guided needle localization. This mammogram illustrates that the mass is not visible in this view even when the location of the mass is marked with a needle.

Ultrasound

Frequency
- 7 MHz

Mass (Fig. 21.5)
- Margin: spiculation/architectural distortion
- Echogenicity: heterogeneous (mixed)
- Retrotumoral acoustic appearance: posterior shadowing distal to mass
- Shape: irregular

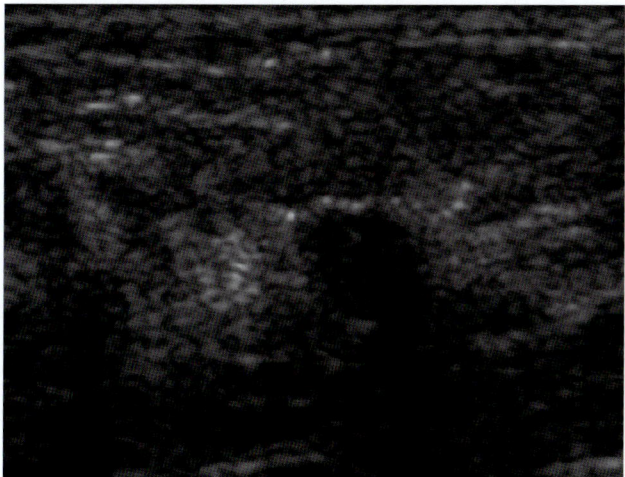

Fig. 21.5 Left breast longitudinal sonogram. At the 3 o'clock position, there is a spiculated irregular mass with heterogeneous echogenicity and posterior acoustic shadowing. This mass corresponds to the mammographic density.

Pathology
- Invasive lobular carcinoma

Management
- BI-RADS assessment category 4, suspicious abnormality; biopsy should be considered.

Pearls and Pitfalls

- Lobular carcinoma is sometimes difficult to identify mammographically because it may appear as an asymmetric density that is visible on only one view. To localize this abnormality, shallow mammographic obliques may be more useful than spot compression views. Lobular carcinoma is commonly easily compressible and may blend into the surrounding parenchymal density.
- Ultrasound is useful to localize suspicious mammographic densities that are visible only on one view.

Suggested Reading

Butler RS, Venta LA, Wiley EL, Ellis RL, Dempsey PJ, Rubin E. Sonographic evaluation of infiltrating lobular carcinoma. AJR Am J Roentgenol 1999;172:325–330

Evans N, Lyons K. The use of ultrasound in the diagnosis of invasive lobular carcinoma of the breast less than 10 mm in size. Clin Radiol 2000;55:261–2631

Case 21.3: Lobular Carcinoma

Case History
A 67-year-old woman, transferred from another medical facility, was evaluated for abdominal pain. Abdominal computed tomography (CT) demonstrated multiple low-density liver masses. Liver biopsy indicated metastatic adenocarcinoma.

Physical Examination
- Normal exam

Mammogram
- Focal asymmetry (**Fig. 21.6**)

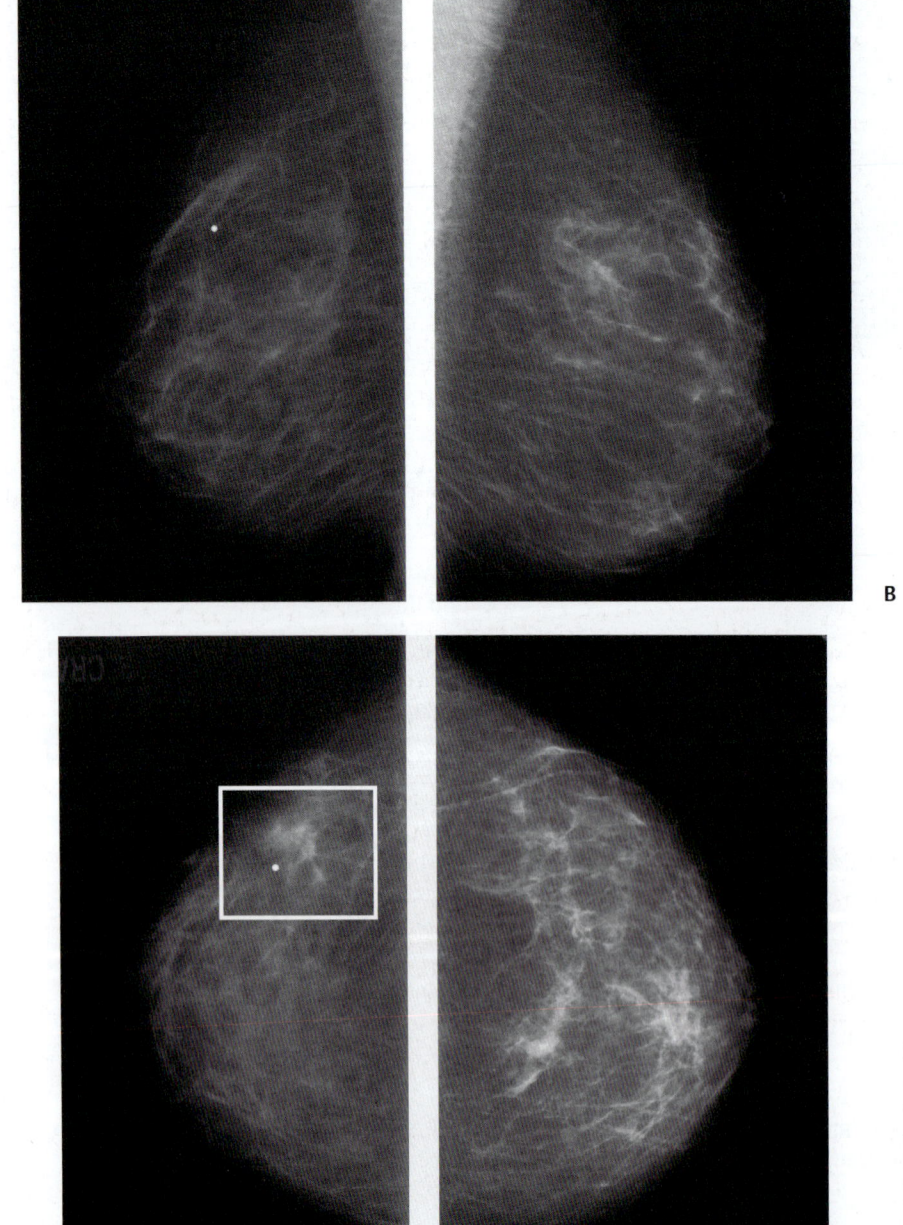

Fig. 21.6 A focal asymmetry (*square*) in the right outer breast is visible only on the CC view. This asymmetry has been unchanged for 5 years. (Radiopaque marker has been placed on skin to aid locating the density on other views.) (**A**) Right MLO mammogram. (**B**) Left MLO mammogram. (**C**) Right CC mammogram. (**D**) Left CC mammogram.

Ultrasound

Low Frequency (Fig. 21.7)

Frequency
- 7 MHz

Mass
- Margin: ill defined
- Echogenicity: hypoechoic
- Retrotumoral acoustic appearance: severe shadowing, mass partially obscured
- Shape: irregular

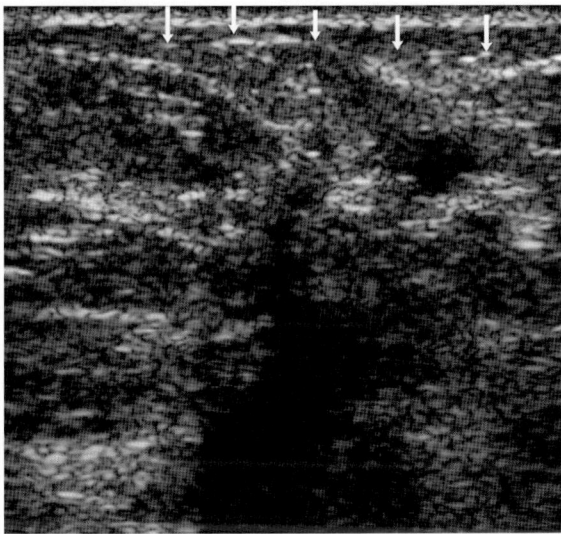

Fig. 21.7 Right radial low-frequency breast sonogram. Mammographic asymmetry demonstrated in **Fig. 21.6** corresponds to an ill-defined hypoechoic mass associated with architectural distortion due to retraction of Cooper's ligaments and the anterior fascial line (*arrows*).

High Frequency (Fig. 21.8)

Frequency
- 10 MHz

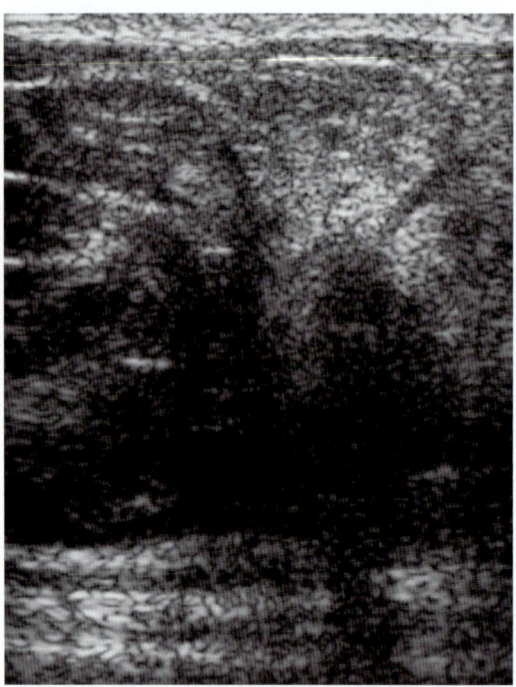

Fig. 21.8 Right radial high-frequency breast sonogram. Sonographic examination of same mass as in **Fig. 21.7**. The architectural distortion, spiculation, and hyperechoic haziness are better defined by this higher-frequency exam compared with the lower-frequency examination (**Fig. 21.7**).

Other Modalities: Computed Tomography (Fig. 21.9)

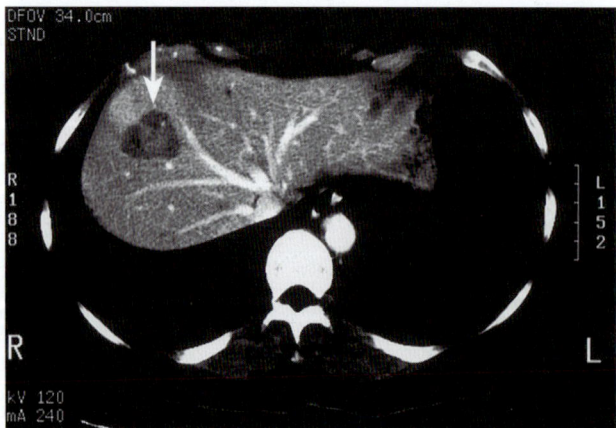

Fig. 21.9 Abdominal CT scan with intravenous contrast. Because the patient's initial chief complaint was abdominal pain, an abdominal CT was the first imaging test performed. In the liver there are multiple low-density solid masses. The largest mass (*arrow*) is in the right lobe of the liver. These masses are metastases from the patient's occult breast cancer.

Pathology
- Invasive lobular carcinoma

Management
- BI-RADS assessment category 4, suspicious abnormality; biopsy should be considered.

> **Pearls and Pitfalls**
>
> - Sonography is useful to identify masses that may be mammographically subtle. Higher-frequency examination improves the conspicuity of malignancies by enhancing visibility of architectural distortion. Sometimes lobular carcinoma is difficult to identify sonographically because the mass is hidden by severe acoustic shadowing. In these cases, architectural distortion is the main clue that differentiates the neoplasm from adjacent dense fibrous tissue.

Suggested Reading
Skaane P, Skjørten F. Ultrasonographic evaluation of invasive lobular carcinoma. Acta Radiol 1999;40:369–375

Architectural Distortion

This is a schematic diagram of the diagnostic approach to architectural distortion masses. For further discussion, see Chapter 1.

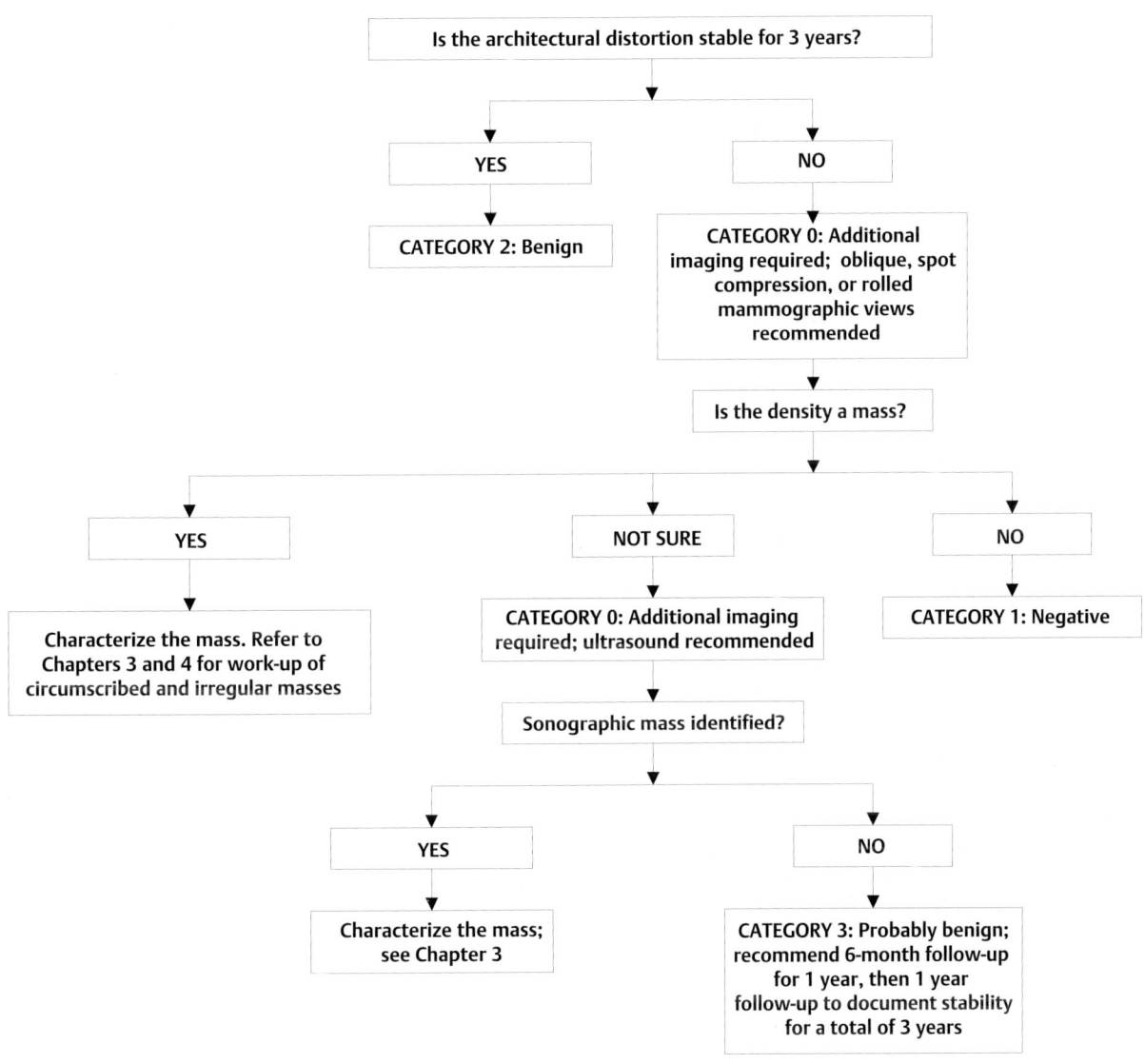

22 Peripheral Architectural Distortion

Case 22.1: Benign Process

Case History
A 62-year-old woman presents for screening mammogram.

Physical Examination
- Normal exam

Mammogram
- Architectural distortion (**Fig. 22.1**)

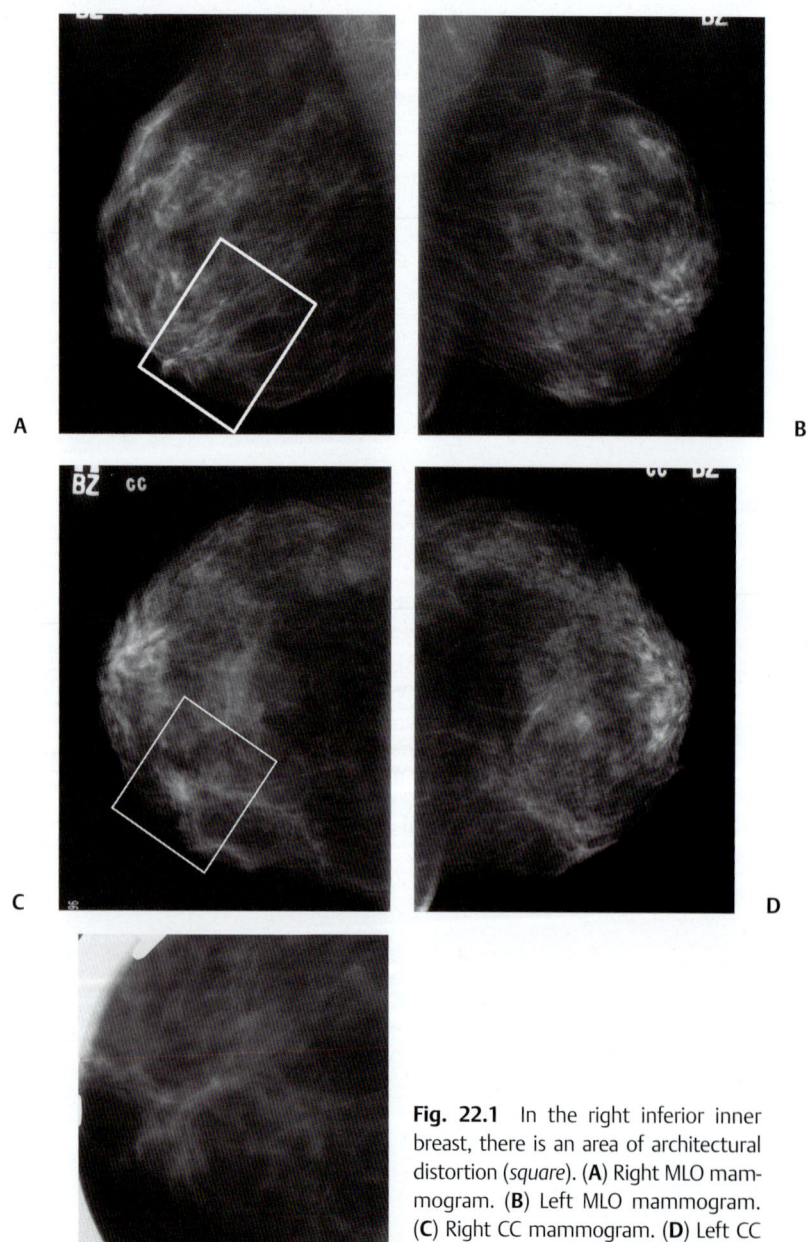

Fig. 22.1 In the right inferior inner breast, there is an area of architectural distortion (*square*). (**A**) Right MLO mammogram. (**B**) Left MLO mammogram. (**C**) Right CC mammogram. (**D**) Left CC mammogram. (**E**) Right MLO spot compression mammogram.

Ultrasound

Frequency
- 13 MHz (**Fig. 22.2**)

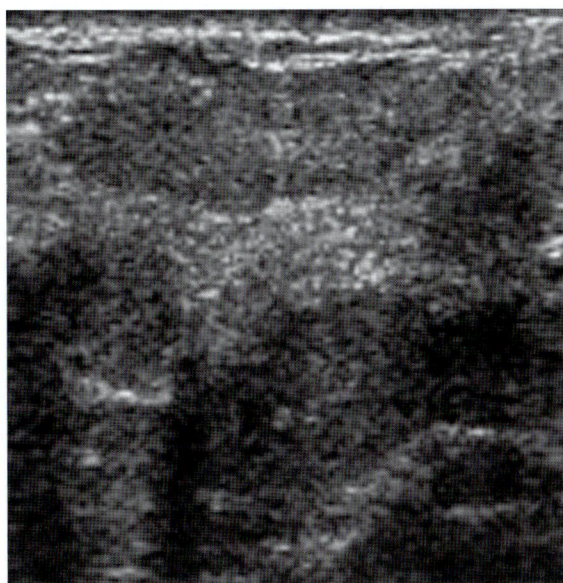

Fig. 22.2 Right antiradial breast sonogram. No sonographic mass is identified in the area of the mammographic architectural distortion. Only normal hyperechoic tissue is present.

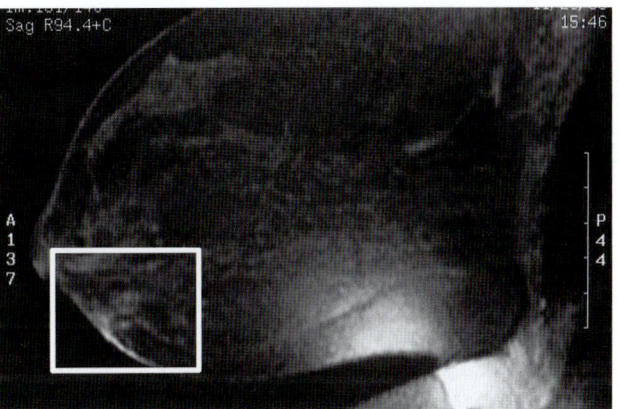

Fig. 22.3 Right sagittal dynamic bolus three-dimensional (3D) volume-gradient series breast MRI. In the area of the mammographic architectural distortion, MRI also demonstrates architectural distortion and skin thickening (*square*). However, there is no associated contrast enhancement of the area.

Other Modalities: MRI (Fig. 22.3)

MRI Findings
Although MRI demonstrates architectural distortion and skin thickening, the lack of contrast enhancement suggests that the architectural distortion is benign.

Pathology
- Fibroadenomatoid hyperplasia

Management
- BI-RADS assessment category 4, suspicious; biopsy should be considered.

Pearls and Pitfalls

- This case illustrates peripheral architectural distortion. The spot compression emphasizes the retraction of the edge of the parenchyma associated with abnormal deviation of the parenchymal lines. Normally, the axis of the parenchymal lines should be toward the nipple. In this case, they are pointing toward the skin away from the nipple.
- The etiologies of architectural distortion are similar to the causes of irregular masses. Benign entities include scar, mastitis, fibrocystic changes, adenosis, mesenchymal lesions (fat necrosis, fibromatosis), and benign neoplasms (e.g., sclerosing papillomas, myofibroblastomas). Malignant entities include infiltrating ductal, invasive lobular, tubular, and occasionally lymphoma.

Suggested Reading
Jones MK. Atlas of Breast Imaging. Malden, MA: Blackwell Science; 1996:108–112

Case 22.2: Radial Scar

Case History
A 54-year-old woman presents for screening mammogram.

Physical Examination
- Normal exam

Mammogram
- Architectural distortion (**Fig. 22.4**)

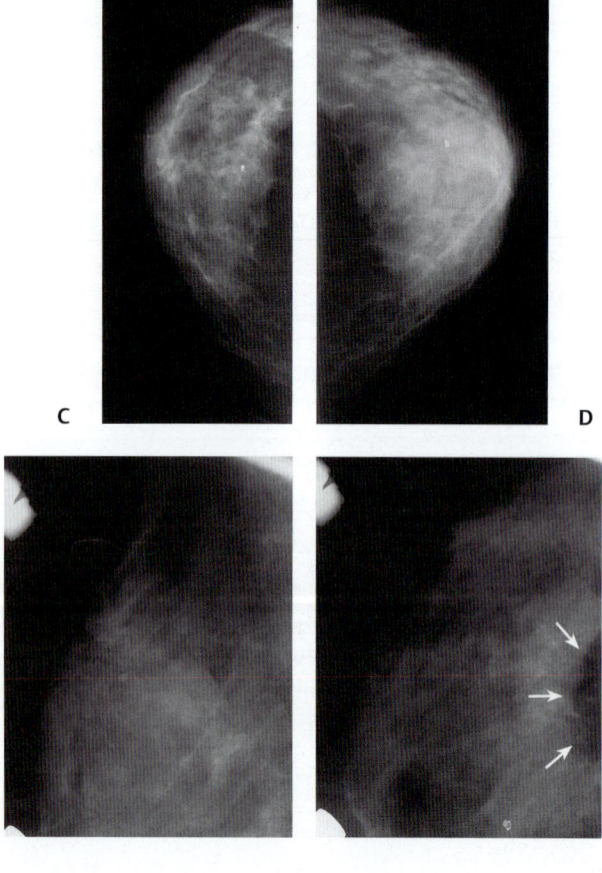

Fig. 22.4 There is architectural distortion of the superior edge of the right breast on the MLO view (*square* in **A**). Posterior parenchymal retraction is present on the right XCCL spot magnification view (*arrows* in **F**). (**A**) Right MLO mammogram. (**B**) Left MLO mammogram. (**C**) Right CC mammogram. (**D**) Left CC mammogram. (**E**) Right MLO spot magnification mammogram. (**F**) Right XCCL spot magnification mammogram.

Ultrasound

Frequency
- 10 MHz

Mass (Fig. 22.5)
- Margin: ill defined
- Echogenicity: hypoechoic
- Retrotumoral acoustic appearance: single edge shadowing
- Shape: irregular

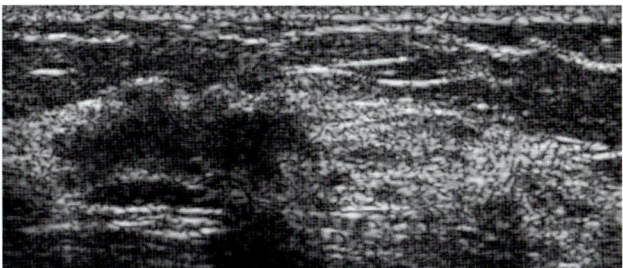

Fig. 22.5 Right radial breast sonogram. In the upper outer quadrant, the mammographic architectural distortion corresponds to an irregular hypoechoic mass.

Pathology
- Radial sclerosing lesion (radial scar)
- Ductal carcinoma in situ
- 0.8 cm ductal carcinoma in situ within the 2.2 cm radial scar

Management
- BI-RADS assessment category 4, suspicious; biopsy should be considered.

Pearls and Pitfalls

- This case illustrates two common areas of architectural distortion in denser breasts: parenchymal retraction of the superior and posterior parenchymal edges. The superior edges of the breast should generally be symmetric in configuration. If there is asymmetry, the superior edge should have a curved or lobulated contour. The parenchymal density should gradually decrease until it blends into the axilla. When a mass produces parenchymal retraction, the superior edge loses the curved or lobular contour and forms a sharp triangular appearance. There is a greater difference between the density of the parenchymal edge and the axillary fat on the abnormal side compared with the normal side.
- When a mass causes retraction of the posterior edge of the breast, the abnormal density forms a V and is termed the "tent" sign.

Suggested Reading
Tabar L, Dean PB. Teaching Atlas of Mammography. 3rd ed. New York: Thieme; 2001:12–13, 119, 137

Case 22.4: Mixed Ductal and Lobular Cancer

Case History

An 81-year-old woman presents for screening mammogram.

Physical Examination
- Normal exam

Mammogram
- Architectural distortion (**Fig. 22.8**)

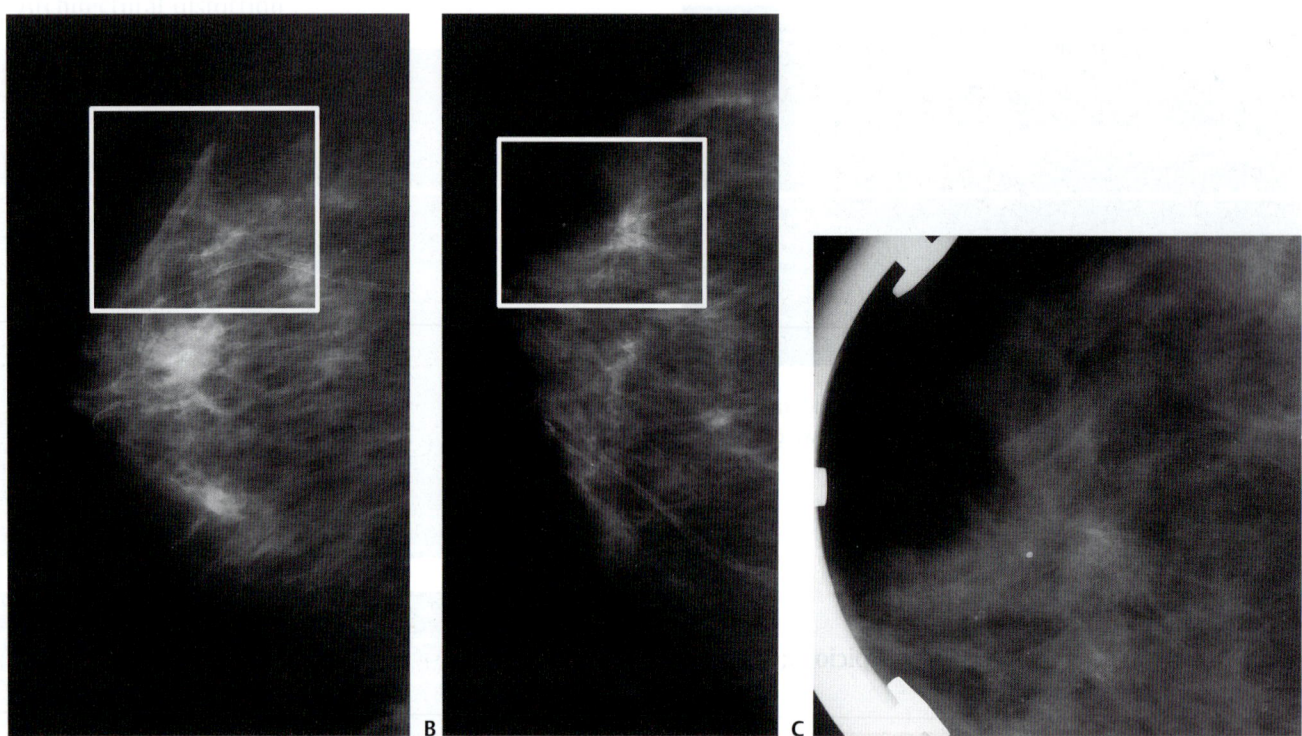

Fig. 22.8 In the right upper outer quadrant there is peripheral architectural distortion (*square*). In the ML view, the superior parenchymal contour is abnormally triangular (**A**), and in the CC view, the anterior parenchymal line is retracted (**B**). (**A**) Right ML mammogram. (**B**) Right CC mammogram. (**C**) Right CC spot compression.

Ultrasound

Low Frequency (Fig. 22.9)

Frequency
- 8 MHz

Mass
- Margin: ill defined
- Echogenicity: hypoechoic
- Retrotumoral acoustic appearance: posterior shadowing distal to mass
- Shape: irregular

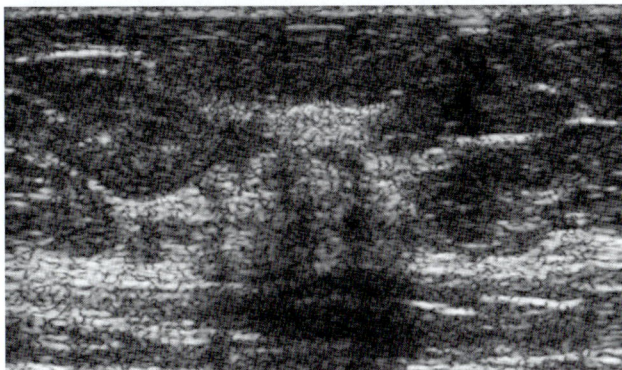

Fig. 22.9 Right antiradial breast sonogram. The mammographic architectural distortion corresponds to an irregular, predominantly hyperechoic mass with irregular shadowing.

High Frequency (Fig. 22.10)

Frequency
- 11.5 MHz

High-Frequency Findings
The higher frequency improves the conspicuity of the mass. With higher frequency, the heavily shadowing mass is easily separated from the surrounding hyperechoic parenchyma.

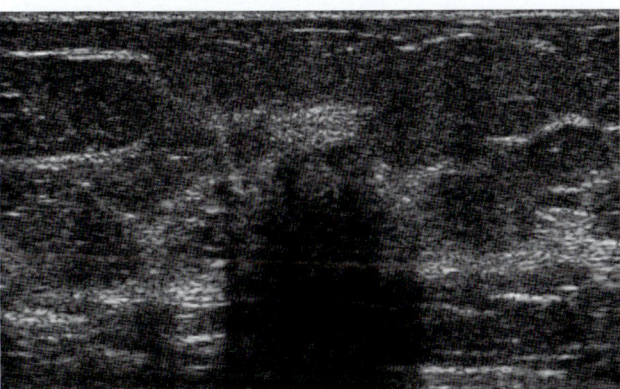

Fig. 22.10 Right antiradial breast sonogram. With a higher frequency, the mass identified in **Fig. 22.9** appears as a focal area of severe acoustic shadowing.

Pathology
- Mixed invasive lobular and ductal carcinoma

Management
- BI-RADS assessment category 4, suspicious; biopsy should be considered.

Pearls and Pitfalls
- This case illustrates a malignant mass producing triangular distortion of the superior parenchymal contour and retraction of the anterior contour.
- For cases of mammographic architectural distortion, sonography is useful to increase diagnostic confidence, clarify the location of the mass, and provide biopsy guidance. However, sonographically identifying the etiology of mammographic architectural distortion is commonly difficult, so sonographic cross-correlation with mammographic anatomy and utilization of high-frequency sonography are important to optimize diagnostic accuracy.

Suggested Reading
Kopans DB. Breast Imaging. 2nd ed. Philadelphia: Lippincott-Raven; 1998:298–302, 384–386

Case 22.5: Mixed Ductal and Lobular Cancer

Case History
A 60-year-old woman presents for screening mammogram.

Physical Examination
- Normal exam

Mammogram
- Architectural distortion (**Fig. 22.11**)

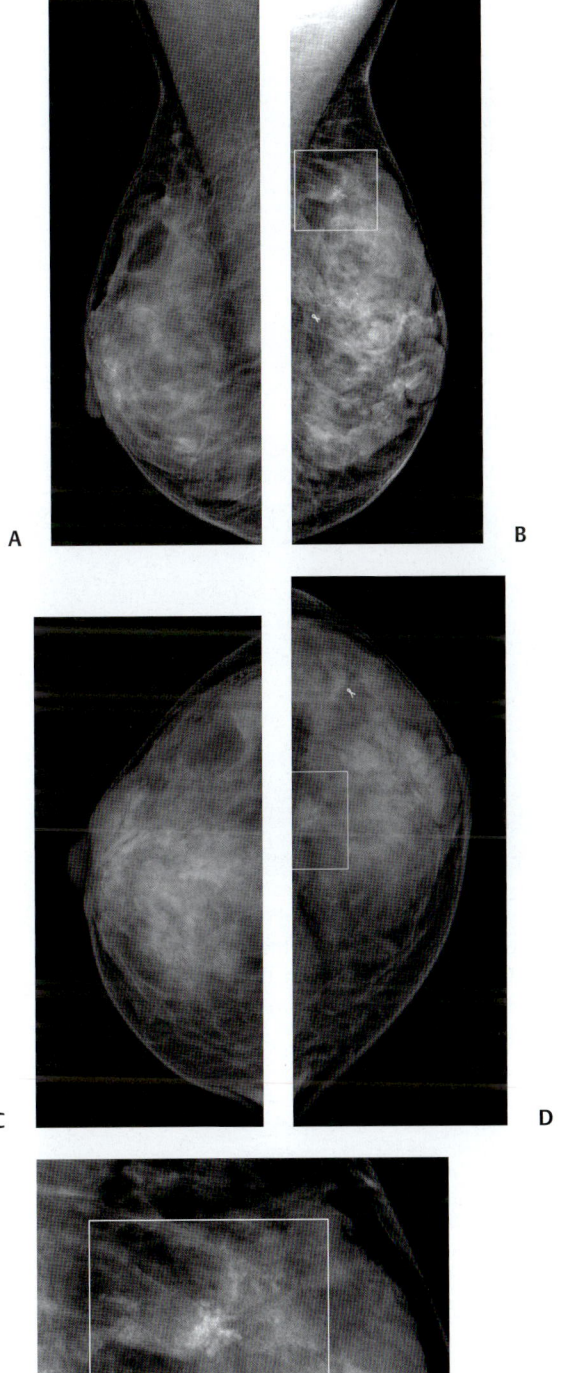

Fig. 22.11 There is new architectural distortion at the 12 o'clock position of the left breast (*square*). Patient has a clip from a previous benign biopsy. Right mammograms are normal. (**A**) Right MLO. (**B**) Left MLO. (**C**) Right CC. (**D**) Left CC. (**E**) Left MLO enlarged.

Ultrasound

Frequency (Fig. 22.12)
- 14 MHz

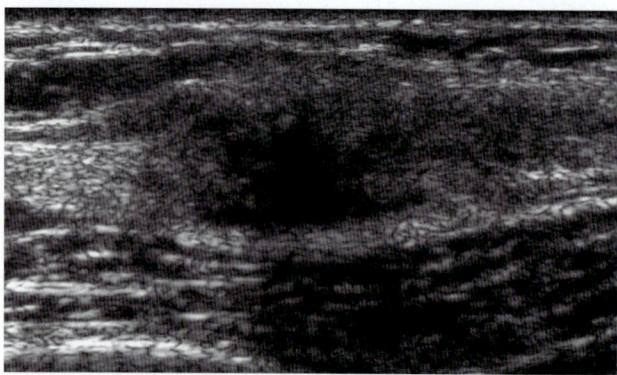

Fig. 22.12 Left radial breast sonogram at the 12 o'clock position. The mammographic architectural distortion corresponds to an irregular hypoechoic solid mass with spiculations. This mass was biopsied sonographically and found to be malignant.

Other Modalities: MRI and Second Look Sonography (Figs. 22.13, 22.14, and 22.15)

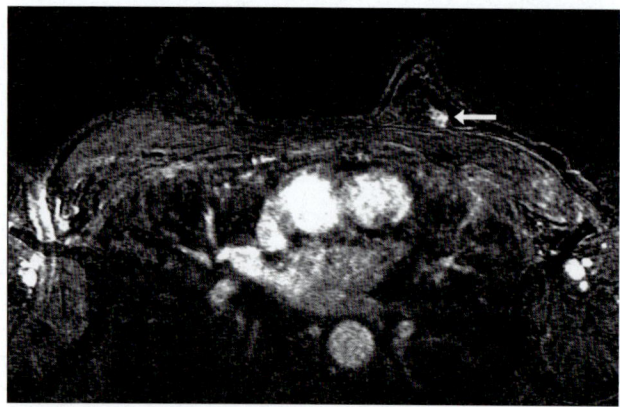

Fig. 22.13 Dynamic bolus T1-weighted 2-minute subtraction axial bilateral breast MRI. Bilateral contrast-enhanced breast MRI. The examination was performed to stage the known malignancy at the left 12 o'clock position and identify any other malignancies. The known malignancy is an irregular rapidly enhancing left breast mass (*arrow*).

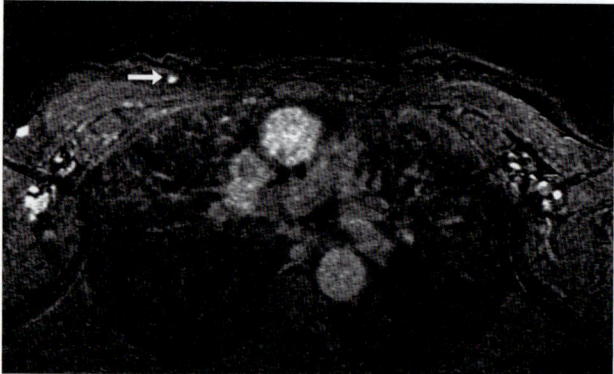

Fig. 22.14 Dynamic bolus T1-weighted 2-minute subtraction axial bilateral breast MRI, 1 cm superior to the image in **Fig. 22.13**. In the right breast at the 1 o'clock position, there is an isolated rapidly enhancing 5 mm focus (*arrow*).

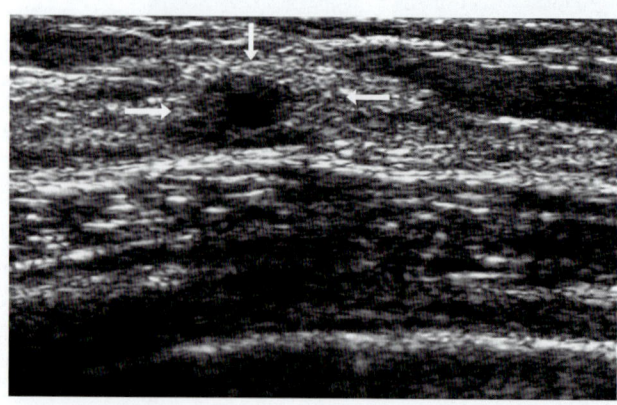

Fig. 22.15 Right radial breast sonogram at the 1 o'clock position performed after MRI. The MRI focus corresponds to a small solid mass (*arrow*) with indistinct margins.

Pathology
- Left breast: lumpectomy: 1.1 cm invasive cancer with ductal and lobular features
- Right breast: lumpectomy: 0.5 cm invasive ductal carcinoma

Management
- Left mammographic and sonographic mass at the 12 o'clock position: BI-RADS assessment category 5, highly suggestive of malignancy
- Right MRI focus at the 12 o'clock position: BI-RADS assessment category 4, suspicious; biopsy should be considered.

Pearls and Pitfalls
- A focus is a tiny (generally < 5 mm) spot of enhancement that is too small to characterize its shape and margins and does not clearly represent a space-occupying mass. One study notes that foci have a low (3%) chance of malignancy compared with larger suspicious masses. However, another group reports that foci associated with a type II kinetic curve (rapid initial enhancement followed by plateau) or type III curve (rapid initial enhancement followed by washout) have a much higher chance of malignancy (37%). Similarly, the likelihood of malignancy is related to the clinical circumstance. Foci are also more likely to be malignant when the MRI is performed to identify the extent of disease of a known primary malignancy. Foci are less likely to be malignant when the MRI is performed for screening.
- Differential diagnosis of MRI-enhancing breast focus: hormonal focal enhancement, fibrocystic change (usually multiple), benign neoplasm (e.g., fibroadenoma), radial scar (usually associated with architectural distortion), atypical ductal hyperplasia, lobular carcinoma in situ, ductal carcinoma in situ (can have segmental, regional, or linear distribution), invasive carcinoma (commonly appears as satellite lesion associated with a dominant invasive carcinoma)

Suggested Reading
Liberman L, Mason G, Morris EA, Dershaw DD. Does size matter? Positive predictive value of MRI-detected breast lesions as a function of lesion size. AJR Am J Roentgenol 2006;186:426–430

Van den Bosch MAAJ, Ikeda DM, Daniel BL. Does size matter? Likelihood of cancer in MRI-detected lesions less than 5 mm. AJR Am J Roentgenol 2007;188:W571

Wang S-C. Foci. In: Berg WA, Birdwell RL, Gombos EC, Wang S-C, Parkinson BT, Raza S, Green GE, Kennedy A, Kettler MD, eds. Diagnostic Imaging Breast. Altona, Manitoba: Friesens; 2006, IV-1-168-169

Case 22.6: Tubular Cancer

Case History
A 70-year-old woman presents for screening mammogram.

Physical Examination
- Normal exam

Mammogram

Mass (Fig. 22.16)
- Margin: indistinct
- Shape: irregular
- Density: equal density
- Architectural distortion

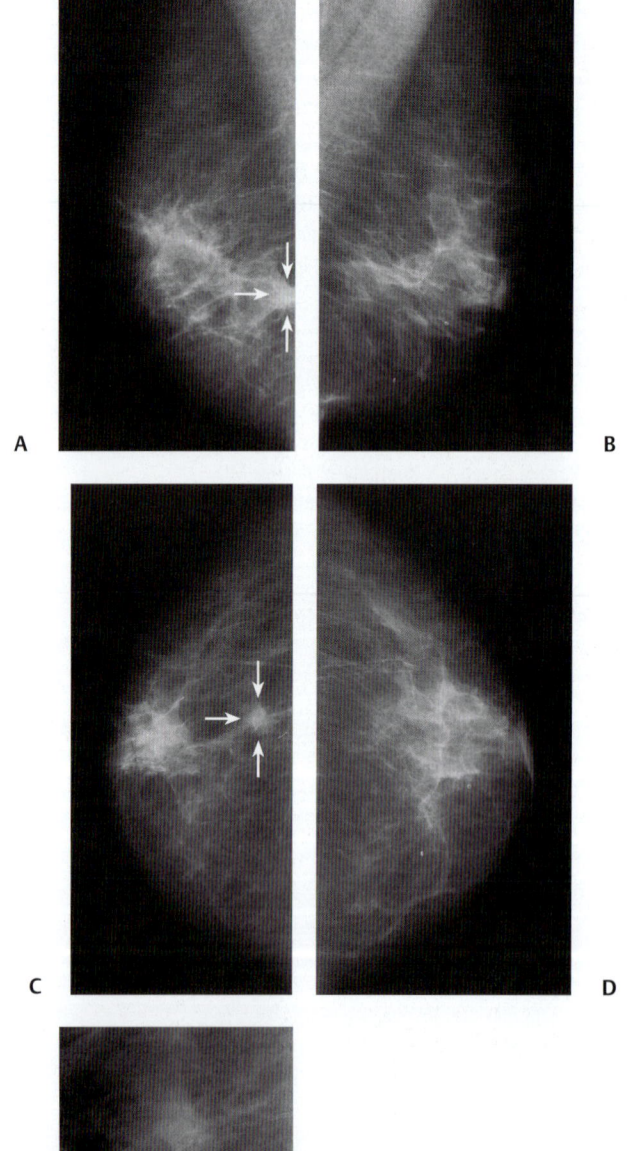

Fig. 22.16 In the 7 o'clock position of the right breast, there is a mass that extends outside the normal posterior parenchymal edge (*arrows*). (**A**) Right MLO mammogram. (**B**) Left MLO mammogram. (**C**) Right CC mammogram. (**D**) Left CC mammogram. (**E**) Right CC spot compression mammogram.

Ultrasound

Low Frequency

Frequency
- 7 MHz

Mass (Fig. 22.17)
- Margin: ill defined
- Echogenicity: hypoechoic
- Retrotumoral acoustic appearance: posterior shadowing distal to mass
- Shape: irregular

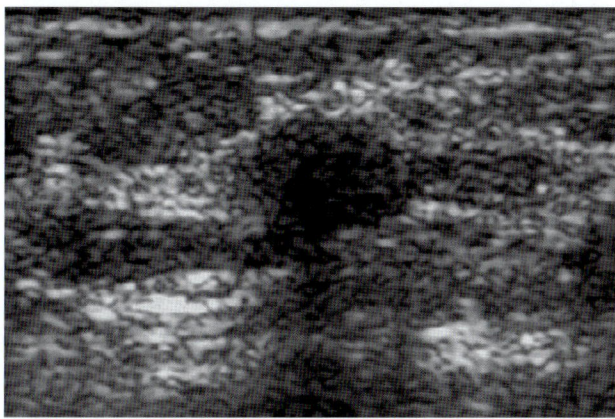

Fig. 22.17 Right radial breast sonogram. The ill-defined mass identified in **Fig 22.16A,C** corresponds to an ill-defined hypoechoic solid mass with posterior acoustic shadowing.

Pathology
- Tubular carcinoma

Management
- BI-RADS assessment category 4, suspicious; biopsy should be considered.

Pearls and Pitfalls

- Besides creating retraction of the parenchymal edge, masses protrude beyond the normal edge. Tubular carcinoma commonly presents mammographically as a small, irregular mass with architectural distortion.

Suggested Reading

Evans AJ, Wilson ARM, Blamey RW, Robertson JFR, Ellis IO, Elston CW. Atlas of Breast Disease Management. Philadelphia: WB Saunders; 1998:98–100

Tabar L, Dean PB. Teaching Atlas of Mammography. 3rd ed. New York: Thieme; 2001:5–9

23 Central Architectural Distortion

Case 23.1: Sclerosing Adenosis

Case History
A 71-year-old woman presents for screening mammogram.

Mammogram
- Architectural distortion (**Fig. 23.1**)

Physical Examination
- Normal exam

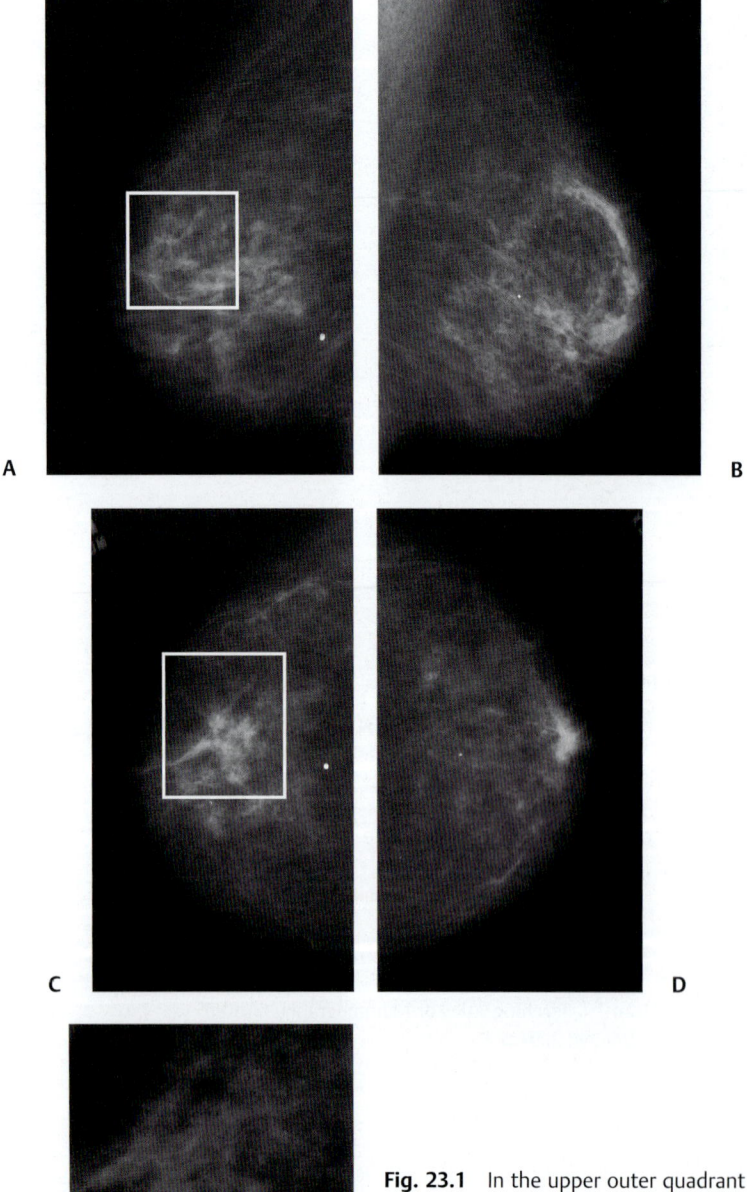

Fig. 23.1 In the upper outer quadrant of the right breast, there is architectural distortion (*square*). Focal increased density was demonstrated only on the CC view. (**A**) Right MLO mammogram. (**B**) Left MLO mammogram. (**C**) Right CC mammogram. (**D**) Left CC mammogram. (**E**) Right CC spot compression mammogram.

Ultrasound

Low Frequency (Fig. 23.2)

Frequency
- 7 MHz

Mass
- Margin: ill defined
- Echogenicity: hypoechoic
- Retrotumoral acoustic appearance: posterior shadowing distal to mass
- Shape: irregular

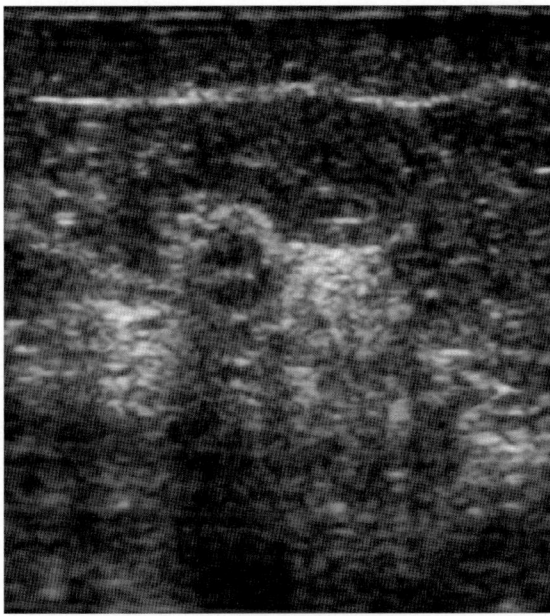

Fig. 23.2 Right antiradial breast sonogram. With lower frequency, the mammographic architectural distortion is an irregular hypoechoic mass with posterior acoustic shadowing.

Architectural Distortion

High Frequency (Fig. 23.3)

Frequency
- 10 MHz

High-Frequency Findings
This case illustrates that weaker penetration with higher frequency causes increased shadowing with benign masses as well as malignant ones. In this case, lower frequency is more useful than high frequency to identify the location of the mass.

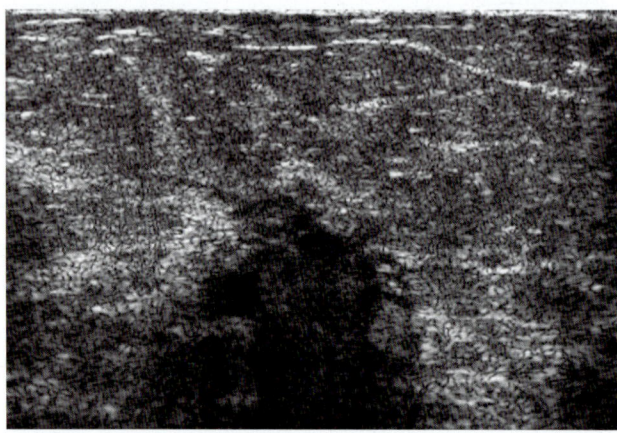

Fig. 23.3 Right antiradial breast sonogram. Higher-frequency examination produces extensive shadowing. The mass identified in **Fig. 23.2** is hidden in the area of shadowing.

Pathology
- Sclerosing adenosis

Management
- BI-RADS assessment category 4, suspicious; biopsy should be considered.

Pearls and Pitfalls

- Sclerosing adenosis is present in 3.1% of breasts. This lesion may present as a palpable mass and is occasionally associated with tenderness.
- Mammographically, sclerosing adenosis produces architectural distortion with or without a focal mass and may simulate malignancy.
- Sonographically, sclerosing adenosis is an irregular hypoechoic mass that cannot be differentiated from malignancy.

Suggested Reading

Tabar L, Dean PB. Teaching Atlas of Mammography. 3rd ed. New York: Thieme; 2001:2–3, 197

Tavassoli FA. Pathology of the Breast. 2nd ed. Stamford: Appleton & Lange; 1999:130–133

Case 23.2: Radial Scar

Case History
A 58-year-old woman presents for screening mammogram.

Physical Examination
- Normal exam

Mammogram
- Architectural distortion (**Fig. 23.4**)

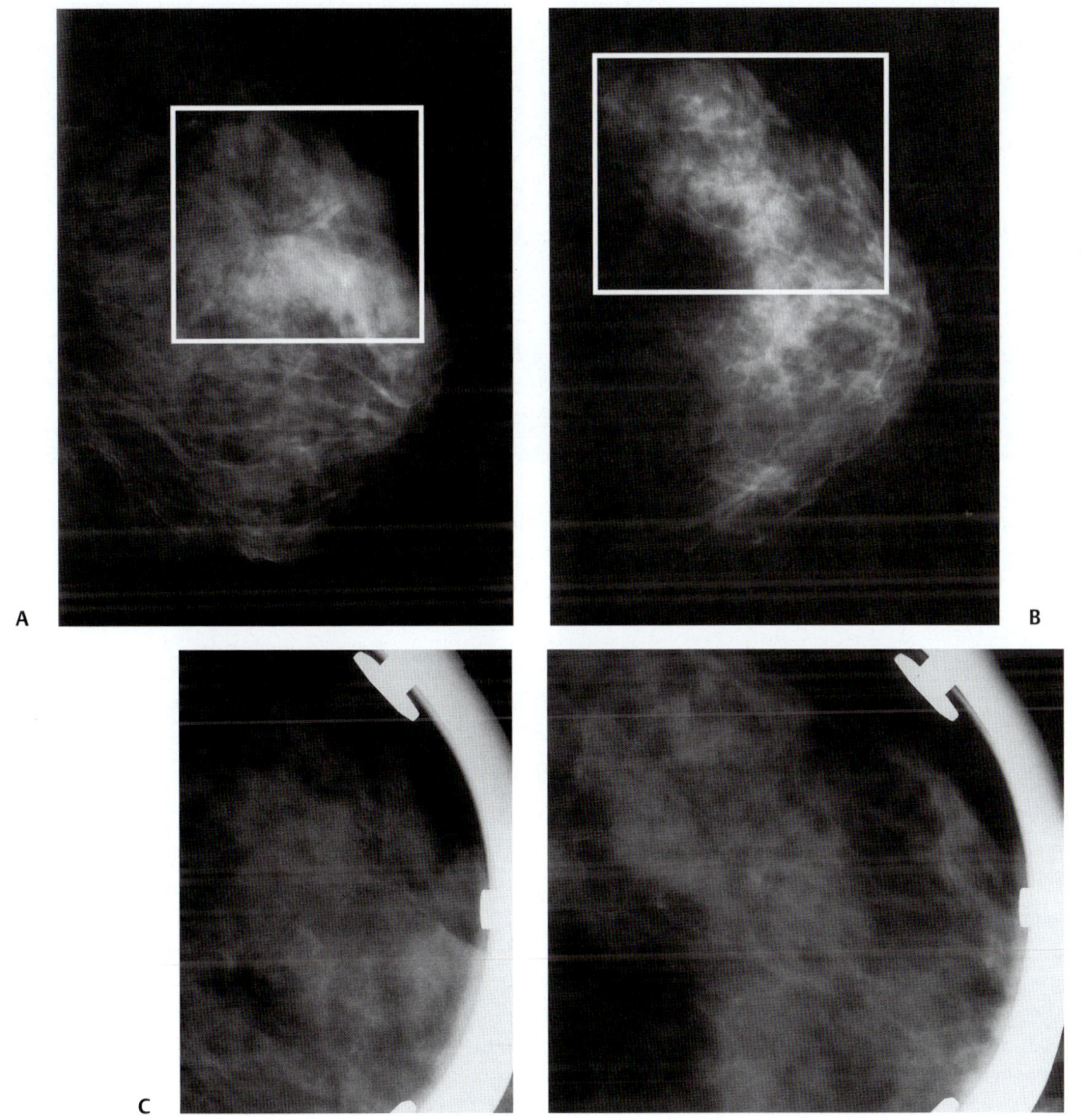

Fig. 23.4 In the left upper outer quadrant, there is a spiculated density on the MLO view, which is less apparent on the CC view. Area of architectural distortion is surrounded by a *square*. (**A**) Left MLO mammogram. (**B**) Left CC mammogram. (**C**) Left MLO spot compression mammogram. (**D**) Left CC spot compression mammogram.

Ultrasound

Frequency
- 7 MHz

Mass (Fig. 23.5)
- Margin: ill defined
- Echogenicity: hypoechoic
- Retrotumoral acoustic appearance: severe shadowing, mass partially obscured
- Shape: irregular

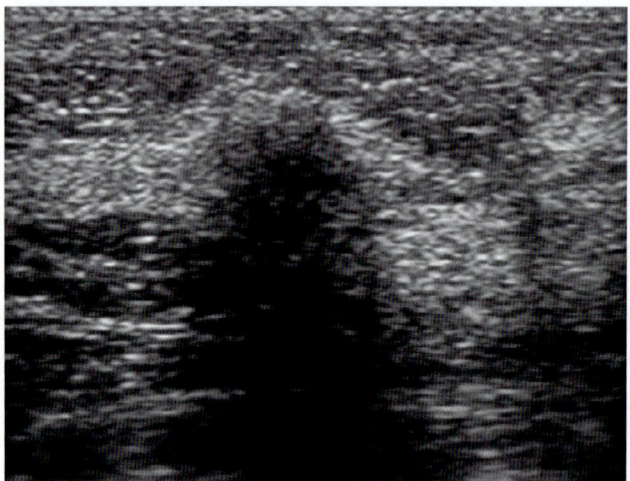 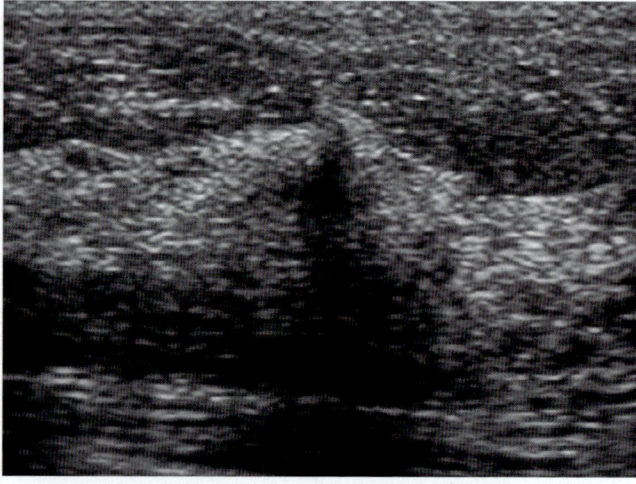

Fig. 23.5 In the left upper outer quadrant, the mammographic architectural distortion corresponds to a lesion exhibiting severe shadowing. The lesion appears wide in the radial view (**A**) and narrow in the antiradial view (**B**). This extreme discrepancy in appearance is characteristic of either posttraumatic or radial scars. (**A**) Left radial breast sonogram. (**B**) Left antiradial breast sonogram.

Pathology
- Radial sclerosing lesion (radial scar)

Management
- BI-RADS assessment category 4, suspicious; biopsy should be considered.

Pearls and Pitfalls
- Clinically, radial scars are generally not palpable.
- Mammographically, radial scars commonly exhibit thin radiating lines without a central dense mass. The abnormality commonly changes appearance from one projection to another.
- Sonographically, radial scars are similar in appearance to surgically produced scars. Radial scars exhibit a large hypoechoic or shadowing area in one view and a thin abnormality in the orthogonal view. The sonographic appearance should not prevent biopsy and excision of this lesion because about one third of radial scars are associated with ductal carcinoma in situ or tubular carcinoma.

Suggested Reading
Evans AJ, Wilson ARM, Blamey RW, Robertson JFR, Ellis IO, Elston CW. Atlas of Breast Disease Management. Philadelphia: WB Saunders; 1998:94–97

Tabar L, Dean PB. Teaching Atlas of Mammography. 3rd ed. New York: Thieme; 2001:93–96, 102–106

Case 23.3: Infiltrating Ductal

Case History
A 63-year-old woman presents with a palpable lump in the left breast.

Mammogram

Mass (Fig. 23.6)
- Margin: spiculated
- Shape: irregular
- Density: equal density
- Architectural distortion

Physical Examination
- Right breast: normal
- Left breast: palpable mass in upper outer quadrant

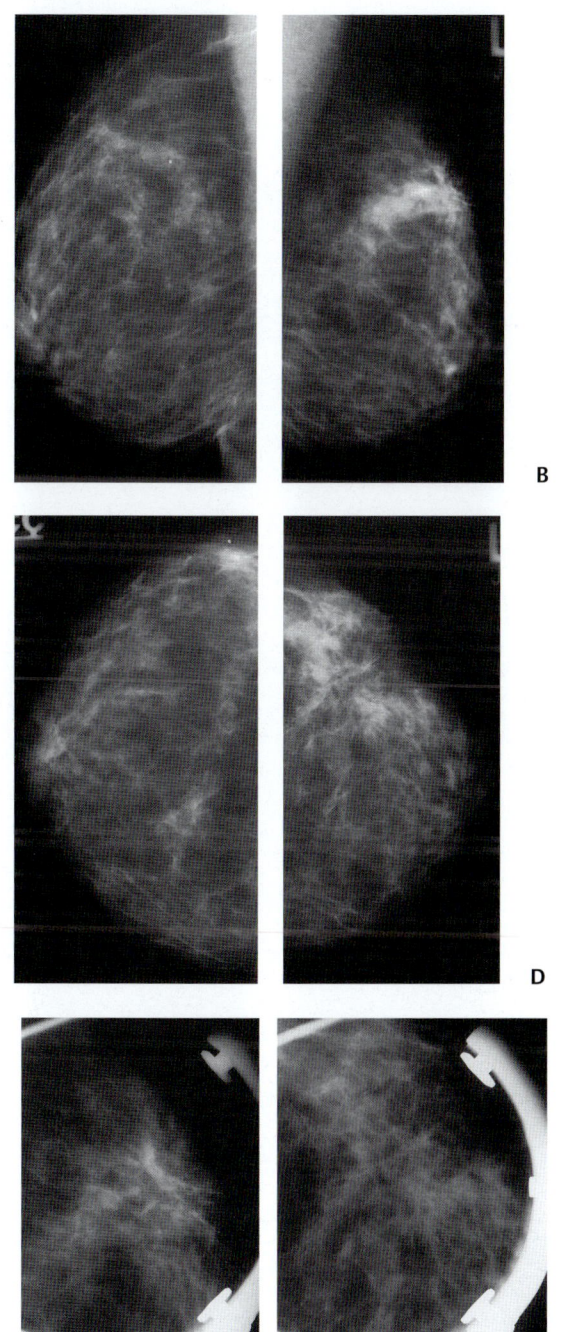

Fig. 23.6 In the upper outer left breast, there is a spiculated mass. (**A**) Right MLO mammogram. (**B**) Left MLO mammogram. (**C**) Right CC mammogram. (**D**) Left CC mammogram. (**E**) Left MLO spot compression mammogram. (**F**) Left CC spot compression mammogram.

Ultrasound

Frequency
- 7 MHz

Mass (Fig. 23.7)
- Margin: ill defined
- Echogenicity: hypoechoic
- Retrotumoral acoustic appearance: severe shadowing, mass partially obscured
- Shape: irregular

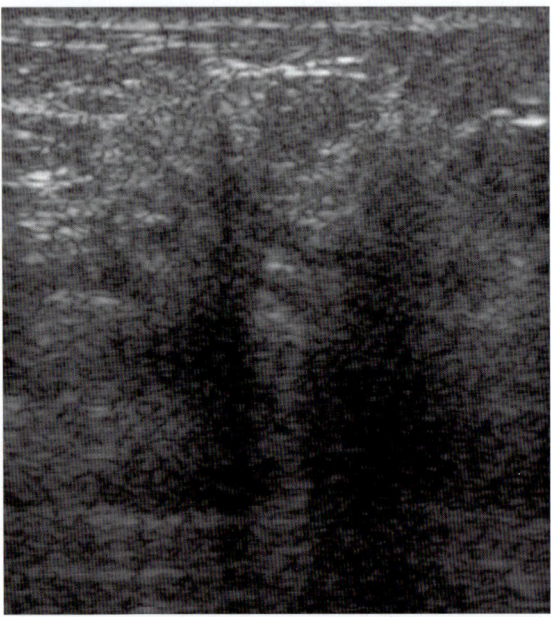

Fig. 23.7 Left radial breast sonogram. The palpable lump in the upper outer quadrant is an ill-defined, irregular, hypoechoic solid mass. This mass corresponds to the spiculated mass on the left mammogram (**Fig. 23.6**).

Pathology
- Invasive ductal carcinoma

Management
- BI-RADS assessment category 4, suspicious; biopsy should be considered,

Pearls and Pitfalls

- Although malignancies commonly produce radiating spiculations, this mass is unusual because it appears more dense on the MLO view compared with the CC view. However, persistent architectural distortion in both views is a suspicious finding if there is no history of trauma or surgery.
- Sonography is useful in this case to confirm that the palpable abnormality corresponds to the mammographic mass and to guide for biopsy.

Suggested Reading
Heywang-Kobrunner SH, Schreer I, Dershaw DD. Diagnostic Breast Imaging. New York: Thieme, 1997:347–357

Case 23.4: Infiltrating Ductal

Case History
A 74-year-old woman presents for screening mammogram.

Physical Examination
- Normal exam

Mammogram
- Architectural distortion (**Fig. 23.8**)

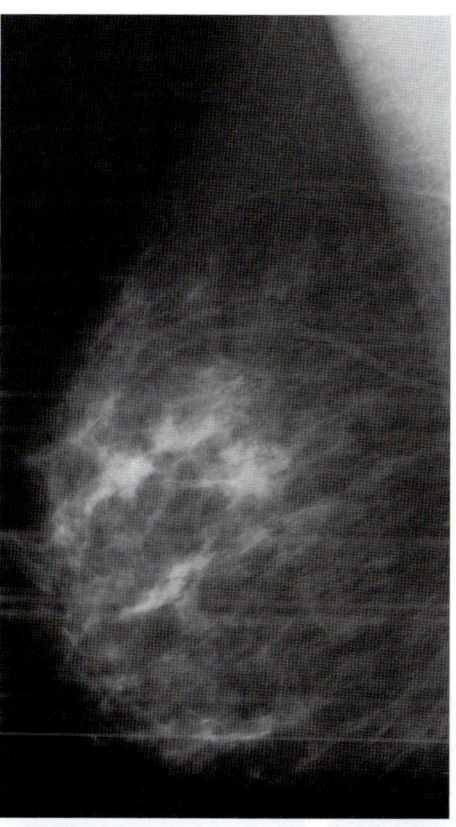
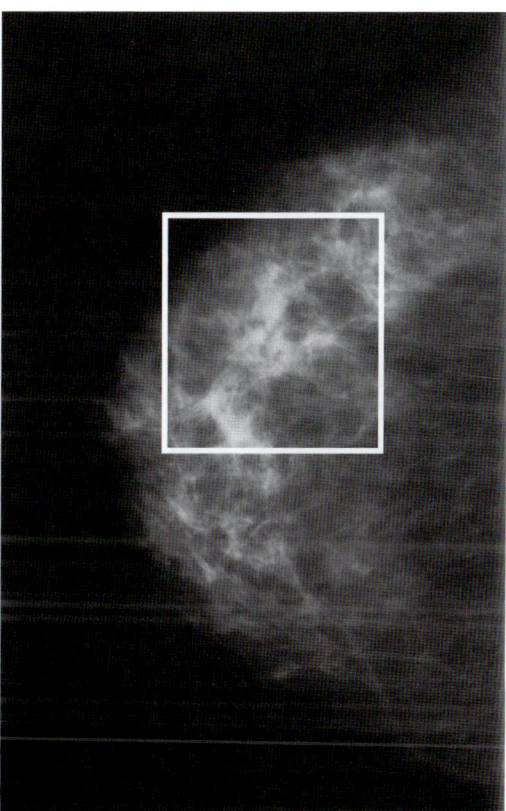
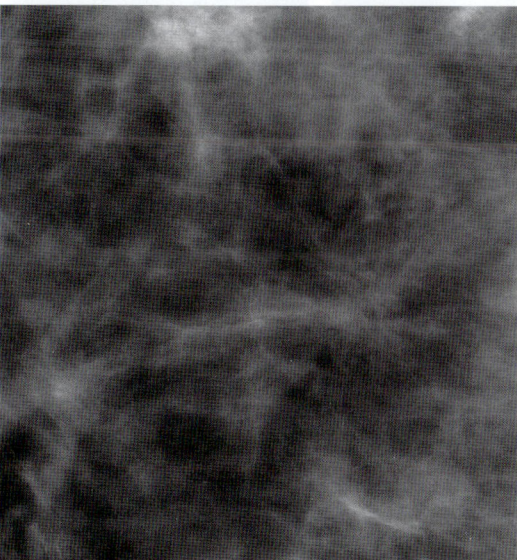

Fig. 23.8 In the outer right breast on the CC view, there is an area of architectural distortion (*square*). The lesion consists of radiating lines. No mass or architectural distortion is identified in any other mammographic view. (**A**) Right MLO mammogram. (**B**) Right CC mammogram. (**C**) Right CC spot magnification mammogram.

Case 23.6: Infiltrating Ductal

Case History
A 77-year-old woman presents for screening mammogram.

Physical Examination
- Normal exam

Mammogram

Mass (Fig. 23.11)
- Margin: indistinct
- Shape: oval
- Density: equal
- Architectural distortion

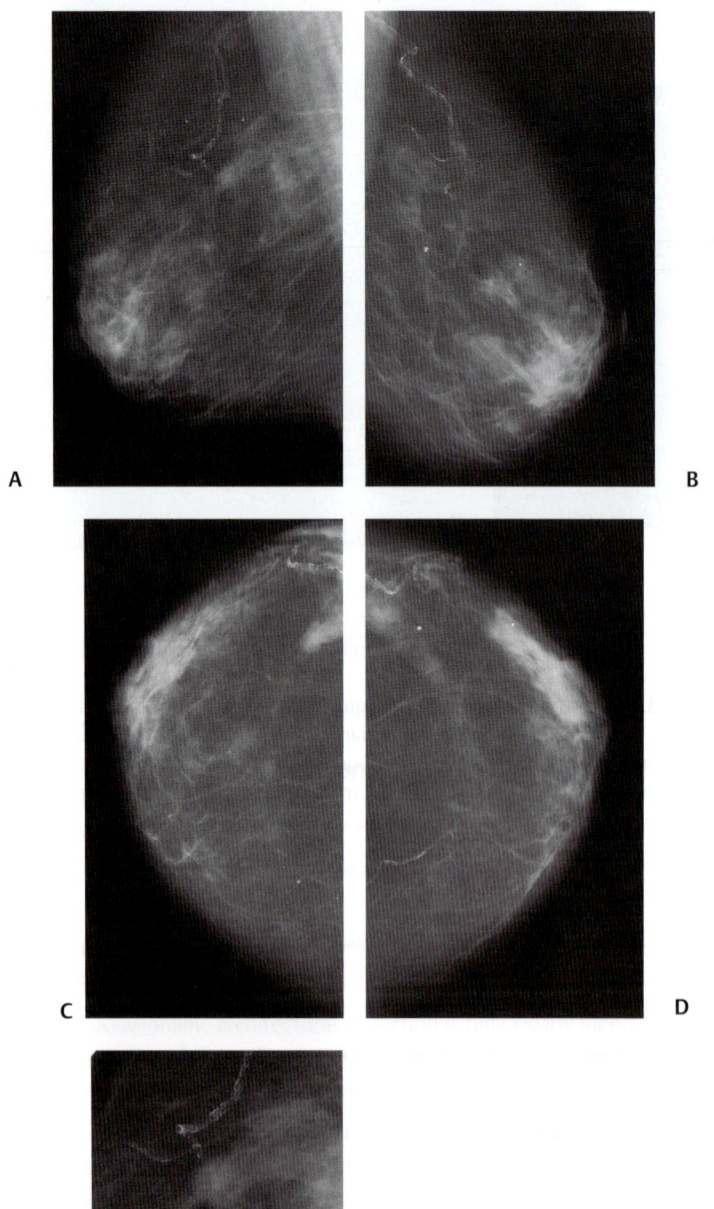

Fig. 23.11 In the right upper outer quadrant, there is a partially obscured oval mass associated with architectural distortion. (**A**) Right MLO mammogram. (**B**) Left MLO mammogram. (**C**) Right CC mammogram. (**D**) Left CC mammogram. (**E**) Right MLO spot compression mammogram.

Ultrasound

Frequency
- 7 MHz

Mass (Fig. 23.12)
- Margin: ill defined
- Echogenicity: hypoechoic
- Retrotumoral acoustic appearance: single edge shadowing
- Shape: ellipsoid

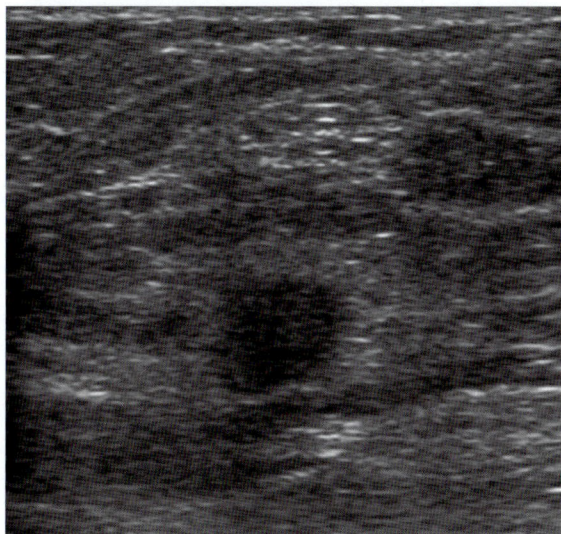

Fig. 23.12 Right breast radial sonogram. The mammographic mass in **Fig. 23.11** corresponds to an ill-defined hypoechoic nodule with posterior acoustic shadowing.

Pathology
- Infiltrating ductal carcinoma

Management
- BI-RADS assessment category 4, suspicious; biopsy should be considered.

Pearls and Pitfalls

- This case demonstrates central architectural distortion due to a malignancy. The tumor is causing retraction of the surrounding density toward the mass. The resulting distorted pattern is readily identified by comparing the abnormal area to the opposite side.

Suggested Reading

Egan RL. Breast Imaging: Diagnosis and Morphology of Breast Diseases. Philadelphia: WB Saunders; 1988:226–240

Kopans DB. Breast Imaging. 2nd ed. Philadelphia: Lippincott-Raven; 1998:382–389

Case 23.7: Infiltrating Ductal

Case History
A 57-year-old woman presents with an inverted nipple.

Mammogram

Mass (Fig. 23.13)
- Margin: spiculated
- Shape: irregular
- Density: high
- Architectural distortion

Physical Examination
- Right breast: inverted right nipple and an 8 cm palpable subareolar mass
- Left breast: normal exam

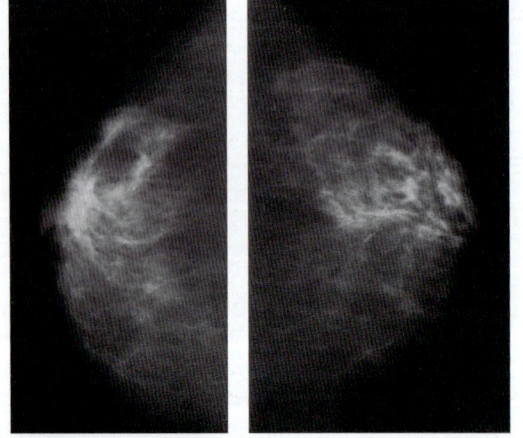

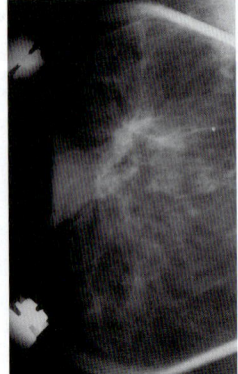

Fig. 23.13 There is a right subareolar spiculated mass associated with nipple retraction and trabecular thickening. (**A**) Right MLO mammogram. (**B**) Left MLO mammogram. (**C**) Right CC mammogram. (**D**) Left CC mammogram. (**E**) Right CC spot compression mammogram.

Pathology
- Invasive ductal carcinoma

Management
- BI-RADS assessment category 5, highly suggestive of malignancy

Pearls and Pitfalls
- Subareolar architectural distortion is sometimes difficult to identify. Even in predominantly fatty breasts, this region may be fairly dense. Spiculations from a subareolar mass may blend into the normal ductal lines that meet at the nipple. Therefore, extra attention should be spent on this region to avoid missing subtle masses or architectural distortion.

Suggested Reading
Heywang-Kobrunner SH, Schreer I, Dershaw DD. Diagnostic Breast Imaging. New York: Thieme; 1997:134–135, 370

Case 23.8: Mixed Ductal and Lobular Cancer

Case History

A 57-year-old woman presents with a new left breast lump.

Mammogram

Mass (Fig. 23.14)
- Margin: indistinct
- Shape: irregular
- Density: high density
- Architectural distortion

Physical Examination
- Left breast: 4 cm mass extending from 2:00 o'clock to 4:00 o'clock
- Right breast: normal exam

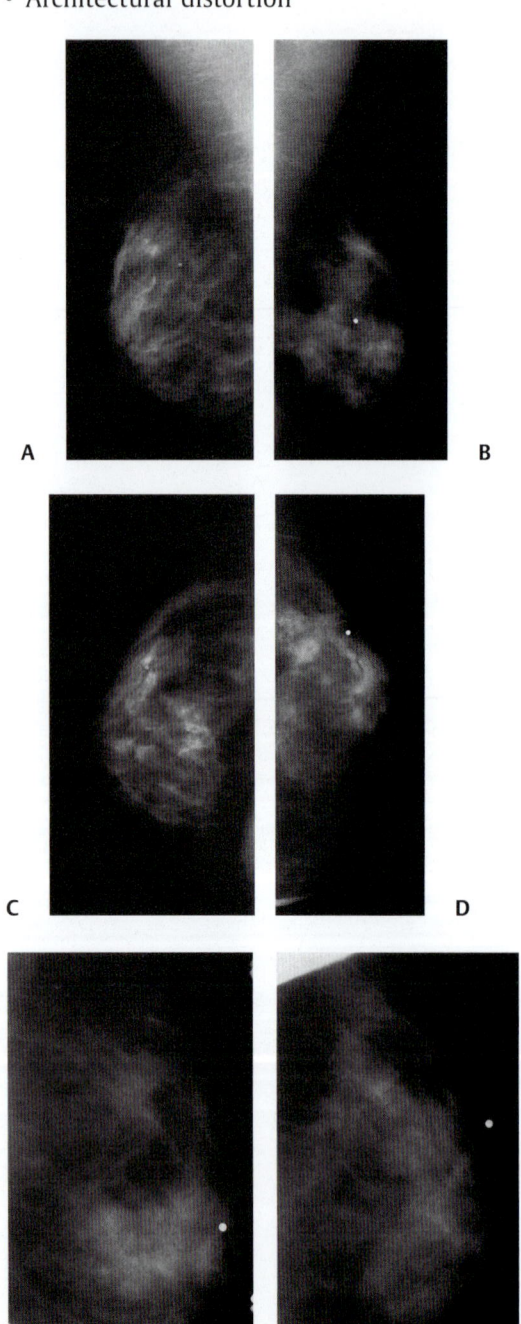

Fig. 23.14 In the left breast, there is an ill-defined mass in the left outer breast. (**A**) Right MLO mammogram. (**B**) Left MLO mammogram. (**C**) Right CC mammogram. (**D**) Left CC mammogram. (**E**) Left MLO spot compression mammogram. (**F**) Left CC spot compression mammogram.

Ultrasound

Frequency
- 10 MHz

Mass (Fig. 23.15)
- Margin: ill defined
- Echogenicity: hypoechoic
- Retrotumoral acoustic appearance: posterior shadowing distal to mass
- Shape: irregular

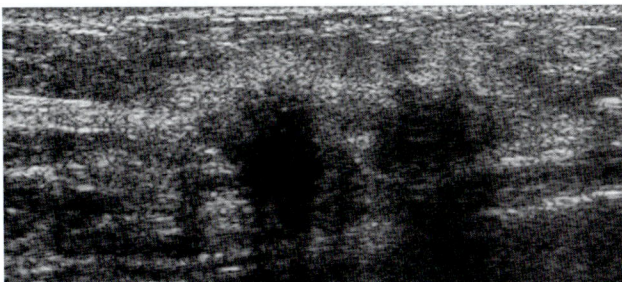

Fig. 23.15 Left radial breast sonogram. The palpable lump is associated with a multilobulated, irregular, hypoechoic mass. This abnormality corresponds to the mammographic mass identified in **Fig. 23.14**.

Other Modalities: MRI (Fig. 23.16)

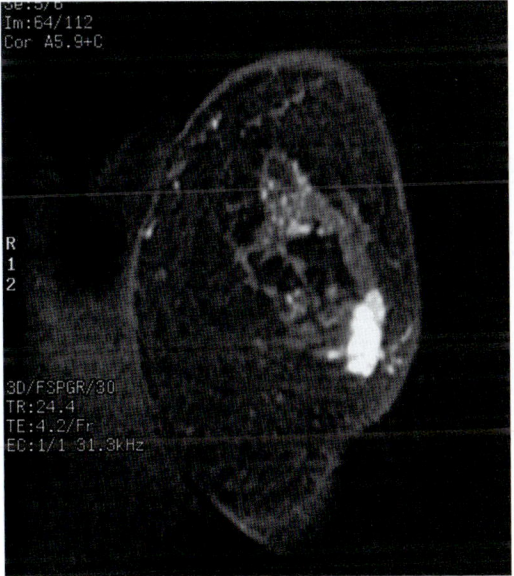

Fig. 23.16 Left coronal dynamic bolus 3D volume-gradient breast MRI. In the outer breast, there is an enhancing, mildly irregular, lobulated mass that corresponds to the mammographic and sonographic mass.

Pathology
- Infiltrating ductal carcinoma

Management
- BI-RADS assessment category 4, suspicious; biopsy should be considered.

Pearls and Pitfalls
- Architectural distortion is a particularly useful sign in denser breasts, as masses are more difficult to identify in these breasts. In this case, the neoplasm causes retraction of the surrounding normal density. This retraction produces a distorted asymmetric parenchymal pattern.
- In this case, sonography was used to correlate the palpable lump with the mammographic abnormality and to provide biopsy guidance. Because of the density of the breast, both sonography and MRI provide better definition of lesion size and location compared with mammography.

Suggested Reading
Bassett LW, Jackson VP, Jahan R, Fu YS, Gold RH. Diagnosis of Diseases of the Breast. Philadelphia: WB Saunders; 1997:116

Case 23.9: Tubular Cancer

Case History
A 55-year-old woman presents with a new right breast lump.

Physical Examination
- Right breast: palpable mass at the 12 o'clock position
- Left breast: normal exam

Mammogram

Mass (Fig. 23.17)
- Margin: spiculated
- Shape: irregular
- Density: high density
- Architectural distortion

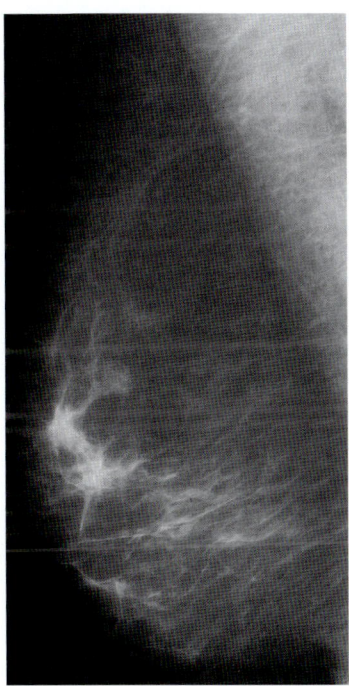
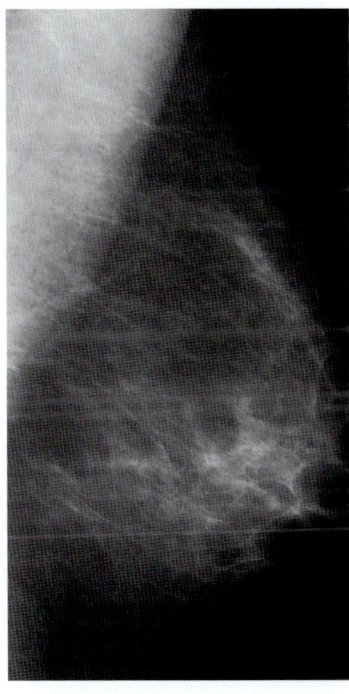

Fig. 23.17 Between the 10 o'clock and the 12 o'clock positions in the right breast, there are at least two irregular spiculated masses. (**A**) Right MLO mammogram. (**B**) Left MLO mammogram.

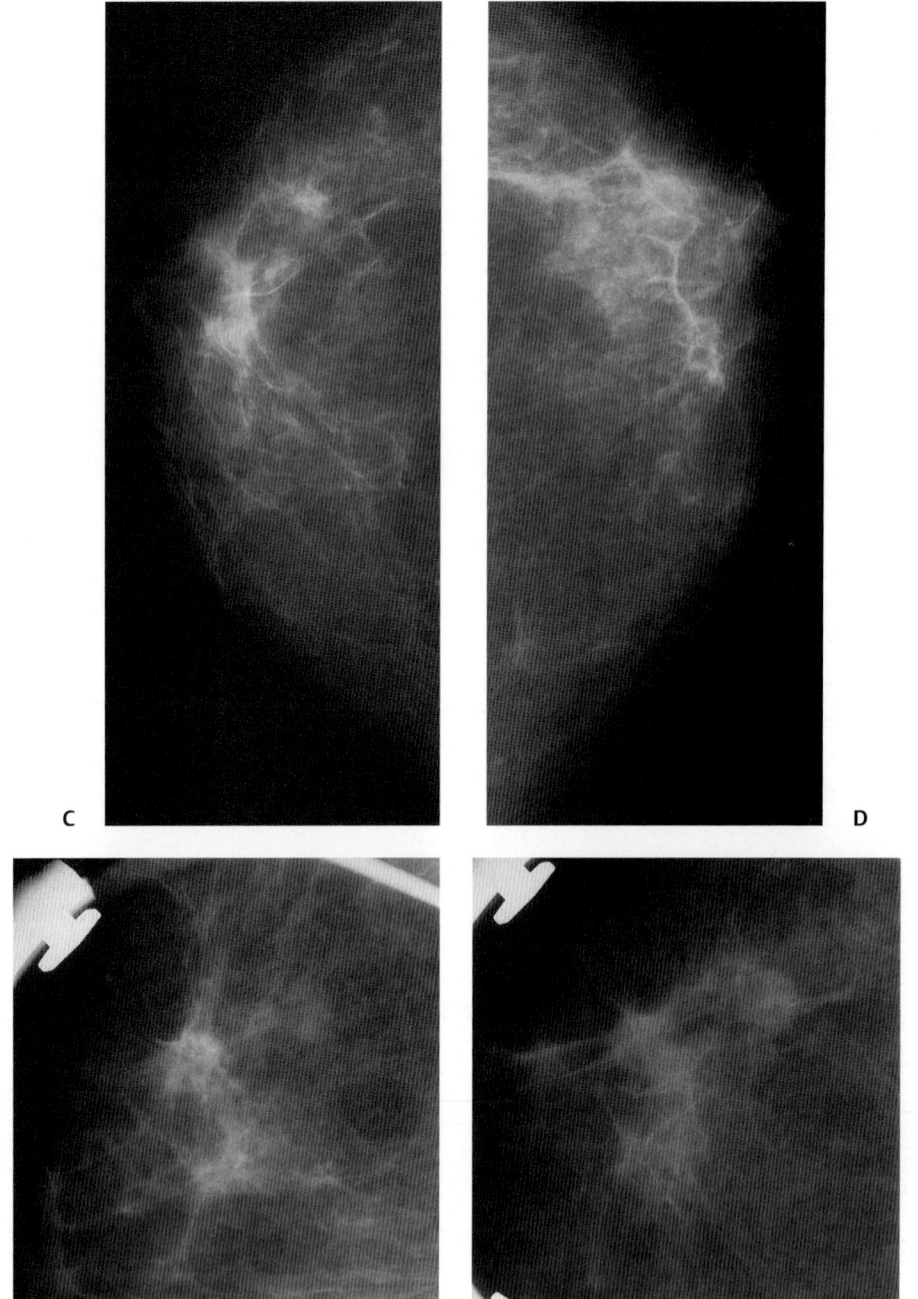

Fig. 23.17 (*continued*) (**C**) Right CC mammogram. (**D**) Left CC mammogram. (**E**) Right MLO spot compression mammogram. (**F**) Right CC spot compression mammogram.

Ultrasound

Frequency
- 7 MHz

Mass (Fig. 23.18)
- Margin: ill defined
- Echogenicity: hypoechoic
- Retrotumoral acoustic appearance: posterior shadowing distal to mass
- Shape: irregular

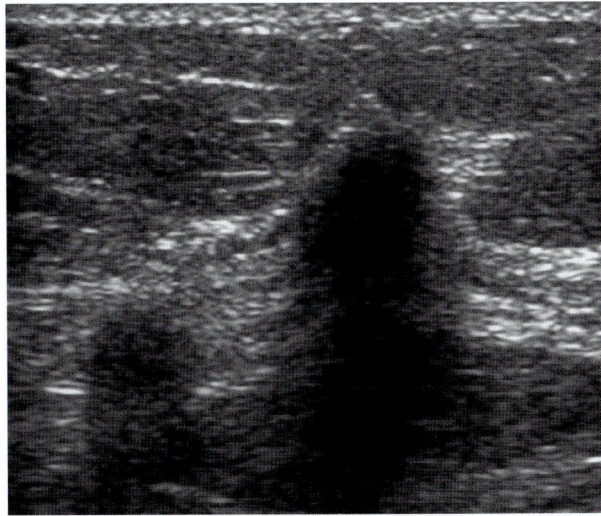

Fig. 23.18 Right radial breast sonogram. In the upper breast, two hypoechoic, irregular shadowing masses are present. The larger mass is palpable. These masses correspond to the mammographic masses.

Pathology
- Infiltrating ductal carcinoma. Both sonographic masses were found to be infiltrating ductal carcinoma, so this is a multifocal neoplasm.

Management
- BI-RADS assessment category 4, suspicious; biopsy should be considered

Pearls and Pitfalls
- For surgical planning, it is important to define the size of the neoplasm within the breast. Architectural distortion of the parenchymal pattern may provide evidence that multifocal disease (multiple lesions within the same quadrant or within 5 cm) is present. With multifocal disease, the parenchymal pattern appears clumped into closely packed irregular or spiculated densities. For small lesions or masses spaced farther apart, magnification views may be useful to identify spiculations connecting the masses.
- Sonography is useful to further confirm the presence of multiple masses and to provide biopsy guidance.

Suggested Reading

Berg WA, Gilbreath PL. Multicentric and multifocal cancer: whole-breast US in preoperative evaluation. Radiology 2000;214:59–66

Gump FE, Shikora S, Habif DV, Kister S, Logerfo P, Estabrook A. The extent and distribution of cancer in breasts with palpable primary tumors. Ann Surg 1986;204:384–390

Male Breast

This is a schematic diagram of the diagnostic approach to mammographic male breast. For further discussion, see Chapter 1.

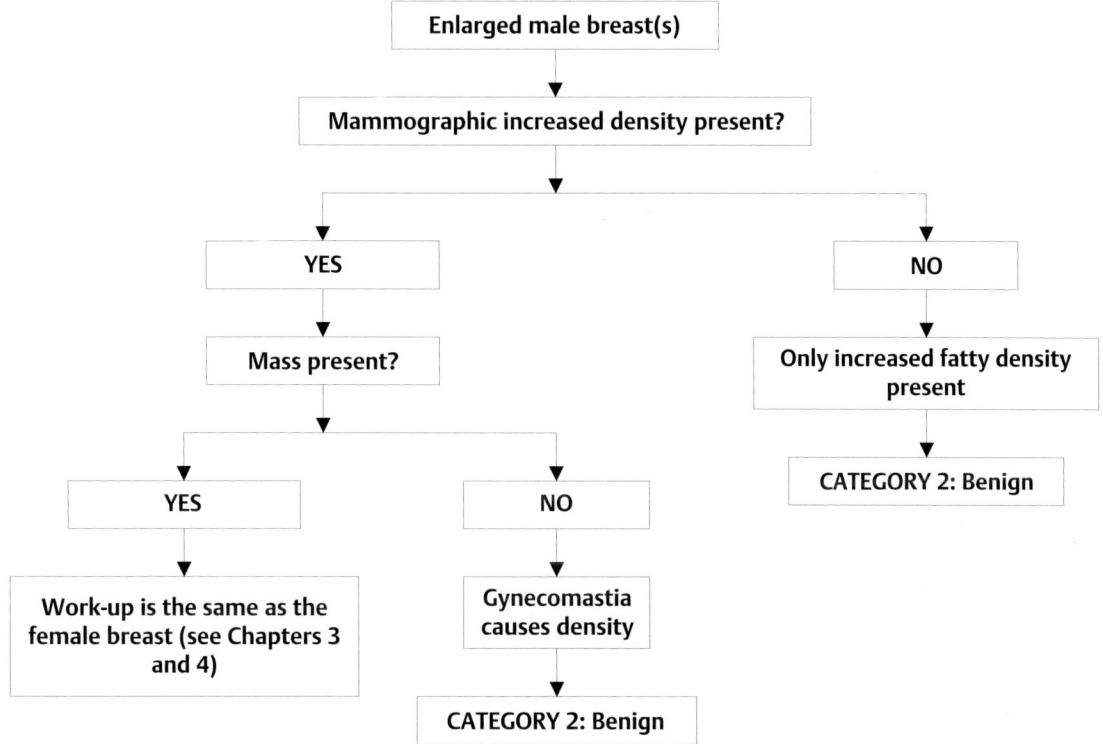

24 Benign Male Breast

Case 24.1: Abscess

Case History
A 64-year-old man presents with a chronic draining sinus tract in the left breast. Two years earlier, he had a hypophysectomy for Cushing's disease, and he has chronic pituitary insufficiency.

Physical Examination
- Left breast: ulcerated nipple with a subareolar mass
- Right breast: enlarged but otherwise normal

Mammogram (Fig. 24.1)

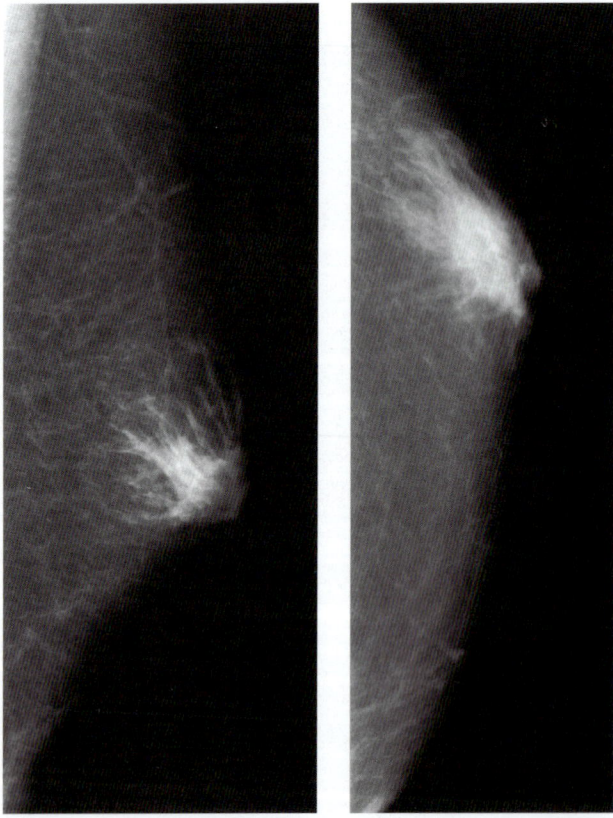

Fig. 24.1 There is ill-defined left subareolar density with coarse linear densities extending into the surrounding fat. (**A**) Left MLO mammogram. (**B**) Left CC mammogram.

Ultrasound

Frequency
- 7.5 MHz

Mass (Fig. 24.2)
- Margin: well defined
- Echogenicity: hypoechoic
- Retrotumoral acoustic appearance: mild acoustic enhancement
- Shape: ellipsoid

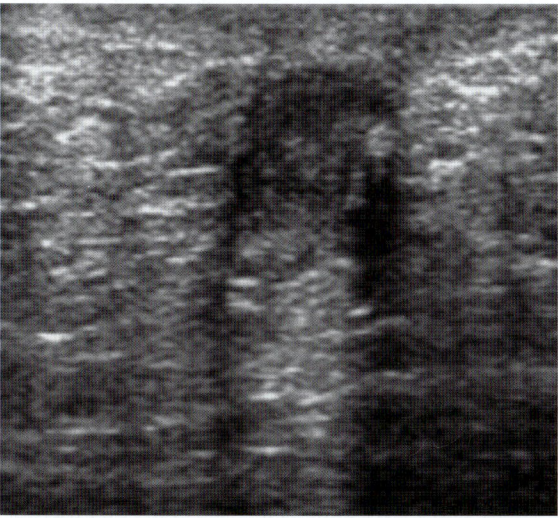

Fig. 24.2 Left transverse breast sonogram. Under the nipple, there is a hypoechoic, well-defined fluid collection with mild posterior acoustic enhancement.

Pathology
- Abscess
- Nipple discharge cultures positive for *Staphylococcus aureus*

Management
- BI-RADS assessment category 3, probably benign; short-interval follow-up

Pearls and Pitfalls

- Because subareolar abscess is a rare lesion of the male breast, there is little previous clinical and radiographic information. In women, the most common infecting organism is *Staphylococcus aureus*. These lesions are commonly recurrent and require excision. This patient failed antibiotic therapy and eventually was treated with excision.
- In females, mammographically, these abscesses produce an ill-defined subareolar mass. Sonographically, there is a hypoechoic fluid collection, which may be mistaken for a solid mass.

Suggested Reading

Appelbaum AH, Evans GFF, Levy KR, Amirkhan RH, Schumpert TD, Schumpert TD. Mammographic appearances of male breast disease. Radiographics 1999;19:559–568

Tavassoli FA. Pathology of the Breast. 2nd ed. Stamford: Appleton & Lange; 1999:792

Case 24.2: Angiolipoma

Case History
A 75-year-old man presents with a new left breast mass.

Physical Examination
- Left breast: palpable, firm, nontender lump at the 9 o'clock position
- Right breast: normal exam

Mammogram

Mass (Fig. 24.3)
- Margin: indistinct
- Shape: irregular
- Density: fat-containing

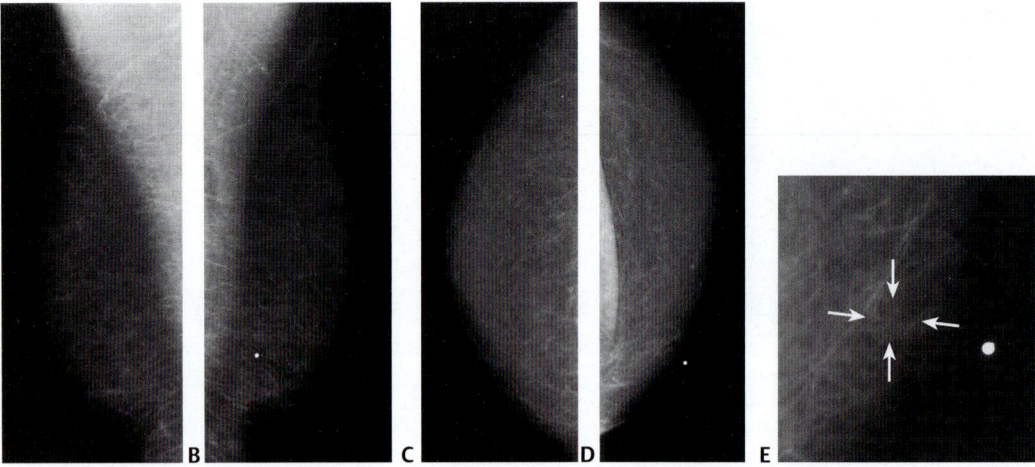

Fig. 24.3 In the left inner breast, the palpable lump corresponds to a small, faint, ill-defined opacity that is partially fat density (*arrows*). (**A**) Right MLO mammogram. (**B**) Left MLO mammogram. (**C**) Right CC mammogram. (**D**) Left CC mammogram. (**E**) Left CC spot magnification mammogram.

Pathology
- Angiolipoma

Management
- BI-RADS assessment category 2, benign finding

Pearls and Pitfalls

- Angiolipomas resemble lipomas. They are encapsulated masses of mature lipocytes with a prominent vascular network. Angiolipomas are commonly found in men. An Armed Forces Institute of Pathology (AFIP) series reported that 17 (24%) of 70 breast angiolipomas were found in men.
- Mammographically, angiolipomas commonly have a benign, fat density appearance.

Suggested Reading
Tavassoli FA. Pathology of the Breast. 2nd ed. Stamford: Appleton & Lange; 1999:695–697

Case 24.3: Fat Necrosis

Case History
A 51-year-old man presents with new left breast lumps.

Physical Examination
- Left breast: two firm nodules between the 12 o'clock and 1 o'clock positions
- Right breast: normal exam

Mammogram

Mass (Fig. 24.4)
- Margin: indistinct
- Shape: oval
- Density: equal density

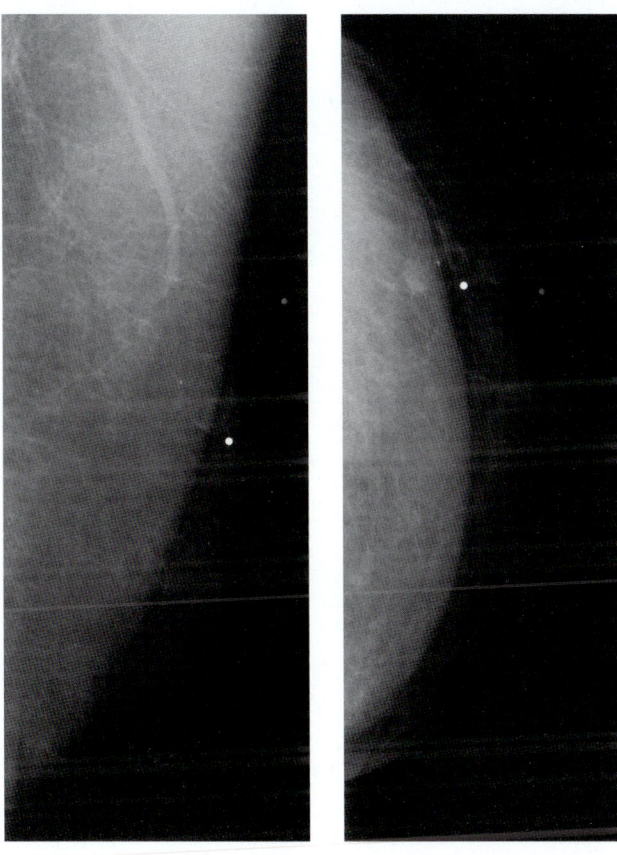

Fig. 24.4 In the left upper breast, there are two palpable lumps that correspond to two ill-defined oval masses. (**A**) Left MLO mammogram. (**B**) Left CC mammogram.

Ultrasound

Frequency
- 13 MHz

Mass (Fig. 24.5)
- Margin: ill defined
- Echogenicity: isoechoic
- Retrotumoral acoustic appearance: no shadowing
- Shape: ellipsoid

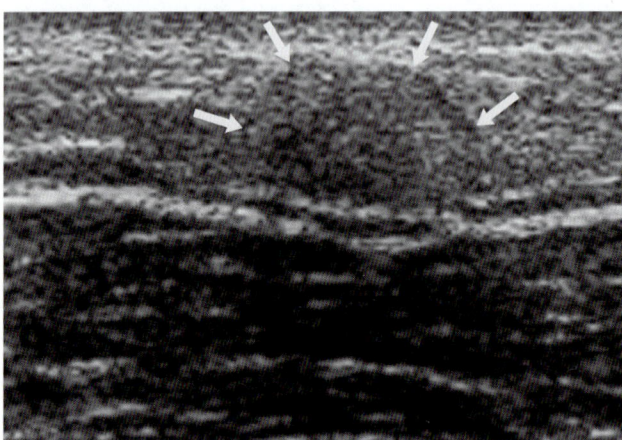 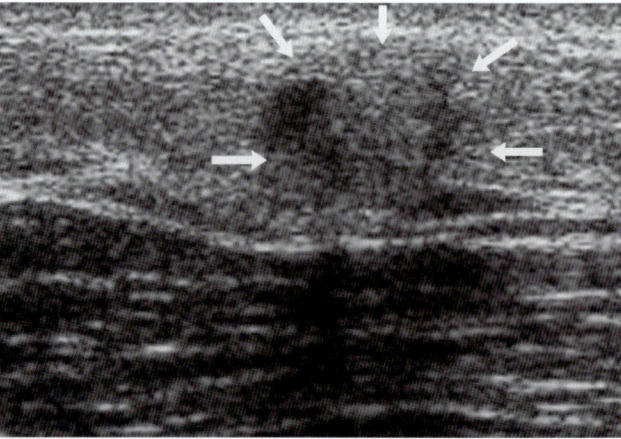

Fig. 24.5 The palpable lumps correspond to two solid masses. One mass (**A**) is an oval, ill-defined, isoechoic mass (*arrows*). The other mass (**B**) is an oval, ill-defined mass with heterogeneous echogenicity (*arrows*). (**A**) Left longitudinal breast sonogram. (**B**) Left longitudinal breast sonogram.

Pathology
- Fat necrosis

Management
- BI-RADS assessment category 4, suspicious; biopsy should be considered.

Pearls and Pitfalls
- Fat necrosis in men is radiographically similar to that in women. Mammographically, fat necrosis produces either a well-defined fat density mass (oil cyst) or an ill-defined irregular mass. The latter abnormality generally cannot be differentiated from malignancy.
- Sonographically, fat necrosis in the male breast is identical to that in the female breast. The mammographic irregular mass generally corresponds to an irregular hypoechoic mass. Occasionally, fat necrosis has a more benign hyperechoic appearance.

Suggested Reading

Chantra PK, So GJ, Wollman JS, Bassett LW. Mammography of the male breast. AJR Am J Roentgenol 1995;164:853–858

Stewart RA, Howlett DC, Hearn FJ. Pictorial review: the imaging features of male breast disease. Clin Radiol 1997;52:739–744

Case 24.4: Gynecomastia—Nodular Pattern/Normal Fatty Male Breast

Case History
A 72-year-old markedly obese male presents with left breast tenderness.

Physical Examination
- Left breast: mildly tender, slightly soft, fullness under the nipple without mass
- Right breast: normal exam

Mammogram (Fig. 24.6)

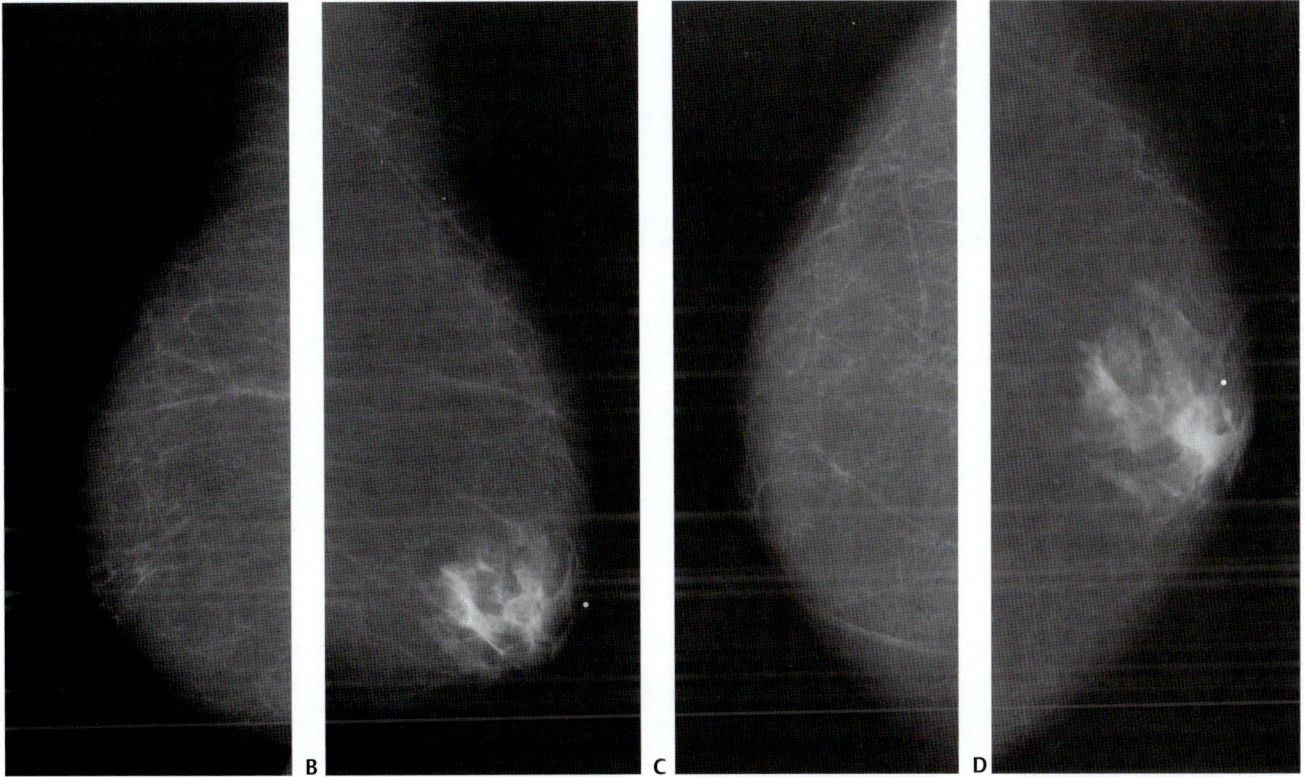

Fig. 24.6 the right breast is completely fatty and normal for an overnweight man. The left breast exhibits mild fan-shaped subareolar density which corresponds to the region of tenderness. (**A**) Right MLO mammogram. (**B**) Left MLO mammogram. (**C**) Right CC mammogram. (**D**) Left CC mammogram.

Ultrasound (Fig. 24.7)

Frequency
- 13 MHz

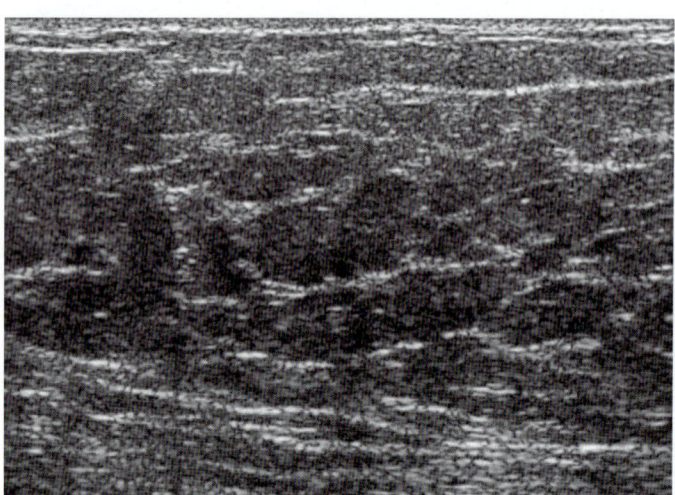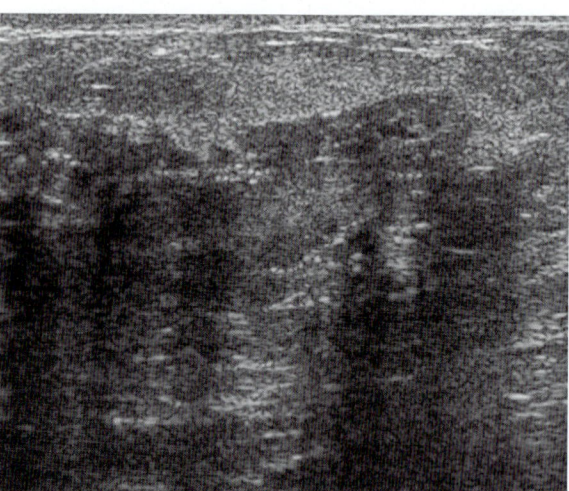

Fig. 24.7 Right breast (**A**) exhibits normal predominately fatty architecture. The tissue of the left breast is heterogeneous echogenicity with random intermittent shadowing. (**A**) Right radial breast sonogram. (**B**) Left radial breast sonogram.

Pathology
- Left gynecomastia

Management
- BI-RADS assessment category 2, benign finding.

> **Pearls and Pitfalls**
>
> - Gynecomastia is clinically defined as more than 2 cm of palpable subareolar tissue in the male breast. In one nonselective autopsy study of 100 men, 55% had gynecomastia. Clinically, most men present with unilateral symptoms. Only 20 to 30% of men note bilateral breast enlargement. The breast enlargement is due to benign ductal and stromal hyperplasia. In this case, the left breast exhibits nodular gynecomastia.
> - When males are overweight, breast enlargement is normal. Radiographically, the normal male breast will be predominately fatty with very little linear or curvilinear density. This patient illustrates a normal right enlarged breast due to obesity.

Suggested Reading
Kapdi CC, Parekh NJ. The male breast. Radiol Clin North Am 1983;21:137–148

Case 24.5: Gynecomastia—Nodular Pattern

Case History
A 38-year-old man presents with new right breast soreness.

Physical Examination
- Right breast: larger than left; no mass
- Left breast: mildly prominent, otherwise normal

Mammogram (Fig. 24.8)

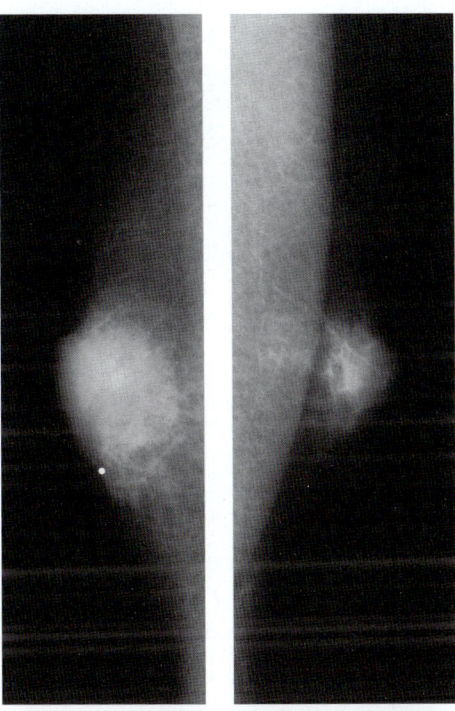

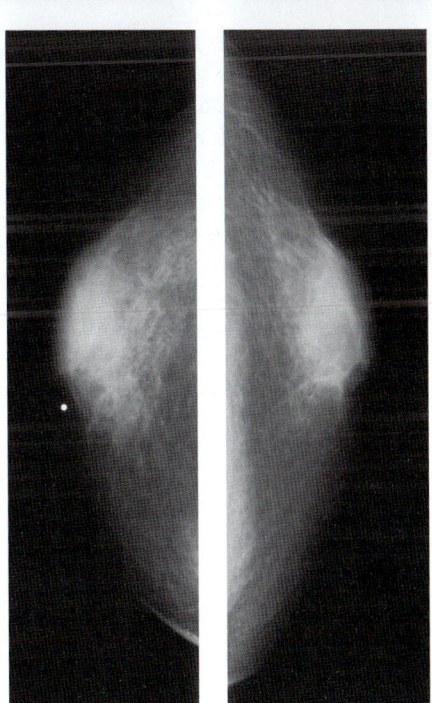

Fig. 24.8 Both breasts exhibit subareolar density. Left breast density is smaller than the right. (**A**) Right MLO mammogram. (**B**) Left MLO mammogram. (**C**) Right CC mammogram. (**D**) Left CC mammogram.

Ultrasound

Frequency
- 11.5 MHz

Mass (Fig. 24.9)
- Margin: ill defined
- Echogenicity: hypoechoic
- Retrotumoral acoustic appearance: no shadowing
- Shape: lobulated

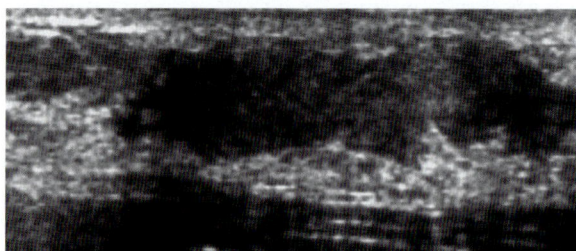 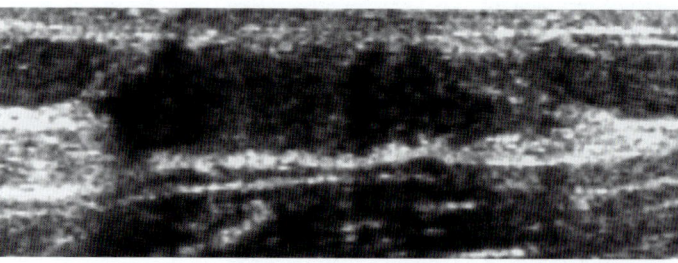

Fig. 24.9 The subareolar mammographic densities correspond to an ellipse of hypoechoic tissue. No separate focal mass is present in the right breast. **(A)** Right radial breast sonogram. **(B)** Left radial breast sonogram.

Pathology
- Gynecomastia

Management
- BI-RADS assessment category 2, benign finding

Pearls and Pitfalls

- Mammographically, there are three patterns of gynecomastia: nodular, dendritic, and diffuse. With the nodular pattern, the subareolar density is spherical with fan-shaped edges. The density is generally centered under the nipple, and the edges blend into the surrounding fat. Dendritic gynecomastia presents a flame-shaped subareolar density that radiates coarse linear or curvilinear densities into the surrounding breast tissue. The diffuse glandular pattern is similar to the heterogeneously dense female parenchymal pattern. This patient illustrates the nodular pattern of gynecomastia.
- Sonographically, the nodular pattern may present with a hypoechoic mass, enlarged ducts, or diffuse heterogeneous changes with no mass. Shadowing may be associated with the hypoechoic mass or heterogeneous echogenicity. However, with the latter situation, the shadowing is random or intermittent. In this patient, because both breasts sonographically appeared similar, gynecomastia was easily confirmed even though a hypoechoic mass was present. Sonographically, the dendritic pattern demonstrates mild linear hyperechoic fibrous tissue without mass.

Suggested Reading

Jackson VP, Gilmor RL. Male breast carcinoma and gynecomastia: comparison of mammography with sonography. Radiology 1983;149:533–536

So GJ, Chantra PK, Wollman JS, Bassett LW. The male breast. In: Bassett LW, Jackson VP, Jahan R, Fu YS, Gold RH, eds. Diagnosis of Diseases of the Breast. Philadelphia: WB Saunders; 1997:501–518

Wigley KD, Thomas JL, Bernardino ME, Rosenbaum JL. Sonography of gynecomastia. AJR Am J Roentgenol 1981;136:927–930

Case 24.6: Gynecomastia—Dendritic Pattern

Case History
A 49-year-old man notes a right breast lump. Eleven years ago, he saw a surgeon for a left breast lump.

Physical Examination
- Right breast: soft, smooth, movable, subareolar lump
- Left breast: normal exam

Mammogram (Fig. 24.10 and 24.11)

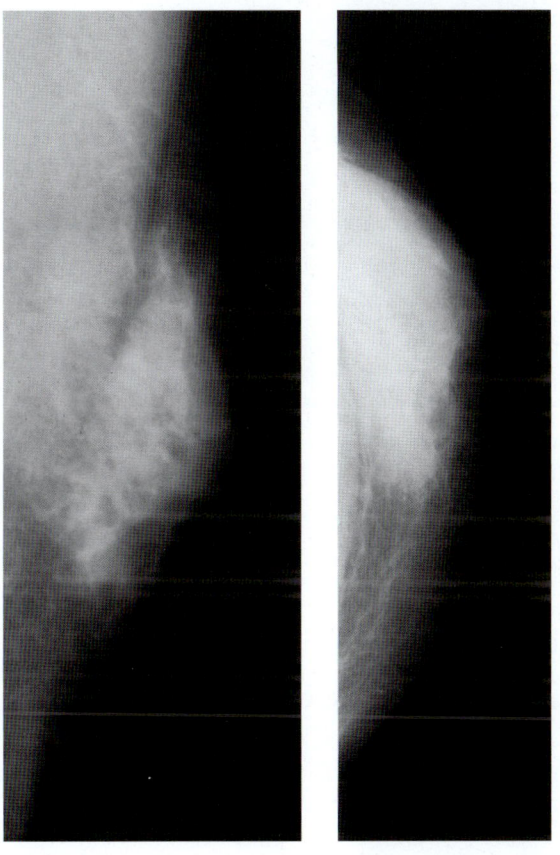

Fig. 24.10 Unilateral left breast mammogram was performed after the patient noted a left breast lump for 2 months. The study demonstrates diffuse increased density of the left breast. (**A**) Left MLO mammogram. (**B**) Left CC mammogram.

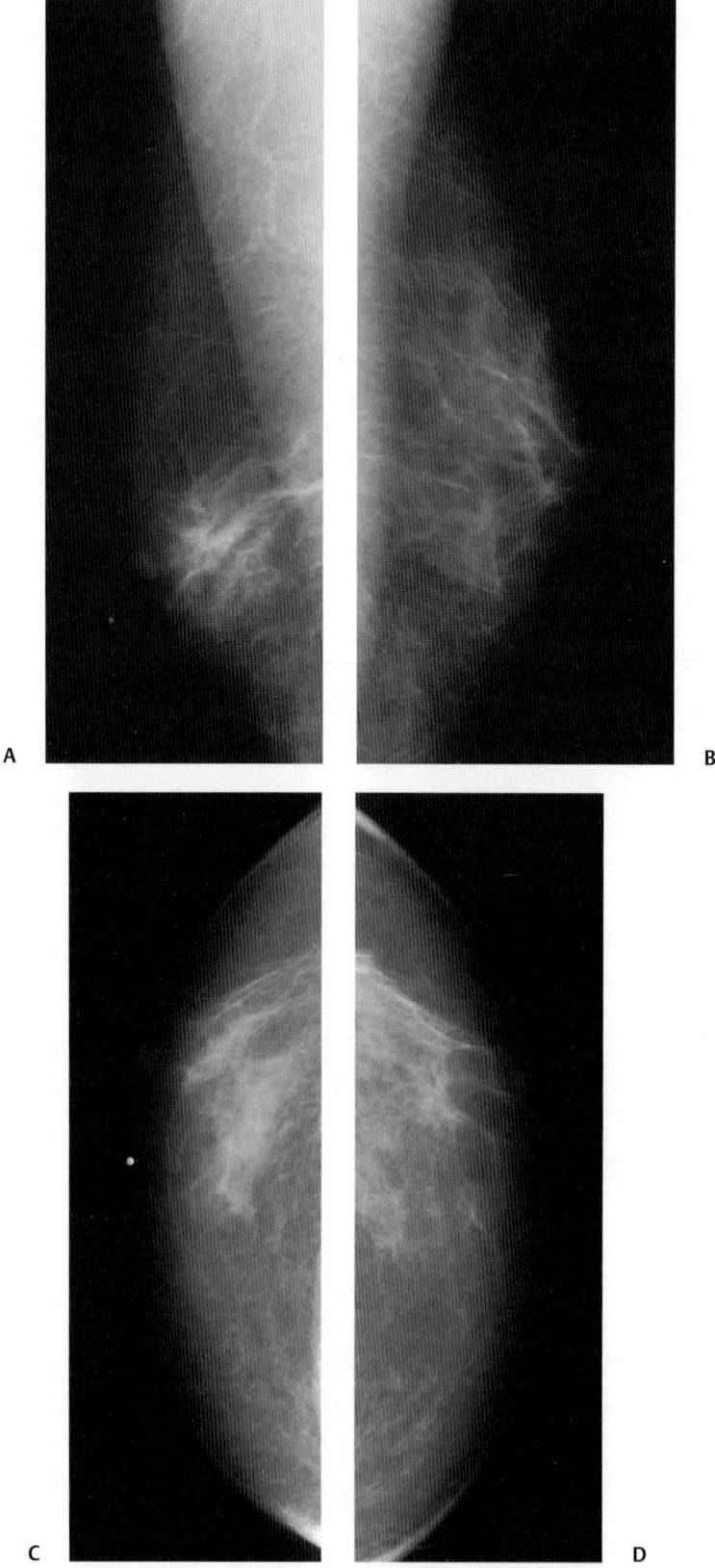

Fig. 24.11 This bilateral study was performed 11 years after that in **Fig. 24.4**. Both breasts exhibit mild coarse subareolar linear densities. (**A**) Right MLO mammogram. (**B**) Left MLO mammogram. (**C**) Right CC mammogram. (**D**) Left CC mammogram.

Pathology
- Gynecomastia

Management
- BI-RADS assessment category 2, benign finding

Pearls and Pitfalls

- The radiographic appearance of gynecomastia is linked to the pathologic findings. Patients with acute symptoms less than 4 months have the florid histology that is associated with the radiographic nodular pattern.
- Patients with gynecomastia longer than 1 year tend to have the fibrous histology that is associated with the dendritic mammographic pattern. This case demonstrates the evolution of nodular (**Fig. 24.10**) to the dendritic (**Fig. 24.11**) pattern.

Suggested Reading

Michels LG, Gold RH, Arndt RD. Radiography of gynecomastia and other disorders of the male breast. Radiology 1977;122:117–122

Tavassoli FA. Pathology of the Breast. 2nd ed. Stamford: Appleton & Lange; 1999:829–855

Case 24.7: Gynecomastia—Diffuse Glandular Pattern

Case History
A 70-year-old man presents with cirrhosis. He is also taking spironolactone.

Physical Examination
- Bilateral breasts: bilaterally enlarged with small subareolar firm nodules

Mammogram (Fig. 24.12)

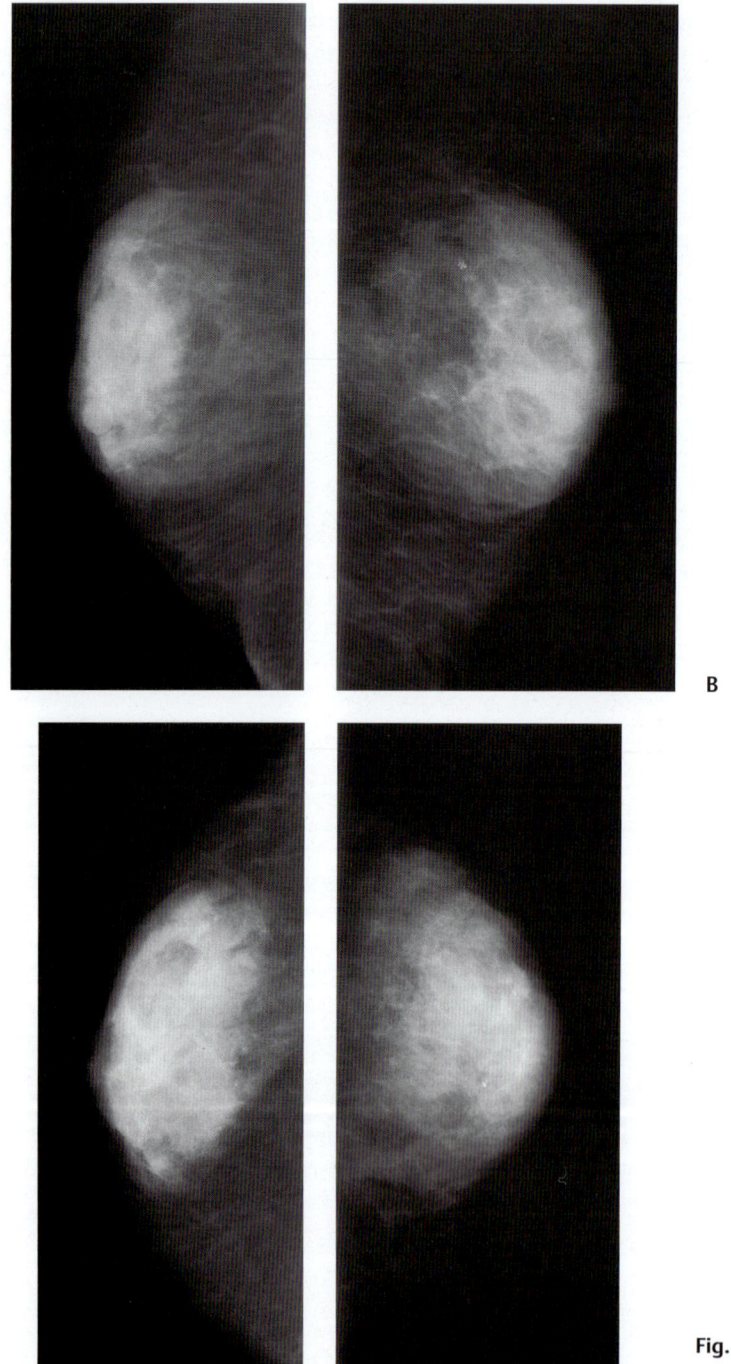

Fig. 24.12 Both breasts are enlarged and exhibit diffusely heterogeneous density. (**A**) Right MLO mammogram. (**B**) Left MLO mammogram. (**C**) Right CC mammogram. (**D**) Left CC mammogram.

Pathology
- Gynecomastia

Management
- BI-RADS assessment category 2, benign finding

Pearls and Pitfalls

- This patient exhibits the diffuse glandular pattern of gynecomastia.
- Gynecomastia is due to increased estrogen, enhanced breast sensitivity to estrogen, decreased testosterone, or reduced breast sensitivity to testosterone. Causes of excess estrogen are the following: (1) puberty, (2) hermaphroditism, (3) testicular tumors, (4) nontesticular tumors (skin, nevus, adrenal, lung, mesothelioma, hepatocellular), (5) endocrine abnormalities, (6) cirrhosis, (7) severe changes in nutrition, and (8) drugs with estrogenic effect (steroids, digitalis estrogens, heroin, tamoxifen, marijuana). Abnormalities that create deficient androgen include (1) senescence, (2) testicular failure (e.g., Klinefelter syndrome, trauma, orchitis), and (3) drugs that inhibit the effect or synthesis of testosterone (antineoplastic agents, cimetidine, diazepam, phenytoin, spironolactone). Idiopathic causes of gynecomastia include (1) drugs (furosemide, methyldopa, reserpine, theophylline, tricyclic antidepressants, verapamil), (2) renal failure, (3) nonneoplastic lung disease, (4) chest wall trauma, (5) pituitary adenoma, and (6) acquired immunodeficiency syndrome [AIDS] and human immunodeficiency virus [HIV] infection.

Suggested Reading
Bland KI, Graves TA, Page DL. Gynecomastia. In: Bland KI, Copeland EM. The Breast. 2nd ed. Philadelphia: WB Saunders; 1998:153–189

Case 24.8: Lipoma

Case History
A 42-year-old man presents with a right breast lump.

Mammogram (Fig. 24.13)

Physical Examination
- Right breast: soft lump in the outer inferior quadrant
- Left breast: normal exam

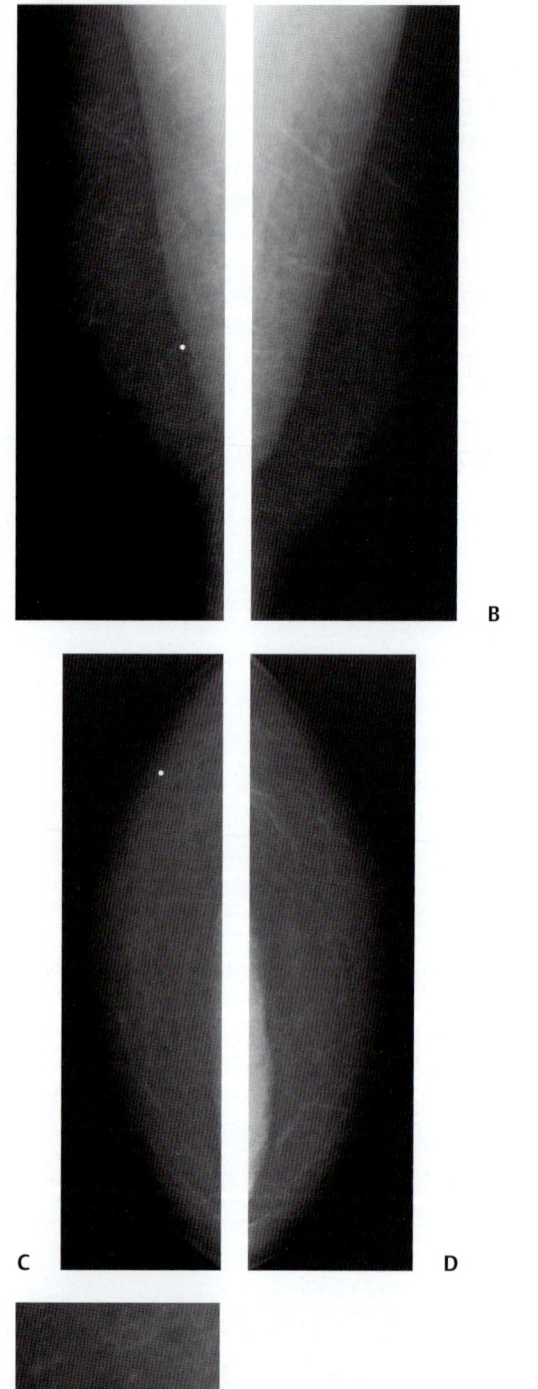

Fig. 24.13 Bilateral normal male mammograms. No mass is identified in the area of the palpable mass. (**A**) Right MLO mammogram. (**B**) Left MLO mammogram. (**C**) Right CC mammogram. (**D**) Left CC mammogram. (**E**) Right MLO spot magnification mammogram.

Ultrasound

Frequency
- 11.5 MHz

Mass (Figs. 24.14 and 24.15)
- Margin: well defined
- Echogenicity: hyperechoic
- Retrotumoral acoustic appearance: no shadowing
- Shape: ellipsoid

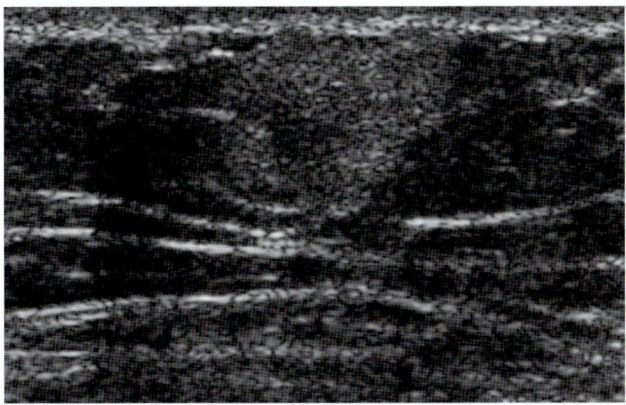

Fig. 24.14 Right radial breast sonogram. The palpable breast lump corresponds to a well-defined hyperechoic oval mass.

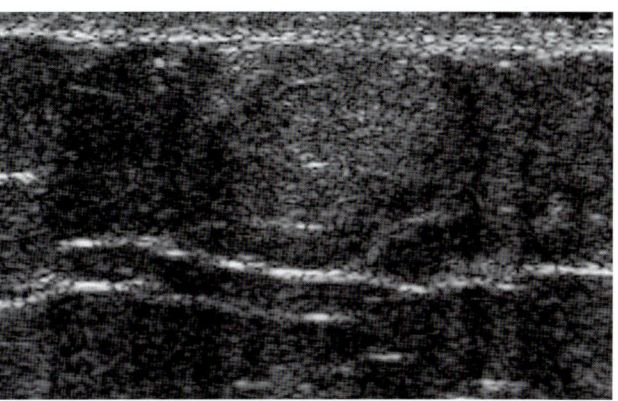

Fig. 24.15 Longitudinal abdominal sonogram. On the anterior abdominal wall, a palpable lump corresponds to a well-defined hyperechoic mass that is similar to the breast mass.

Pathology
- Lipoma

Management
- BI-RADS assessment category 2, benign finding

Pearls and Pitfalls

- Lipomas are composed of mature lipocytes that are surrounded by a fibrous capsule. Lipomas are present in any organ containing fat and are commonly multiple.
- Mammographically, lipomas are well-circumscribed fat density masses. If the capsule is thin, the capsule may not be radiographically evident as in this case.
- Sonographically, the lipoma is a well-defined mass that is isoechoic, hypoechoic, hyperechoic, or heterogeneous echogenicity compared with subcutaneous fat.

Suggested Reading

Stewart RA, Howlett DC, Hearn FJ. Pictorial review: the imaging features of male breast disease. Clin Radiol 1997;52:739–744

Case 24.9: Lymph Node

Case History
An 84-year-old obese man has a palpable lump in the right breast.

Physical Examination
- Right breast: firm, movable nodule in the peripheral right upper outer quadrant
- Left breast: normal exam

Mammogram

Mass (Fig. 24.16)
- Margin: circumscribed
- Shape: lobular
- Density: equal

Associated Mammographic Findings
- Lymph node accounting for palpable lump in a male patient with pseudogynecomastia

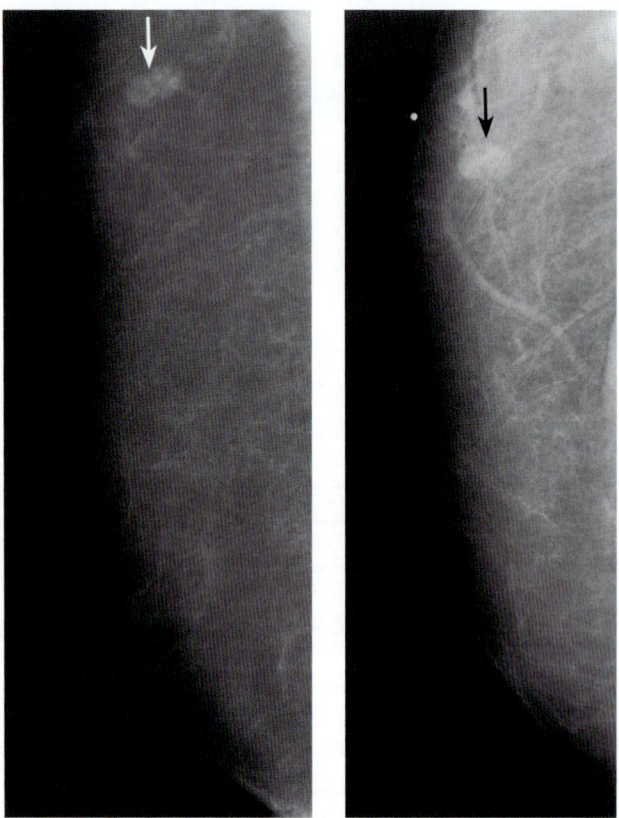

Fig. 24.16 Right breast is primarily fatty. The palpable lump corresponds to a lobulated mass (*arrow*) in the extreme upper outer quadrant (**B**). (**A**) Right MLO mammogram. (**B**) Right XCCL mammogram.

Pathology
- Intramammary lymph node/pseudogynecomastia

Management
- BI-RADS assessment category 2, benign finding

Pearls and Pitfalls
- This patient demonstrates pseudogynecomastia or enlarged fatty breast associated with obesity. This condition is not true gynecomastia.
- The palpable mammographic nodule has the characteristic central lucency consistent with a lymph node.

Suggested Reading
Michels LG, Gold RH, Arndt RD. Radiography of gynecomastia and other disorders of the male breast. Radiology 1977;122:117–122

Case 24.10: Myofibroblastoma

Case History
A 61-year-old man presents with fullness of the right breast.

Physical Examination
- Right breast: vague firm area in the 11 o'clock position
- Left breast: normal exam

Mammogram

Mass (Fig. 24.17)
- Margin: circumscribed
- Shape: lobular
- Density: high density

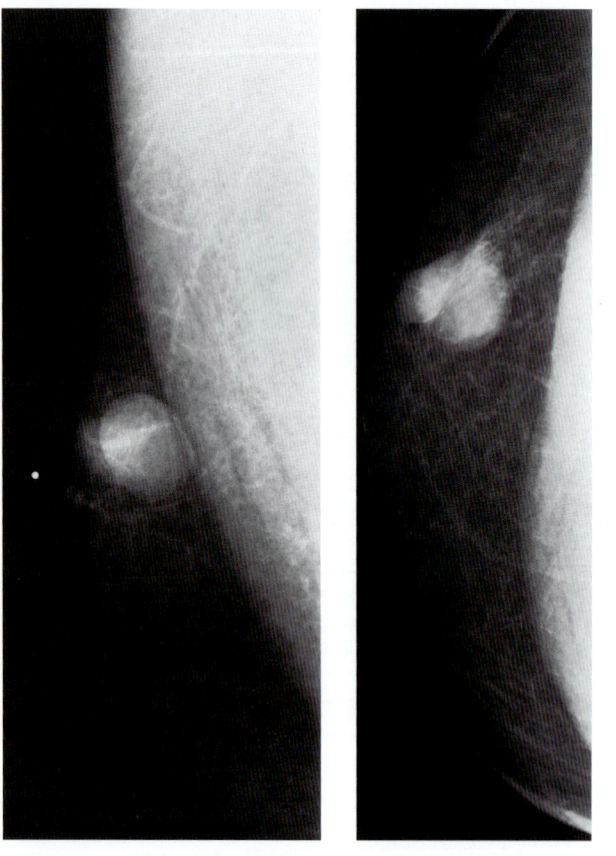

Fig. 24.17 A circumscribed lobulated mass is present in the right upper outer breast. (**A**) Right MLO mammogram. (**B**) Right CC mammogram.

Ultrasound

Frequency
- 14 MHz

Mass (Fig. 24.18)
- Margin: well defined
- Echogenicity: hypoechoic
- Retrotumoral acoustic appearance: increased posterior acoustic enhancement
- Shape: lobulated

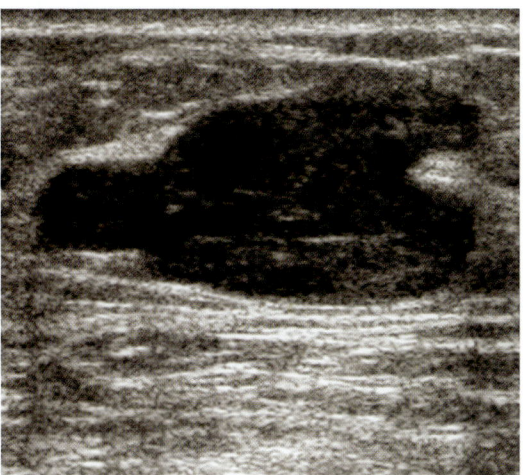 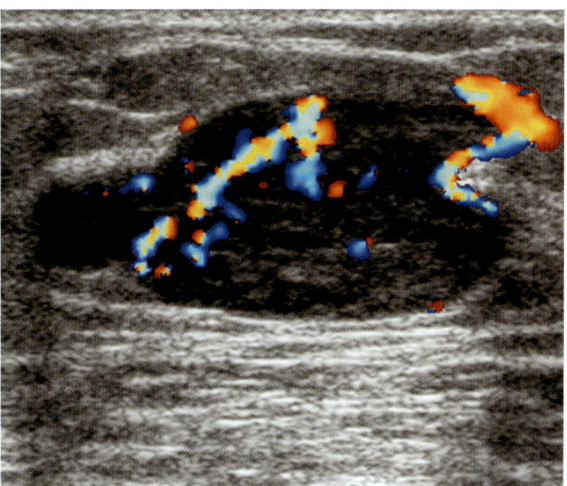

Fig. 24.18 The palpable firmness in the right upper outer quadrant corresponded to a well-defined, lobulated, hypoechoic mass. (**A**) Right radial breast sonogram. (**B**) Right radial color Doppler breast sonogram.

Pathology
- Myofibroblastoma

Management
- BI-RADS assessment category 4, suspicious; biopsy should be considered.

Pearls and Pitfalls

- Myofibroblastoma is a benign mass consisting of proliferating spindle-shaped cells. This tumor primarily affects men in their late 50s or early 60s. The lesion presents as a nontender, solitary, firm, movable mass.
- Mammographically, myofibroblastomas are noncalcified, well-defined, lobulated masses.
- Sonographically, these tumors are well-defined, lobulated, hypoechoic solid masses that may or may not shadow. Mammographically and sonographically, these tumors resemble fibroadenomas.

Suggested Reading

Greenberg JS, Kaplan SS, Grady C. Myofibroblastoma of the breast in women: imaging appearances. AJR Am J Roentgenol 1998;171:71–72

Miller JA, Levine C, Simmons MZ. Imaging characteristics of giant myofibroblastoma of the breast diagnosed by ultrasound-guided core biopsy. J Clin Ultrasound 1997;25:395–397

Rebner M, Faju U. Myofibroblastoma of the male breast. Breast Dis 1993;6:157–160

Tavassoli FA. Pathology of the Breast. 2nd ed. Stamford: Appleton & Lange; 1999:686–691

Case 24.11: Sebaceous Cyst

Case History
A 73-year-old man has a right breast mass, which has been present for many years.

Physical Examination
- Right breast: mildly enlarged; small, firm area in the outer breast
- Left breast: normal exam

Mammogram

Mass (Fig. 24.19)
- Margin: circumscribed
- Shape: oval
- Density: equal density

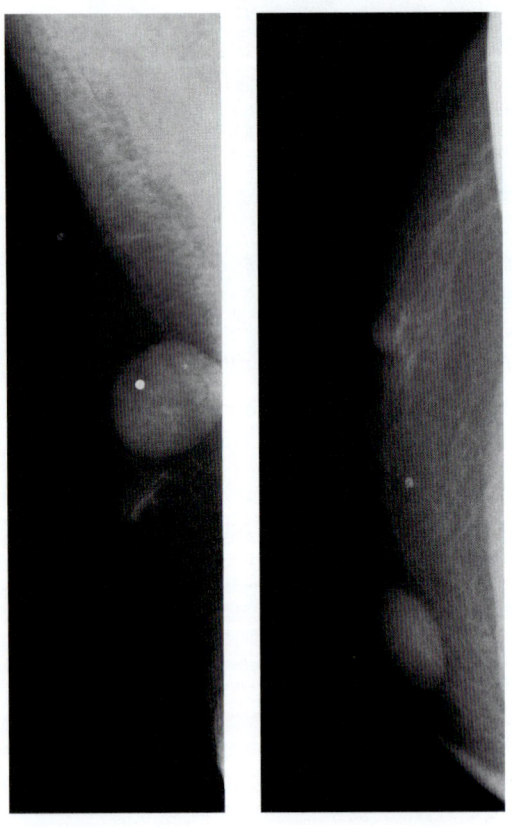

Fig. 24.19 In the right upper outer quadrant, there is a well-circumscribed oval subcutaneous mass. (**A**) Right MLO mammogram. (**B**) Right CC mammogram.

Ultrasound

Frequency
- 11.5 MHz

Mass (Fig. 24.20)
- Margin: well defined
- Echogenicity: hypoechoic
- Retrotumoral acoustic appearance: increased posterior acoustic transmission
- Shape: ellipsoid

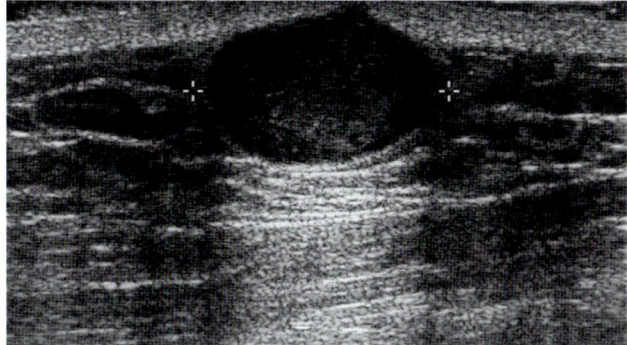

Fig. 24.20 Right antiradial breast sonogram. The mammographic mass corresponds to a well-circumscribed, hypoechoic oval mass with strong acoustic enhancement. The mass demonstrates continuity with the dermis through a small "beak" in its anterior margin.

Pathology
- Sebaceous cyst

Management
- BI-RADS assessment category 2, benign finding

Pearls and Pitfalls

- Epidermal inclusion and sebaceous cysts occur in cutaneous or subcutaneous tissues. Epidermal inclusion cysts usually arise from either hair follicles or squamous metaplasia of sweat ducts. Sebaceous cysts result from obstructed sebaceous glands.
- Sebaceous cysts and epidermal inclusion cysts have similar mammographic findings. They are both circumscribed round masses. The appearance of these entities is the same as in women. Occasionally, the cyst may rupture and cause an inflammatory mass, which is indistinguishable from malignancy.
- Sonographically, these cysts appear as well-defined, anechoic, or hypoechoic fluid collections with increased posterior acoustic transmission.

Suggested Reading

Appelbaum AH, Evans GFF, Levy KR, Amirkhan RH, Schumpert TD. Mammographic appearances of male breast disease. Radiographics 1999;19:559–568

Jackson VP, Jahan R, Fu YS. Benign breast lesions. In: Bassett LW, Jackson VP, Jahan R, Fu YS, Gold RH, eds. Diagnosis of the Diseases of the Breast. Philadelphia: WB Saunders; 1997:357–443

Wigley KD, Thomas JL, Bernardino ME, Rosenbaum JL. Sonography of gynecomastia. AJR Am J Roentgenol 1981;136:927–930

25 Malignant Male Breast

Case 25.1: Ductal Carcinoma in Situ

Case History
A 77-year-old man presents with right bloody nipple discharge.

Mammogram (Fig. 25.1)

Physical Examination
- Right breast: bloody discharge easily expressed from nipple at the 2 o'clock position; normal nipple and areola
- Left breast: normal exam

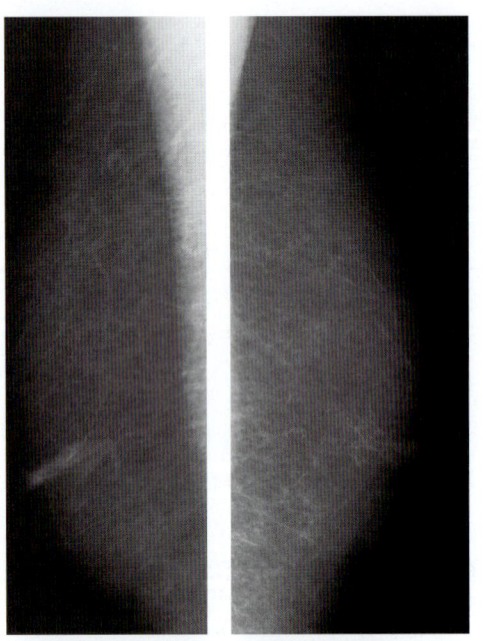
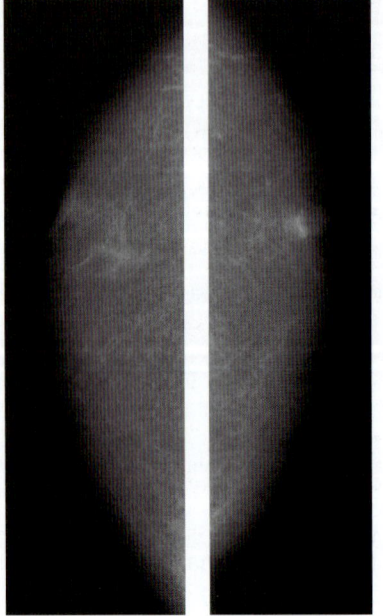

Fig. 25.1 There is mild prominence of a right subareolar duct. The left breast is normal. (**A**) Right MLO mammogram. (**B**) Left MLO mammogram. (**C**) Right CC mammogram. (**D**) Left CC mammogram.

Pathology
- Ductal carcinoma in situ

Management
- BI-RADS assessment category 0; need additional imaging

Pearls and Pitfalls

- Male breast cancer consists of less than 1% of all new breast cancer cases and only 0.2% of all newly discovered cancers in men. Infiltrating ductal carcinoma is the most common histology (approximately 85% of cases). Ductal carcinoma in situ comprises 5% of male breast cancers. Men develop ductal carcinoma in situ and invasive cancer later than women. Mean age at presentation is in the mid-60s. These tumors generally present with a nontender palpable mass. Nipple discharge is relatively common and is present in approximately 35% of patients with ductal carcinoma in situ and in 10 to 20% of those with invasive tumors. Other associated findings include skin thickening, nipple retraction, and axillary adenopathy.
- Mammographically, invasive malignancies have a wide variety of appearances. They may be either well or ill defined. Their shapes include round, oval, lobulated, and irregular. Microcalcifications are present in 25 to 30% of tumors. Commonly, these calcifications are coarser than the ones found in female breast cancer.
- Sonographically, male invasive malignancies have the same appearances as female tumors. However, male ductal carcinoma in situ differs from female ductal carcinoma in situ. The papillary subtype predominates in men, so male ductal carcinoma in situ lesions sonographically commonly appear associated with fluid collections or ducts.
- Bloody discharge, a prominent duct, and no palpable mass suggest that ductography may be useful to identify the intraductal abnormality. Sonography may also be used to identify a focally dilated ductal system and guide intraoperative excision. However, this patient had no further imaging. The patient's ducts were initially surgically excised. When ductal carcinoma in situ was identified, a mastectomy was performed.

Suggested Reading

American Cancer Society. Cancer Facts and Figures: 2001. Atlanta: ACS; 2001

Appelbaum AH, Evans GFF, Levy KR, Amirkhan RH, Schumpert TD, Schumpert TD. Mammographic appearances of male breast disease. Radiographics 1999;19:559–568

Camus MG, Joshi MG, Mackarem G, et al. Ductal carcinoma in situ of the male breast. Cancer 1994;74:1289–1293

Hittmair AP, Lininger RA, Tavassoli FA. Ductal carcinoma in situ (DCIS) in the male breast: a morphologic study of 84 cases of pure DCIS and 30 cases of DCIS associated with invasive carcinoma—a preliminary report. Cancer 1998;83:2139–2149

Quimet-Oliva D, Hebert G, Ladouceur J. Radiographic characteristics of male breast cancer. Radiology 1978;129:37–40

Scott-Conner CEH, Jochimsen PR, Menck HR, Winchester DJ. An analysis of male and female breast cancer treatment and survival among demographically identical pairs of patients. Surgery 1999;126:775–780, discussion 780–781

Case 25.2: Inflammatory Carcinoma

Case History
A 68-year-old man presents with left breast swelling and shortness of breath.

Physical Examination
- Left breast: entire breast is hard and lumpy; diffuse skin thickening and erythema are present; palpable nodes are present in the left axillary and supraclavicular areas.
- Right breast: normal exam
- Chest: decreased breath sounds bilaterally at bases

Mammogram

Mass (Fig. 25.2)
- Margin: indistinct
- Shape: irregular
- Density: high density
- Skin thickening
- Trabecular thickening

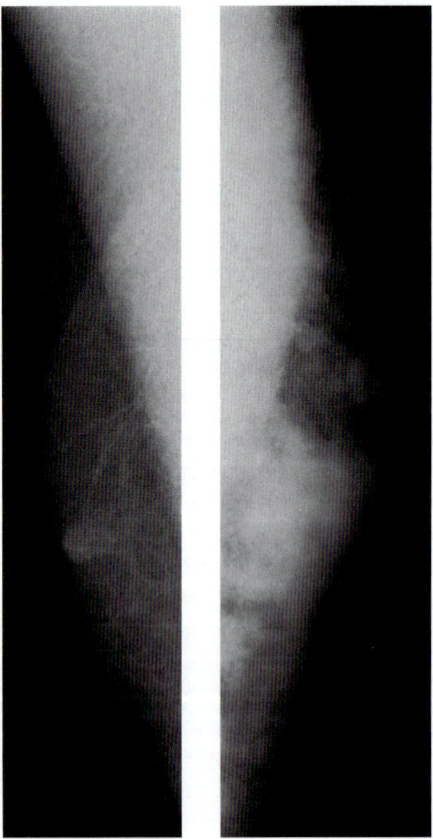

Fig. 25.2 The left breast shows marked, diffuse increase in density compared with the right breast. There is associated skin thickening and diffuse nodularity throughout the left breast. (**A**) Right MLO mammogram. (**B**) Left MLO mammogram.

Other Modalities: Chest Radiography and Bone Scan (Figs. 25.3 and 25.4)

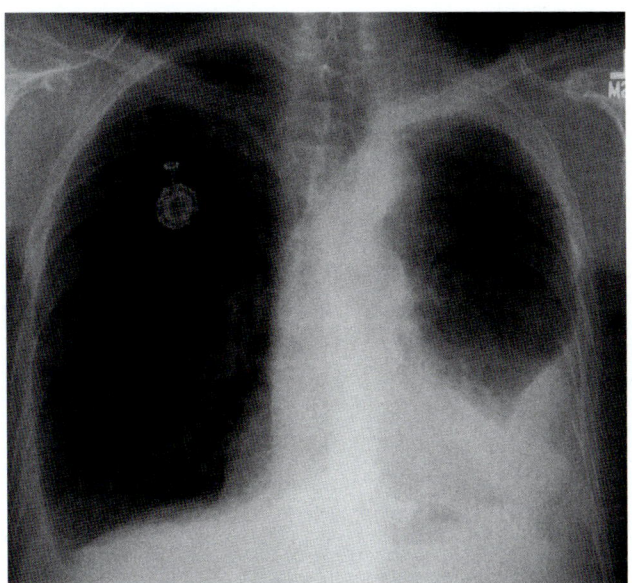

Fig. 25.3 Posterior anterior (PA) chest radiograph. There are bilateral pleural effusions and mild right lower lobe increased interstitial densities.

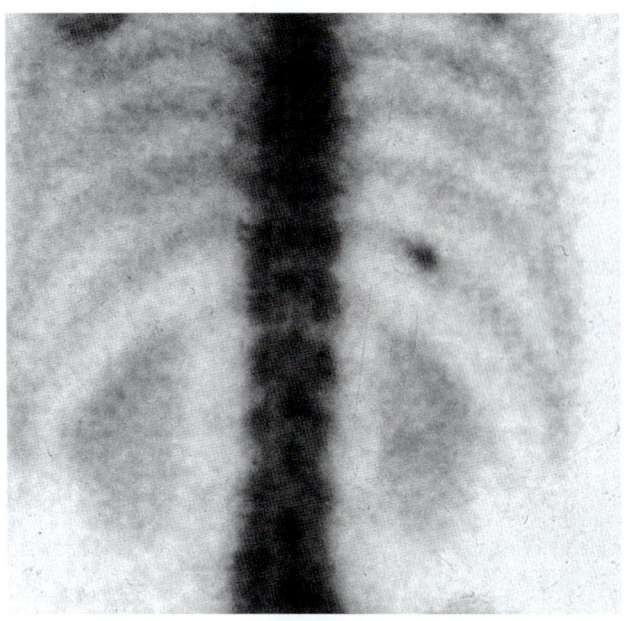

Fig. 25.4 Bone scan, technetium 99m MDP (methylene diphosphonate). There is a focal area of increased radionuclide uptake in the right 11th posterior rib.

Pathology
- Inflammatory carcinoma

Management
- BI-RADS assessment category 5, highly suggestive of malignancy

Pearls and Pitfalls
- Inflammatory breast cancer comprises 0.5 to 2.0% of male breast malignancies. The number of men presenting with inflammatory breast cancer is extremely small, but they appear to have a poor prognosis.
- Like female breast cancer, the prognosis of male breast cancer is related to tumor, node, metastases (TNM) stage, as well as tumor histologic grade. Although there is conflicting data, it appears that male survival is comparable to female survival for similar-stage disease. Five-year survival rates are the following: stage I, 82 to 100%; stage II, 63 to 83%; stage III, 74%. Unfortunately, men commonly present later than do women and have more advanced disease. Besides axillary and supraclavicular adenopathy, this patient had pulmonary and bony metastatic disease. He died approximately 3 years after initial presentation.

Suggested Reading

Donegan WL, Redlich PN, Lang PJ, Gall MT. Carcinoma of the breast in males: a multiinstitutional survey. Cancer 1998; 83:498–509

Joshi MG, Lee AK, Loda M, et al. Male breast carcinoma: an evaluation of prognostic factors contributing to a poorer outcome. Cancer 1996;77:490–498

Tavassoli FA, Fattaneh A. Pathology of the Breast. 2nd ed. Stamford: Appleton & Lange; 1999:837–843

Wilhelm MC, Langenburg SC, Wanebo HJ. Cancer of the male breast. In: Bland KI, Copeland EM, eds. The Breast. 2nd ed. Philadelphia: WB Saunders; 1998:1416–1420

Case 25.3: Metastatic Tumor

Case History
A 55-year-old presents with right areolar ulcer and bloody nipple discharge. The patient was initially sent for breast sonogram because of areolar induration. He has had removal of two previous squamous cell carcinomas on his face.

Mammogram

Mass
- Margin: circumscribed
- Shape: oval
- Density: high density

Physical Examination
- Right breast: the nipple areolar complex is replaced by a large ulceration; the area is also indurated and erythematous.
- Left breast: normal exam
- Neck: large left supraclavicular mass

Calcifications (Fig. 25.5)
- Type: pleomorphic/heterogeneous
- Distribution: grouped/clustered

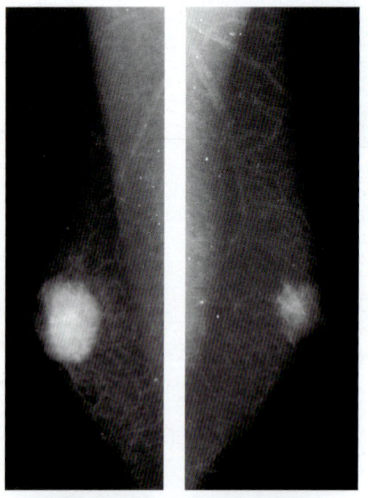
A
B

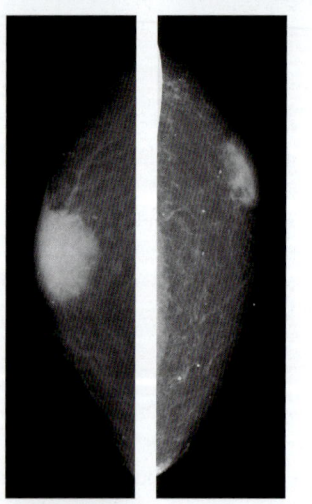
C
D

E

Fig. 25.5 The sonographic mass corresponds to a right oval subareolar mammographic mass with heterogeneous calcifications. Although the mass appears circumscribed on the routine views (**A,C**), the spot compression image (**E**) demonstrates that the mass has ill-defined margins. (**A**) Right MLO mammogram. (**B**) Left MLO mammogram. (**C**) Right CC mammogram. (**D**) Left CC mammogram. (**E**) Right CC spot compression mammogram.

Ultrasound

Frequency
- 10 MHz

Mass (Fig. 25.6)
- Margin: well defined
- Echogenicity: hypoechoic
- Retrotumoral acoustic appearance: increased acoustic transmission
- Shape: ellipsoid

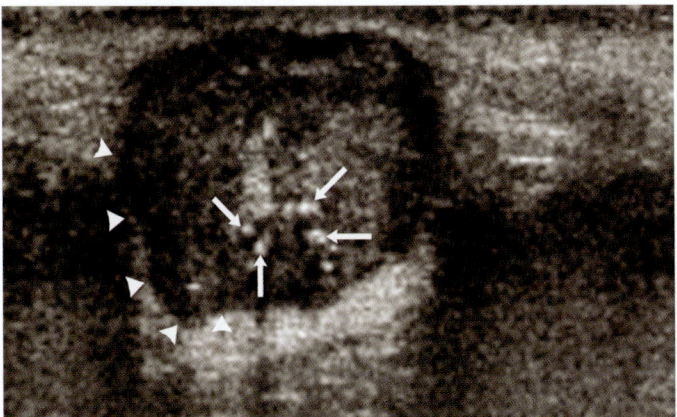 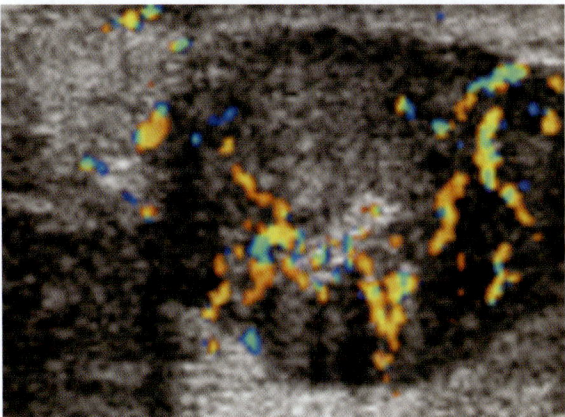

Fig. 25.6 In the right subareolar area, there is an oval, hypoechoic solid mass with calcifications (*arrows*). Although the margins are generally well defined, there is mild irregularity of the contour of the mass (*arrowheads*). (**A**) Right radial breast sonogram. (**B**) Right radial color Doppler breast sonogram.

Other Modalities: CT (Figs. 25.7 and 25.8)

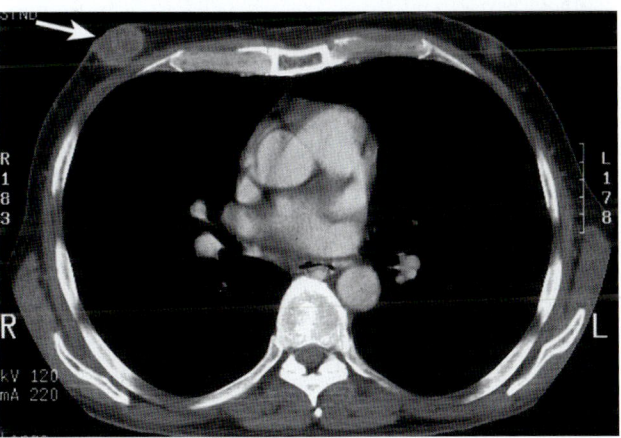

Fig. 25.7 Transverse contrast-enhanced computed tomography. Right breast subareolar soft tissue mass is evident (*arrow*).

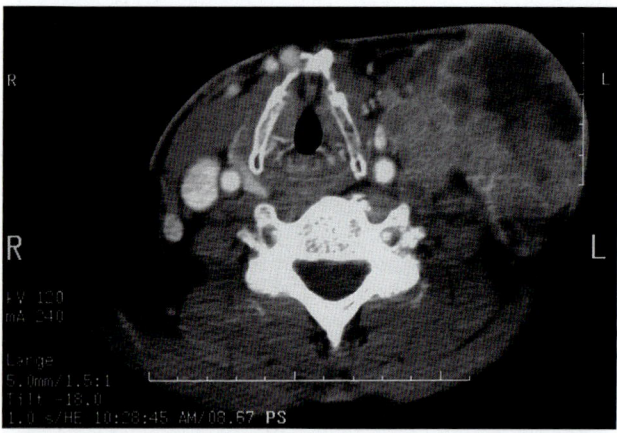

Fig. 25.8 Transverse contrast-enhanced neck computed tomography. There is a large partially enhancing solid mass in the left neck, which extends to the clavicle.

Pathology
- Metastases
- Biopsy of right areola and neck mass: poorly differentiated squamous carcinoma

Management
- BI-RADS assessment category 4, suspicious; biopsy should be considered.

Pearls and Pitfalls

- This patient had metastatic squamous carcinoma to the breast. The most common metastatic tumor to the male breast is prostate carcinoma. Clinically, patients present with a palpable tumor. Nipple discharge or retraction is unusual.
- The imaging appearance of metastatic tumors in men is the same as in women. Mammographically, these masses are superficial, circumscribed, oval or lobulated masses. Sonographically, they are hypoechoic and generally do not shadow.

Suggested Reading

Cappabianca S, Grassi R, D'Alessandro P, Del Vecchio A, Maioli A, Donofrio V. Metastasis to the male breast from carcinoma of the urinary bladder. Br J Radiol 2000;73:1326–1328

Demirkazik FB, Başkan O, Aydingöz U, Tacal T, Firat P. Case report: squamous cell carcinoma of the skin metastasizing to the breast—imaging findings. Br J Radiol 1996;69:678–680

Salyer WR, Salyer DC. Metastases of prostatic carcinoma to the breast. J Urol 1973;109:671–675

Yang WT, Muttarak M, Ho LWC. Nonmammary malignancies of the breast: ultrasound, CT, and MRI. Semin Ultrasound CT MR 2000;21:375–394

Case 25.4: Intracystic Papillary Carcinoma

Case History
A 57-year-old man presents with bloody nipple discharge. He has a long history of primary testicular failure and gynecomastia.

Physical Examination
- Right breast: firm, small, subareolar nodule
- Left breast: normal exam

Mammogram

Mass (Fig. 25.9)
- Margin: circumscribed
- Shape: oval
- Density: equal density

Calcifications
- Type: pleomorphic/heterogeneous
- Distribution: grouped/clustered

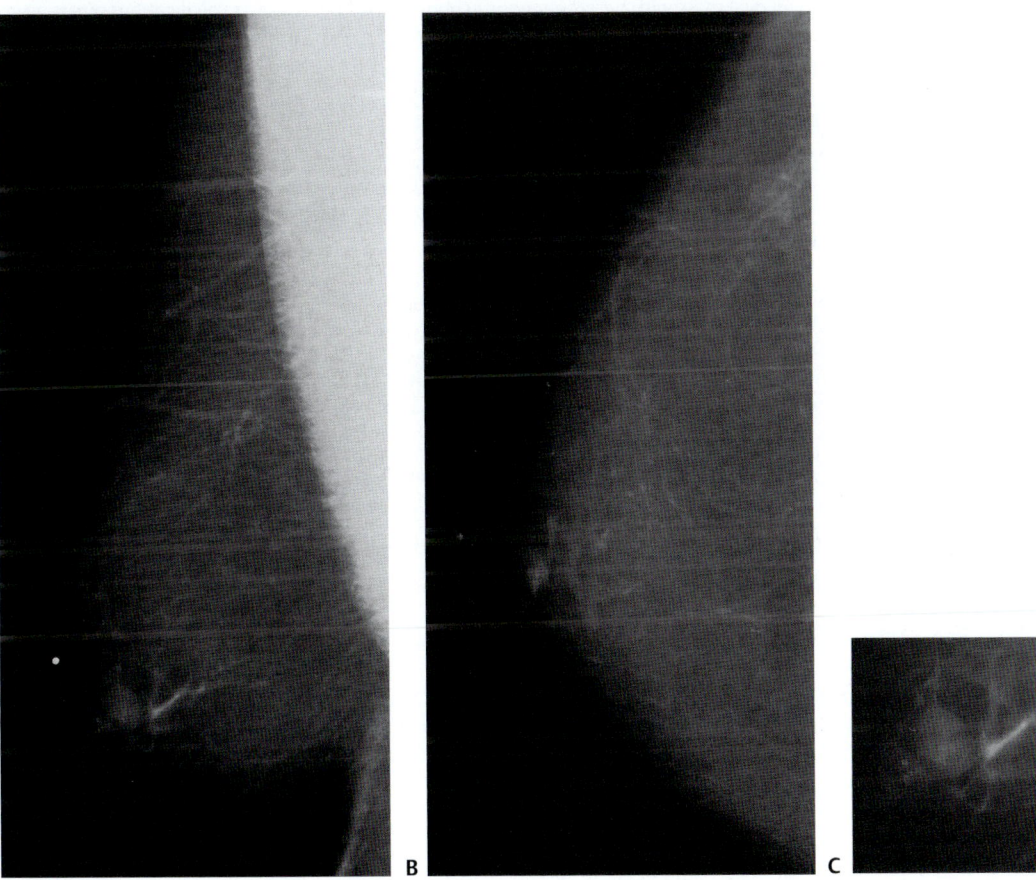

Fig. 25.9 In the subareolar area, the palpable mass corresponds to an oval mass with heterogeneous calcifications. (**A**) Right MLO mammogram. (**B**) Right CC mammogram. (**C**) Right MLO mammogram (lesion enlarged).

Ultrasound

Frequency
- 11.5 MHz

Mass (Fig. 25.10)
- Margin: well defined
- Echogenicity: heterogeneous
- Retrotumoral acoustic appearance: bilateral edge shadowing
- Shape: ellipsoid

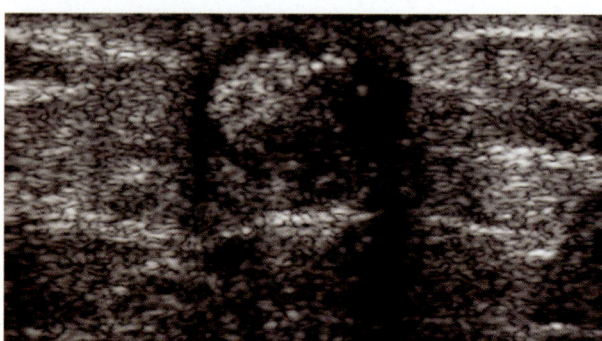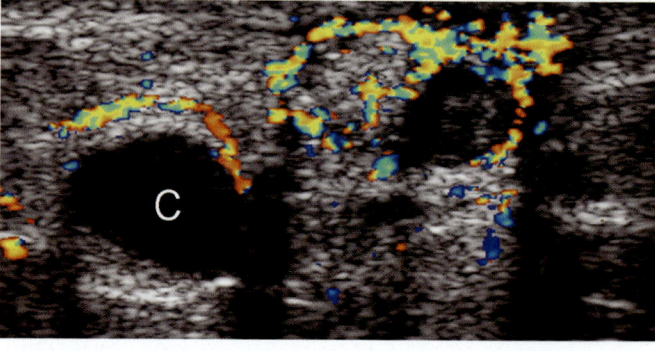

Fig. 25.10 The mammographic mass corresponds to an oval mass with heterogeneous echogenicity. The mass has calcifications and is asymmetrically bordered by a cyst (C). (**A**) Right longitudinal breast sonogram. (**B**) Right transverse color Doppler sonogram.

Pathology
- Intracystic papillary carcinoma

Management
- BI-RADS assessment category 4, suspicious; biopsy should be considered.

Pearls and Pitfalls

- Male nipple discharge has been reported in 2% of benign lesions and approximately 4 to 20% of malignancies. Half of the benign masses presenting with nipple discharge were papillomas. Serosanguinous discharge is strongly associated with malignancy.
- Complex cysts are more likely to be malignant in men than in women. Therefore, any cystic mass should be carefully sonographically examined. Any cyst with a thick wall or intracystic mass should be biopsied. Besides papillary carcinoma, the papillary subtype of ductal carcinoma in situ has been reported to present as a complex cystic mass.

Suggested Reading

Amoroso WL Jr, Robbins GF, Treves N. Serous and serosanguineous discharge from the male nipple. AMA Arch Surg 1956;73:319–329

Fallentin E, Rothman L. Intracystic carcinoma of the male breast. J Clin Ultrasound 1994;22:118–120

Goss PE, Reid C, Pintilie M, Lim RK, Miller N. Male breast carcinoma: a review of 229 patients who presented to the Princess Margaret Hospital during 40 years: 1955–1996. Cancer 1999;85:629–639

Madden CM, Reynolds HE. Intracystic papillary carcinoma of the male breast. AJR Am J Roentgenol 1995;165:1011–1012

So GJ, Chantra PK, Wollman JS, Bassett LW. The male breast. In: Bassett LW, Jackson VP, Jahan R, Fu YS, Gold RH, eds. Diagnosis of Diseases of the Breast. Philadelphia: WB Saunders; 1997:501–518

Stebbings WS, George BD, Boyle S, Plowman PN, Gilmore OJ. Malignant cysts of the male breast. Postgrad Med J 1987;63:985–987

Yang WT, Whitman GJ, Yuen EHY, Tse GMK, Stelling CB. Sonographic features of primary breast cancer in men. AJR Am J Roentgenol 2001;176:413–416

Postsurgical Findings

This is a schematic diagram of the diagnostic approach to mammographic postsurgical findings: augmentation mammoplasty. For further discussion, see Chapter 1.

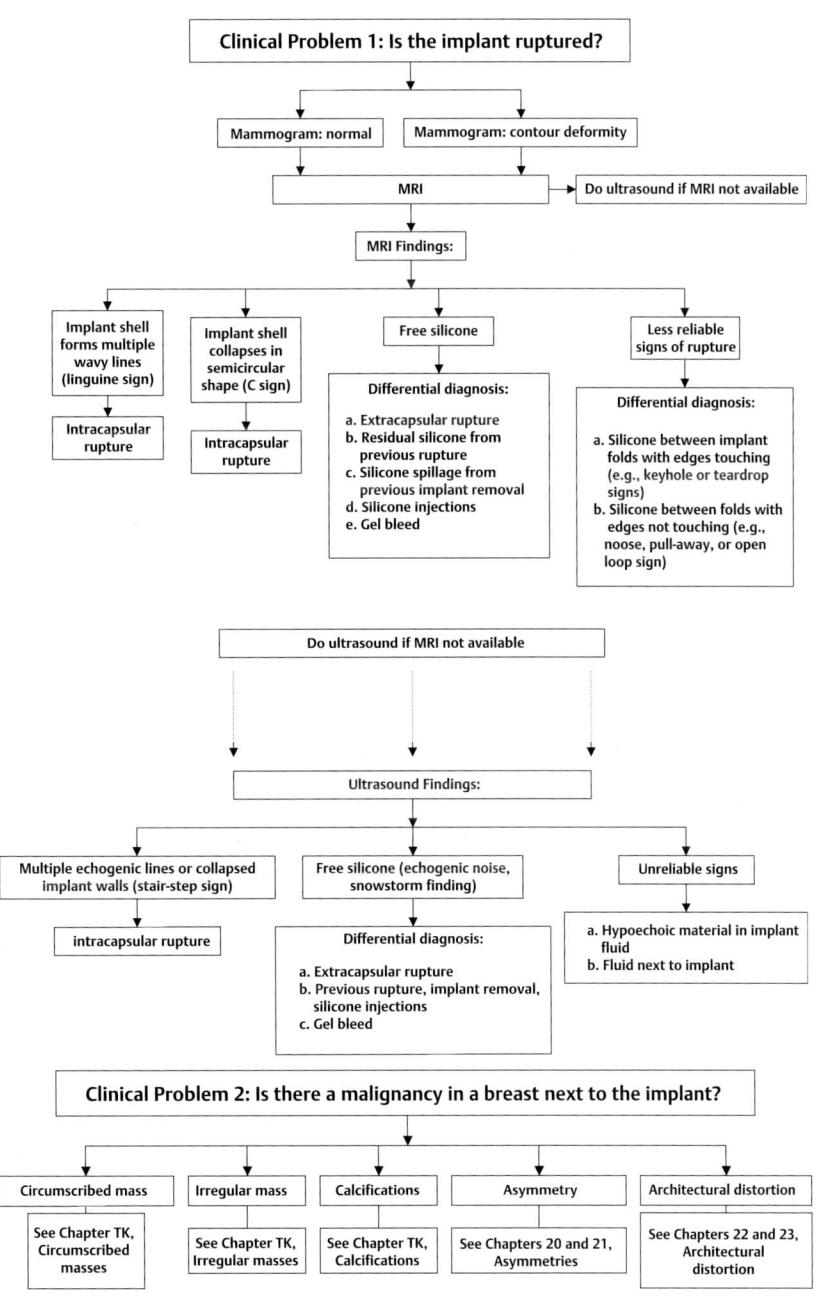

26 Augmentation Mammoplasty

Case 26.1: Subglandular Implants—Infected Fluid

Case History

A 47-year-old woman presents with right breast pain. She had undergone bilateral breast augmentation 20 years prior to evaluation.

Physical Examination
- Right breast: swollen and firm
- Left breast: normal exam

Mammogram (Fig. 26.1)

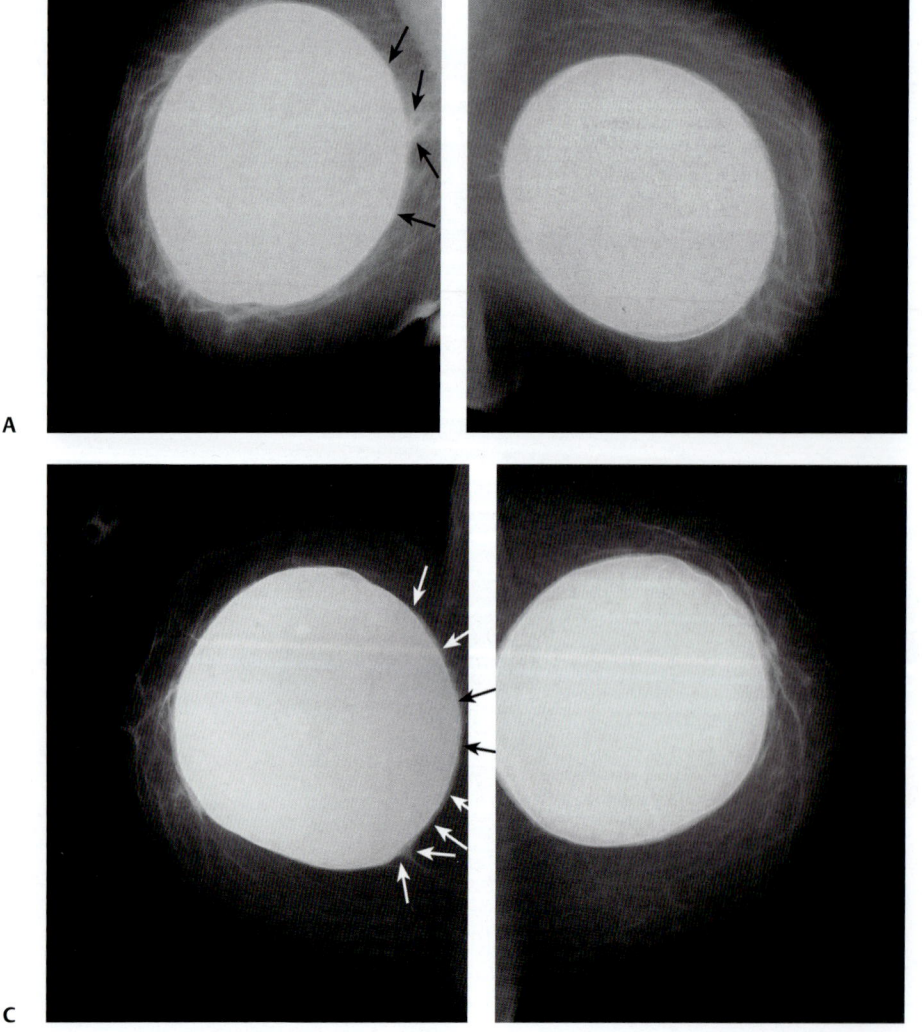

Fig. 26.1 Bilateral subglandular implants are present. There is increased density associated with the posterior deep margin of the right implant (arrows). (**A**) Right MLO mammogram. (**B**) Left MLO mammogram. (**C**) Right CC mammogram. (**D**) Left CC mammogram.

Ultrasound

Frequency
- 7 MHz

Mass (Fig. 26.2)
- Echogenicity: hypoechoic
- Retrotumoral acoustic appearance: increased acoustic enhancement

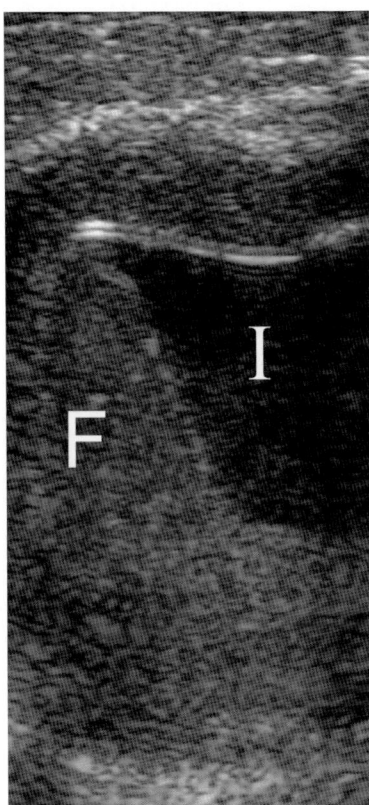

Fig. 26.2 Right transverse breast sonogram at the 10 o'clock position. The density identified in **Fig. 26.1** corresponds to a complex hypoechoic fluid collection (F). The adjacent implant is anechoic (I).

Pathology
- Infected fluid

Management
- BI-RADS assessment category 2, benign finding

> **Pearls and Pitfalls**
>
> - Implants are generally located either deep to the pectoralis muscle (retropectoral) or within the breast glandular tissue anterior to the pectoralis (subglandular). Subglandular implants generally obscure more breast parenchyma than subpectoral implants. To improve visualization of the parenchyma, Eklund or implant-displaced views should be routinely done in patients with implants. Although we always perform implant-displaced views, these views are not shown in this book unless they provide specific information for the case.
> - The main complications associated with implants include bleeding or hematoma, infection, capsule contracture, rupture, and silicone granulomas.

Suggested Reading

Steinbach BG, Hardt NS, Abbitt PL, Lanier L, Caffee HH. Breast implants, common complications, and concurrent breast disease. Radiographics 1993;13:95–118

Case 26.2: Subpectoral Implants

Case History
A 47-year-old woman presents for screening mammogram.

Physical Examination
- Normal exam

Mammogram (Fig. 26.3)

Fig. 26.3 Bilateral implant views. The subpectoral implants are normal. (**A**) Right MLO implant view. (**B**) Left MLO implant view. (**C**) Right CC implant view. (**D**) Left CC implant view.

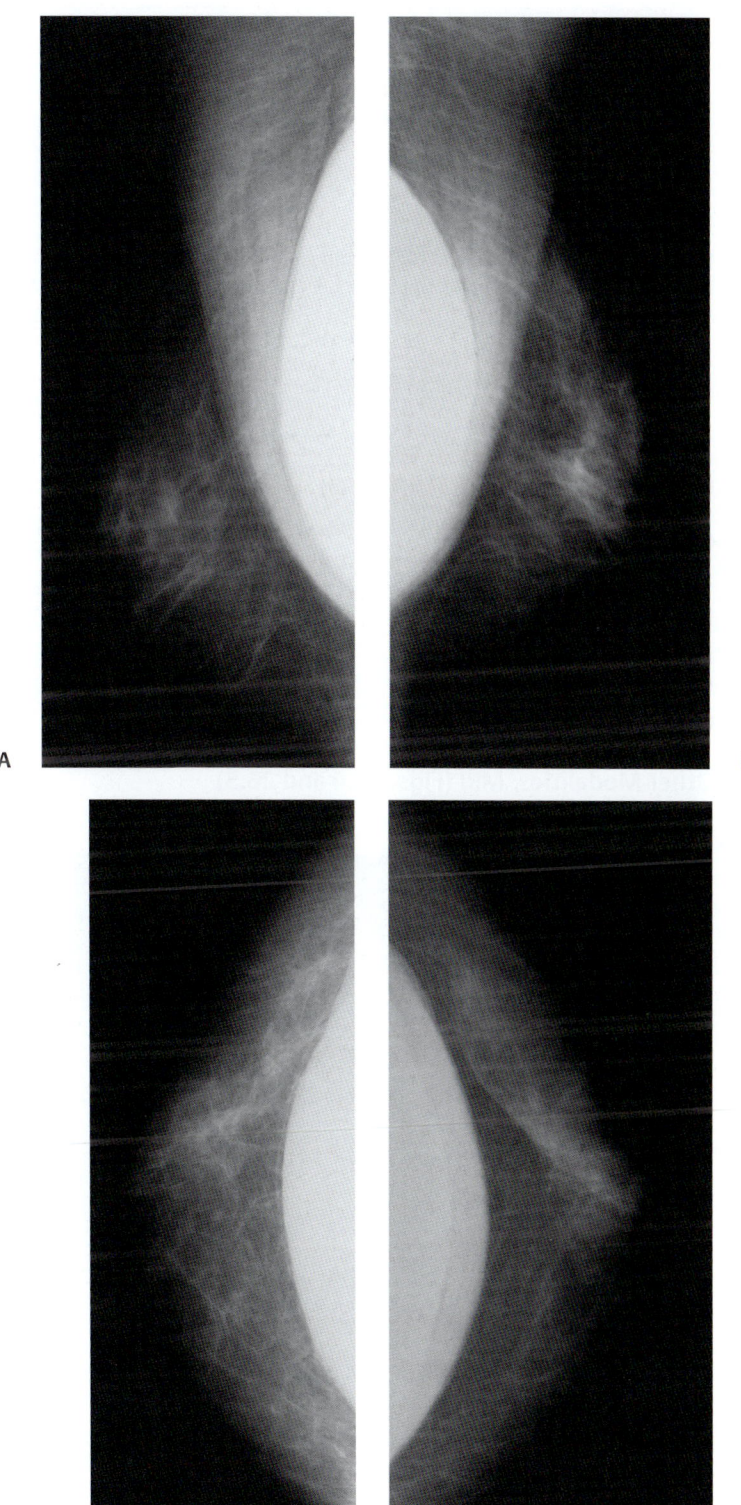

Pathology
- Normal implant

Management
- BI-RADS assessment category 1, negative

> **Pearls and Pitfalls**
>
> - The advantage of subpectoral implants is that they interfere less with imaging the breast parenchyma and are associated with a lower rate of capsular contraction.

Suggested Reading

Biggs TM, Yarish RS. Augmentation mammaplasty: retropectoral versus retromammary implantation. Clin Plast Surg 1988;15:549–555

Vazquez B, Given KS, Houston GC. Breast augmentation: a review of subglandular and submuscular implantation. Aesthetic Plast Surg 1987;11:101–105

Case 26.3: Subpectoral Implants

Case History
A 49-year-old woman presents with chronic pain in her left breast. She received breast augmentation 10 years prior to evaluation.

Physical Examination
- Normal exam

Other Modalities: MRI (Figs. 26.4 and 26.5)

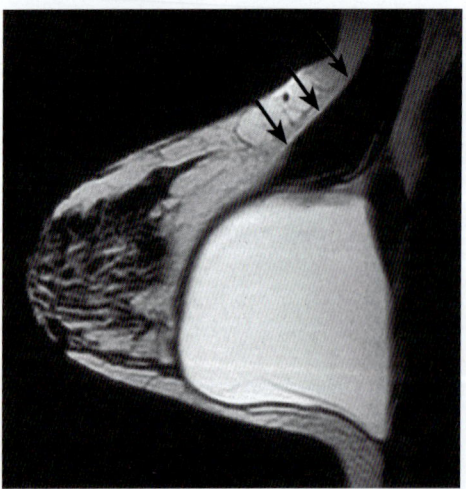
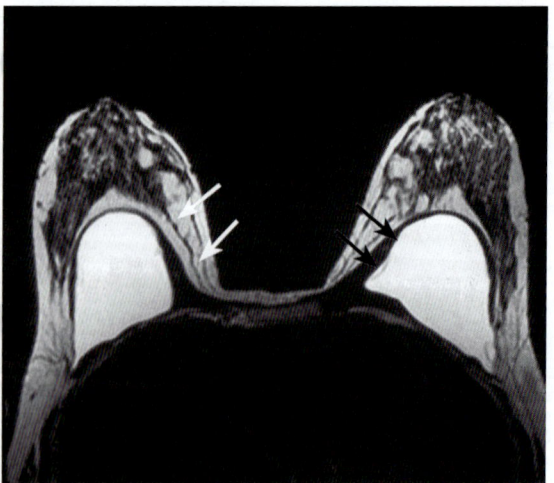

Fig. 26.4 The implants are subpectoral in location and normal in appearance. Pectoralis muscle (*arrows*). (**A**) Right breast T2-weighted with water saturation longitudinal MRI. (**B**) Bilateral breasts T2-weighted with water saturation transverse MRI.

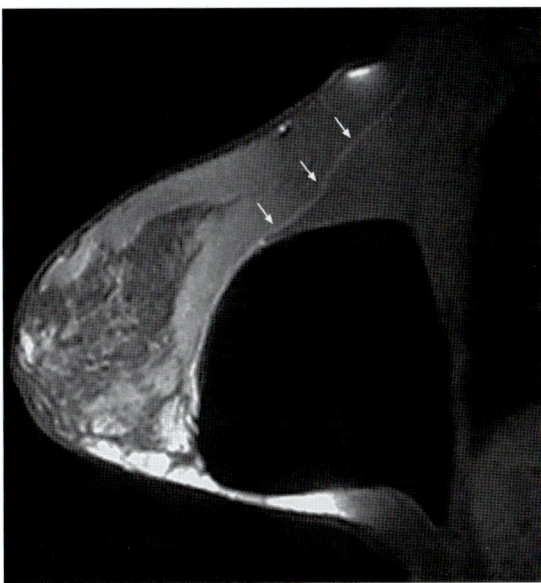

Fig. 26.5 Right breast T1-weighted with fat saturation longitudinal MRI. Pectoralis (*arrows*) is not well identified on this sequence. This sequence is excellent for identifying free silicone due to extracapsular rupture.

Pathology
- Normal implant

Management
- BI-RADS assessment category 1, negative

Pearls and Pitfalls

- MRI is an excellent method to identify implant rupture. With an MRI T2-weighted series, the fibrous capsule and the implant shell are dark lines, which are normally inseparable except for normal folds of the shell. Silicone and water are bright on T2 series. If water saturation is added to the T2 sequence, then silicone will be brighter than water. This T2 method displays intracapsular rupture well. An alternative technique is an STIR series with water saturation which causes silicone to be bright. The silicone is easily identified either as free silicone or between the layers of the fibrous capsule and the shell of the prosthesis.

Suggested Reading
Middleton MS. Breast implants and soft tissue silicone. In: Stark DD, Bradley WG, eds. Magnetic Resonance Imaging. 3rd ed. St. Louis: Mosby; 1999:335–353

Case 26.4: Silicone Injections

Case History
A 66-year-old woman who had silicone injections over 40 years ago presents for annual mammogram.

Physical Examination
- Bilateral breasts: lobulated pattern in both breasts, which is more prominent in the upper outer quadrants

Mammogram (Fig. 26.6)

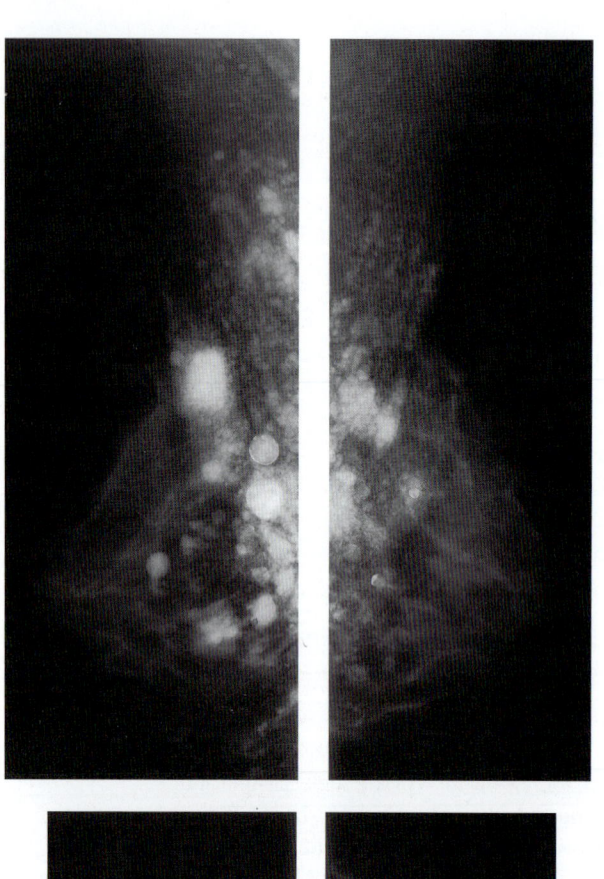

Fig. 26.6 Both breasts exhibit high-density material posteriorly in breast parenchyma, in the lymph nodes, and within the pectoralis muscles. (**A**) Right MLO mammogram. (**B**) Left MLO mammogram. (**C**) Right CC mammogram. (**D**) Left CC mammogram.

Pathology
- Free silicone

Management
- BI-RADS assessment category 1, negative

Pearls and Pitfalls
- Silicone was developed in the 1940s and injected into breasts for augmentation in the 1950s and 1960s. Unfortunately, silicone injections resulted in painful hardening of the breast, sloughing of skin, granulomatous hepatitis, and pulmonary embolism. The U.S. Food and Drug Administration banned these injections in 1965.
- Mammographically, silicone injections result in high-density round or oval masses and architectural distortion. In the areas containing silicone, neoplasms may be hidden by the silicone masses.

Suggested Reading
Ganott MA, Harris KM, Ilkhanipour ZS, Costa-Greco MA. Augmentation mammoplasty: normal and abnormal findings with mammography and US. Radiographics 1992;12:281–295

Leibman AJ, Sybers R. Mammographic and sonographic findings after silicone injection. Ann Plast Surg 1994;33:412–414

Case 26.5: Normal Findings—Bulge

Case History
A 66-year-old woman presents with right breast pain and increasing "dimpling" at the edge of her augmentation scar.

Physical Examination
- Right breast: tenderness and subtle nodularity in the upper outer quadrant
- Left breast: normal exam

Mammogram (Fig. 26.7)

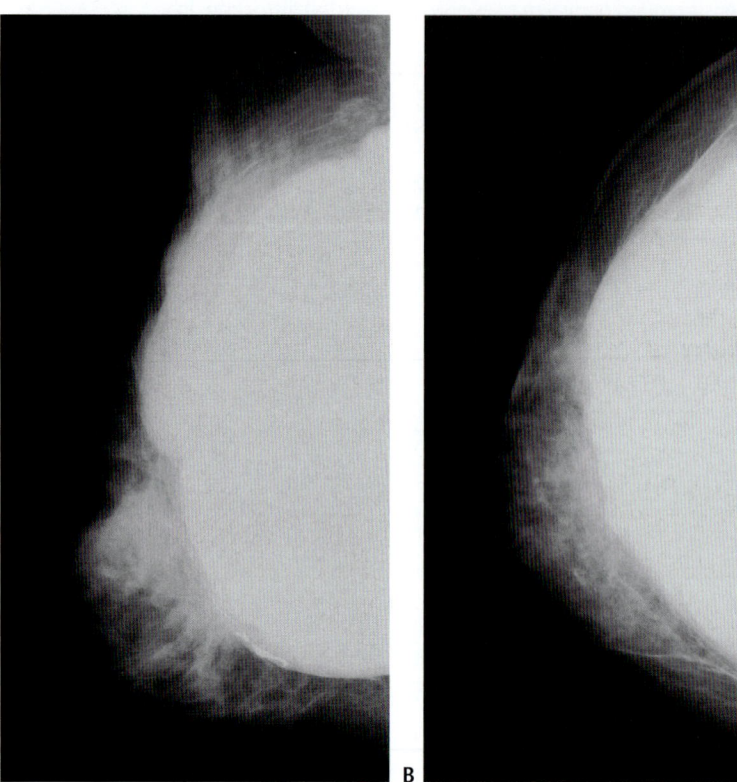

Fig. 26.7 In the upper outer quadrant of the right breast, there is a contour bulge, which is visible only on the MLO view. (**A**) Right MLO implant mammogram. (**B**) Right CC implant mammogram.

Other Modalities: MRI (Fig. 26.8)

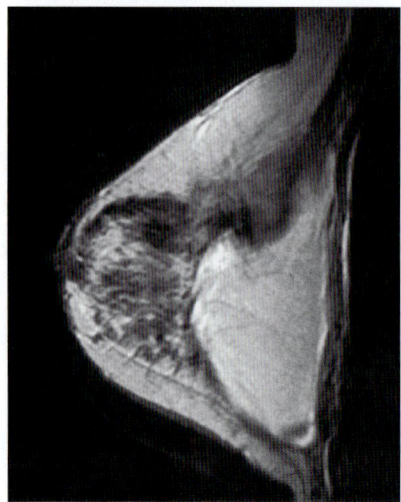
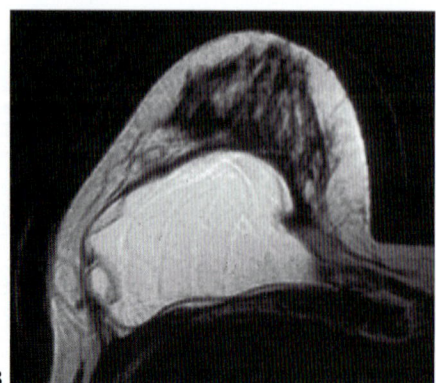

Fig. 26.8 (**A**) Right breast T2-weighted longitudinal MRI. The superior edge of the implant demonstrates a contour deformity that corresponds to the mammographic abnormality. There is no evidence of capsular rupture. (**B**) Right breast T2-weighted transverse MRI. Normal folds extend from the lateral aspect of the implant.

Pathology
- Normal implant

Management
- BI-RADS assessment category 1, negative

Pearls and Pitfalls
- About half of all implants demonstrate small focal contour deformities without rupture. Wrinkling is more common with saline implants compared with silicone prostheses. The most common location for contour deformities in silicone implants is the superior edge of the implant in the MLO view, as illustrated in this case.
- Contour deformities should be differentiated from implant herniation. Both contour deformities and implant folds are normal findings of an intact implant. Herniation is when an intact implant shell is extruded through the fibrous capsule. Capsular herniation is distinguished from a contour bulge by identifying bunching of the implant at the location of the ruptured capsule.

Suggested Reading

Destouet JM, Monsees BS, Oser RF, Nemecek JR, Young VL, Pilgram TK. Screening mammography in 350 women with breast implants: prevalence and findings of implant complications. AJR Am J Roentgenol 1992;159:973–978, discussion 979–981

Ganott MA, Harris KM, Ilkhanipour ZS, Costa-Greco MA. Augmentation mammoplasty: normal and abnormal findings with mammography and US. Radiographics 1992;12:281–295

Middleton MS. Breast implants and soft tissue silicone. In: Stark DD, Bradley WG, eds. Magnetic Resonance Imaging. 3rd ed. St. Louis: Mosby; 1999:335–353

Case 26.6: Normal Findings—Fluid

Case History
A 57-year-old woman who had a right mastectomy 5 years ago with breast reconstruction using a subpectoral silicone implant is worried about her implant.

Physical Examination
- Right breast: implant smaller than left breast, otherwise normal
- Left breast: normal exam

Ultrasound

Frequency
- 7 MHz (**Fig. 26.9**)

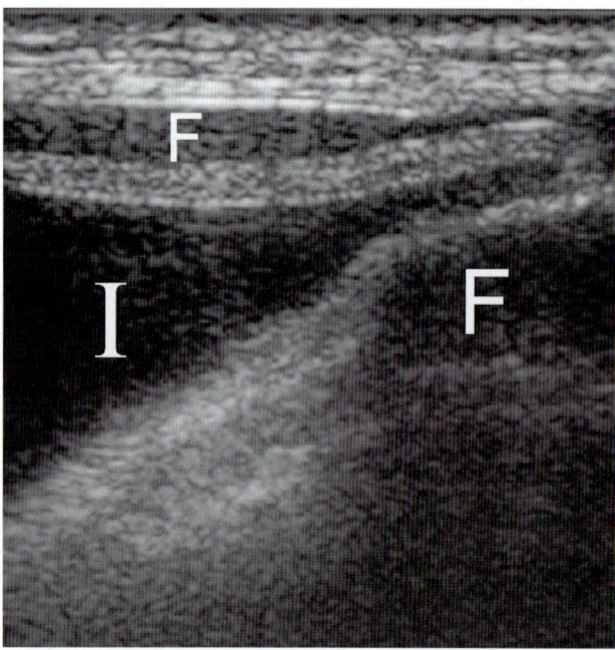

Fig. 26.9 Right transverse breast sonogram. The implant (I) wall is intact, but there is a thin fluid collection (F) outside the implant.

Pathology
- Normal implant

Management
- BI-RADS assessment category 1, negative

Pearls and Pitfalls
- Small fluid collections of water may form outside the nonruptured implant. These collections are identifiable by sonography or MRI and should not be mistaken for signs of extracapsular rupture.

Suggested Reading

Caskey CI, Hamper UM. Sonographic evaluation of breast implants. In: Sohn C, Blohmer JU, Hamper UM eds. Breast Ultrasound. New York: Thieme; 1999:143–165

Middleton MS. Breast implants and soft tissue silicone. In: Stark DD, Bradley WG, eds. Magnetic Resonance Imaging. 3rd ed. St. Louis: Mosby; 1999:335–353

Reynolds HE. Evaluation of the augmented breast. Radiol Clin North Am 1995;33:1131–1145

Case 26.7: Implant Calcifications

Case History
A 66-year-old woman presents with angina. She has had breast implants for over 20 years.

Physical Examination
- Bilateral breasts: normal exam

Mammogram (Fig. 26.10)

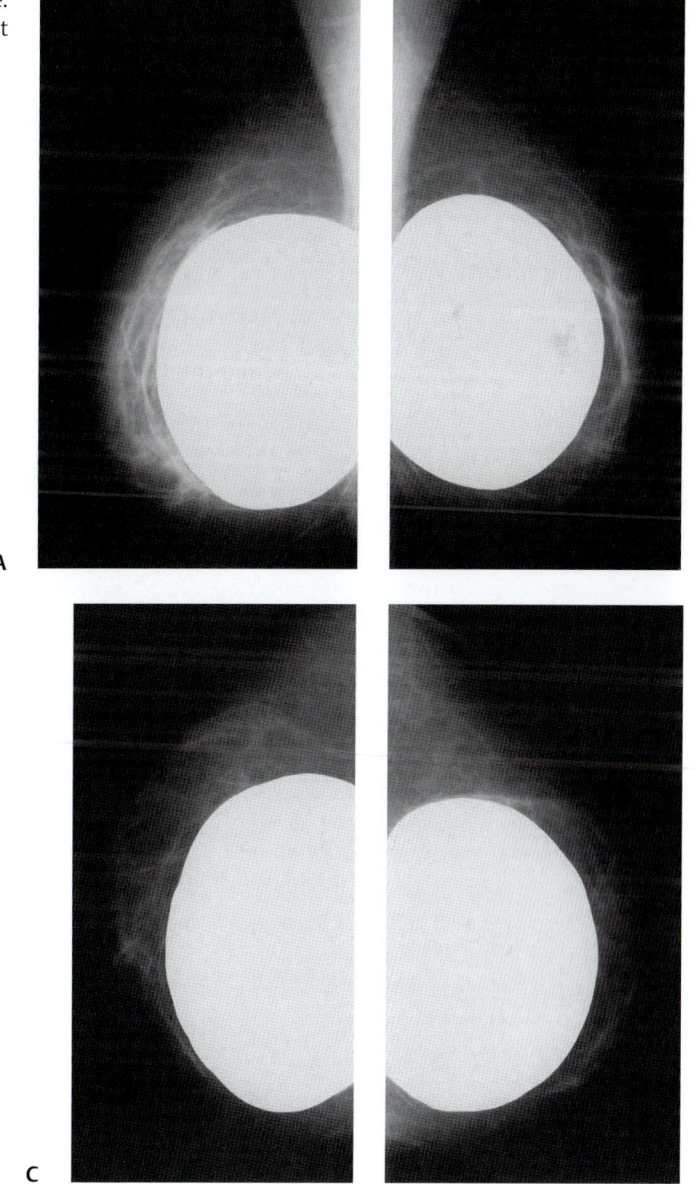

Fig. 26.10 Bilateral implants exhibit normal contours and shape. (**A**) Right MLO mammogram. (**B**) Left MLO mammogram. (**C**) Right CC mammogram. (**D**) Left CC mammogram.

Other Modalities: Chest Radiography (Fig. 26.11)

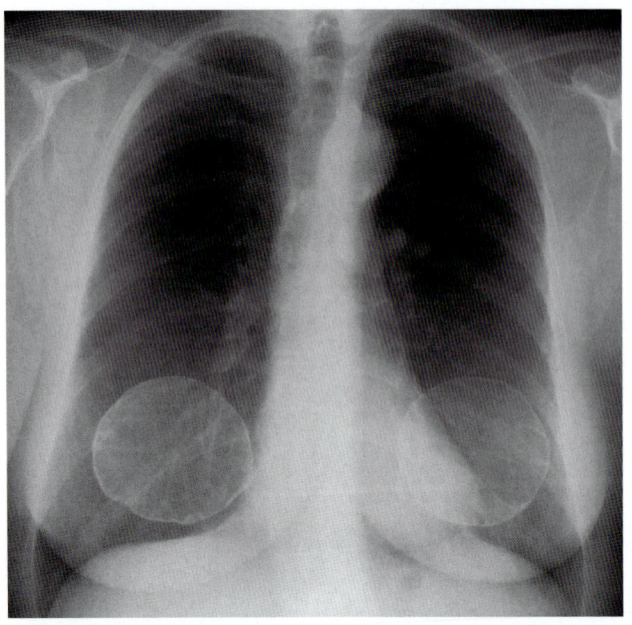 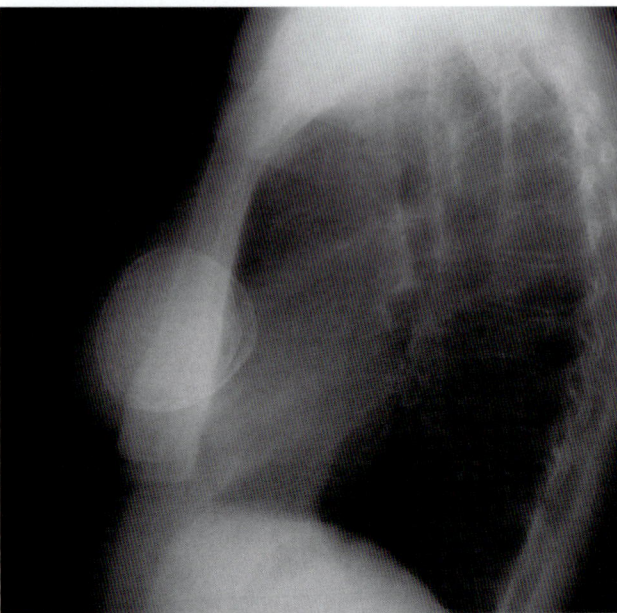

Fig. 26.11 Chest radiograph demonstrates round densities within the breasts, which represent the patient's calcified implants. (**A**) Posteroanterior (PA) chest radiograph. (**B**) Lateral chest radiograph.

Pathology
- Calcified implants

Management
- BI-RADS assessment category 2, benign finding

Pearls and Pitfalls
- Implant calcification is common and generally not associated with a significant clinical problem. About 20% of all types of implants demonstrate at least a small amount of calcification. In a few cases, heavy calcification has been associated with severe capsular contracture, which has been labeled the Krakatau syndrome. This syndrome is named after the famous volcano in Indonesia because when this abnormal implant is removed, the breast exhibits a craterlike depression.

Suggested Reading

Ganott MA, Harris KM, Ilkhanipour ZS, Costa-Greco MA. Augmentation mammoplasty: normal and abnormal findings with mammography and US. Radiographics 1992;12:281–295

Koide T, Katayama H. Calcification in augmentation mammoplasty. Radiology 1979;130:337–340

Steinbach BG, Hardt NS, Abbitt PL. Mammography: breast implants—types, complications, and adjacent breast pathology. Curr Probl Diagn Radiol 1993;22:39–86

Vuursteen PJ. The Krakatau syndrome; a late complication of retroglandular mammary augmentation. Br J Plast Surg 1992;45:34–37

Case 26.8: Changes after Implant Renewal—Residual Silicone

Case History
A 64-year-old woman has a history of implant rupture 28 years ago. She removed her implants 15 years ago.

Physical Examination
- Bilateral breasts: multilobulated but stable

Mammogram (Fig. 26.12)

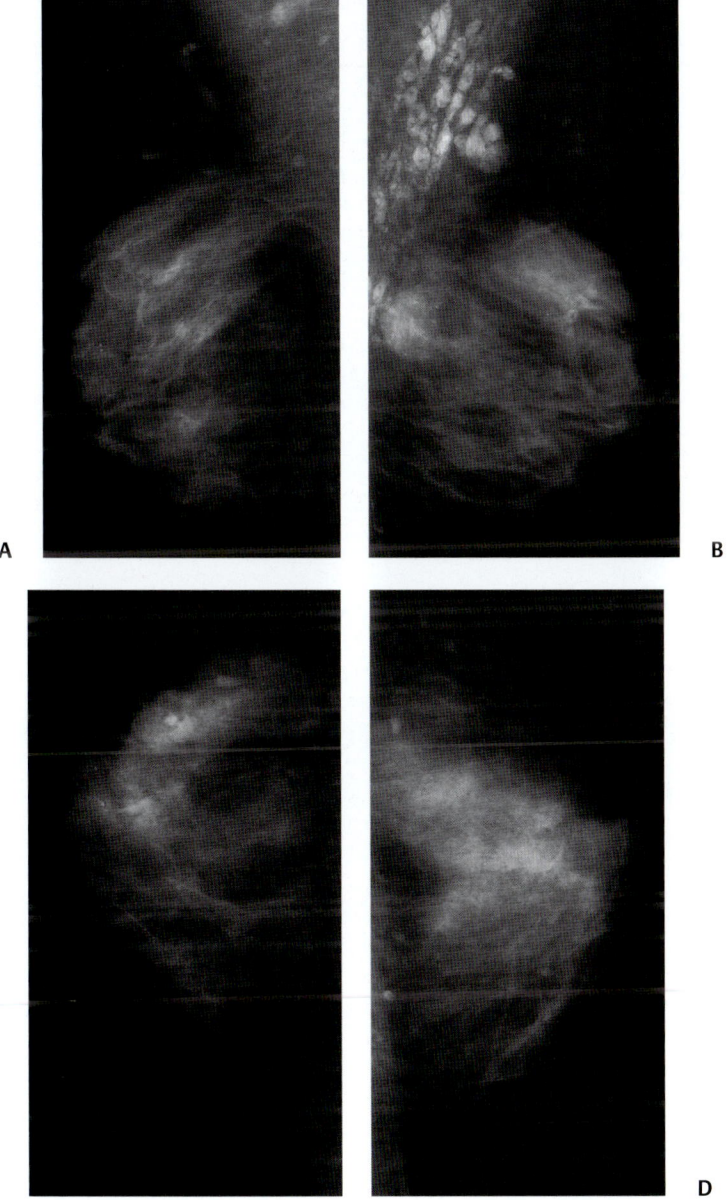

Fig. 26.12 There are scattered small, oval, high-density masses in the breast parenchyma and numerous densities in the axilla. (**A**) Right MLO mammogram. (**B**) Left MLO mammogram. (**C**) Right CC mammogram. (**D**) Left CC mammogram.

Pathology
- Free silicone

Management
- BI-RADS assessment category 2, benign finding

> **Pearls and Pitfalls**
>
> - Reasons for free silicone in the breast include silicone injections, ruptured implant, and escape of silicone from an intact implant elastomer shell (gel bleed). The elastomer shell is a semiporous membrane that allows silicone to flow into the surrounding tissues without rupture of the shell. The most common migration of free silicone is to the upper outer or upper medial soft tissues. Rarely, silicone will migrate to the breast or axilla from a distal injection site, such as the arm.

Suggested Reading

Hayes MK, Gold RH, Bassett LW. Mammographic findings after the removal of breast implants. AJR Am J Roentgenol 1993;160:487–490

Middleton MS. Magnetic resonance evaluation of breast implants and soft-tissue silicone. Top Magn Reson Imaging 1998;9:92–137

Roux SP, Bertucci GM, Ibarra JA, Blatt G, Ashworth CR. Unilateral axillary adenopathy secondary to a silicone wrist implant: report of a case detected at screening mammography. Radiology 1996;198:345–346

Case 26.9: Changes after Implant Renewal—Calcifications

Case History
A 60-year-old woman who has had removal of bilateral implants presents for her annual mammogram.

Physical Examination
- Normal exam

Mammogram

Calcifications (Fig. 26.13)
- Type: dystrophic

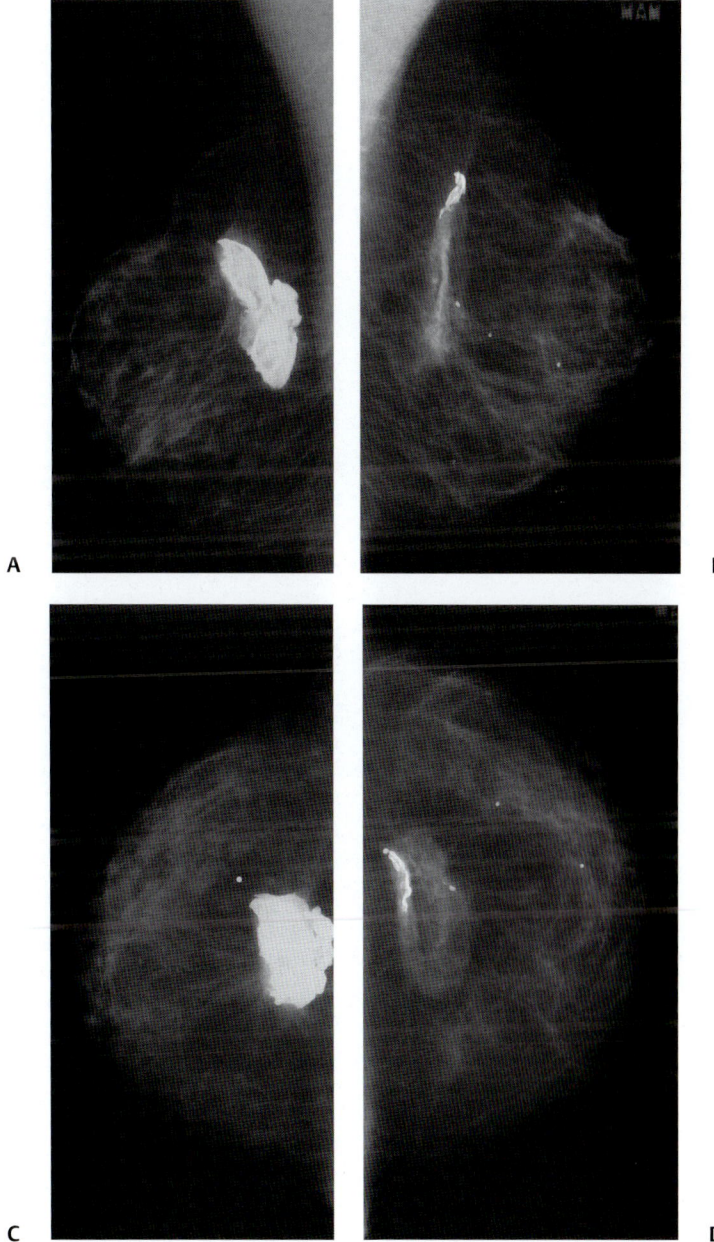

Fig. 26.13 There are large dystrophic calcifications and scarring in the areas of the patient's previous implants. (**A**) Right MLO mammogram. (**B**) Left MLO mammogram. (**C**) Right CC mammogram. (**D**) Left CC mammogram.

Pathology
- Scar

Management
- BI-RADS assessment category 2, benign finding

Pearls and Pitfalls
- The appearance and location of the large coarse calcifications, architectural distortion, and oval densities are characteristic of mammographic changes after implant removal. The abnormalities in this case may also be due to retained portions of the fibrous capsule that previously surrounded the patient's implants.

Suggested Reading
Hayes MK, Gold RH, Bassett LW. Mammographic findings after the removal of breast implants. AJR Am J Roentgenol 1993;160:487–490

Augmentation Mammoplasty 419

Case 26.10: Changes after Implant Renewal—Pseudocapsule

Case History
A 38-year-old woman removed her implants 1 year ago.

Physical Examination
- Normal exam

Mammogram (Figs. 26.14 and 26.15)

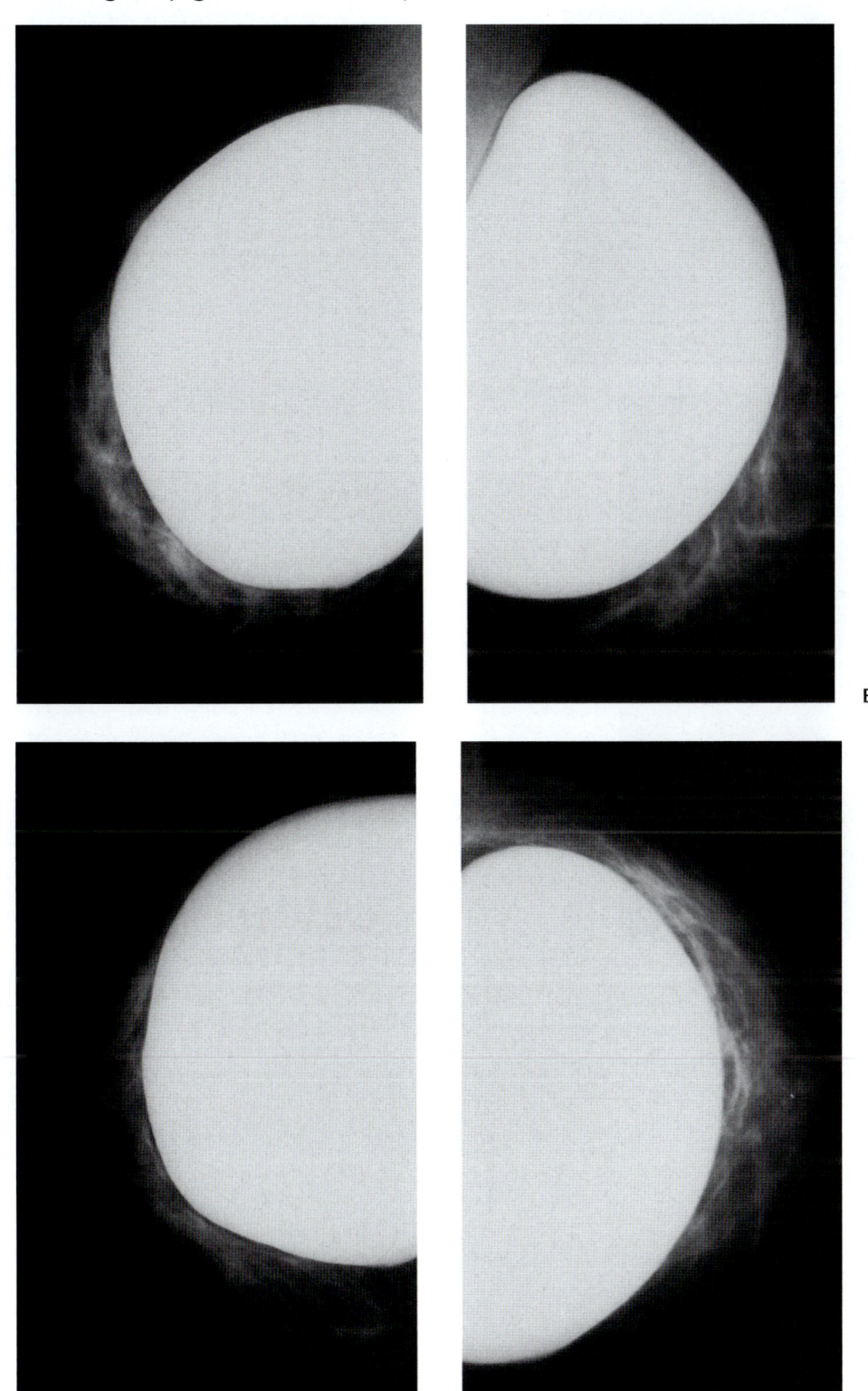

Fig. 26.14 Normal bilateral breast implant views. (**A**) Right MLO implant mammogram. (**B**) Left MLO implant mammogram. (**C**) Right CC implant mammogram. (**D**) Left CC implant mammogram.

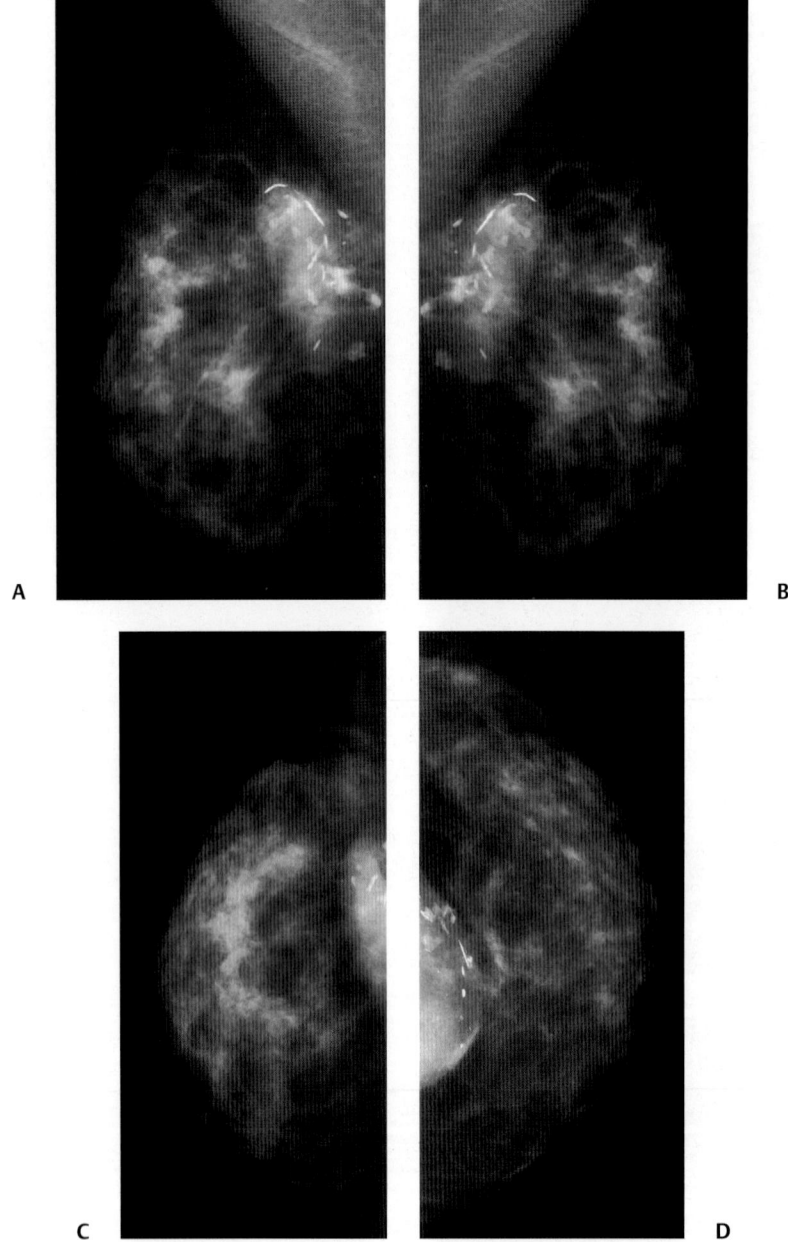

Fig. 26.15 This mammographic exam was performed 4 years after the mammograms in **Fig. 26.14** and 1 year after removal of implants. There are oval densities with calcifications in the areas of the previous implants. (**A**) Right MLO mammogram. (**B**) Left MLO mammogram. (**C**) Right CC mammogram. (**D**) Left CC mammogram.

Pathology
- Scar

Management
- BI-RADS assessment category 2, benign finding

Pearls and Pitfalls

- Mammographic findings after removal of breast implants include fat necrosis, scarring, architectural distortion, skin thickening, silicone in the breast parenchyma and axilla, and calcifications. Usually the fibrous capsule surrounding the implants is removed with the implants. In this case, some or all of the fibrous capsule was left within the breast. These fibrous capsules were subsequently removed.

Suggested Reading

Hayes MK, Gold RH, Bassett LW. Mammographic findings after the removal of breast implants. AJR Am J Roentgenol 1993;160:487–490

Case 26.11: Implant Rupture—Implant Collapse or Rupture

Case History
A 52-year-old woman has had the same saline implants for over 25 years. After partial mastectomy for breast cancer, the woman noticed that her left breast is larger than her right, and there is a new thickening in the lumpectomy site.

Physical Examination
- Right breast: mild nodularity of healing scar in the inner inferior breast; right breast smaller than left breast
- Left breast: normal exam

Mammogram (Fig. 26.16)

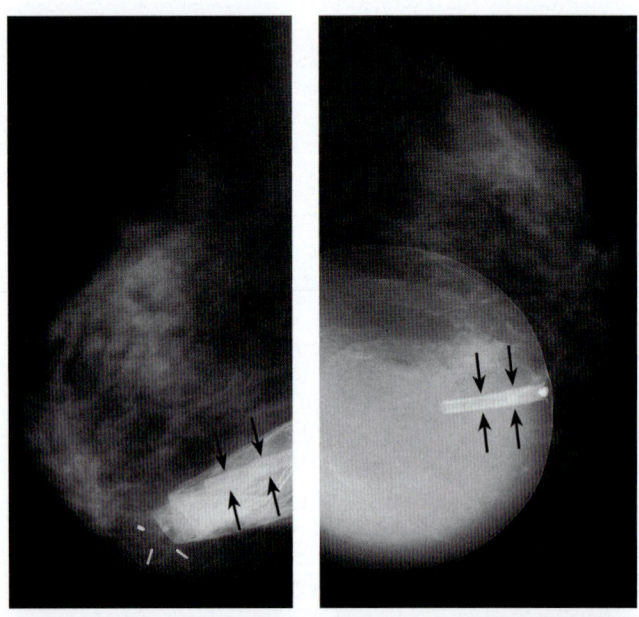

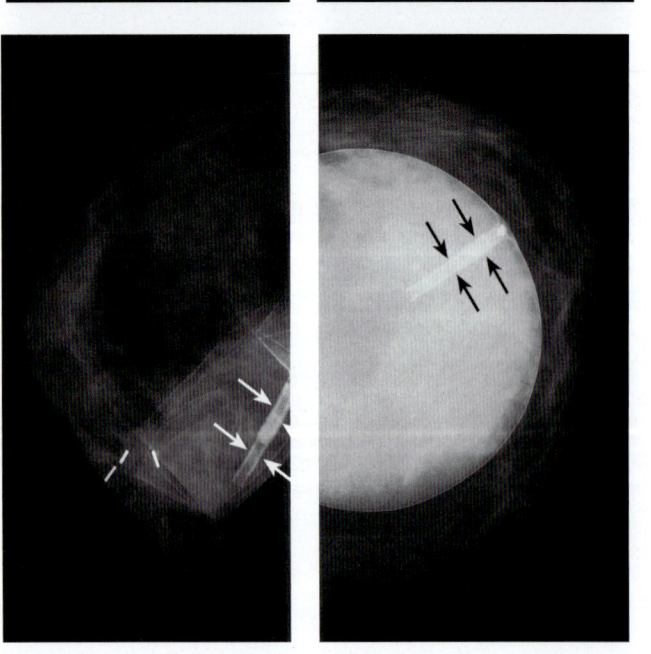

Fig. 26.16 Patient has bilateral saline implants. The tubular structure (*arrows*) is the valve that was used to fill the implant. The right implant has ruptured and completely collapsed. The clips mark the location of the recent lumpectomy. (**A**) Right MLO mammogram. (**B**) Left MLO mammogram. (**C**) Right CC mammogram. (**D**) Left CC mammogram.

Ultrasound (Figs. 26.17 and 26.18)

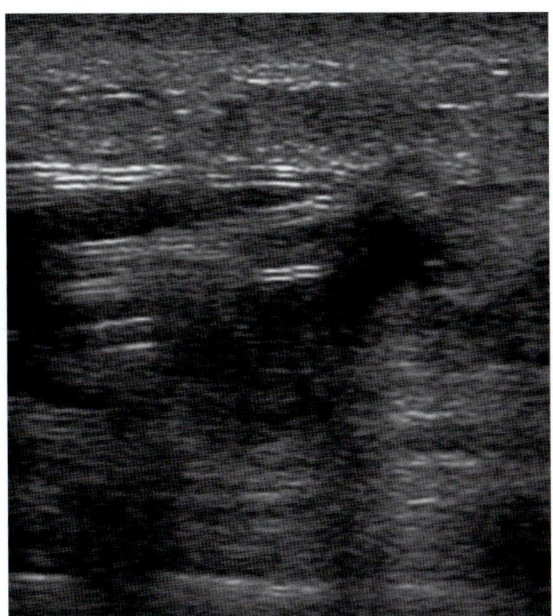

Fig. 26.17 Right breast sonogram. The breast sonogram was performed before the mammograms to investigate the palpable abnormality in the lumpectomy scar. The palpable thickening corresponds sonographically to a deformed, collapsed implant.

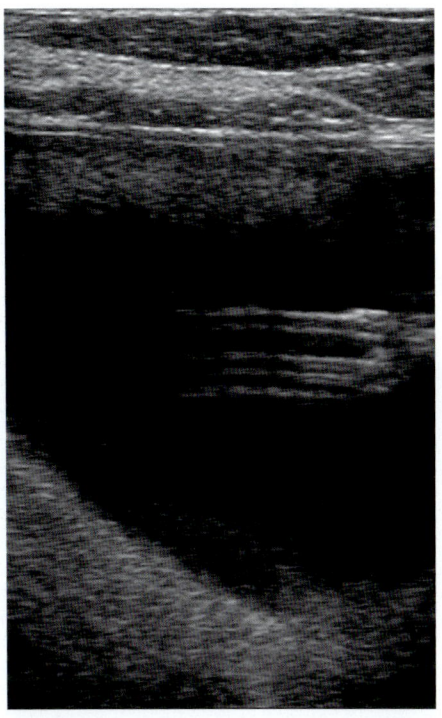

Fig. 26.18 Left breast sonogram. The left implant is normal without evidence of rupture. The linear lines within the implant correspond to the valve identified in **Fig. 26.16**.

Pathology
- Ruptured implant

Management
- BI-RADS assessment category 2, benign finding

Pearls and Pitfalls

- When an implant is inserted, a fibrous capsule develops around the implant elastomer shell. There are two types of implant failure: intracapsular and extracapsular. Intracapsular failure involves rupture of the implant elastomer shell without rupture of the surrounding fibrous capsule. With intracapsular rupture, the liquid contents of the implant are contained within the fibrous capsule. Extracapsular failure is when both the implant elastomer shell and the fibrous capsule have been ruptured. As a result of this type of rupture, the internal contents of the implant (silicone or water) are extruded outside the capsule into the surrounding tissues.
- Saline implants have a higher rate of leakage and a less natural feel than silicone implants. The advantages of saline are that they have a lower reported incidence of contracture and that leakage from the implant is undesirable but harmless.

Suggested Reading

Ganott MA, Harris KM, Ilkhanipour ZS, Costa-Greco MA. Augmentation mammoplasty: normal and abnormal findings with mammography and US. Radiographics 1992;12:281–295

Lavine DM. Saline inflatable prostheses: 14 years' experience. Aesthetic Plast Surg 1993;17:325–330

Newman J. Mammographic evaluation of the augmented breast. Radiol Technol 1998;69:319–338, quiz 339–342

Steinbach BG, Hardt NS, Abbitt PL. Mammography: breast implants—types, complications, and adjacent breast pathology. Curr Probl Diagn Radiol 1993;22:39–86

Case 26.12: Implant Rupture—Implant Collapse or Rupture

Case History
A 39-year-old woman who has had breast augmentation with saline implants notes a new palpable abnormality in her left breast.

Physical Examination
- Left breast: deformed and small implant
- Right breast: normal exam

Mammogram (Fig. 26.19)

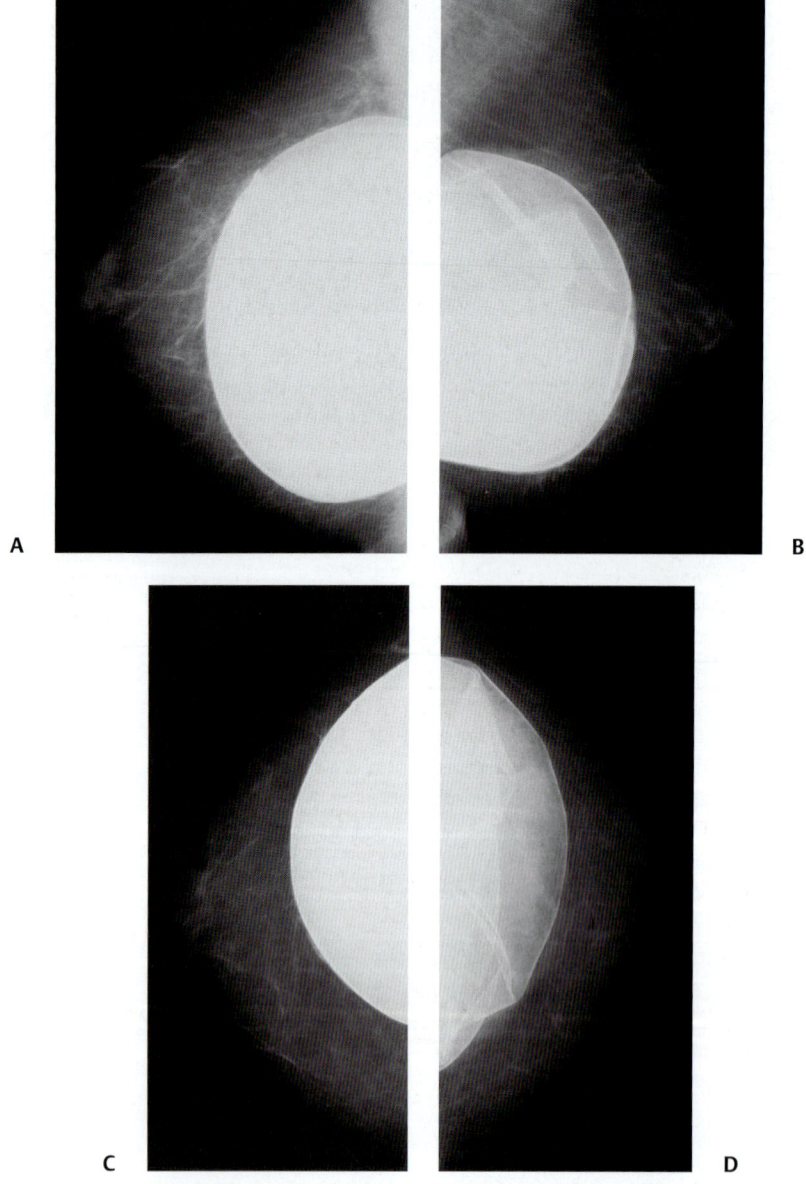

Fig. 26.19 The left implant is deformed and smaller than the right. (**A**) Right MLO mammogram. (**B**) Left MLO mammogram. (**C**) Right CC mammogram. (**D**) Left CC mammogram.

Ultrasound

Frequency
- 11.5 MHz (**Figs. 26.20** and **26.21**)

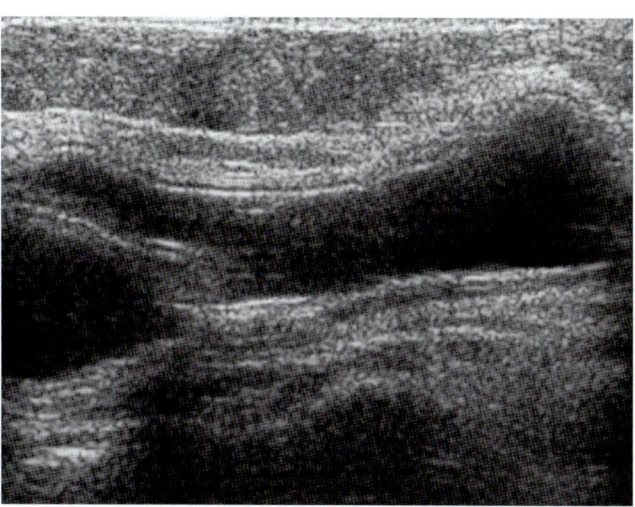 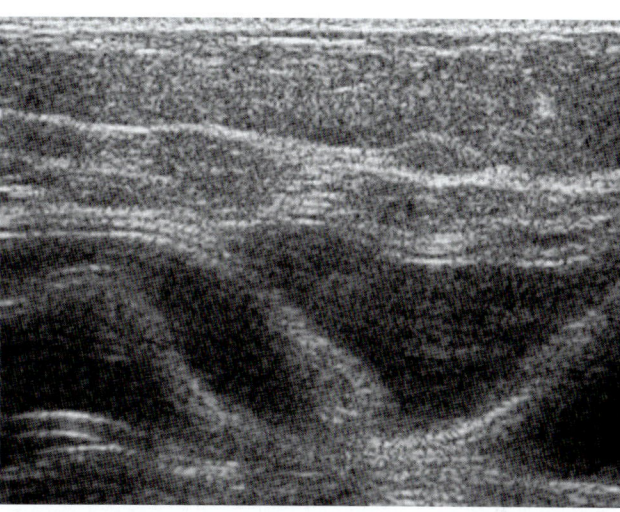

Fig. 26.20 Sonography of the left implant demonstrates a distorted, small implant with multiple linear invaginations, suggesting implant rupture. (**A**) Left radial breast implant sonogram. (**B**) Left antiradial implant sonogram.

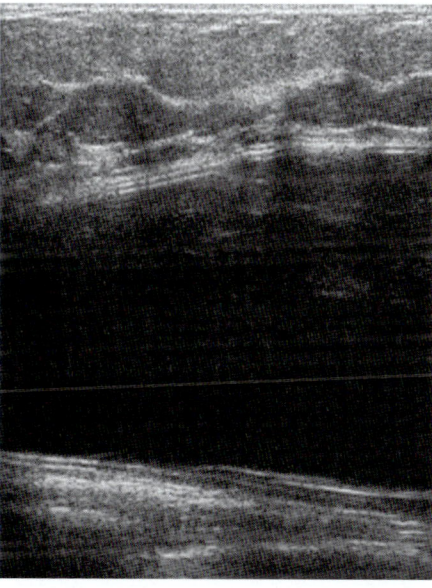

Fig. 26.21 Right radial implant sonogram. Right implant is normal.

Pathology
- Deflation of saline implant

Management
- BI-RADS assessment category 2, benign finding

Pearls and Pitfalls

- Sonography is better than mammography but not as accurate as MRI in identifying implant rupture. One article reviewing the literature found that mammography has a sensitivity of 28.4% and specificity of 92.9%. Ultrasound's sensitivity and specificity are 59.0% and 76.8%, respectively. MRI's sensitivity and specificity are 78.1% and 80.0%, respectively.
- The main pitfalls of sonographically identifying implant rupture include mistaking normal implant folds for collapsed walls, confusing normal peri-implant fluid for abnormal leakage, and identifying silicone collections or nodes that are due to normal seepage of silicone through an intact implant shell or due to a previously ruptured implant.

Suggested Reading

Goodman CM, Cohen V, Thornby J, Netscher D. The life span of silicone gel breast implants and a comparison of mammography, ultrasonography, and magnetic resonance imaging in detecting implant rupture: a meta-analysis. Ann Plast Surg 1998;41:577–585, discussion 585–586

Samuels JB, Rohrich RJ, Weatherall PT, Ho AM, Goldberg KL. Radiographic diagnosis of breast implant rupture: current status and comparison of techniques. Plast Reconstr Surg 1995;96:865–877

Case 26.13: Implant Rupture—Implant Collapse or Rupture

Case History
A 46-year-old woman has had subglandular silicone gel implants for 13 years.

Physical Examination
- Bilateral breasts: both implants feel irregular in shape

Mammogram (Fig. 26.22)

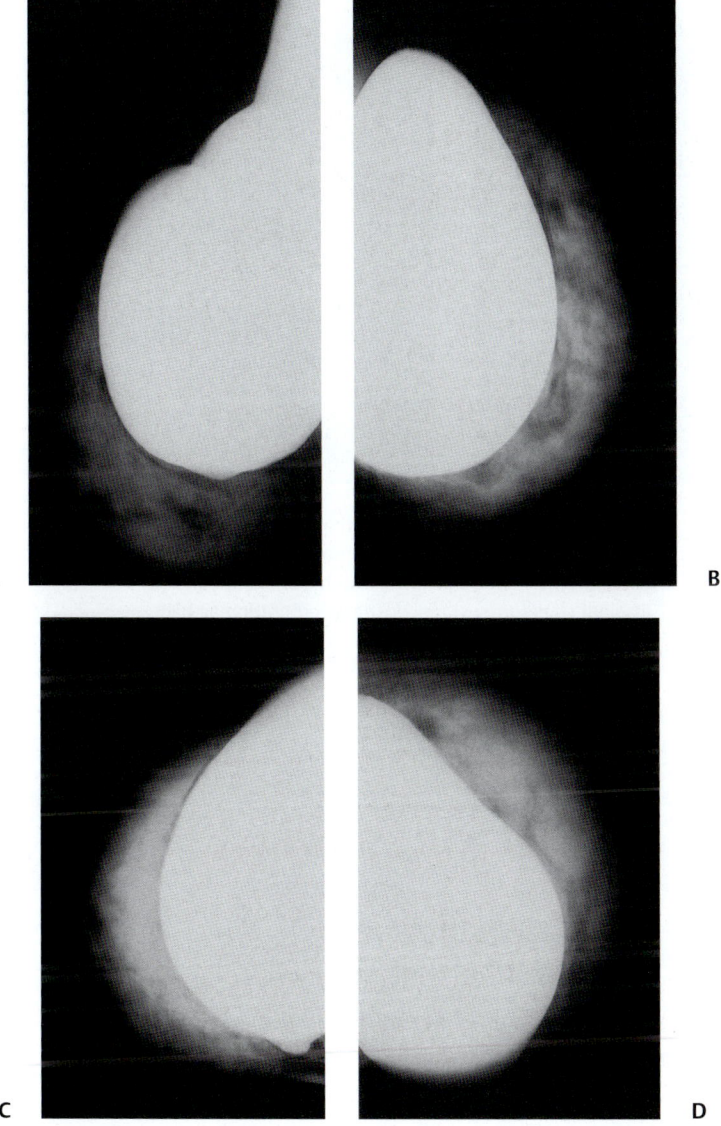

Fig. 26.22 There is asymmetric extension of the right implant in the right upper outer quadrant. There is also a focal contour bulge in the medial aspect of the implant on the CC view. (**A**) Right MLO mammogram. (**B**) Left MLO mammogram. (**C**) Right CC mammogram. (**D**) Left CC mammogram.

428 Postsurgical Findings

Ultrasound (Fig. 26.23)

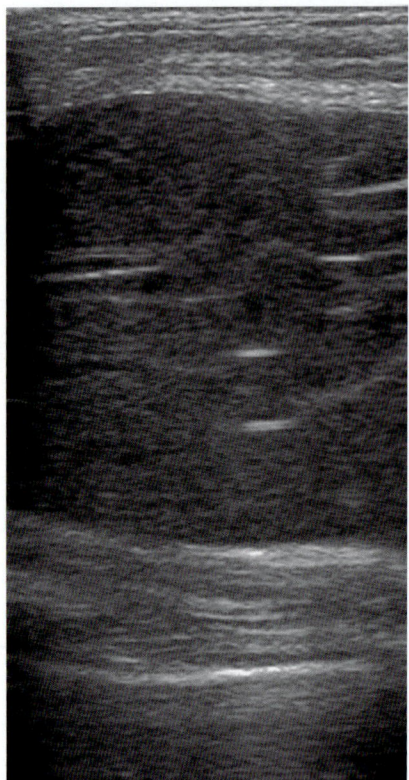
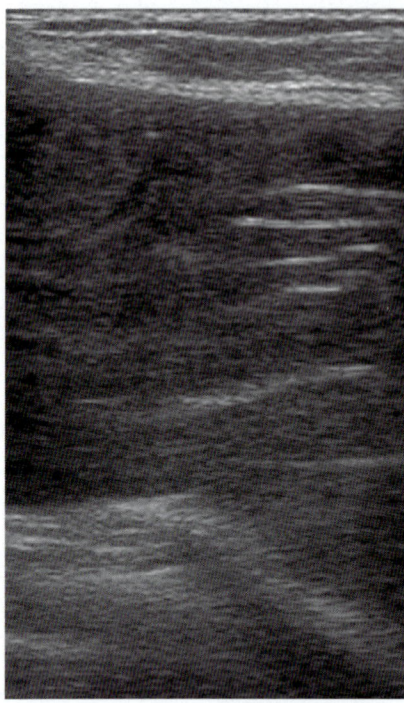
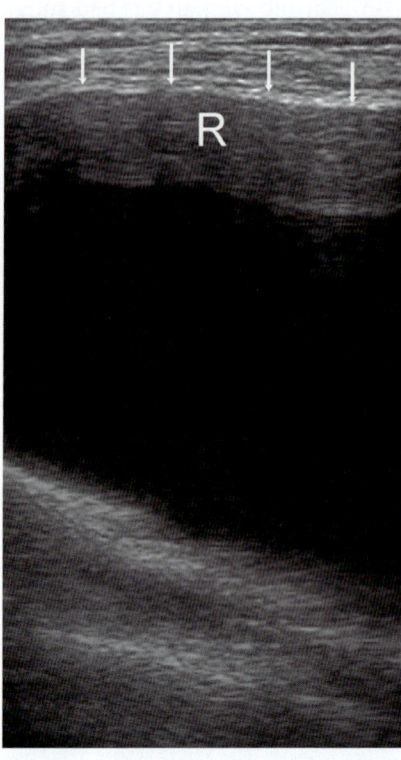

Fig. 26.23 (**A**) Transverse right breast implant sonogram. The right implant is filled with hypoechoic fluid and exhibits multiple echogenic lines within it. (**B**) Transverse right breast implant sonogram, which illustrates the "stepladder" sign created by the echogenic lines. This is a different position from that in **A**. (**C**) Transverse left breast sonogram. Left implant appears normal. The fluid is anechoic, and there are no echogenic lines. The hypoechoic band (R) next to the implant shell (*arrows*) is acoustic reverberation artifact.

Pathology
- Ruptured right implant

Management
- BI-RADS assessment category 2, benign finding

Pearls and Pitfalls

- Implant rupture increases with increasing prosthesis age. A review of over 1000 silicone gel implants found that the median life span for those implants was 16.4 years. About 79% of silicone implants were intact at 10 years. Only 49% were unruptured by 15 years.
- With experienced operators, sonography is a useful method to identify implant rupture. The most reliable sign of rupture is identification of multiple horizontal, straight, or curvilinear lines ("stepladder" sign) within the silicone gel. This sonographic finding corresponds to the MRI "linguine" sign. The lines represent the collapsed walls of the implant. Another important sonographic sign of rupture is the presence of "echodense noise" (snowstorm appearance), which indicates free silicone. Hypoechoic debris within the implant is a less reliable finding of rupture.

Suggested Reading

DeBruhl ND, Gorczyca DP, Ahn CY, Shaw WW, Bassett LW. Silicone breast implants: US evaluation. Radiology 1993;189:95–98

Goodman CM, Cohen V, Thornby J, Netscher D. The life span of silicone gel breast implants and a comparison of mammography, ultrasonography, and magnetic resonance imaging in detecting implant rupture: a meta-analysis. Ann Plast Surg 1998;41:577–585, discussion 585–586

Case 26.14: Implant Rupture—Intracapsular Rupture

Case History
A 31-year-old woman is concerned that her implants feel asymmetric.

Physical Examination
- Right breast: implant is irregular in shape
- Left breast: normal exam

Other Modalities: MRI (Figs. 26.24 and 26.25)

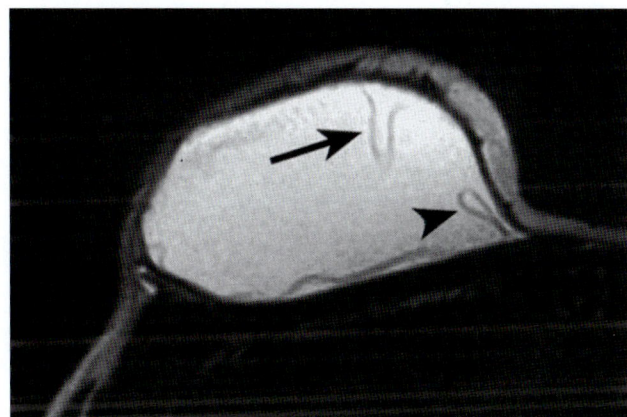
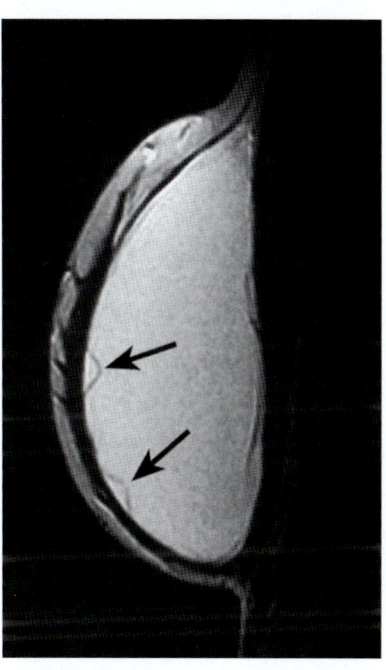

Fig. 26.24 Right breast T2-weighted transverse MRI. This image illustrates mild collapse of the implant shell with silicone on both sides of the collapsing walls. Two mild or indirect signs of intracapsular rupture are the "keyhole" sign (*arrow*) and the "noose" sign (*arrowhead*).

Fig. 26.25 Right breast T2-weighted longitudinal MRI. This image demonstrates more small areas (*arrows*) where the implant shell has separated from the fibrous capsule.

Pathology
- Intracapsular implant rupture

Management
- BI-RADS assessment category 2, benign finding

> **Pearls and Pitfalls**
>
> - MRI findings of intracapsular rupture include multiple wavy lines ("linguine" sign) and curvilinear lines that form a semicircular shape with the fibrous capsule (C sign). The least reliable signs of rupture are the group that demonstrates silicone on both sides of the folded implant wall. When the edges of the fold are touching, the sign is called the "keyhole" or "teardrop" sign. When the walls are not touching, the abnormality has a variety of names, including "noose," "pull-away," and open loop sign. The reason that these signs may be misleading is that these findings are also present when nonruptured silicone is against the wall. Furthermore, complex normal implant folds may also be misinterpreted as representing one of these findings.

Suggested Reading

Soo MS, Kornguth PJ, Walsh R, Elenberger CD, Georgiade GS. Complex radial folds versus subtle signs of intracapsular rupture of breast implants: MR findings with surgical correlation. AJR Am J Roentgenol 1996;166:1421–1427

Gorczyca, DP, Gorczyca, SM, Gorczyca, KL. The diagnosis of silicone breast implant rupture. Plast Reconstr Surg 2007;120 (Suppl 1): 49S–61S.

Case 26.15: Implant Rupture—Intracapsular Rupture

Case History
A 57-year-old woman presents for screening mammogram. She has no breast symptoms.

Physical Examination
- Breast exam: normal exam

Mammogram (Fig. 26.26)

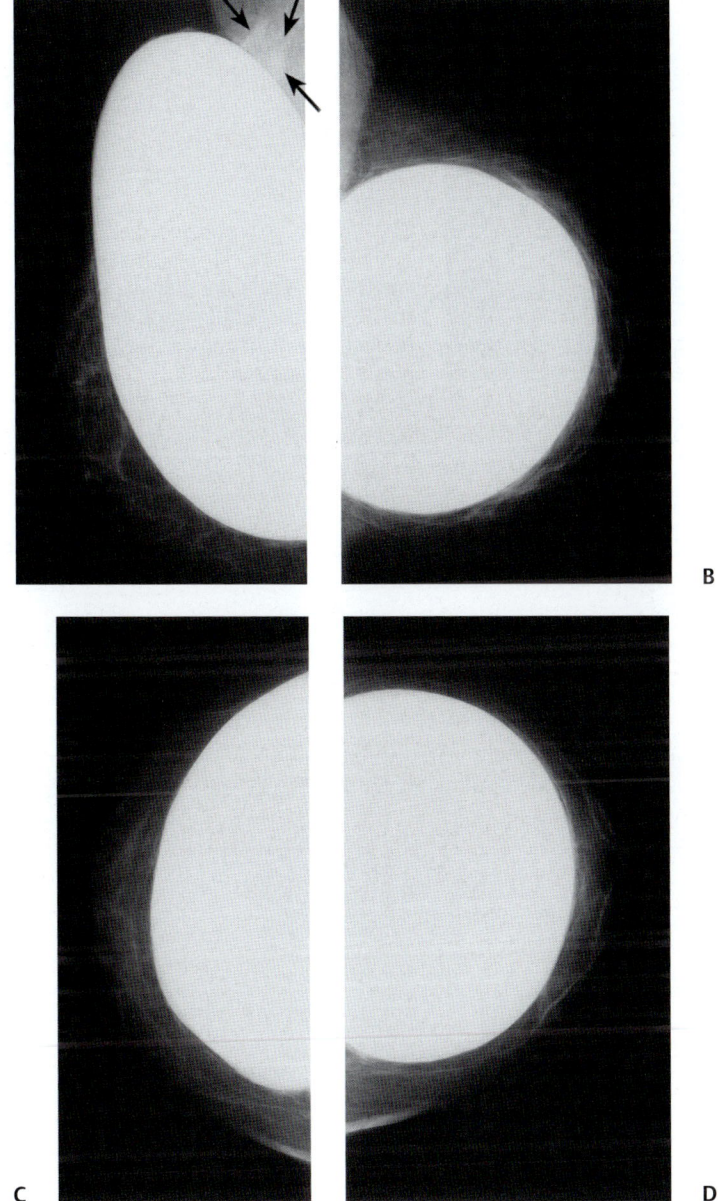

Fig. 26.26 In the right axilla, there are some oval high-density collections (*arrows*) consistent with silicone. These collections have been present for at least 7 years. (**A**) Right MLO mammogram. (**B**) Left MLO mammogram. (**C**) Right CC mammogram. (**D**) Left CC mammogram.

Other Modalities: MRI (Fig. 26.27)

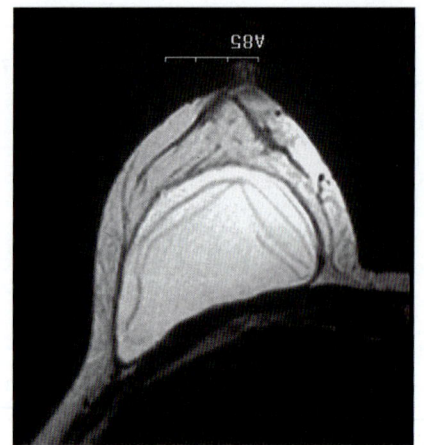 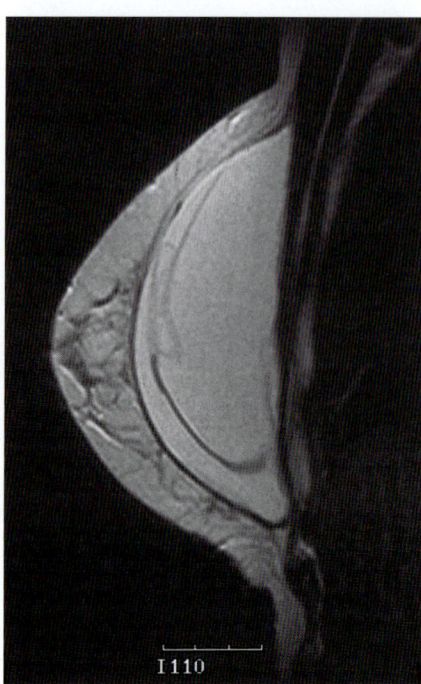

Fig. 26.27 There are multiple curvilinear lines consistent with implant shell rupture. (**A**) Right breast T2 transverse MRI. (**B**) Right breast T2 longitudinal MRI.

Pathology
- Implant rupture

Management
- BI-RADS assessment category 2, benign finding

Pearls and Pitfalls

- Only an intracapsular rupture was identified by MRI. The right axillary silicone identified mammographically may be either the result of an occult capsular rupture or due to passage of silicone through the fibrous capsule without a rupture in the capsule. This patient elected not to remove the implants.

Suggested Reading
Middleton MS. Magnetic resonance evaluation of breast implants and soft-tissue silicone. Top Magn Reson Imaging 1998;9:92–137

Case 26.16: Implant Rupture—Extracapsular Rupture

Case History
A 40-year-old woman had implants for 20 years. She notes an enlarging bulge in the lateral side of her right implant.

Physical Examination
- Right breast: implant is contracted and irregular in contour.
- Left breast: normal exam

Mammogram (Fig. 26.28)

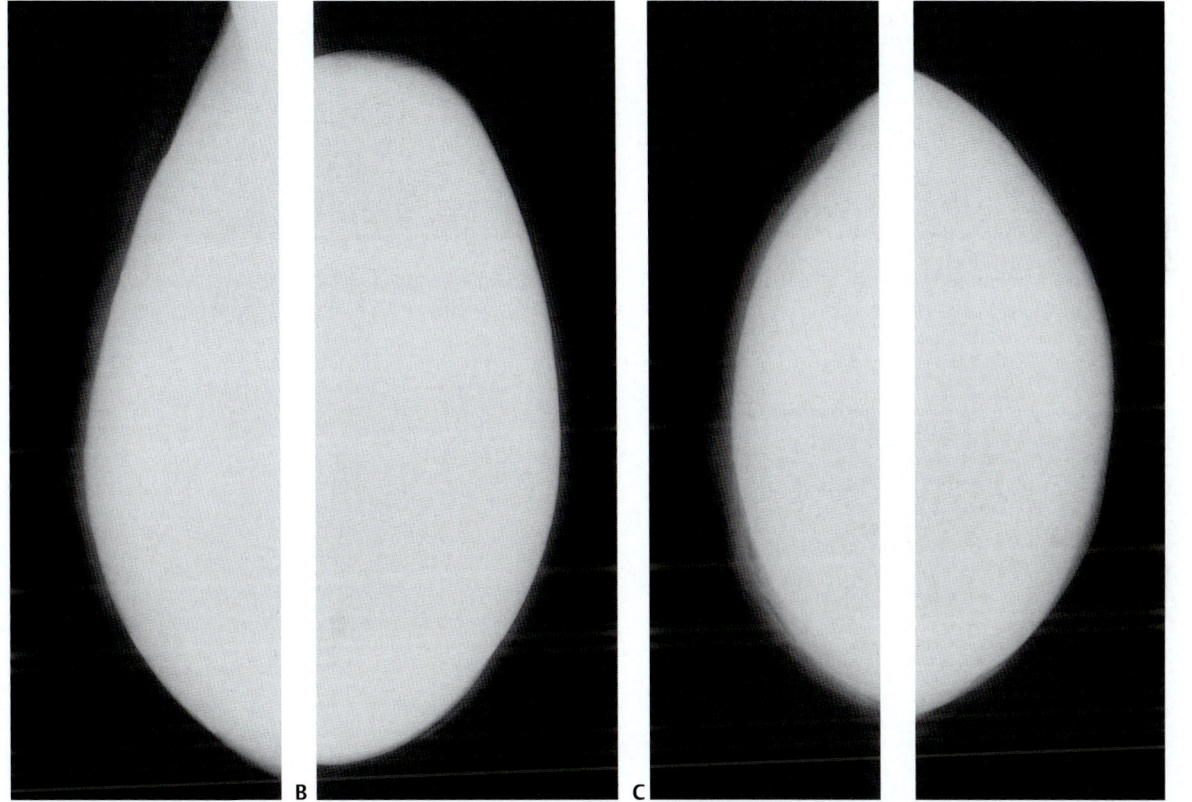

Fig. 26.28 There is mild asymmetry in the shape of the implants. Otherwise the exam is normal. (**A**) Right MLO implant mammogram. (**B**) Left MLO implant mammogram. (**C**) Right CC implant mammogram. (**D**) Left CC implant mammogram.

Other Modalities: MRI (Figs. 26.29, 26.30, and 26.31)

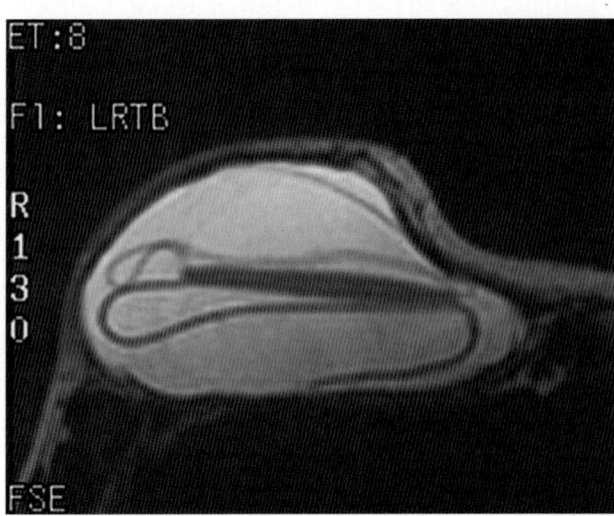

Fig. 26.29 Right breast T2-weighted transverse MRI. Right breast implant demonstrates multiple wavy lines ("linguine" sign), which represent the collapse of the implant shell.

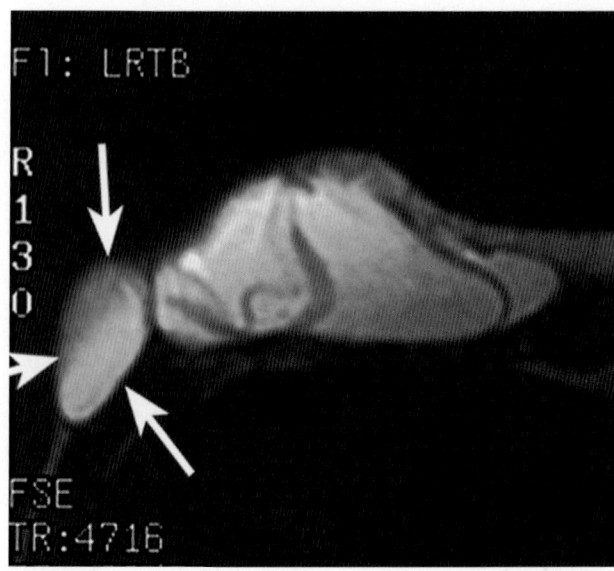

Fig. 26.30 Right breast T2-weighted transverse MRI. An oval collection of silicone is present lateral to the edge of the implant (*arrows*).

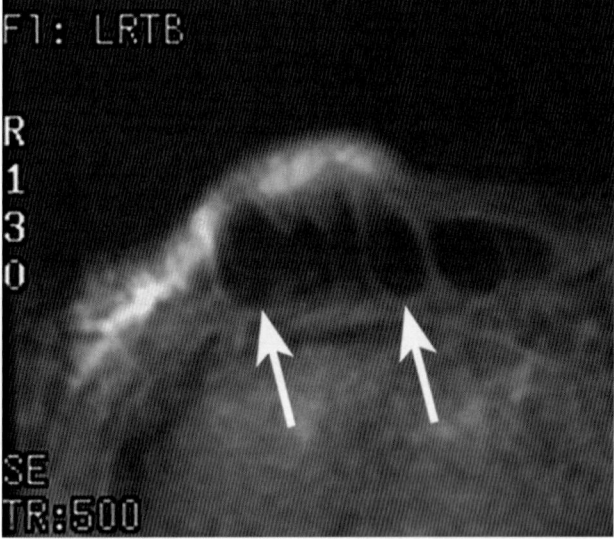

Fig. 26.31 Right breast T1-weighted transverse MRI. Oval collections of extracapsular silicone (which is dark with this technique) are present superior to the fibrous capsule (*arrows*).

Pathology
- Extracapsular rupture

Management
- BI-RADS assessment category 2, benign finding

> **Pearls and Pitfalls**
>
> - The most dramatic and reliable MRI sign of capsular rupture is the demonstration of multiple curvilinear low-signal lines that correspond to the collapsed elastomer shell ("linguine sign"). The collapsed ruptured shell and the free silicone are strong evidence of extracapsular rupture.

Suggested Reading
Orel SG. MR imaging of the breast. Radiol Clin North Am 2000;38:899–913

Case 26.17: Implant Rupture—Extracapsular Rupture

Case History
A 56-year-old woman presents with a new right breast lump. She has bilateral breast implants.

Physical Examination
- Right breast: implant irregular; palpable lump at the 6 o'clock position adjacent to implant
- Left breast: normal exam

Mammogram (Fig. 26.32)

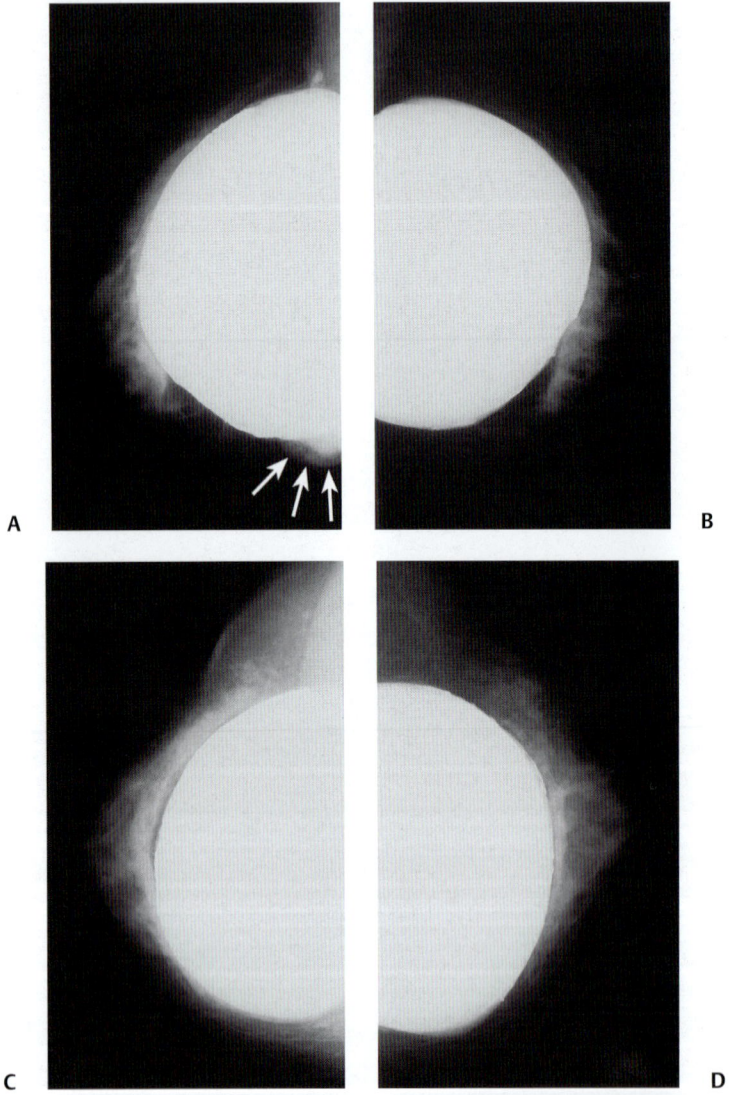

Fig. 26.32 An oval density is present in the right inferior breast adjacent to the implant (*arrows*). It corresponds to the palpable lump. (**A**) Right MLO mammogram. (**B**) Left MLO mammogram. (**C**) Right CC mammogram. (**D**) Left CC mammogram.

Augmentation Mammoplasty

Ultrasound

Frequency
- 13 MHz (**Fig. 26.33**)

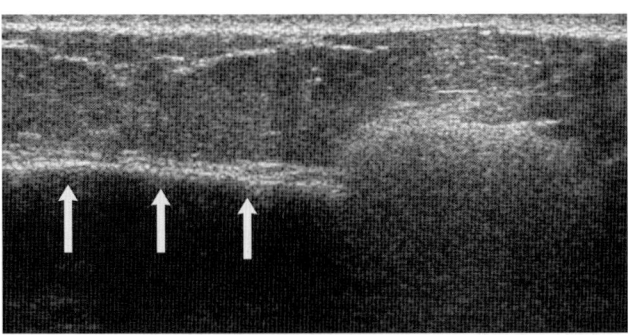
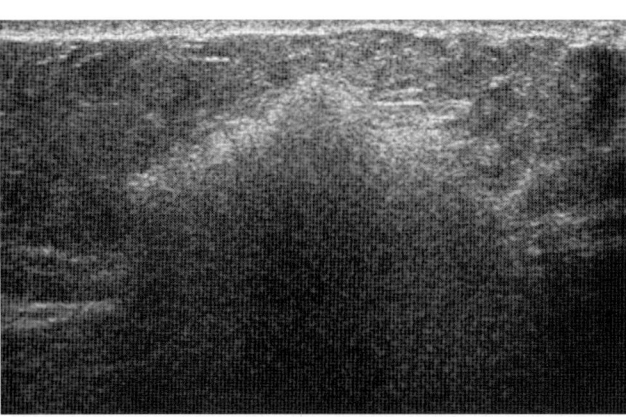

Fig. 26.33 The right palpable lump at the 6 o'clock position corresponds to a focal area of echogenic noise. The wall of the implant and the fibrous capsule form a well-defined hyperechoic line (*arrows*) adjacent to this mass. (**A**) Right longitudinal breast sonogram. (**B**) Right transverse breast sonogram.

Other Modalities: MRI (Figs. 26.34 and 26.35)

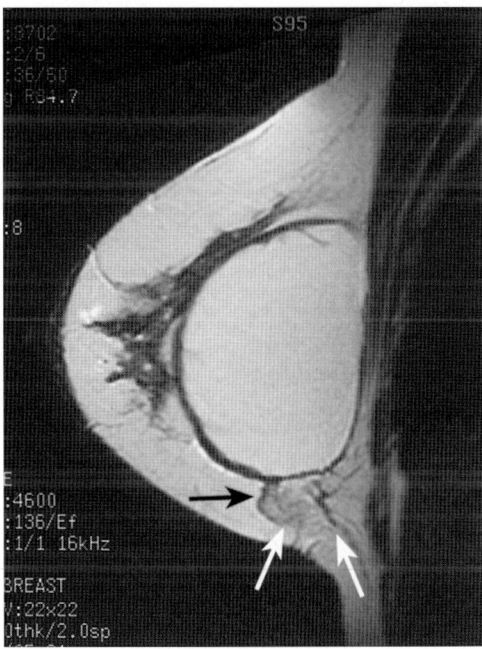
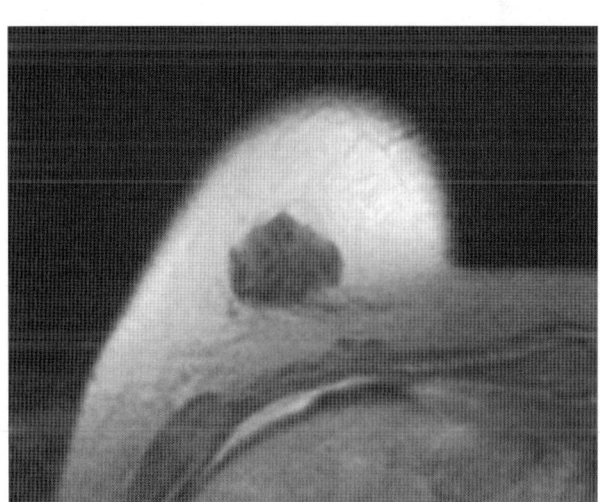

Fig. 26.34 Right breast T2-weighted longitudinal MRI. Inferior to the breast (in the areas of the palpable mass) there is a faint mass (*arrows*). It does not appear as bright as the intracapsular silicone.

Fig. 26.35 Right breast T1-weighted with fat saturation transverse MRI. The extracapsular silicone identified sonographically corresponds to the low signal intensity (dark) focus in the breast.

Pathology
- Extracapsular ruptured implant
- Grossly ruptured right implant when removed
- Palpable lump corresponded microscopically to a silicone granuloma.

Management
- BI-RADS assessment category 2, benign finding

Pearls and Pitfalls

- Five appearances of extracapsular silicone have been described with MRI: (1) cyst, (2) granuloma, (3) infiltration of fatty breast parenchyma, (4) infiltration of muscle, and (5) globules in muscle. If the silicone forms a fluid collection, it will appear as a cystic mass that has the same high intensity on T2-weighted sequences as intracapsular silicone. If the silicone becomes infiltrated with scar (granuloma formation), then the intensity will vary depending upon the concentration of silicone within the granuloma. Less than 5 to 15% silicone concentration is probably not detectable with current MRI techniques. Irregular, lacy silicone infiltration of both breast tissue and muscle will be bright on T2-weighted sequences. Usually this pattern is due to previous silicone injection. Silicone muscle globules are similar in appearance to silicone cysts in the breast. Globules are a rarer presentation of silicone migration to muscle.

Suggested Reading

Caskey CI, Berg WA, Hamper UM, Sheth S, Chang BW, Anderson ND. Imaging spectrum of extracapsular silicone: correlation of US, MR imaging, mammographic, and histopathologic findings. Radiographics 1999;19(Spec. No.):S39–S51, quiz S261–S262

Middleton MS. Breast implants and soft tissue silicone. In: Stark DD, Bradley WG, eds. Magnetic Resonance Imaging. 3rd ed. St. Louis: Mosby; 1999:335–353

Case 26.18: Implant Rupture—False Positive for Intra- and Extracapsular Rupture

Case History
A 47-year-old woman with left axillary lumps and a breast lump. She had bilateral augmentation mammoplasties with silicone implants 25 years ago. Seven years ago, they became contractured, and the right implant ruptured, so both were replaced at that time.

Physical Examination
- Left breast: palpable mass at the 3 o'clock position. Three palpable lymph nodes are identified.
- Right breast: normal exam

Mammogram (Fig. 26.36)

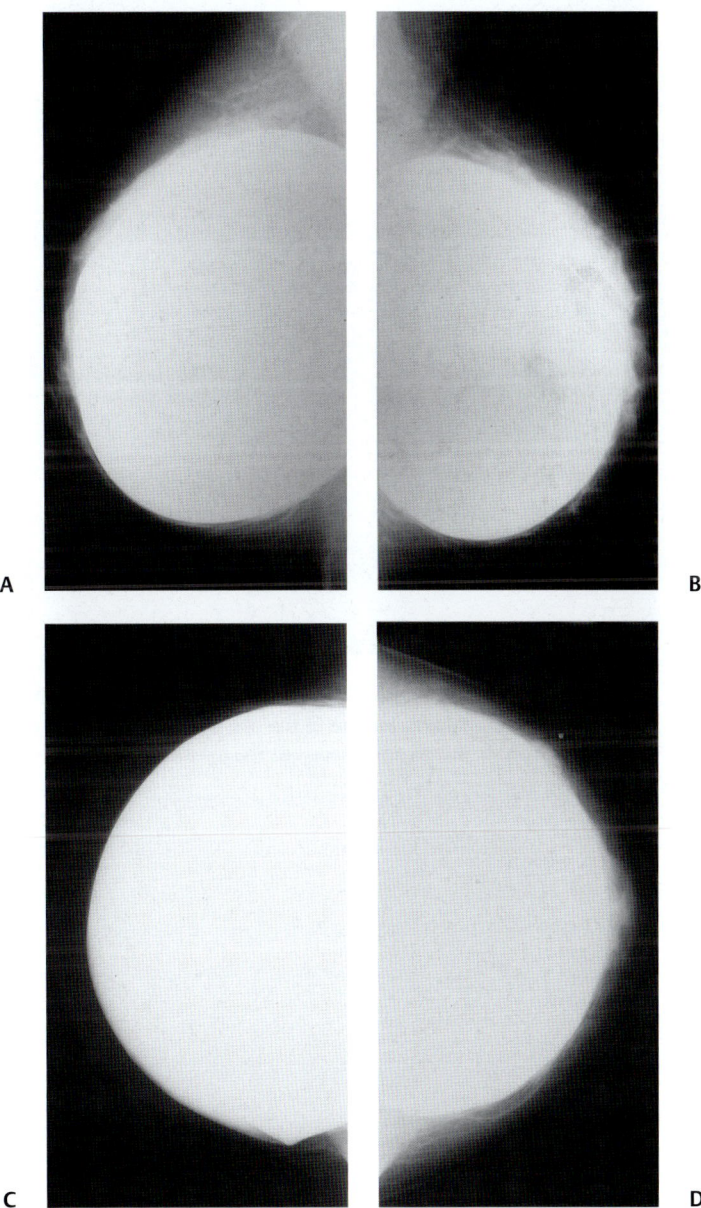

Fig. 26.36 There is a mass in the left outer breast, which corresponds to the palpable lump. A high-density lymph node is present in the left axilla. (**A**) Right MLO mammogram. (**B**) Left MLO mammogram. (**C**) Right CC mammogram. (**D**) Left CC mammogram.

Postsurgical Findings

Ultrasound

Frequency
- 13 MHz (**Figs. 26.37** and **26.38**)

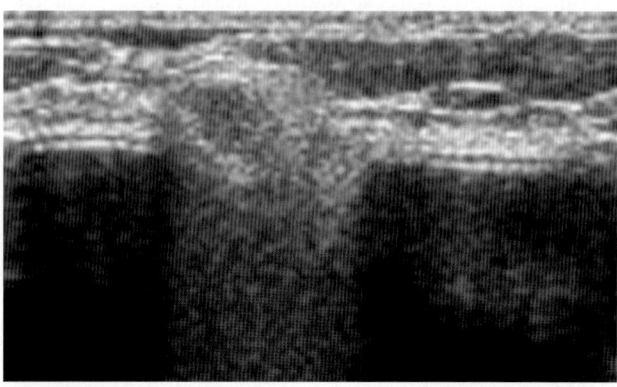

Fig. 26.37 Left transverse breast sonogram. The palpable lump corresponds to a hyperechoic mass with echogenic noise characteristic of silicone.

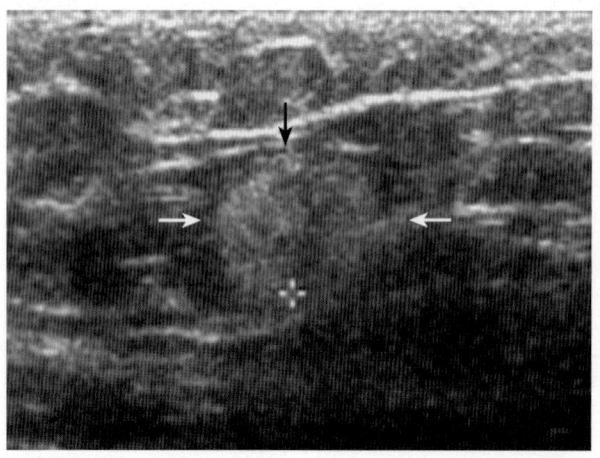

A

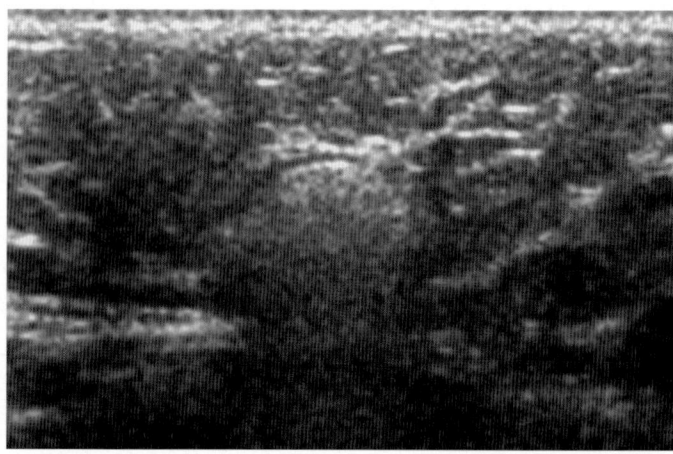

B

Fig. 26.38 Within the axilla, two abnormal hyperechoic masses were identified. The internal architecture of the mass (*arrows* in **A**) is suggestive of silicone within a lymph node. (**B**) The mass could either be a silicone-laden node or a granuloma. (**A**) Longitudinal left axillary sonogram of mass 1. (**B**) Longitudinal left axillary sonogram of mass 2.

Other Modalities: MRI (Fig. 26.39)

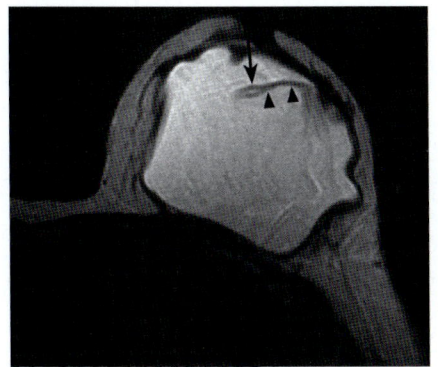
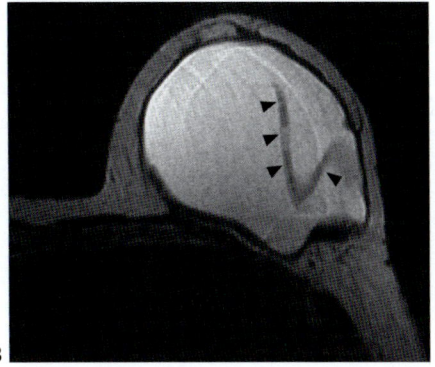
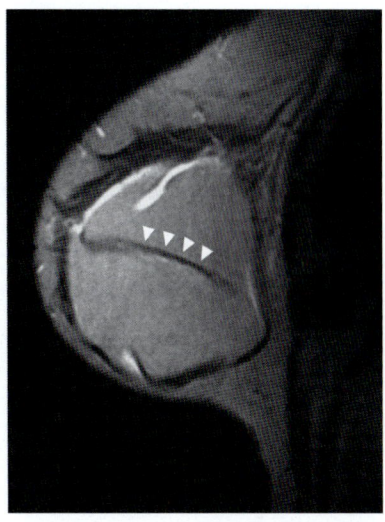

Fig. 26.39 These T2-weighted images demonstrate a pseudo-keyhole sign (*arrow*) that is created by a complex normal fold of the implant. (**A,B**) In the transverse plane, the fold (*arrowheads*) forms an S-shaped line that ends with the pseudo-keyhole (*arrow*). (**C**) In the longitudinal plane, the sheetlike configuration of this fold (*arrowheads*) is confirmed. This fold meets the surface of the implant close to the region of the palpable lump. (**A**) Left breast T2-weighted transverse MRI. (**B**) Left breast T2-weighted transverse MRI. This image is inferior to that in **A**. (**C**) Left breast T2-weighted longitudinal MRI.

Pathology
- Intact implant, extracapsular silicone

Management
- BI-RADS assessment category 2, benign finding

Pearls and Pitfalls
- The left breast implant was removed, and no rupture was identified. The palpable breast lump was histologically found to be a silicone granuloma. The patient also had silicone axillary adenopathy. This case demonstrates some pitfalls in the identification of implant rupture. In this case, complex implant folds (radial folds) simulated collapse of the ruptured implant shell. Furthermore, silicone outside the capsule was not a result of extracapsular rupture. In this patient, the free silicone may be due to either silicone that leaked during the previous replacement surgery or silicone that has seeped through an intact implant shell (gel bleed).

Suggested Reading
Caskey CI, Berg WA, Hamper UM, Sheth S, Chang BW, Anderson ND. Imaging spectrum of extracapsular silicone: correlation of US, MR imaging, mammographic, and histopathologic findings. Radiographics 1999;19(Spec. No.):S39–S51, quiz S261–S262

442 Postsurgical Findings

Case 26.19: Neoplasm and Implants

Case History
A 55-year-old woman presents with a left breast lump. She has had bilateral augmentation mammoplasty. This is her baseline examination.

Physical Examination
- Left breast: mass on medial breast
- Right breast: normal exam

Mammogram

Mass
- Margin: spiculated
- Shape: irregular
- Density: equal density

Calcifications (Fig. 26.40)
- Type: pleomorphic/heterogeneous
- Distribution: grouped/clustered

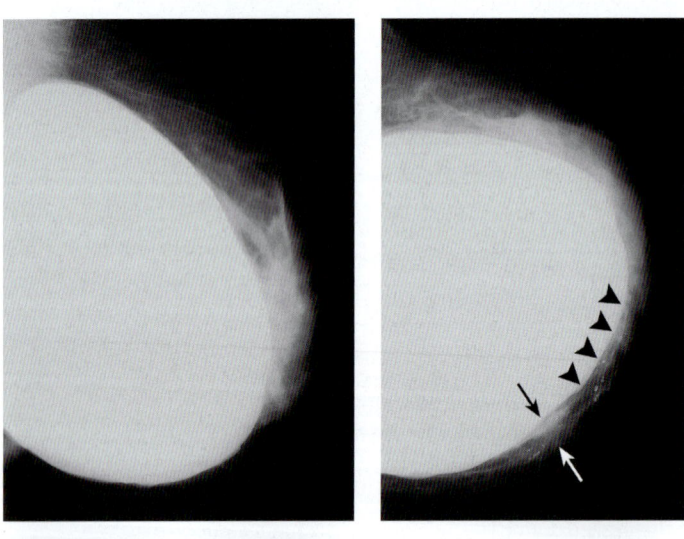

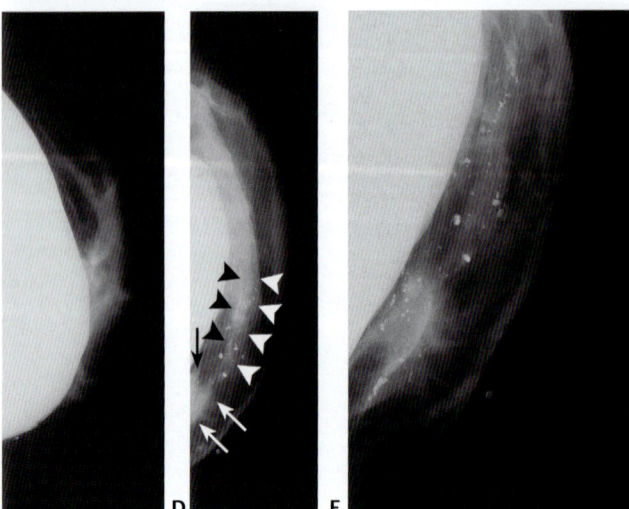

Fig. 26.40 In the left medial breast, there is an irregular density (*arrows*) containing heterogeneous calcifications. Adjacent to the mass are more heterogeneous calcifications (*arrowheads*). (**A**) Left MLO implant mammogram. (**B**) Left CC implant mammogram. (**C**) Left MLO implant displaced mammogram. (**D**) Left CC implant displaced mammogram. (**E**) Close-up of left medial breast.

Ultrasound

Low Frequency (Fig. 26.41)

Frequency
- 7.5 MHz

Mass
- Margin: ill defined
- Echogenicity: hypoechoic
- Retrotumoral acoustic appearance: no shadowing
- Shape: irregular

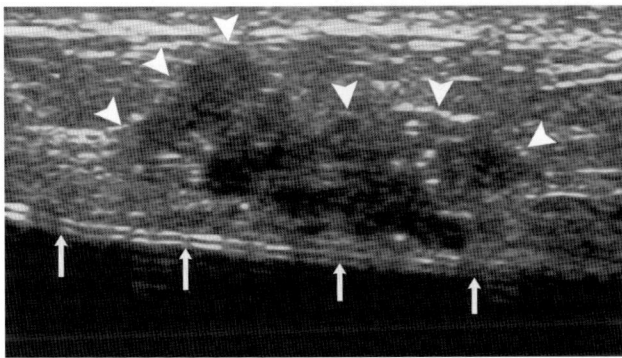

Fig. 26.41 Left radial low-frequency breast sonogram. The mammographic spiculated density and palpable mass (*arrowheads*) correspond to an irregular hypoechoic mass with calcifications. With the lower frequency, the mass does not shadow. No second mass is identified. Implant shell (*arrows*).

High Frequency
- 13 MHz (**Fig. 26.42**)

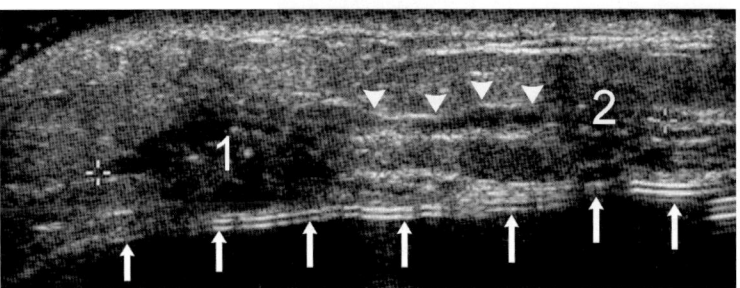

Fig. 26.42 Left radial high-frequency breast sonogram. With higher frequency, two masses are identified. One mass (labeled 1) corresponds to the mass previously identified with the lower-frequency exam. The second mass (labeled 2) is closer to the nipple and connected to the first mass with a dilated duct (*arrowheads*). Implant shell (*arrows*).

446 Postsurgical Findings

Mammogram (Fig. 26.45)

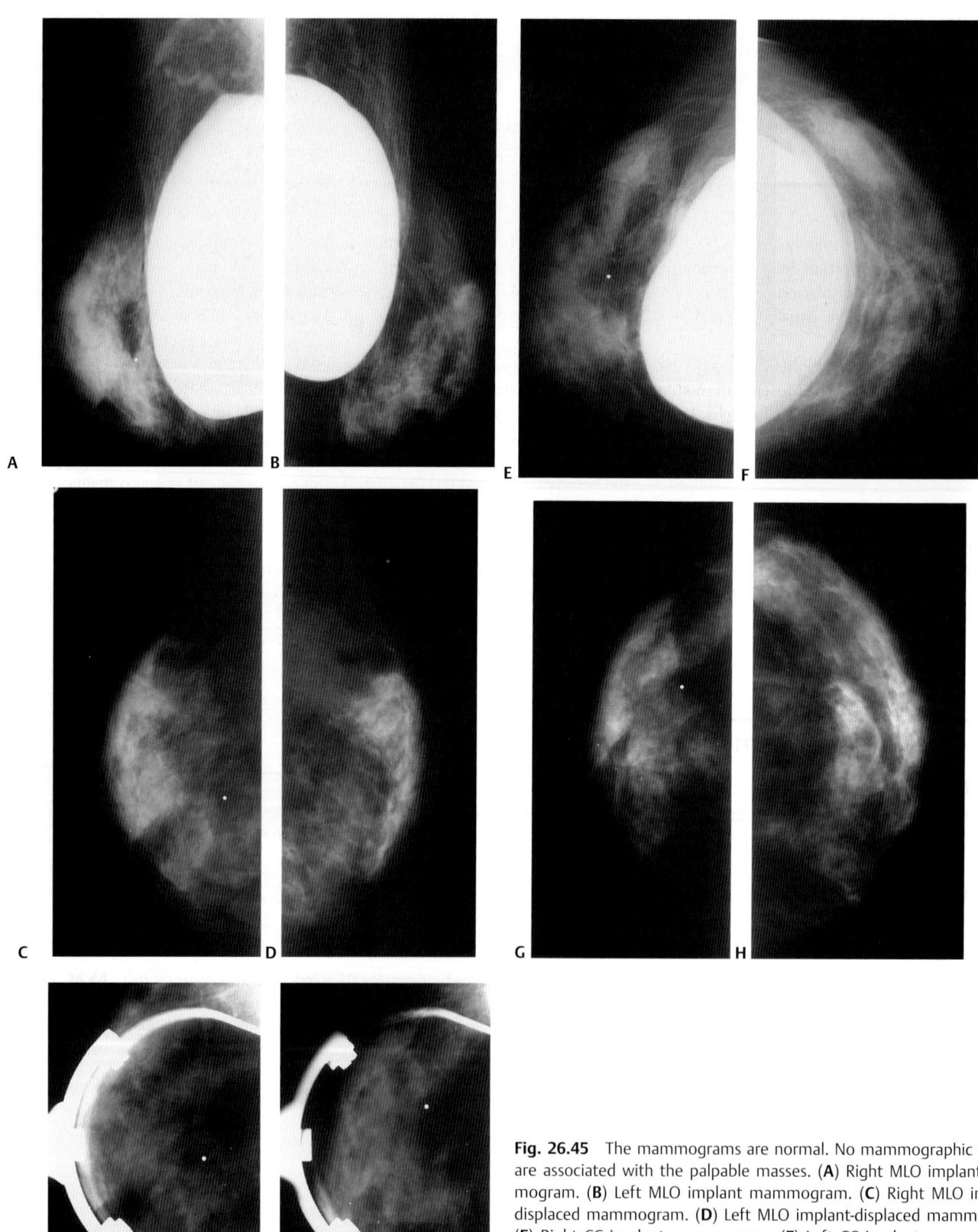

Fig. 26.45 The mammograms are normal. No mammographic masses are associated with the palpable masses. (**A**) Right MLO implant mammogram. (**B**) Left MLO implant mammogram. (**C**) Right MLO implant-displaced mammogram. (**D**) Left MLO implant-displaced mammogram. (**E**) Right CC implant mammogram. (**F**) Left CC implant mammogram. (**G**) Right CC implant-displaced mammogram. (**H**) Left CC implant-displaced mammogram. (**I**) Right MLO spot compression mammogram. (**J**) Right CC spot compression mammogram.

Ultrasound

Frequency
- 10 MHz

Mass (Figs. 26.46 and 26.47)
- Margin: irregular
- Echogenicity: hypoechoic
- Retrotumoral acoustic appearance: no shadowing
- Shape: lobulated

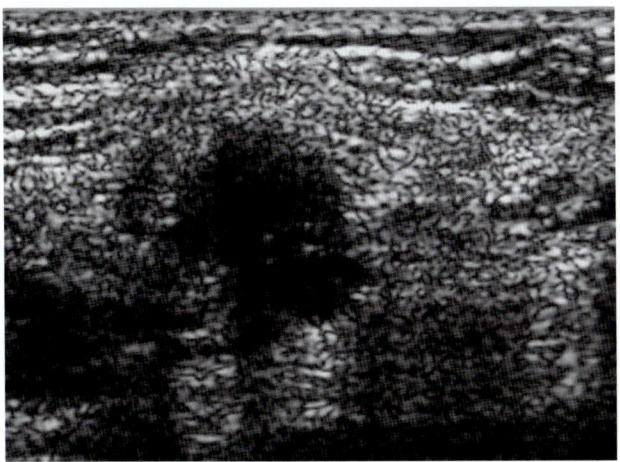

Fig. 26.46 Right antiradial breast sonogram. At the 7 o'clock position, a palpable lump corresponds to an irregular, hypoechoic mass with calcifications.

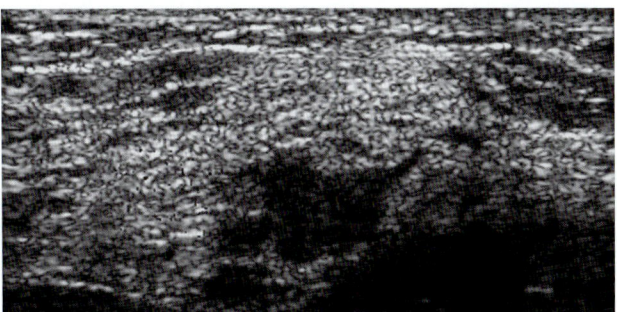

Fig. 26.47 Right antiradial breast sonogram. At the 10 o'clock position, the second palpable mass corresponds to another irregular, hypoechoic mass.

Pathology
- Infiltrating ductal carcinoma
- Two separate but histologically similar nodules of infiltrating ductal carcinoma. A mass at the 7 o'clock position has < 25% ductal carcinoma in situ, and a mass at the 10 o'clock position has no ductal carcinoma in situ.

Management
- BI-RADS assessment category 4, suspicious; biopsy should be considered.

Pearls and Pitfalls

- The risk of breast cancer is not increased in patients with breast augmentation. Palpable lumps should be examined in a manner similar to patients without augmentation. In this case, sonography was useful to identify multicentric disease.

Suggested Reading

Berkel H, Birdsell DC, Jenkins H. Breast augmentation: a risk factor for breast cancer? N Engl J Med 1992;326:1649–1653

Leibman AJ, Kruse B. Breast cancer: mammographic and sonographic findings after augmentation mammoplasty. Radiology 1990;174:195–198

Leibman AJ, Kruse BD. Imaging of breast cancer after augmentation mammoplasty. Ann Plast Surg 1993;30:111–115

Postsurgical Findings: Reduction Mammoplasty

This is a schematic diagram of the diagnostic approach to mammographic postsurgical findings: reduction mammoplasty. For further discussion, see Chapter 1.

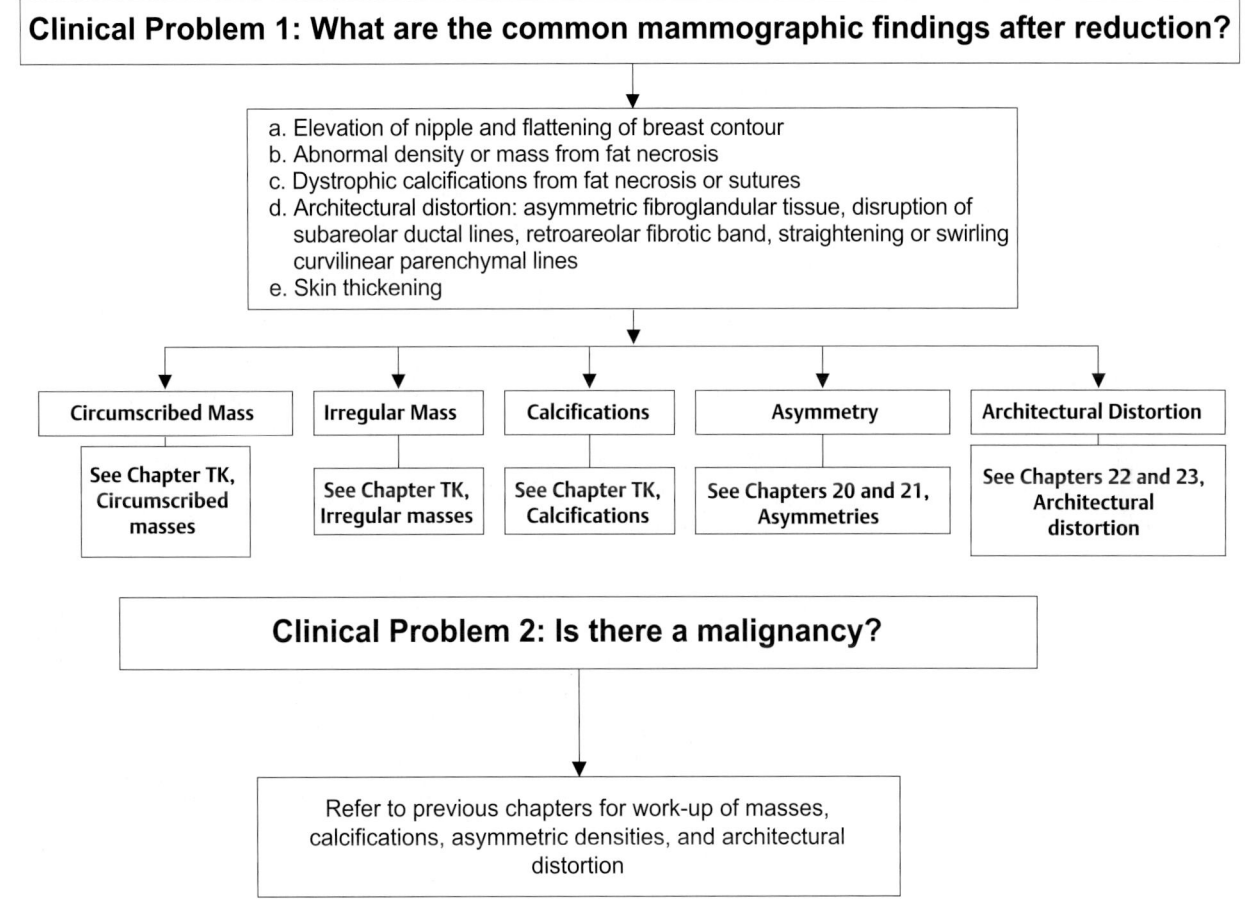

27 Reduction Mammoplasty

Case 27.1: Architectural Distortion

Case History
A 61-year-old woman had reduction mammoplasty 2 years ago.

Physical Examination
- Bilateral breasts: bilateral reduction scars, otherwise normal

Mammogram (Figs. 27.1 and 27.2)

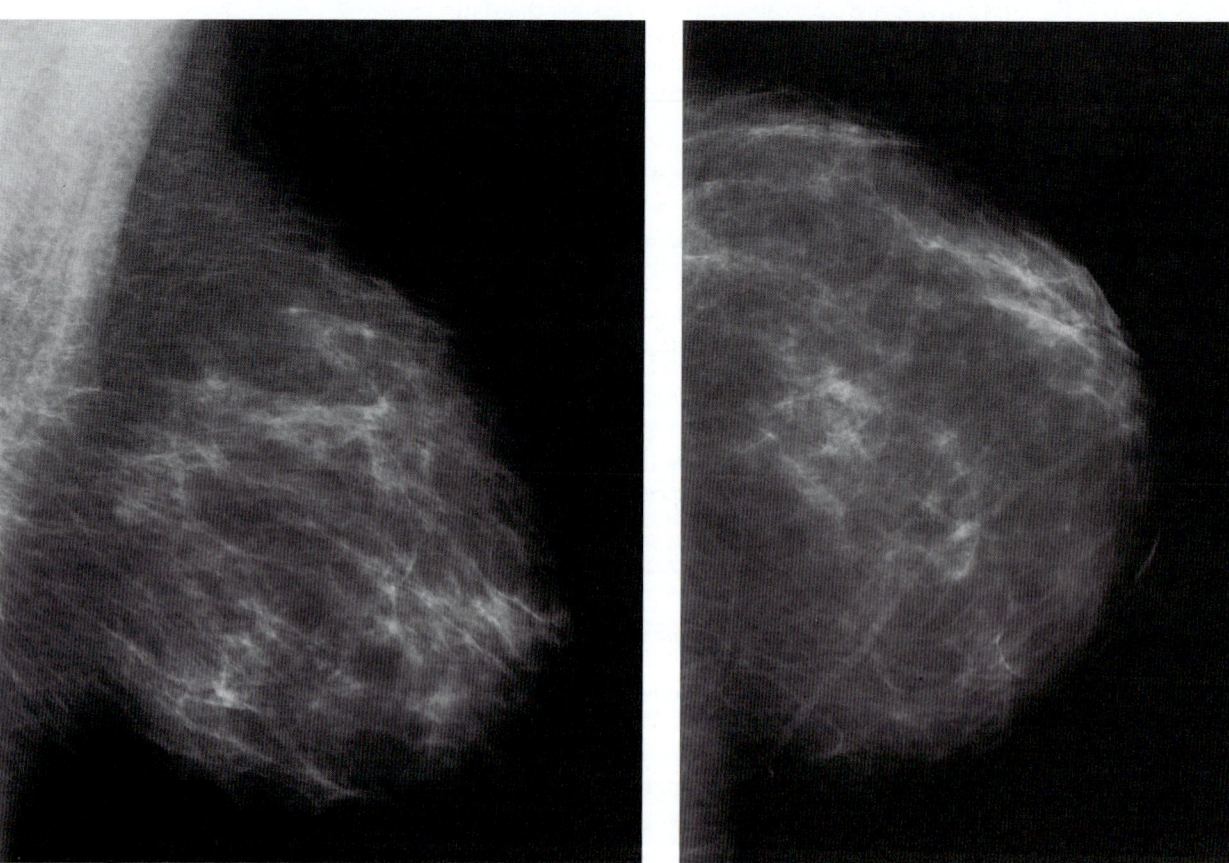

Fig. 27.1 Normal mammogram prior to reduction mammoplasty. (**A**) Left MLO mammogram. (**B**) Left CC mammogram.

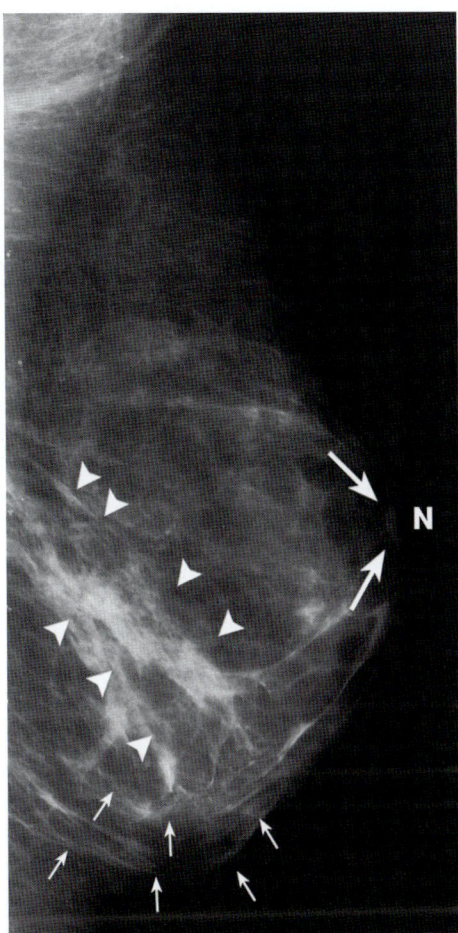 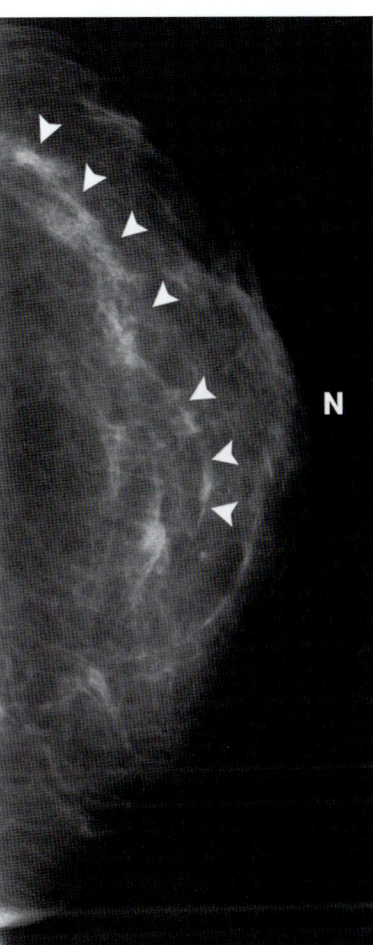

Fig. 27.2 Normal mammogram 2 years after reduction mammoplasty. The nipple (N) is higher in position, and the contour of the breast is flatter. Architectural distortion has resulted in swirled lines (*small arrows*); disruption of the normal subareolar ductal lines (*large arrows*); and increase in the density of the inferior breast, which in this patient is associated with straight parenchymal bands (*arrowheads*). (**A**) Left MLO mammogram. (**B**) Left CC mammogram.

Pathology
- Changes from reduction mammoplasty

Management
- BI-RADS assessment category 2, benign finding

Pearls and Pitfalls

- The various reduction mammoplasty procedures involve removing tissue from the inferior breast. The residual upper breast tissue is brought together in the midline to reform a smaller breast, and the nipple areolar complex is transposed superiorly. After these procedures, mammograms exhibit the following findings: (1) elevation of the nipple with flattening of the breast contour, (2) architectural distortion, (3) fat necrosis, (4) dystrophic calcifications, and (5) skin thickening.

Suggested Reading
Jackson VP. Reduction mammoplasty. In: Bassett LW, Jackson VP, Jahan R, Fu YS, Gold RH, eds. Diagnosis of Diseases of the Breast. Philadelphia: WB Saunders; 1997:581–587

Case 27.2: Architectural Distortion

Case History
An 85-year-old woman presents for screening mammogram.

Physical Examination
- Bilateral breasts: reduction mammoplasty scars, otherwise normal

Mammogram (Fig. 27.3)

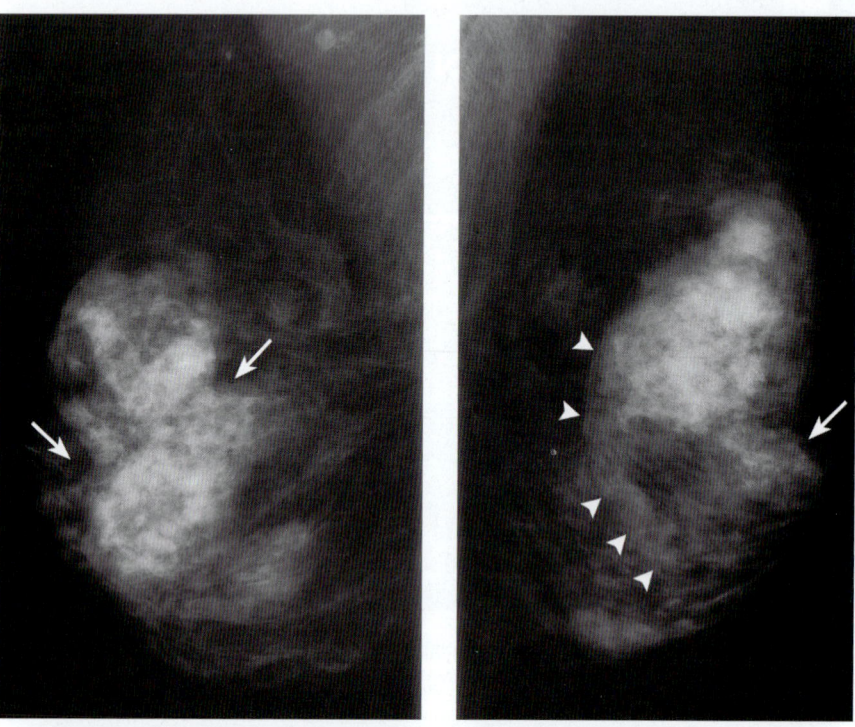

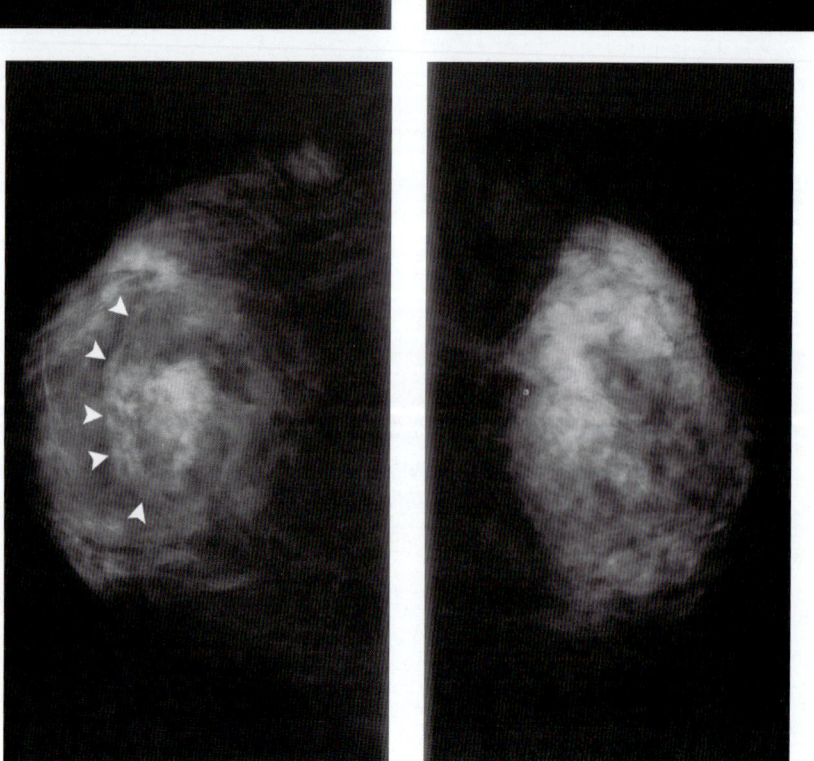

Fig. 27.3 Bilateral normal mammograms after reduction. Architectural distortion from reduction has resulted in asymmetry in both the anterior and posterior contours of the breasts. There are unusual indentations in the parenchymal outline (*arrows*). There are also linear and curvilinear parenchymal bands (*arrowheads*). (**A**) Right MLO mammogram. (**B**) Left MLO mammogram. (**C**) Right CC mammogram. (**D**) Left CC mammogram.

Pathology
- Changes from reduction mammoplasty

Management
- BI-RADS assessment category 2, benign finding

Pearls and Pitfalls
- Architectural distortion from reduction includes unusual straight linear or swirling curvilinear parenchymal lines, loss of the normal subareolar ductal pattern, retroareolar fibrotic band, asymmetric parenchymal contours, and asymmetric parenchymal density.

Suggested Reading
Miller CL, Feig SA, Fox JW IV. Mammographic changes after reduction mammoplasty. AJR Am J Roentgenol 1987;149:35–38

Case 27.3: Architectural Distortion

Case History
A 65-year-old woman presents with a palpable lump or thickening at the right 12 o'clock periareolar position. One year ago, she had reduction mammoplasty.

Physical Examination
- Right breast: ill-defined subareolar thickening at the 12 o'clock position
- Left breast: less prominent but similar subareolar thickening

Mammogram (Figs. 27.4 and 27.5)

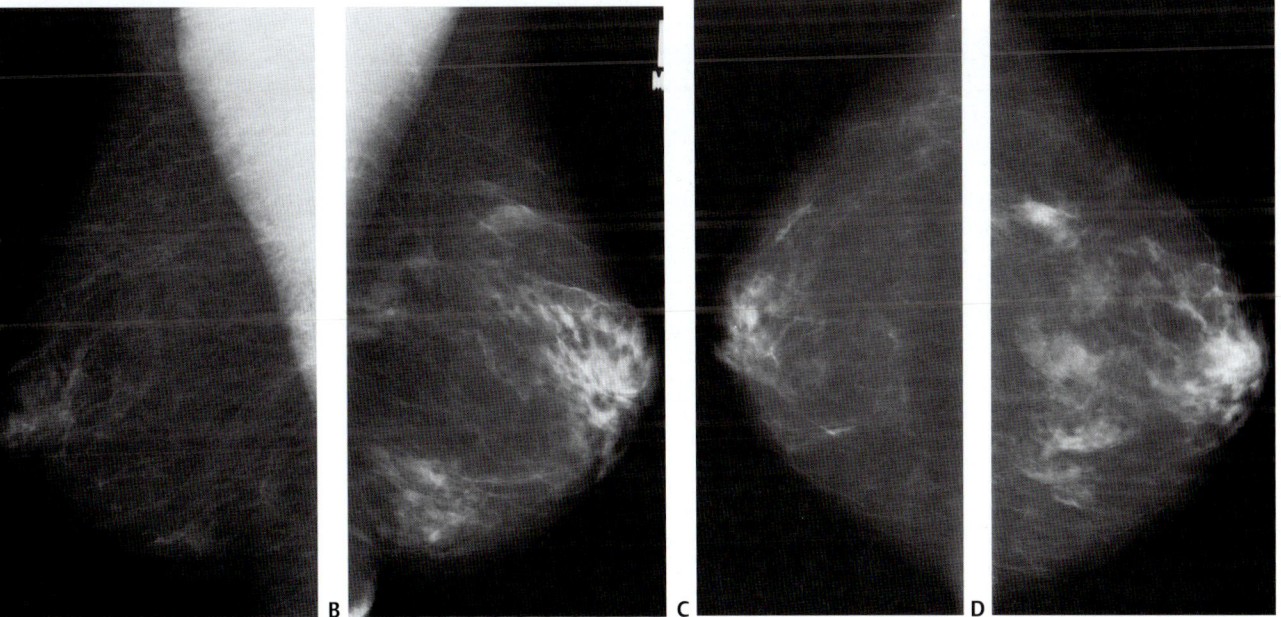

Fig. 27.4 The mammograms demonstrate changes due to previous reduction. The left breast exhibits asymmetric parenchymal densities, particularly in the inferior breast. This breast also demonstrates parenchymal swirls. Right breast does not exhibit any abnormal mass. (**A**) Right MLO mammogram. (**B**) Left MLO mammogram. (**C**) Right CC mammogram. (**D**) Left CC mammogram.

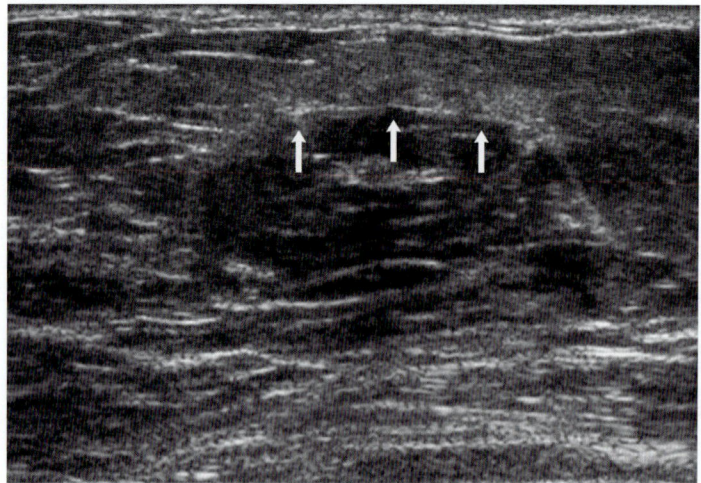 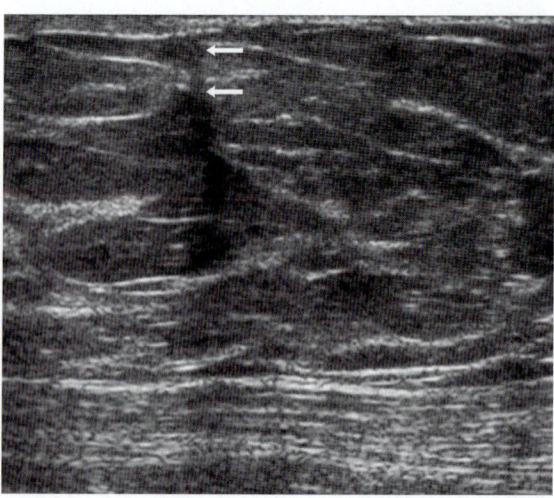

Fig. 27.5 Sonographic examination of the right breast demonstrates that the periareolar thickening corresponds to an irregular hyperechoic line. This line represents a scar (*arrows*), which is wider in the antiradial view (**A**) compared with the radial view (**B**). In the radial view, the scar (*arrows*) appears as a thin, straight line associated with shadowing. (**A**) Right antiradial breast sonogram. (**B**) Right radial breast sonogram.

Ultrasound (Fig. 27.5)

Pathology
- Scar

Management
- BI-RADS assessment category 2, benign finding

Pearls and Pitfalls
- After the acute postsurgical changes have resolved, the most common palpable masses that develop after breast reduction are scar, fat necrosis, and carcinoma. The mammographic and sonographic identification of palpable masses in these women is similar to that in women who have not had reduction. Sonographically, scars may be differentiated from carcinoma if there is no mass associated with the architectural distortion (as in this case).

Suggested Reading
Beer GM, Kompatscher P, Hergan K. Diagnosis of breast tumors after breast reduction. Aesthetic Plast Surg 1996;20:391–397

Case 27.4: Fat Necrosis

Case History

A 50-year-old woman presents for screening mammogram.

Physical Examination
- Bilateral breasts: bilateral reduction mammoplasty scars, otherwise normal

Mammogram (Figs. 27.6 and 27.7)

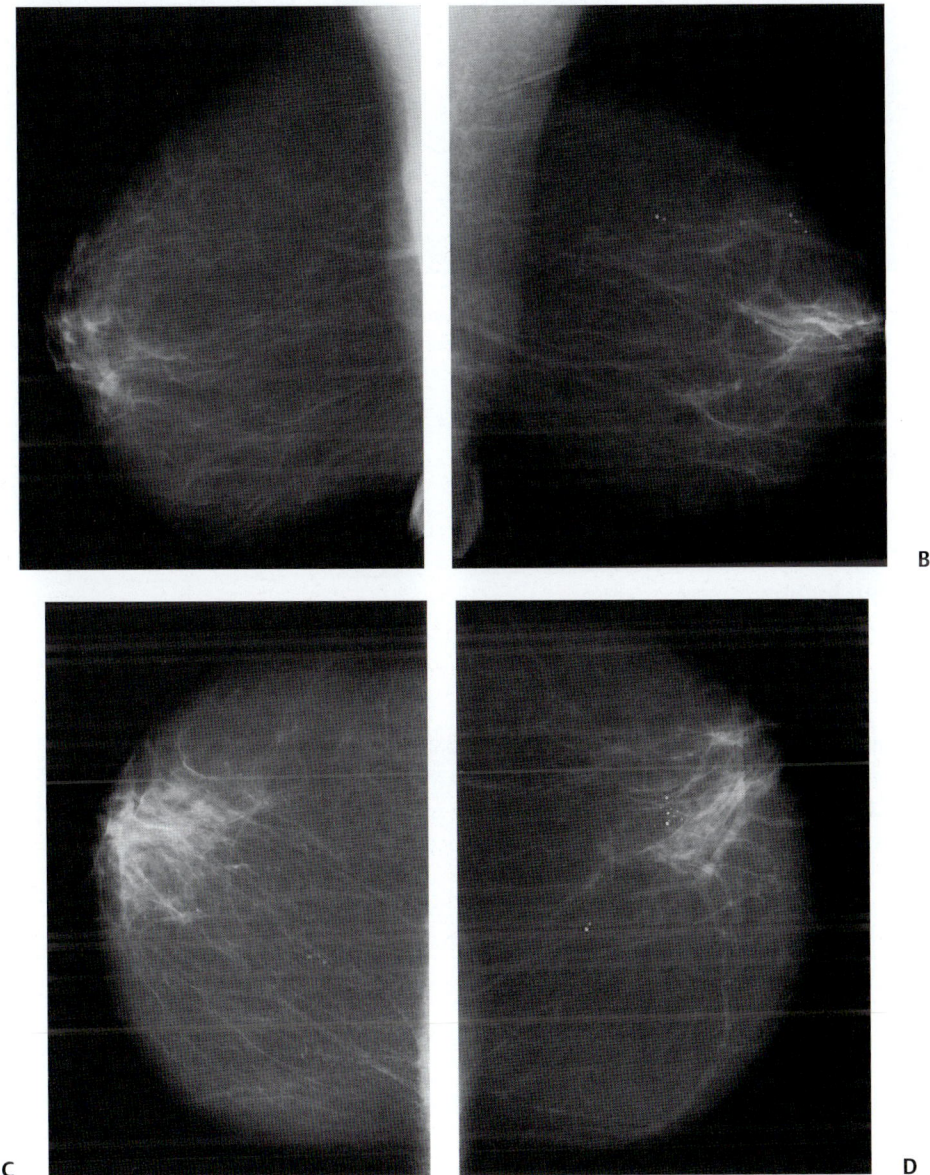

Fig. 27.6 These normal bilateral mammograms were performed prior to reduction mammoplasty. (**A**) Right MLO mammogram. (**B**) Left MLO mammogram. (**C**) Right CC mammogram. (**D**) Left CC mammogram.

Postsurgical Findings

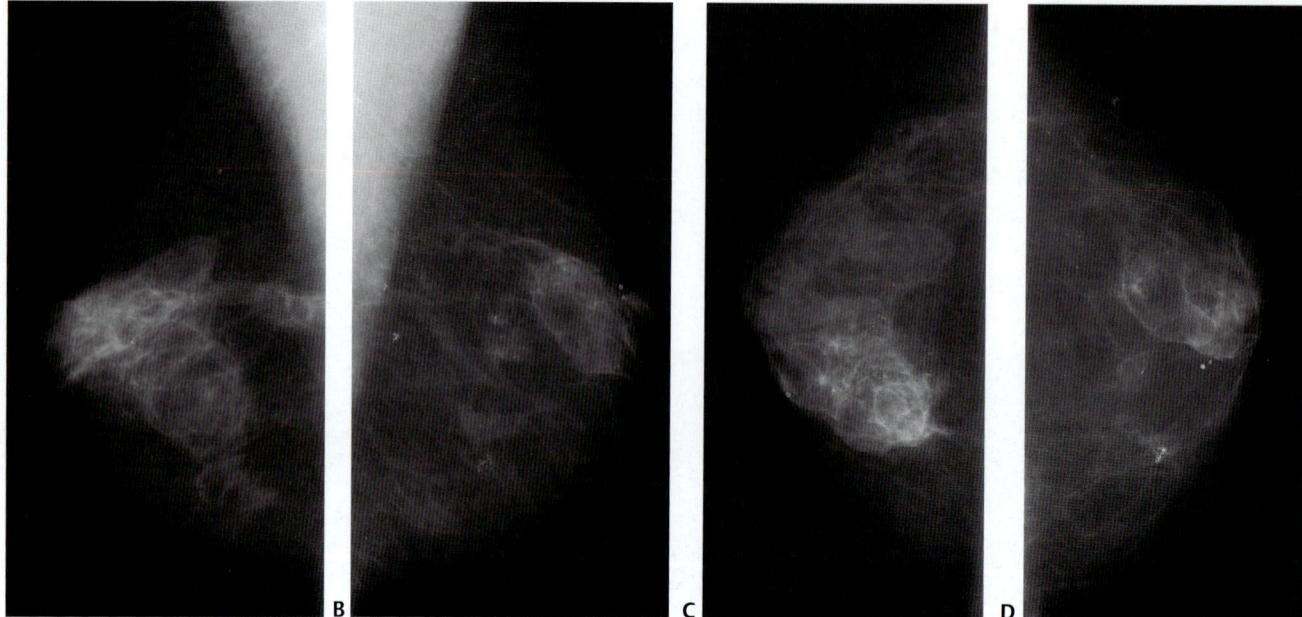

Fig. 27.7 Bilateral mammograms after reduction mammoplasty. Both breasts exhibit new dystrophic calcifications. There are also multiple rounded lucencies indicating fat necrosis. (**A**) Right MLO mammogram. (**B**) Left MLO mammogram. (**C**) Right CC mammogram. (**D**) Left CC mammogram.

Pathology
- Fat necrosis

Management
- BI-RADS assessment category 2, benign finding

Pearls and Pitfalls

- Benign calcifications are a common finding after breast reduction: 20 to 50% of patients develop new calcifications, and most of these calcifications develop 2 years after the patient's reduction mammoplasty. The most common benign calcifications either are characteristic of oil cysts or are large, coarse, and dystrophic in appearance. Less commonly, suture calcifications may appear. Calcifications are commonly located in the periareolar or inferior aspect of the breast.
- Fat necrosis is mammographically evident in approximately 10% of patients after breast reduction. Although fat necrosis is generally easily identifiable mammographically, occasionally fat necrosis will produce an irregular mass or heterogeneous calcifications that simulate malignancy.

Suggested Reading

Brown FE, Sargent SK, Cohen SR, Morain WD. Mammographic changes following reduction mammaplasty. Plast Reconstr Surg 1987;80:691–698

Miller JA, Festa S, Goldstein M. Benign fat necrosis simulating bilateral breast malignancy after reduction mammoplasty. South Med J 1998;91:765–767

Mitnick JS, Roses DF, Harris MN, Colen SR. Calcifications of the breast after reduction mammoplasty. Surg Gynecol Obstet 1990;171:409–412

Postsurgical Findings: After Diagnostic or Therapeutic Procedures for Neoplasm

This is a schematic diagram of the diagnostic approach to mammographic postsurgical findings: diagnostic or therapeutic procedures for neoplasm. For further discussion, see Chapter 1.

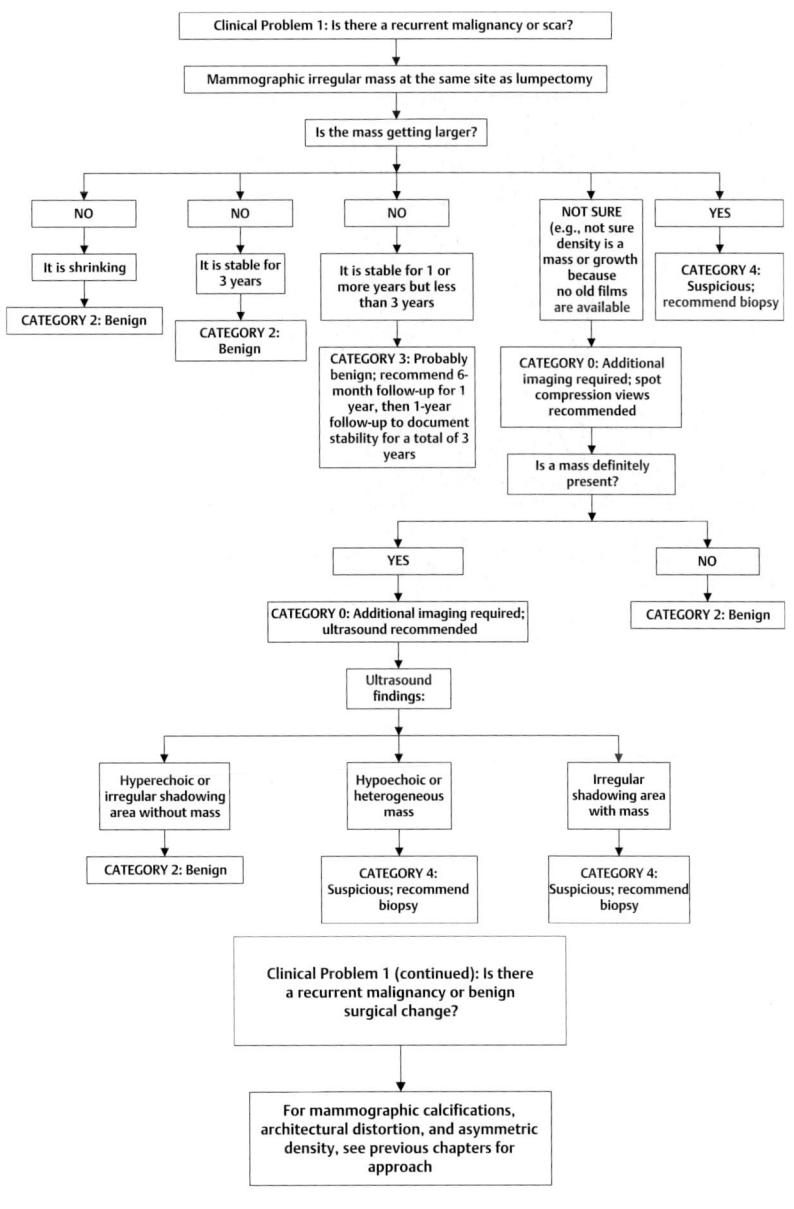

28 After Diagnostic or Therapeutic Procedures for Neoplasm

Case 28.1: Scar—Architectural Distortion

Case History

A 77-year-old woman presents for screening right breast mammogram. She had a left mastectomy for neoplasm and a benign right excisional biopsy several years ago.

Physical Examination
- Normal exam

Mammogram (Fig. 28.1)

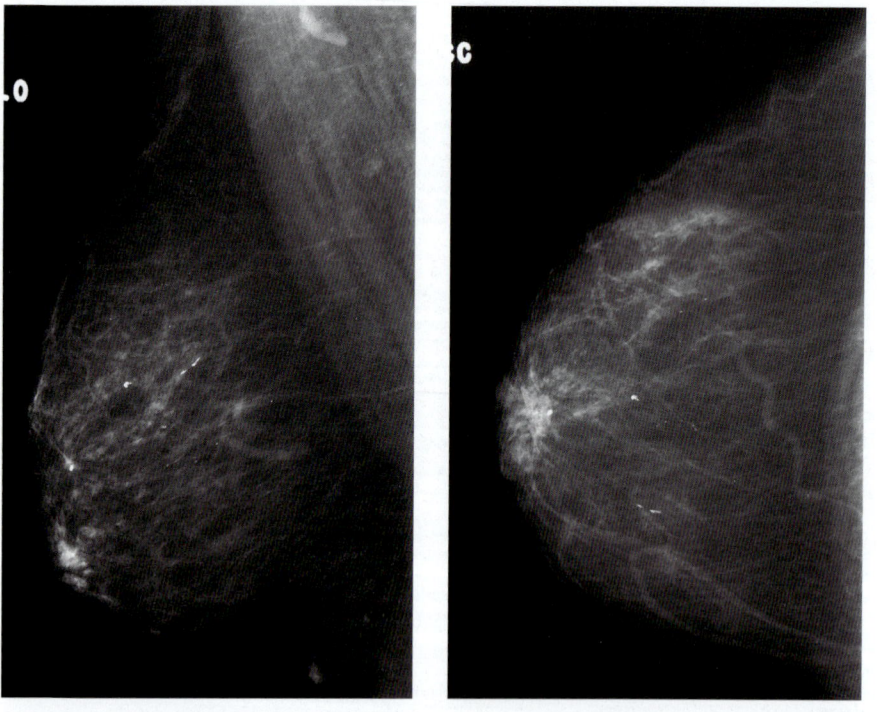

Fig. 28.1 In the right subareolar area, there are disruption and distortion of the ductal system. This architectural distortion resulted from the patient's benign excisional biopsy and has been stable for at least 10 years. (**A**) Right MLO mammogram. (**B**) Right CC mammogram.

Pathology
- Scar

Management
- BI-RADS assessment category 2, benign finding

Pearls and Pitfalls

- Mammographically, a scar presents as architectural distortion or irregular density. Patients treated for malignancy demonstrate scarring more often than those treated for benign lesions. One year after surgery, more than 90% of patients treated with lumpectomy and radiation therapy have mammographically detectable scars compared with less than 50% for those experiencing benign excisional biopsies. Five years after surgery, architectural distortion is mammographically evident in 70 and 20%, respectively.

Suggested Reading

Brenner RJ, Pfaff JM. Mammographic features after conservation therapy for malignant breast disease: serial findings standardized by regression analysis. AJR Am J Roentgenol 1996;167:171–178

Mendelson EB. Evaluation of the postoperative breast. Radiol Clin North Am 1992;30:107–138

Sickles EA, Herzog KA. Mammography of the postsurgical breast. AJR Am J Roentgenol 1981;136:585–588

Case 28.2: Scar—Architectural Distortion

Case History
A 66-year-old woman had left breast lumpectomy and radiation therapy 6 months ago.

Physical Examination
- Left breast: large scar; otherwise normal exam
- Right breast: normal exam

Mammogram

Mass (Fig. 28.2)
- Margin: spiculated
- Shape: irregular
- Density: high

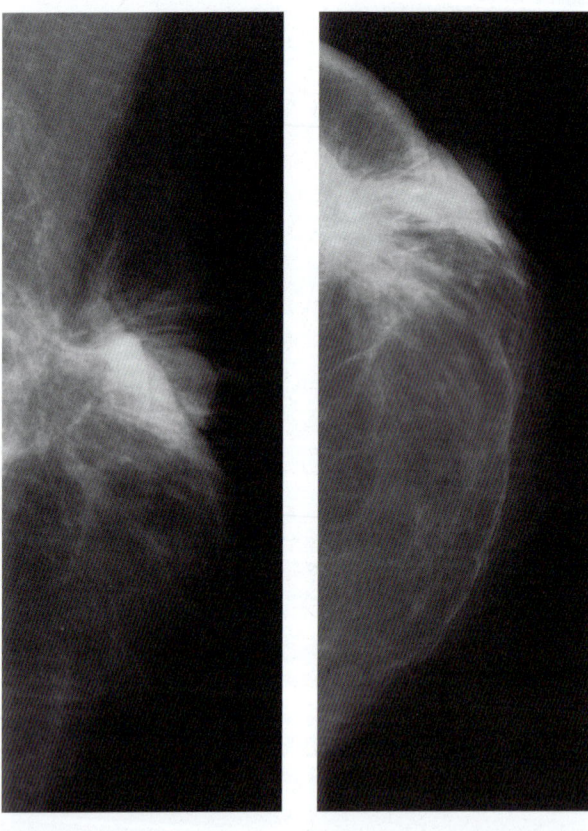

Fig. 28.2 In the site of a previous lumpectomy, there are irregular density, architectural distortion, spiculation, skin thickening, and retraction. (**A**) Left MLO mammogram. (**B**) Left CC mammogram.

Pathology
- Scar

Management
- BI-RADS assessment category 2, benign finding

Pearls and Pitfalls

- Within the first year, the density associated with breast excision is a combination of hematoma, fat necrosis, and scar. The combination of these abnormalities will produce either an ill-defined regional density or a focal irregular mass. When the postoperative lesion is a regional density, the density may decrease in size, but it tends to persist even after 5 years. However, when the postsurgical abnormality is a mass, it tends to completely resolve.

Suggested Reading

Brenner RJ, Pfaff JM. Mammographic features after conservation therapy for malignant breast disease: serial findings standardized by regression analysis. AJR Am J Roentgenol 1996;167:171–178

Case 28.3: Scar—Irregular Density

Case History
A 77-year-old woman had a right lumpectomy and radiation 2 years ago.

Physical Examination
- Right breast: lumpectomy scar; otherwise normal exam
- Left breast: normal exam

Mammogram

Mass (Figs. 28.3 and 28.4)
- Margin: spiculated
- Shape: irregular
- Density: equal density

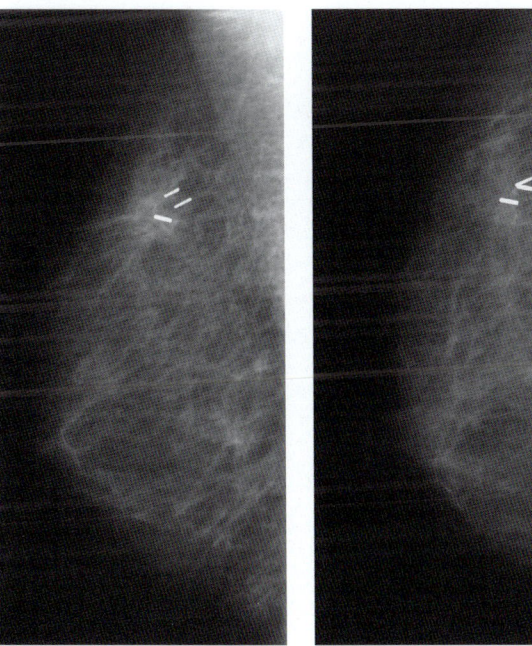

Fig. 28.3 These mammograms were performed 1 year after a lumpectomy and radiation therapy. There is an ill-defined density associated with the clips from the previous lumpectomy. (**A**) Right MLO mammogram. (**B**) Right exaggerated CC mammogram.

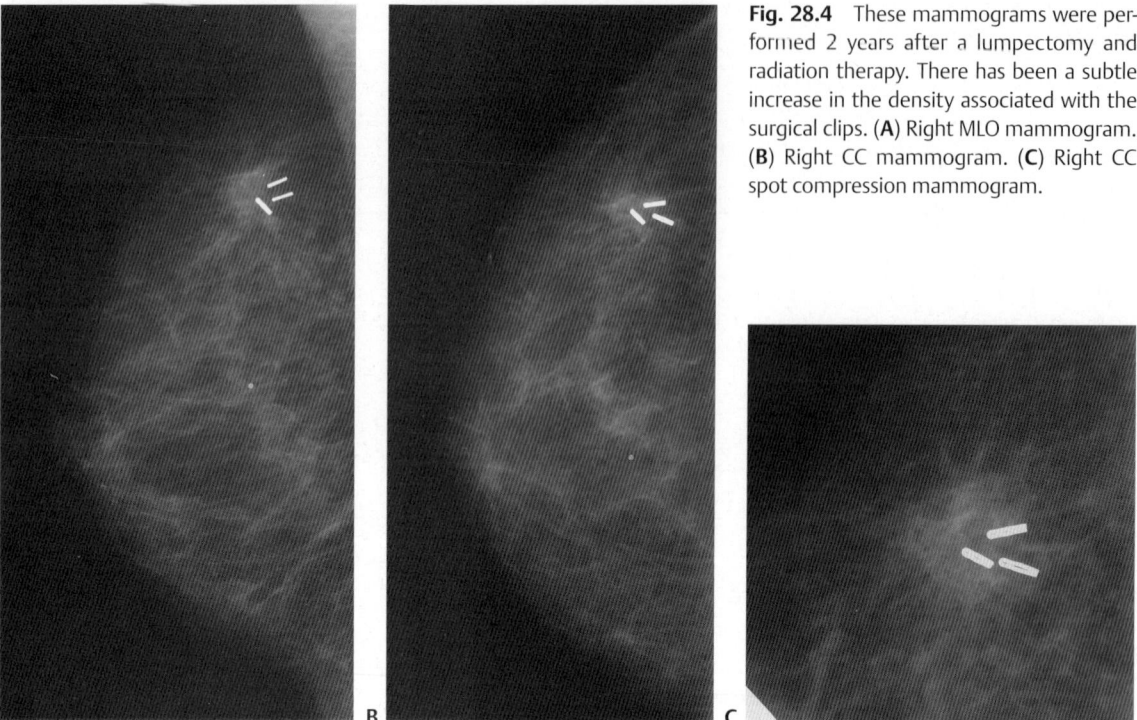

Fig. 28.4 These mammograms were performed 2 years after a lumpectomy and radiation therapy. There has been a subtle increase in the density associated with the surgical clips. (**A**) Right MLO mammogram. (**B**) Right CC mammogram. (**C**) Right CC spot compression mammogram.

Ultrasound

Low Frequency

Frequency
- 7 MHz

Mass (Fig. 28.5)
- Margin: spiculation/architectural distortion
- Echogenicity: hypoechoic
- Retrotumoral acoustic appearance: severe shadowing, mass completely obscured
- Shape: irregular

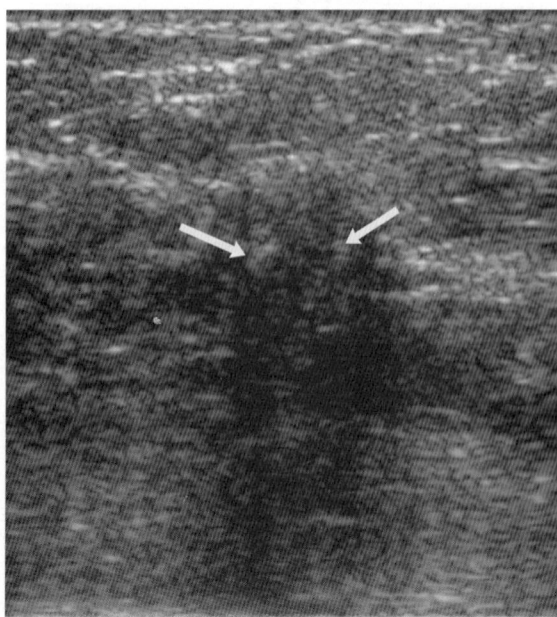

Fig. 28.5 Right breast radial sonogram. With lower frequency sonography, the lumpectomy site still exhibits an irregular, hypoechoic solid mass. Surgical clips (*arrows*).

High Frequency

Frequency
- 11.5 MHz (**Fig. 28.6**)

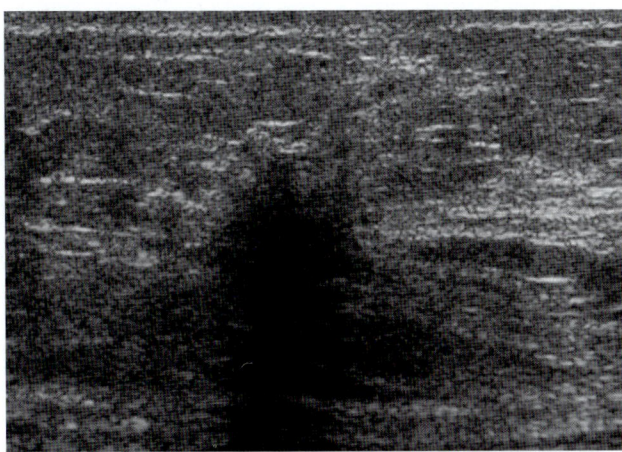

Fig. 28.6 Right breast radial sonogram. With high-frequency sonography, the lumpectomy site is an irregular hypoechoic, heavily shadowing mass.

Pathology
- Scar

Management
- BI-RADS assessment category 4, suspicious; biopsy should be considered.

> **Pearls and Pitfalls**
> - Usually, scars remain unchanged or diminish in mammographic density and size. However, if the mammographic density of an excisional site increases and the site exhibits a sonographic mass, then biopsy is indicated.
> - Sonographically, scars commonly cause severe posterior acoustic shadowing. If this shadowing is present when using a high frequency, switch to low frequency. A benign scar produces a hyperechoic irregularity without a mass. However, this case illustrates that some scars appear identical to malignancies.

Suggested Reading
Mendelson EB. Imaging the post-surgical breast. Semin Ultrasound CT MR 1989;10:154–170

Case 28.4: Scar—Sonographic Technique

Case History
A 61-year-old woman has had 6 months of left breast pain. She had a benign left breast biopsy 20 years ago.

Physical Examination
- Left breast: scar in left upper outer quadrant; also extremely tender to palpation in the upper outer quadrant
- Right breast: diffusely mildly tender, otherwise normal exam

Mammogram (Fig. 28.7)

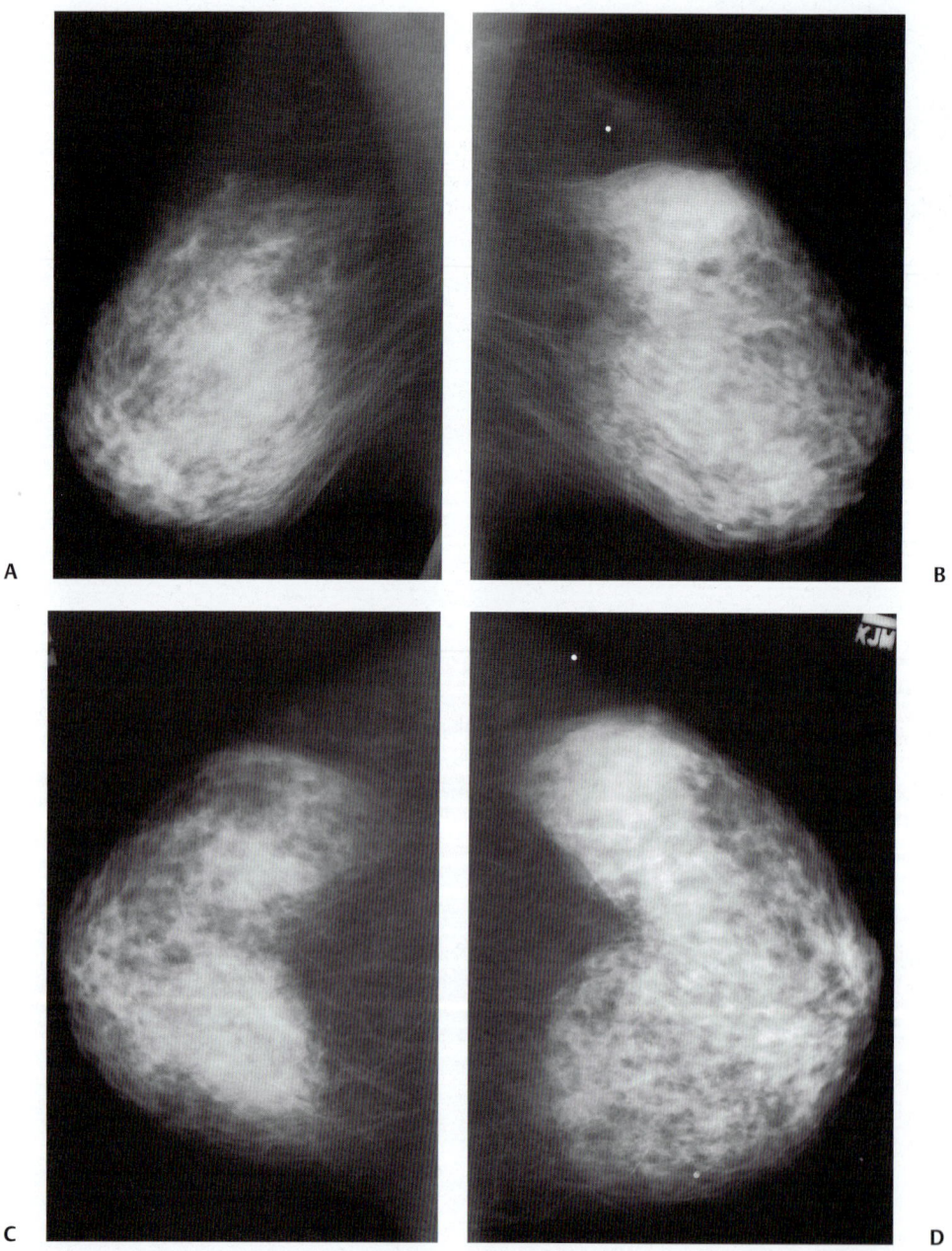

Fig. 28.7 Bilateral normal mammograms. (**A**) Right MLO mammogram. (**B**) Left MLO mammogram. (**C**) Right CC mammogram. (**D**) Left CC mammogram.

Ultrasound

Low Frequency

Frequency
- 10 MHz (**Fig. 28.8**)

Fig. 28.8 With lower frequency in the radial view (**A**), the scar appears to be a hypoechoic area, but the antiradial view (**B**) demonstrates that the lesion corresponds to a thin line of architectural distortion associated with shadowing (*arrows*). (**A**) Left radial breast sonogram. (**B**) Left antiradial breast sonogram.

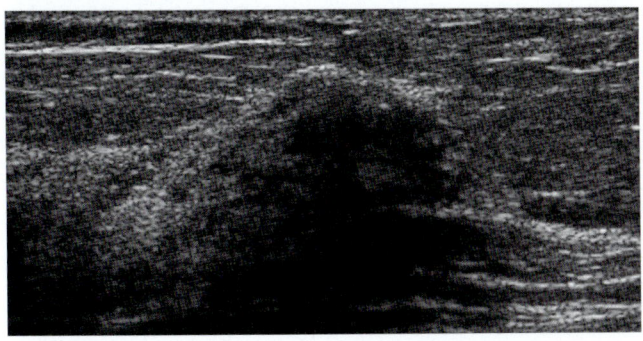

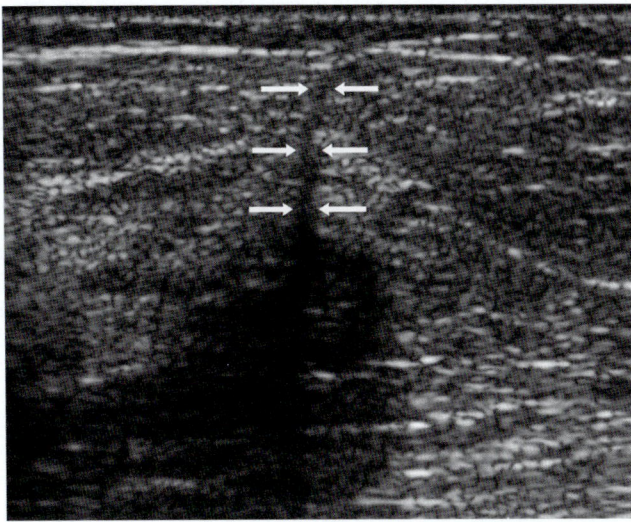

High Frequency

Frequency
- 13 MHz (**Fig. 28.9**)

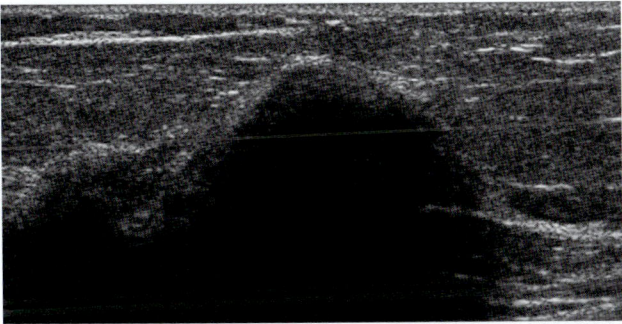

Fig. 28.9 Left radial breast sonogram. The patient's scar was in the middle of the area of tenderness. With high frequency, the scar creates severe shadowing, so the benign nature of this lesion is not visible.

Pathology
- Scar

Management
- BI-RADS assessment category 2, benign finding

Pearls and Pitfalls

- In an area of surgical excision, a scar can be mammographically differentiated from a neoplasm in the following ways: (1) identify lucencies within the center of the scar, (2) observe that the scar changes in appearance with different views, and (3) note decreases in size or density of the lesion on sequential exams.
- Sonographically, scars have the following characteristics: (1) scars are hyperechoic, (2) they exhibit different appearances with different angles, and (3) benign scars have no associated hypoechoic mass (which is visible on two views). Because scars strongly attenuate sound, lower-frequency sonography is generally better than higher-frequency sonography in characterizing scars.

Suggested Reading

Mendelson EB. Evaluation of the postoperative breast. Radiol Clin North Am 1992;30:107–138

Case 28.5: Hematoma

Case History

A 63-year-old woman presents 3 months after right lumpectomy for breast cancer. She now has a lump in her surgical site.

Physical Examination

- Right breast: tender, palpable lump in the lumpectomy site
- Left breast: normal exam

Mammogram

Mass (Figs. 28.10 and 28.11)
- Margin: circumscribed
- Shape: oval
- Density: equal density

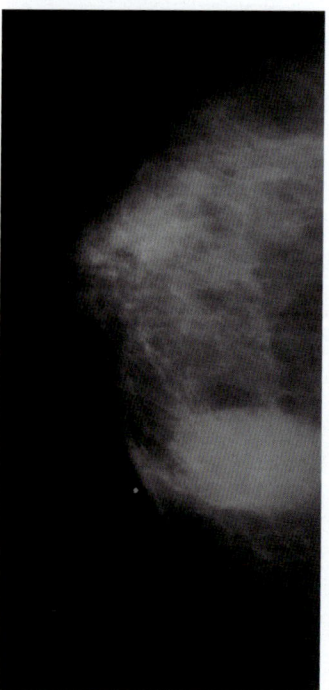
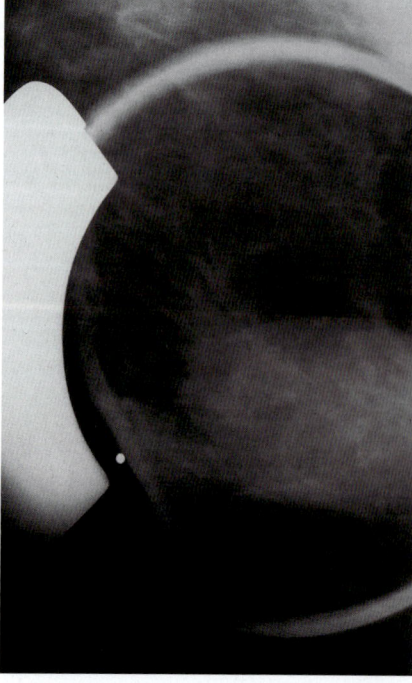

Fig. 28.10 Three months after the patient's right lumpectomy, there is an ill-defined oval mass associated with the lumpectomy site. The palpable lump corresponds to this mass. (**A**) Right CC mammogram. (**B**) Right CC spot compression mammogram.

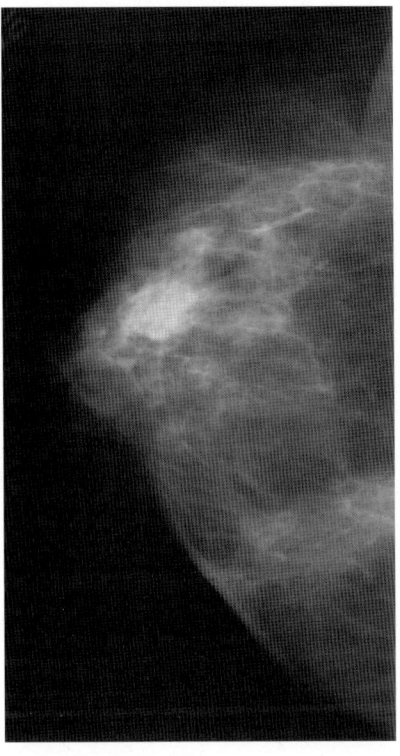

Fig. 28.11 Right CC mammogram. Ten months after the patient's surgery, the oval mass has decreased in size and density.

Ultrasound

Frequency
- 7 MHz

Mass (Figs. 28.12 and 28.13)
- Margin: well defined
- Echogenicity: heterogeneous (mixed)
- Retrotumoral acoustic appearance: increased acoustic transmission
- Shape: ellipsoid

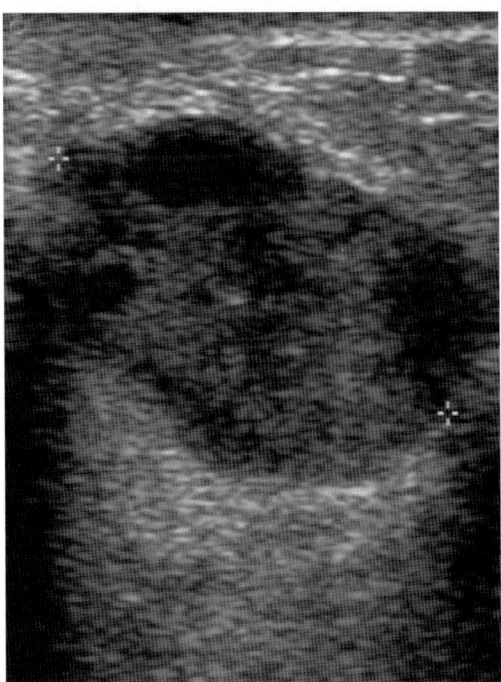

Fig. 28.12 Right transverse breast sonogram. Three months after surgery, the palpable lump is a sonographically complex, well-defined fluid collection with heterogeneous echogenicity and increased acoustic transmission.

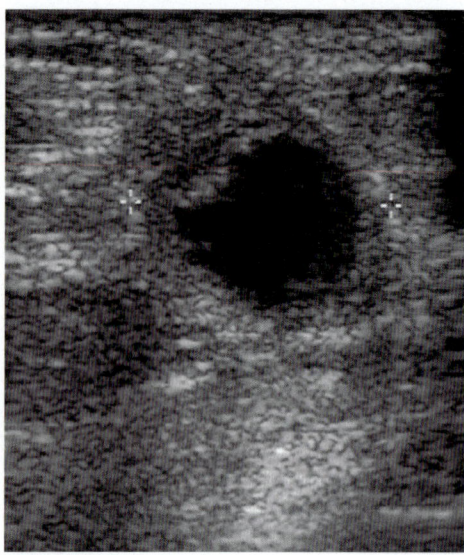

Fig. 28.13 Right transverse breast sonogram. Sonographic examination 10 months after surgery demonstrates that the fluid collection has greatly decreased in size. The fluid is anechoic and surrounded by thick walls. Anterior to the fluid, there is architectural distortion with skin thickening.

Pathology
- Hematoma

Management
- BI-RADS assessment category 2, benign finding

Pearls and Pitfalls

- Hematomas or seromas have been observed in 50% of patients 1 month after surgery. These lesions tend to resolve, so only 25% of patients exhibit fluid collections 6 months after excision. However, rarely patients will have persistent seromas years later.
- Mammographically, the hematoma/seroma typically appears as an oval mass of water density. Sometimes, the mass may demonstrate fat-fluid layering on 90-degree lateral views. The margins may be well defined, ill defined, or spiculated.
- Sonographically, the hematoma/seroma is a hypoechoic, anechoic, or heterogeneous fluid collection. Internal septations and dependent solid material may be present.

Suggested Reading
Soo MS, Williford ME. Seromas in the breast: imaging findings. Crit Rev Diagn Imaging 1995;36:385–440

Case 28.6: Fat Necrosis

Case History
A 59-year-old woman had excision of ductal carcinoma in situ (DCIS) and radiation therapy 4 months ago. She now notes a ridge next to her lumpectomy site.

Physical Examination
- Left breast: vague ridge of tissue in the axilla near healing scar
- Right breast: normal exam

Mammogram
- Asymmetric density (**Fig. 28.14**)

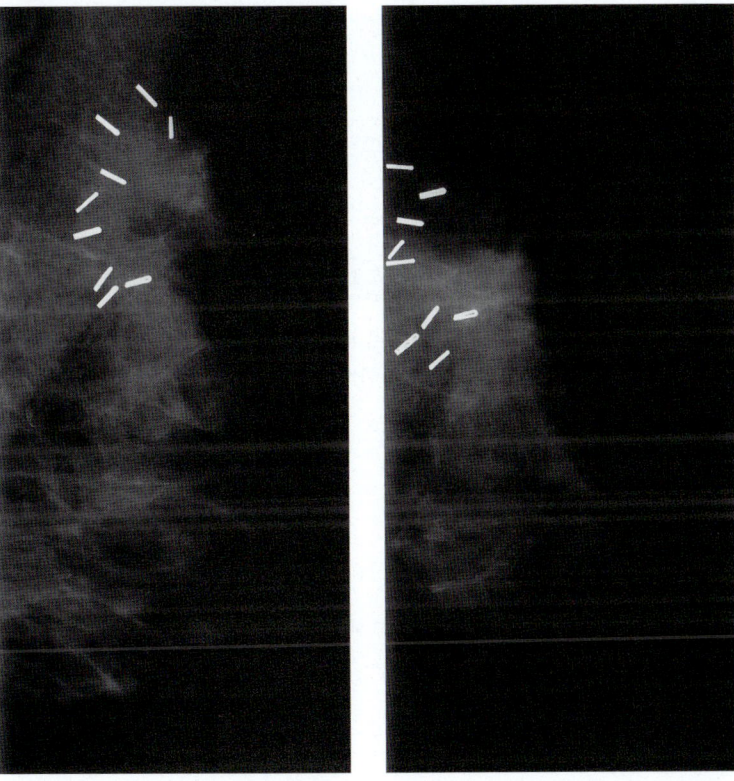

Fig. 28.14 In the left upper outer breast, there are clips and ill-defined density in the lumpectomy site. (**A**) Left MLO mammogram. (**B**) Left exaggerated CC mammogram.

Postsurgical Findings

Ultrasound

Frequency
- 14 MHz

Mass (Figs. 28.15 and 28.16)
- Margin: ill defined
- Echogenicity: hypoechoic
- Retrotumoral acoustic appearance: single edge shadowing
- Shape: irregular

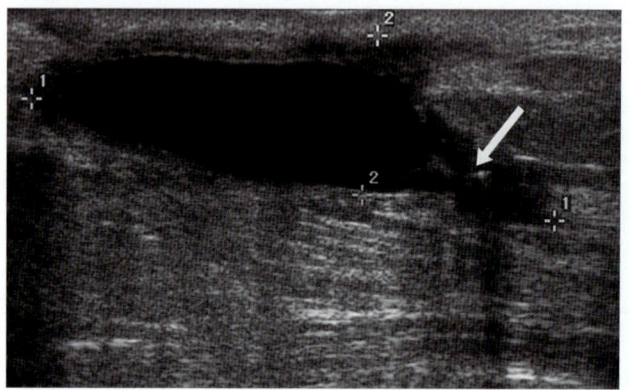

Fig. 28.15 Left radial breast sonogram. Within the lumpectomy site, there is a well-defined anechoic fluid collection that is characteristic of a hematoma or seroma. Anteriorly, there are architectural distortion and skin thickening. At the edge of the fluid is a hyperechoic, shadowing focus (*arrow*), which is one of the clips.

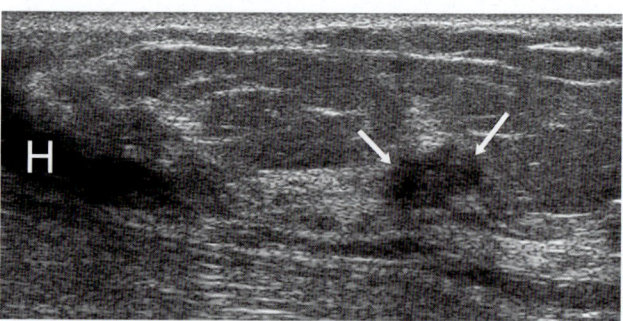

Fig. 28.16 Left radial breast sonogram. Next to the hematoma (H), there is a small irregular, hypoechoic mass (*arrows*).

Pathology
- Fat necrosis

Management
- BI-RADS assessment category 4, suspicious; biopsy should be considered.

Pearls and Pitfalls

- When surgical trauma ruptures adipocytes, the released fat may incite a fibrotic response, which produces an ill-defined, irregular mass. This type of fat necrosis cannot be differentiated mammographically or sonographically from neoplasm.

Suggested Reading

Bassett LW, Gold RH, Cove HC. Mammographic spectrum of traumatic fat necrosis: the fallibility of "pathognomonic" signs of carcinoma. AJR Am J Roentgenol 1978;130:119–122

Tohno D, Cosgrove DO, Sloane JP, eds. Ultrasound Diagnosis of Breast Diseases. New York: Churchill Livingstone; 1994:140–143

Case 28.7: Fat Necrosis

Case History
A 52-year-old woman presents for diagnostic postoperative mammogram. She had lumpectomy and radiation therapy 2 years prior for primary breast lymphoma. She currently has no symptoms.

Physical Examination
- Left breast: well-healed scar; otherwise normal
- Right breast: normal exam

Mammogram

Mass (Figs. 28.17 and 28.18)
- Margin: circumscribed
- Shape: oval
- Density: fat-containing

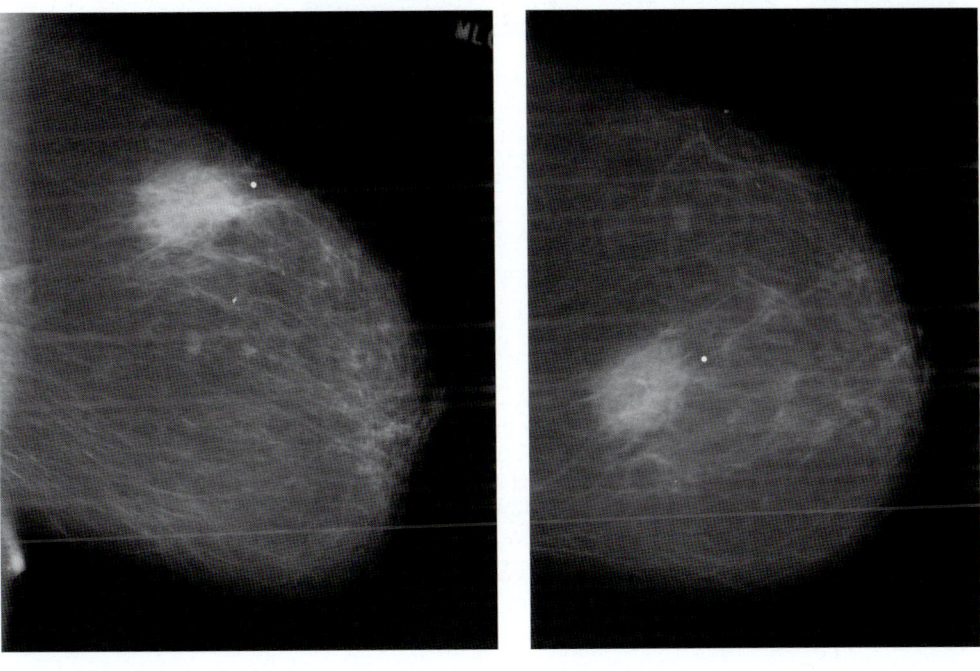

Fig. 28.17 This mammogram was performed 6 months after the lumpectomy. Ill-defined increased density, multiple lucencies, and skin retraction are within the area of the excision. (**A**) Left MLO mammogram. (**B**) Left CC mammogram.

472   Postsurgical Findings

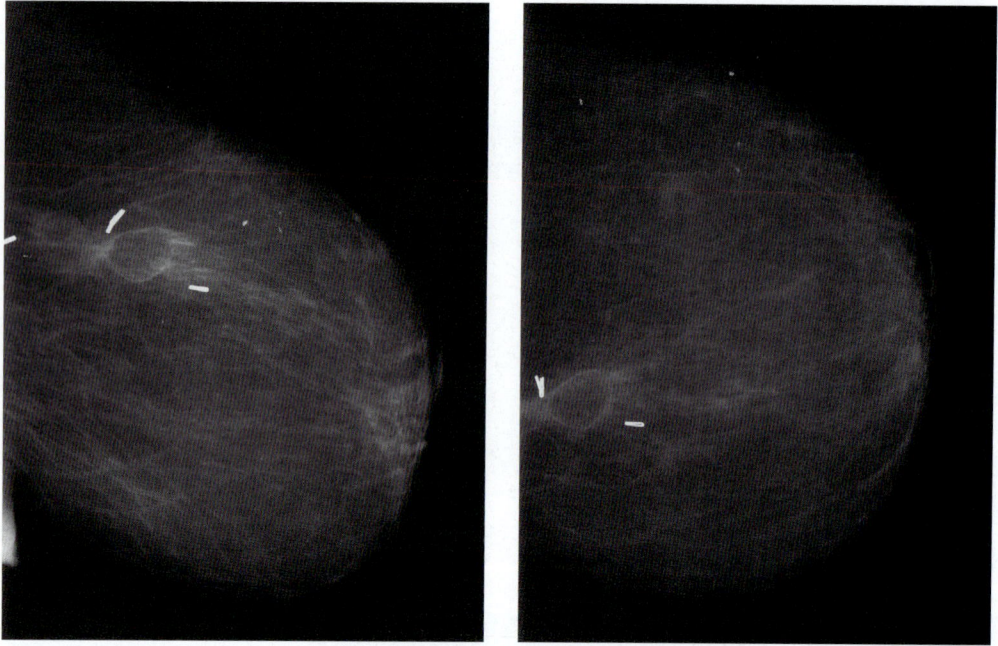

Fig. 28.18 This study was done 2 years after the lumpectomy. In the area of the excision, the density has decreased, and an oil cyst has formed. (**A**) Left MLO mammogram. (**B**) Left CC mammogram.

Pathology
- Fat necrosis

Management
- BI-RADS assessment category 2, benign finding

> **Pearls and Pitfalls**
>
> - When fat necrosis results, a release of lipid occurs, which does not cause a fibrotic reaction. The material forms an oil cyst. The mammographic appearance of this round or oval, circumscribed, fat density mass is characteristic of this lesion.

Suggested Reading
Morgan CL, Trought WS, Peete W. Xeromammographic and ultrasonic diagnosis of a traumatic oil cyst. AJR Am J Roentgenol 1978;130:1189–1190

Case 28.8: Pseudoaneurysm

Case History
A 45-year-old woman presents for preoperative evaluation for sentinel node biopsy. Her left breast tumor was biopsied with sonographic guidance 3 weeks ago.

Physical Examination
- Left breast: healed biopsy incision in upper outer quadrant; otherwise normal exam
- Right breast: normal exam

Mammogram (Fig. 28.19)

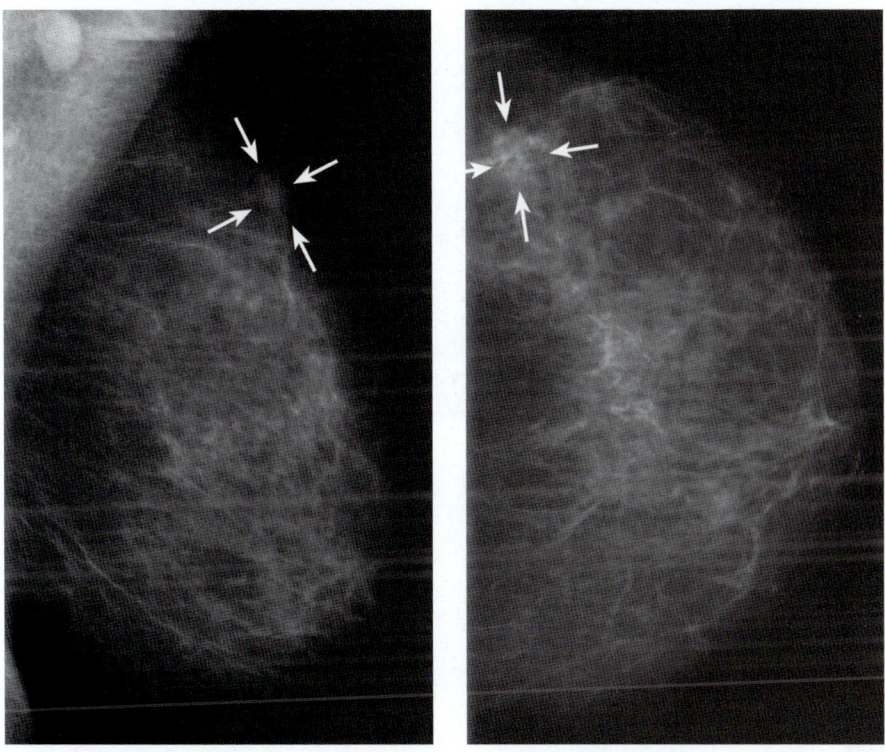

Fig. 28.19 In the upper outer quadrant, there is an ill-defined mass (*arrows*). After this mammogram was performed, the mass was biopsied and found to be infiltrating ductal carcinoma. (**A**) Left MLO mammogram. (**B**) Left CC mammogram.

474 Postsurgical Findings

Ultrasound

Frequency
- 10 MHz

Mass (Fig. 28.20)
- Margin: well defined
- Echogenicity: heterogeneous
- Retrotumoral acoustic appearance: increased acoustic enhancement
- Shape: ellipsoid

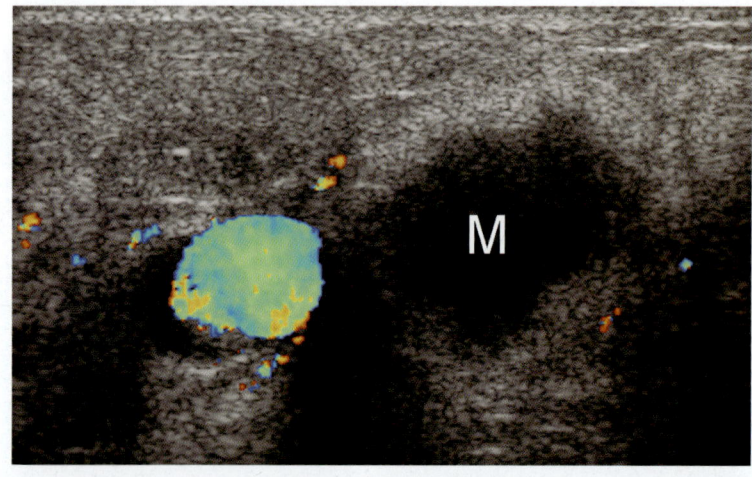
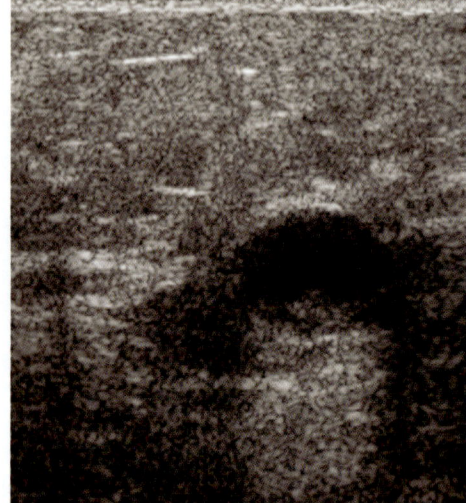
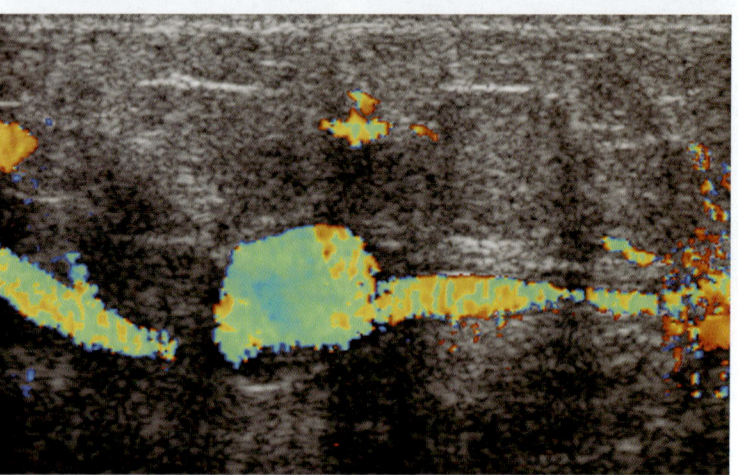

Fig. 28.20 In the left upper outer quadrant, there was an ill-defined hypoechoic mass (M) that corresponded to the tumor (**B**). Adjacent to the tumor was an oval fluid collection, which was predominantly anechoic except for its hypoechoic inferior rim (**A**). Color Doppler demonstrates that the hypoechoic lesion is filled with high-velocity swirling blood flow characteristic of a pseudoaneurysm. (**A**) Left antiradial breast sonogram. Pseudoaneurysm without color Doppler. (**B**) Left antiradial color Doppler breast sonogram. Pseudoaneurysm next to mass (M). (**C**) Left antiradial color Doppler breast sonogram. Pseudoaneurysm with feeding and draining vessels.

Pathology
- Pseudoaneurysm

Management
- BI-RADS assessment category 2, benign finding

Pearls and Pitfalls

- As a result of core needle biopsies, breast imagers have reported breast pseudoaneurysms. Researchers have described treatments including manual compression and placement of coils. Because this pseudoaneurysm was adjacent to a malignancy, it was removed with the tumor.

Suggested Reading

Beres RA, Harrington DG, Wenzel MS. Percutaneous repair of breast pseudoaneurysm: sonographically guided embolization. AJR Am J Roentgenol 1997;169:425–427

Smith SM. Breast pseudoaneurysm after core biopsy. AJR Am J Roentgenol 1996;167:817

Case 28.9: Lymphedema

Case History

A 74-year-old woman with left breast swelling. She had lumpectomy and axillary dissection 3 years ago. She had no symptoms until after she had coronary artery revascularization 3 months ago. During that procedure, her left internal mammary artery was harvested.

Physical Examination

- Left breast: healed upper outer scar; entire breast is rock hard with diffuse skin thickening; no warmth or erythema; no arm edema
- Right breast: normal exam

Mammogram (Fig. 28.21)

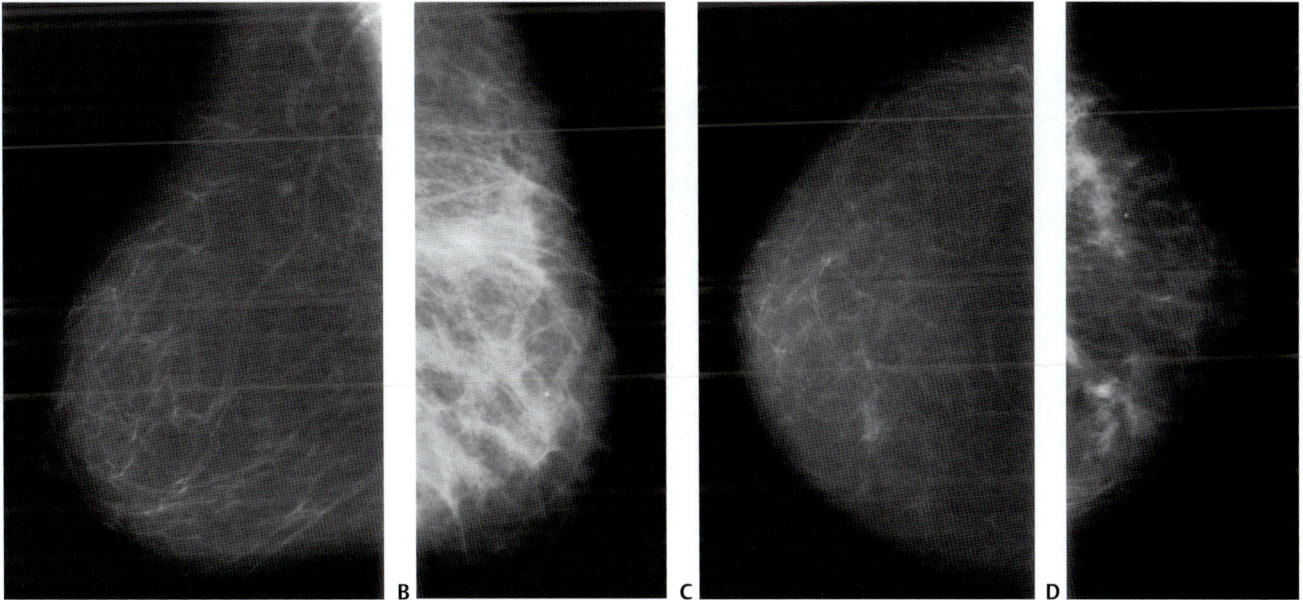

Fig. 28.21 The right breast is normal. The left breast is small and exhibits diffuse increased density. Lumpectomy site is in upper outer quadrant and is only partially evident on the left MLO view. (**A**) Right MLO mammogram. (**B**) Left MLO mammogram. (**C**) Right CC mammogram. (**D**) Left CC mammogram.

Ultrasound

Low Frequency

Frequency
- 8 MHz (**Fig. 28.22**)

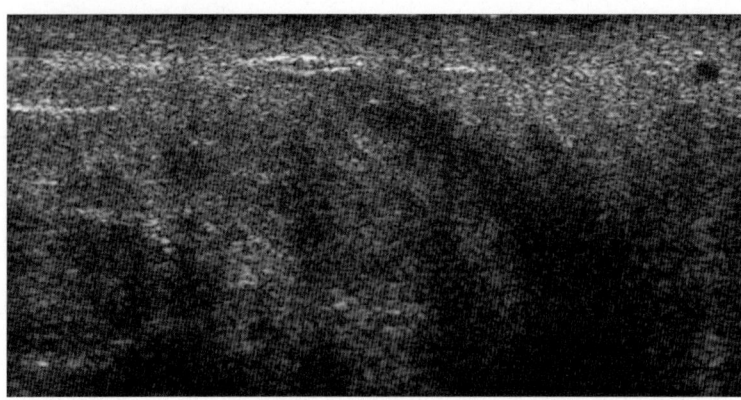

Fig. 28.22 Left radial breast sonogram. There is diffuse thickening of the parenchymal tissues with loss of normal architecture. The edematous tissue produces indistinct, random shadowing.

High Frequency

Frequency
- 13 MHz (**Fig. 28.23**)

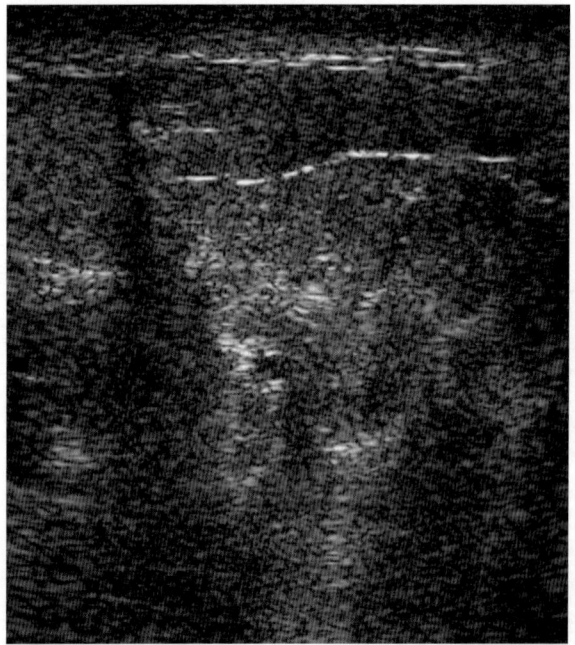

Fig. 28.23 Left radial breast sonogram. Sonographic examination of the breast demonstrates irregular skin thickening. There is also intermittent loss of the border between the skin and the hyperechoic subcutaneous fat.

Pathology
- Lymphedema

Management
- BI-RADS assessment category 3, probably benign; short-interval follow-up

Pearls and Pitfalls

- Lymphedema is due to lymphatic obstruction (see Chapters 20 and 21). In this case, the patient's axillary lymphatic drainage had been damaged after the axillary dissection, and the internal mammary drainage was compromised by a combination of the median sternotomy and trauma from dissecting the internal mammary artery.

Suggested Reading
Tabar L, Dean PB. Teaching Atlas of Mammography. 3rd ed. New York: Thieme; 2001:239–246

Case 28.10: Radiation Changes

Case History
A 47-year-old woman presents for first postlumpectomy mammogram 6 months after the procedure.

Physical Examination
- Right breast: healing excision site
- Left breast: normal exam

Mammogram

Mass (Figs. 28.24 and 28.25)
- Margin: spiculated

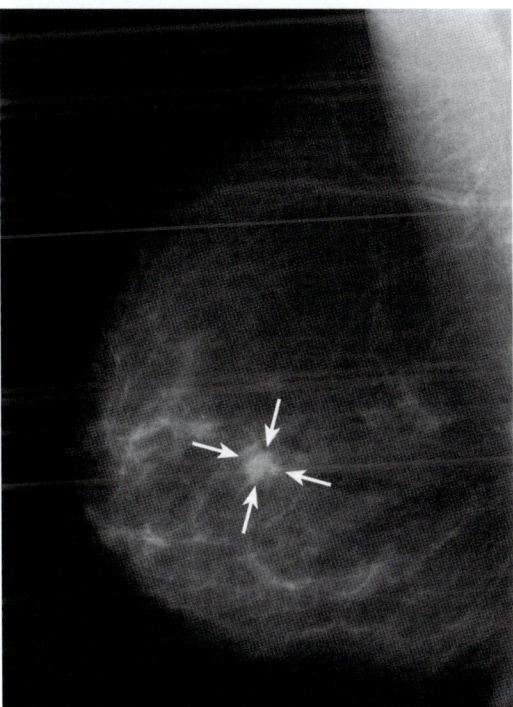
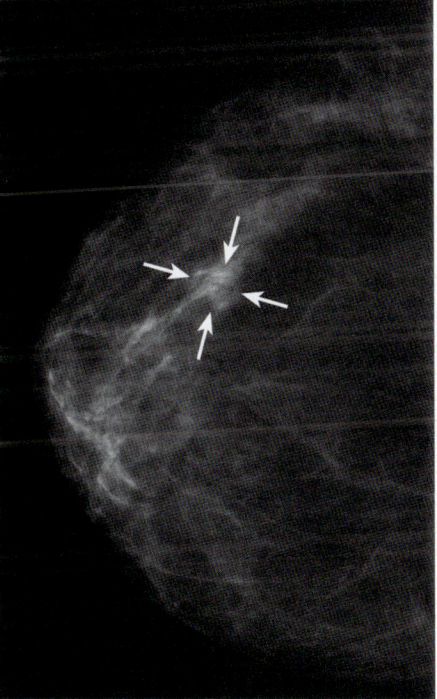

Fig. 28.24 This is the patient's screening mammogram prior to surgery. An ill-defined mass is present in the right outer breast (*arrows*). (**A**) Right MLO mammogram. (**B**) Right CC mammogram.

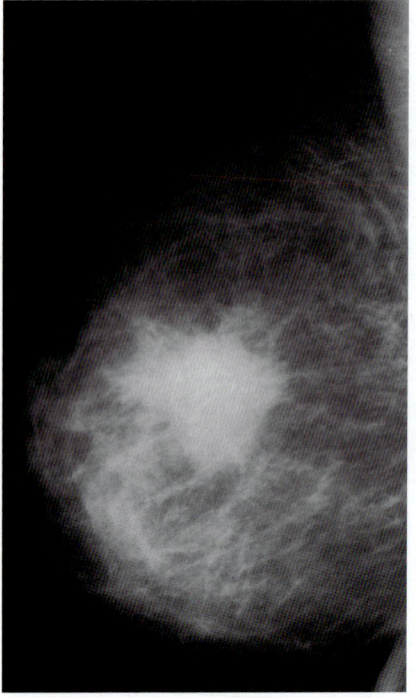 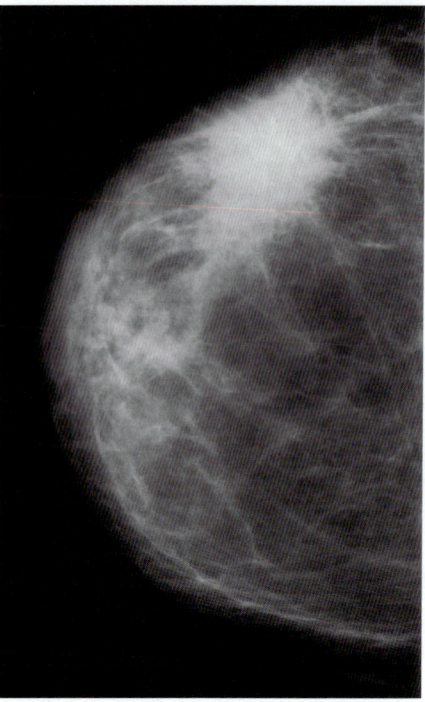

Fig. 28.25 This study was performed 6 months after lumpectomy and radiation therapy. The right breast exhibits diffuse increased density. A large spiculated mass is present in the lumpectomy site. (**A**) Right MLO mammogram. (**B**) Right CC mammogram.

Pathology
- Scar, lymphedema, seroma

Management
- BI-RADS assessment category 2, benign finding

Pearls and Pitfalls

- Skin thickening and tissue edema are mammographically evident in 50 to 95% of patients 1 year after lumpectomy and radiation therapy. These abnormalities gradually diminish and stabilize between 2 and 3 years after treatment. After 5 years, 40 to 50% of patients still demonstrate either thickened skin or increased glandular density.

Suggested Reading

Brenner RJ, Pfaff JM. Mammographic features after conservation therapy for malignant breast disease: serial findings standardized by regression analysis. AJR Am J Roentgenol 1996;167:171–178

Dershaw DD, Shank B, Reisinger S. Mammographic findings after breast cancer treatment with local excision and definitive irradiation. Radiology 1987;164:455–461

Destouet JM. Mammography of the altered breast. Curr Opin Radiol 1990;2:734–740

Case 28.11: Recurrent Neoplasm

Case History
A 57-year-old woman presents with left nipple inversion. She had a left lumpectomy for infiltrating ductal carcinoma 3 years ago. She refused postoperative radiation and chemotherapy.

Physical Examination
- Left breast: healed incision in upper outer quadrant, no masses, inverted nipple, mild periareolar erythema, and peau d'orange.
- Right breast: normal exam

Mammogram

Mass (Figs. 28.26, 28.27, and 28.28)
- Margin: spiculated

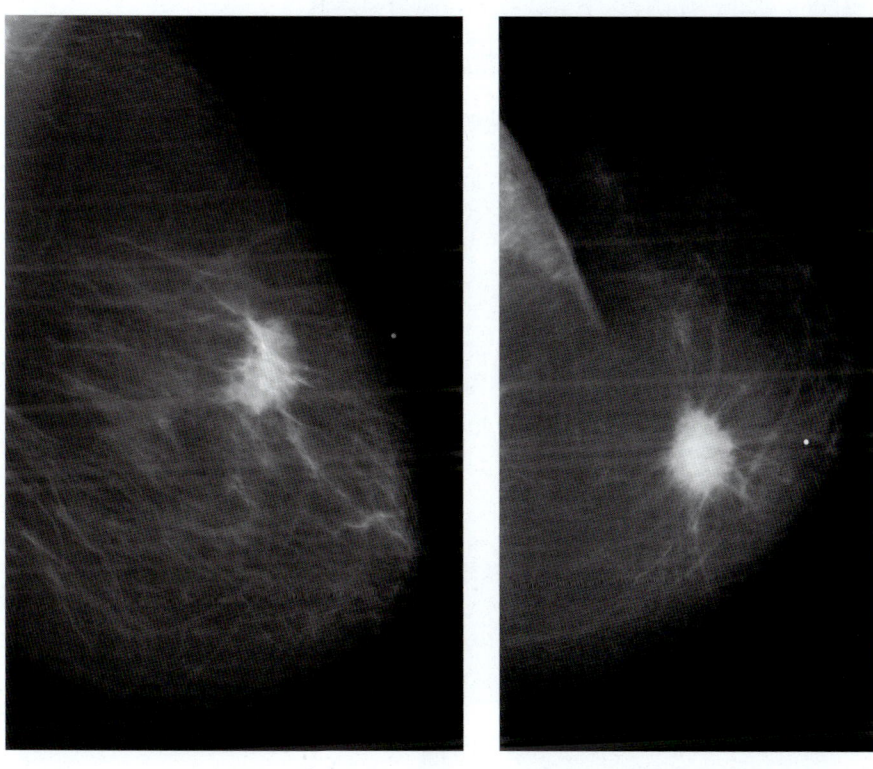

Fig. 28.26 Screening mammogram prior to lumpectomy demonstrated a dense spiculated mass in the upper inner left breast. (**A**) Left MLO mammogram. (**B**) Left CC mammogram.

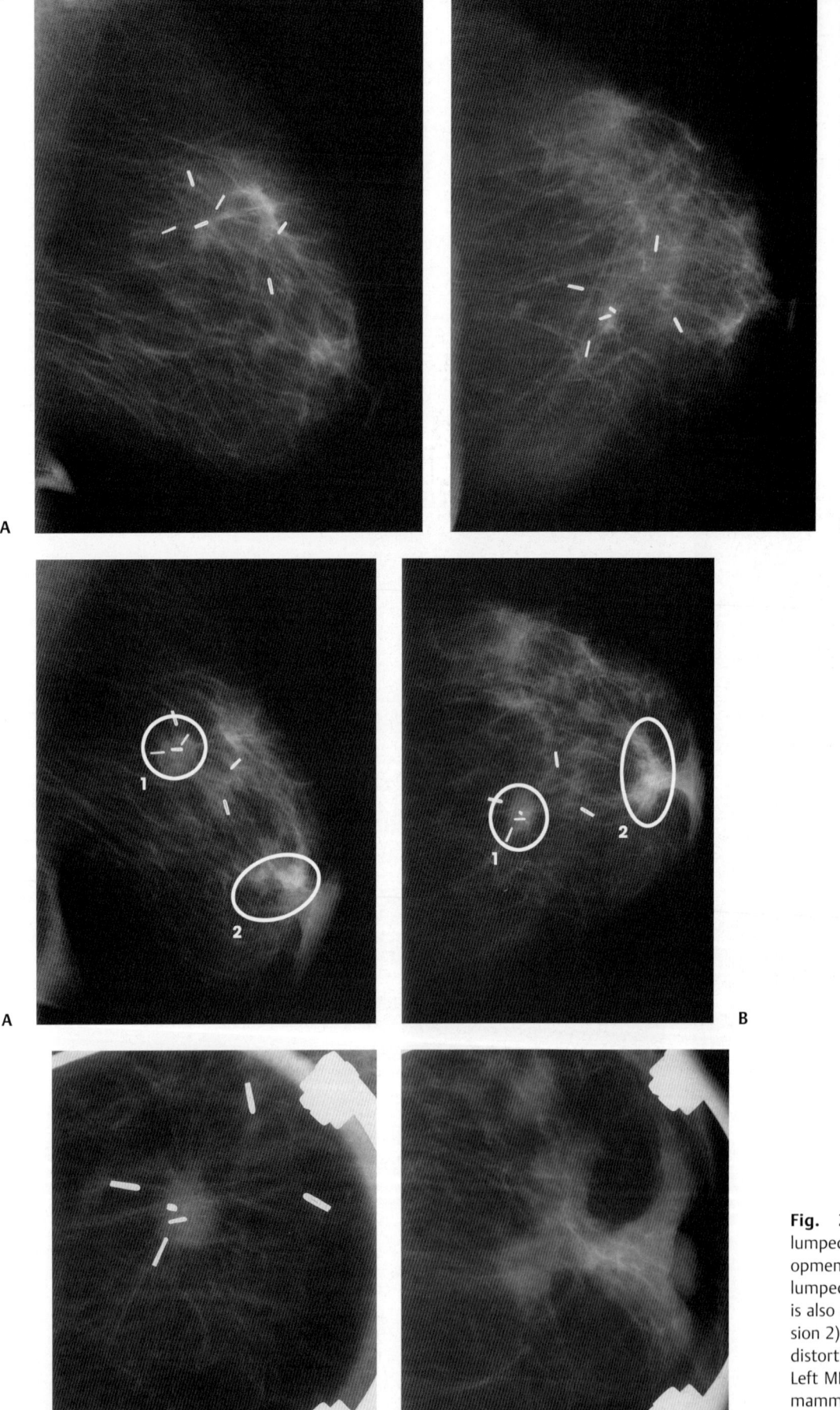

Fig. 28.27 Two years after lumpectomy, there is mild ill-defined increased density and skin thickening and retraction associated with the lumpectomy site. This appearance had been stable for 1 year. (**A**) Left MLO mammogram. (**B**) Left CC mammogram.

Fig. 28.28 Three years after lumpectomy, there has been development of a spiculated mass in the lumpectomy site (lesion 1). There is also a subareolar lobular mass (lesion 2) associated with architectural distortion and skin thickening. (**A**) Left MLO mammogram. (**B**) Left CC mammogram. (**C**) Left CC spot compression of lesion 1. (**D**) Left CC spot compression of lesion 2.

Ultrasound

Frequency
- 7 MHz

Mass (Figs. 28.29 and 28.30)
- Margin: spiculation/architectural distortion
- Echogenicity: hypoechoic
- Retrotumoral acoustic appearance: posterior shadowing distal to mass
- Shape: irregular

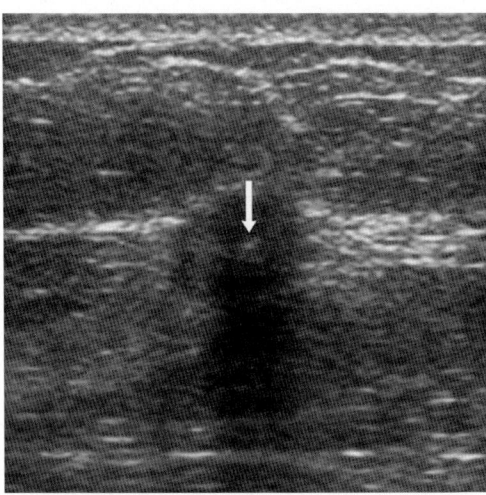

Fig. 28.29 Left transverse breast sonogram. At the 11 o'clock position, there is a hypoechoic ill-defined mass that corresponds to the mammographic lesion 1. In the center of the mass is a hyperechoic focus, which is a clip (*arrow*).

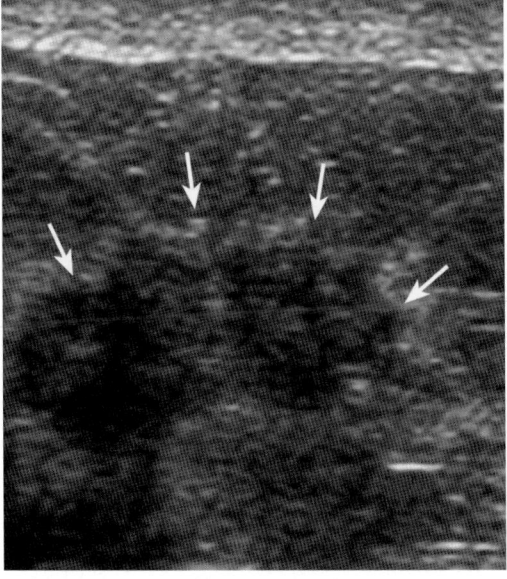

Fig. 28.30 Left transverse breast sonogram. In the subareolar area, there is a hypoechoic, ill-defined lobular mass (*arrows*) that corresponds to the mammographic lesion 2.

Pathology
- Infiltrating ductal carcinoma

Management
- BI-RADS assessment category 5, highly suggestive of malignancy

Pearls and Pitfalls

- Although lumpectomy with radiation therapy for small tumors has the same clinical result as mastectomy, multiple studies have shown that lumpectomy alone has a higher recurrence rate compared with lumpectomy with radiation therapy. After 5 years, the local recurrence rate for lumpectomy and radiation therapy is approximately 3 to 5%, but for lumpectomy alone, the rate is between 12 and 19%.
- Mammographically, the findings of recurrence include new calcifications, mass or enlarging density, architectural distortion, and inflammatory changes.

Suggested Reading

Orel SG, Troupin RH, Patterson EA, Fowble BL. Breast cancer recurrence after lumpectomy and irradiation: role of mammography in detection. Radiology 1992;183:201–206

Stomper PC, Recht A, Berenberg AL, Jochelson MS, Harris JR. Mammographic detection of recurrent cancer in the irradiated breast. AJR Am J Roentgenol 1987;148:39–43

Veronesi U. Conservation surgery and irradiation in stages I and II disease: the European experience. In: Bland KI, Copeland EM, eds. The Breast. 2nd ed. Philadelphia: WB Saunders; 1998:1191–1196

Case 28.12: Recurrent Neoplasm

Case History
A 67-year-old woman is referred for a new left breast lump. She was treated for left breast cancer 15 years ago with left lumpectomy, axillary node dissection, and radiation therapy.

Physical Examination
- Left breast: diffusely erythematous, thickened skin; no dominant masses; slightly inverted nipple
- Right breast: single enlarged axillary node; otherwise normal exam

Mammogram (Fig. 28.31)

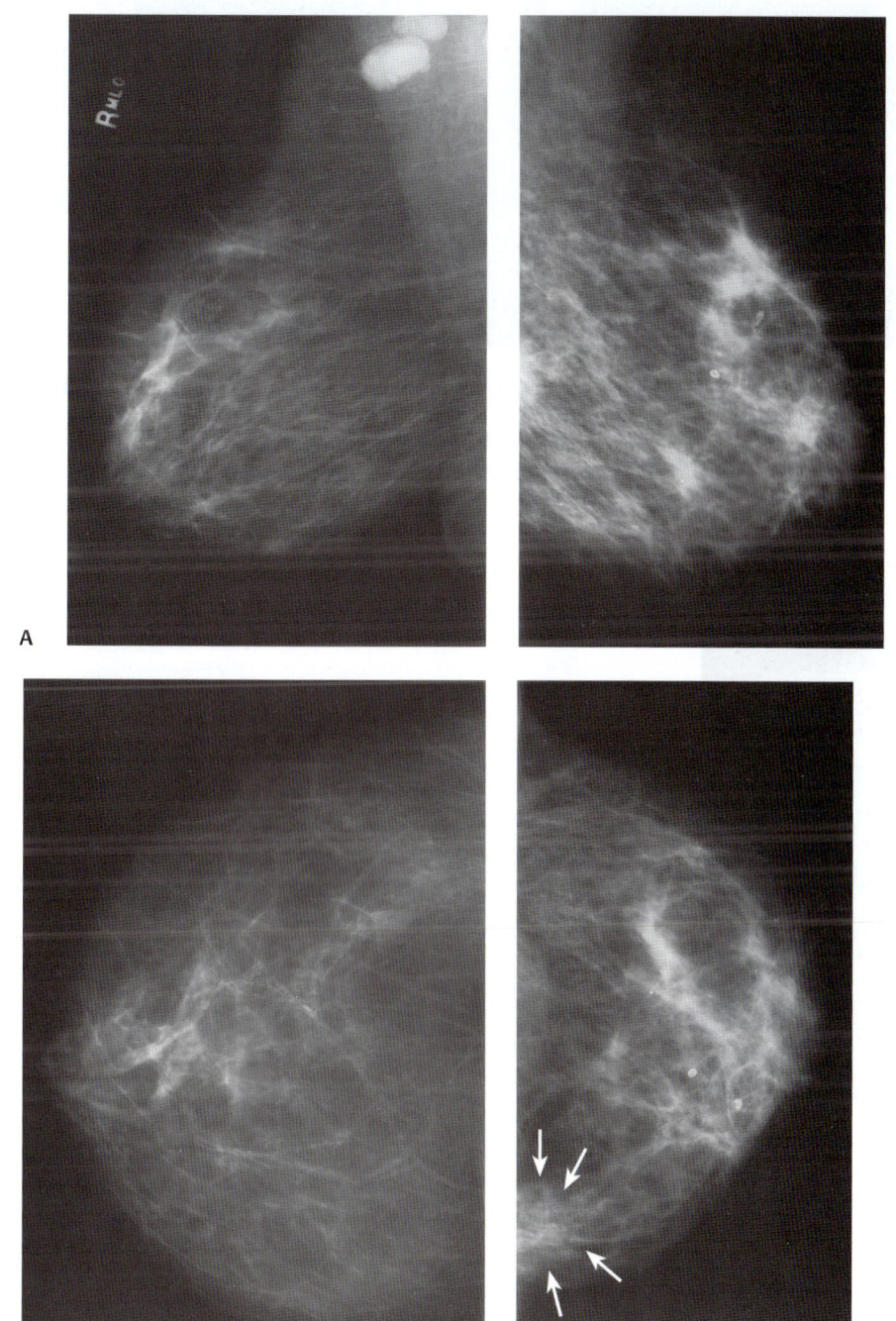

Fig. 28.31 Old lumpectomy site is in the left axilla. There is diffuse increased density of the left breast with skin and trabecular thickening. An asymmetric density is present in the left medial breast (*arrows*). Multiple enlarged, dense nodes are present in the right axilla. (**A**) Right MLO mammogram. (**B**) Left MLO mammogram. (**C**) Right CC mammogram. (**D**) Left CC mammogram.

Case 28.14: Recurrent Neoplasm

Case History
A 54-year-old woman initially presents for screening mammography. Mammography demonstrates left breast heterogeneous calcifications in a linear pattern at the 12 o'clock position. Biopsy of the calcifications reveals high-grade ductal carcinoma in situ (DCIS). The patient is treated with partial mastectomy, which removes all of the mammographic calcification, but the margins of the mastectomy are histologically positive for DCIS. Breast MRI is performed to identify the location and extent of residual malignancy.

Physical Examination
- Left breast: unremarkable exam; normally healing partial mastectomy site

Mammogram

Calcifications (Fig. 28.38)
- Type: heterogeneous/pleomorphic
- Distribution: linear

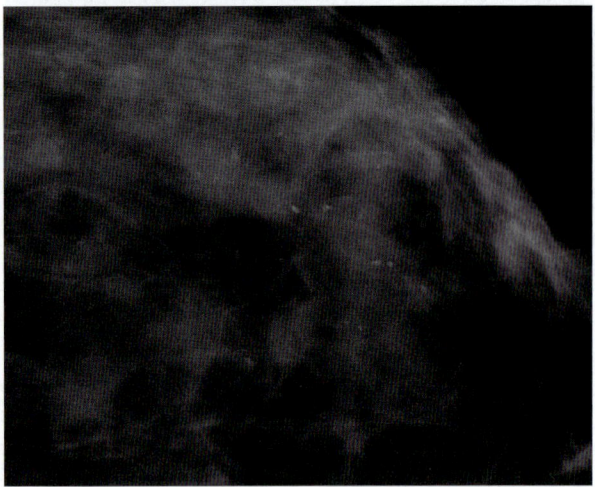

Fig. 28.38 Left ML magnification mammogram. Heterogeneous calcifications in a linear pattern are present at the 12 o'clock position.

Other Modalities: MRI and Second Look Sonography (Fig. 28.39, 28.40, and 28.41)

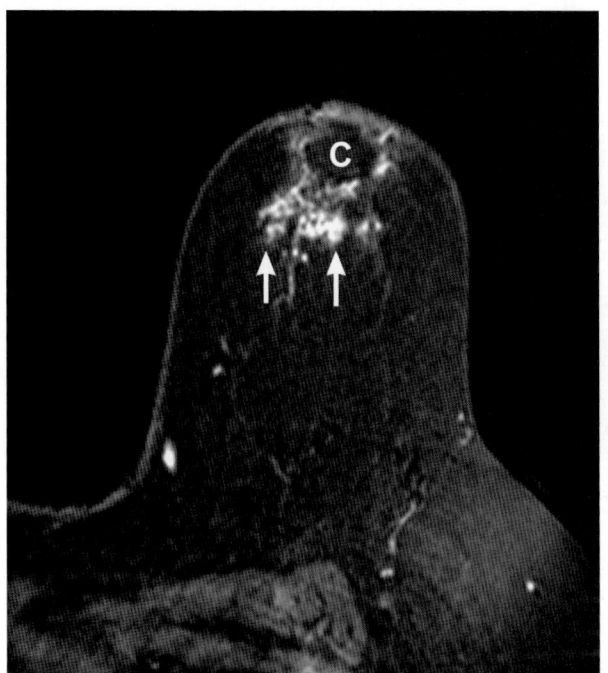
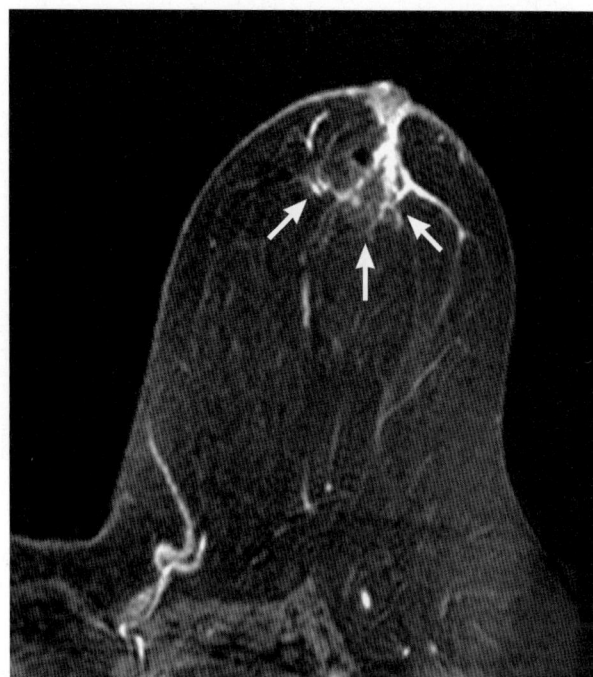

Fig. 28.39 Bilateral transverse breast MRI fat-suppressed T1-weighted spoiled rotating delivery of excitation off resonance (RODEO) images immediately after intravenous contrast administration. There is abnormal irregular enhancement both superior (**A**) and inferior (**B**) to the left partial mastectomy cavity. Abnormal enhancement (*arrows*). Partial mastectomy cavity (**C**). (**A**) Transverse image of superior edge of cavity. (**B**) Transverse image of inferior edge of cavity.

Ultrasound

Frequency (Figs. 28.40 and 28.41)
- 14 MHz

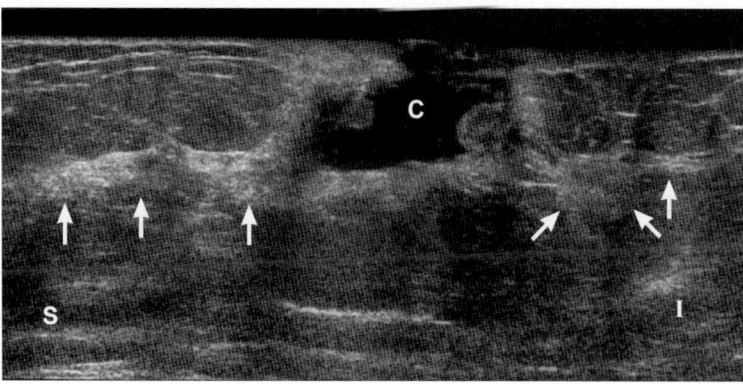

Fig. 28.40 Left longitudinal extended field of view breast sonogram. This extended field of view image demonstrates that there is hyperechoic breast tissue (*arrows*) both superior and inferior to the partial mastectomy cavity (C). Although this hyperechoic tissue appears sonographically normal, the location of this tissue matches the areas of abnormal MRI enhancement. S, superior; I, inferior.

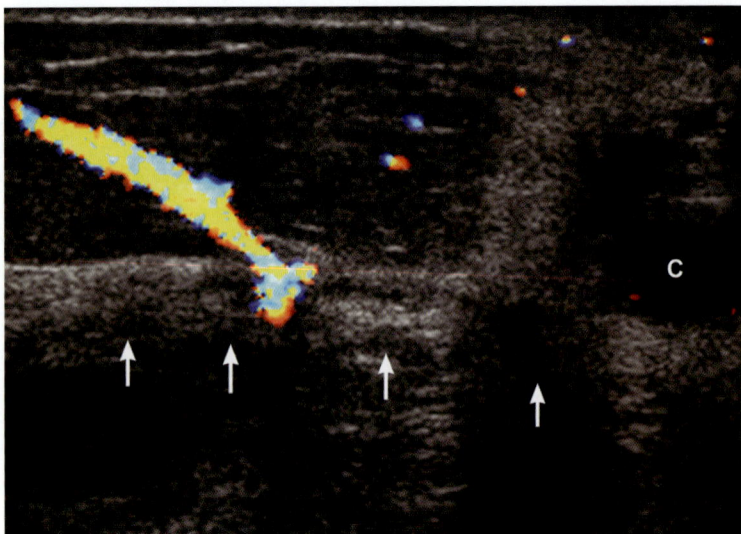

Fig. 28.41 Left longitudinal breast color Doppler sonogram. This is a sonogram of the hyperechoic tissue associated with the superior edge of the partial mastectomy cavity (C). This tissue exhibits increased color flow Doppler, which further confirms that this "normal"-appearing hyperechoic tissue (*arrows*) probably corresponds to the area of MRI enhancement. This tissue is sonographically biopsied to confirm residual malignancy.

Pathology
- Left breast calcifications: high-grade DCIS
- Left breast hyperechoic tissue surrounding the partial mastectomy cavity: high-grade DCIS

Management
- Left breast MRI enhancement around partial mastectomy site: BI-RADS assessment category 5, highly suggestive of malignancy

Pearls and Pitfalls

- When patients are treated with breast conservation surgery, 32 to 63% of them are found to have residual malignancy within the breast. Factors that predispose to residual malignancy include younger patient age (younger than 45 years of age), residual mammographic microcalcifications, tumors consisting of either invasive lobular carcinoma or extensive intraductal component, as well as microscopically positive or close margins associated with the surgical specimen. Furthermore, patients with positive or close margins that are not reexcised are at higher risk for recurrent malignancy. The rate of local recurrence for these patients has been reported to be between 10 and 25%, compared with 2 to 8% for those patients with negative margins.
- Researchers have reported that breast MRI may be an excellent method to identify residual tumor after breast conservation. Furthermore, Frei et al[1] noted that the sensitivity (95%), specificity (75%), and positive (92%) and negative (86%) predictive values for MRI detection of residual malignancy were optimally obtained 28 to 35 days after surgical intervention. The main factors associated with false-negative MRI results are postoperative enhancement, which obscures small residual tumors, and the presence of primary tumors consisting of invasive lobular or DCIS histologies.
- When ultrasound is used for biopsy guidance of suspicious MRI lesions, the goal of the sonographic exam is to identify the same anatomical location as the MRI finding. As this case illustrates, many suspicious MRI abnormalities appear as sonographically "normal" structures. Because the MRI is suspicious, the sonographic exam is not necessary to characterize or assess the abnormality. Even if the breast tissue appears "normal," as long as it represents the same structure as the suspicious MRI finding, sonographically guided biopsy should be performed. Color Doppler is sometimes useful to provide additional diagnostic confidence that the sonographically "normal" tissue matches the MRI lesion.

Reference

1. Frei KA, Kinkel K, Bonel HM, Lu Y, Esserman LJ, Hylton NM. MR imaging of the breast in patients with positive margins after lumpectomy: influence of the time interval between lumpectomy and MR imaging. AJR Am J Roentgenol 2000;175:1577–1584

Suggested Reading

Aziz D, Rawlinson E, Narod SA, et al. The role of reexcision for positive margins in optimizing local disease control after breast-conserving surgery for cancer. Breast J 2006;12:331–337

Morrow M, Harris JR. Local management of invasive cancer: breast. In: Harris JR, Lippman ME, Morrow M, Osborne CK, eds. Diseases of the Breast. 3rd ed. Philadelphia: Lippincott Williams & Wilkins; 2004:719-744

Orel SG, Reynolds C, Schnall MD, Solin LJ, Fraker DL, Sullivan DC. Breast carcinoma: MR imaging before re-excisional biopsy. Radiology 1997;205:429–436

Smitt MC, Horst K. Association of clinical and pathologic variables with lumpectomy surgical margin status after preoperative diagnosis or excisional biopsy of invasive breast cancer. Ann Surg Oncol 2007;14:1040–1044

Smitt MC, Nowels K, Carson RW, Jeffrey SS. Predictors of reexcision findings and recurrence after breast conservation. Int J Radiat Oncol Biol Phys 2003;57:979–985

Soderstrom CE, Harms SE, Farrell RS Jr, Pruneda JM, Flamig DP. Detection with MR imaging of residual tumor in the breast soon after surgery. AJR Am J Roentgenol 1997;168:485–488

Tartter PI, Kaplan J, Bleiweiss I, et al. Lumpectomy margins, reexcision, and local recurrence of breast cancer. Am J Surg 2000;179:81–85

Masses Poorly Identified Mammographically

Any benign or malignant mass may be poorly identified mammographically. Visualization depends upon mammographic technique, breast radiographic density, and lesion location. The cases presented in this chapter are presented because of the following reasons: (1) The mass commonly presents as a palpable mass. (2) The case has a teaching point about the disease process that has not been illustrated in the rest of the book. (3) The mass is an unusual histology that is not illustrated in the rest of the book.

29 Patient Unable to Tolerate Mammogram

Case 29.1: Patient Unable to Tolerate Mammogram

Case History

A 35-year-old woman is admitted for severe disseminated encephalomyelitis of unknown origin. She is comatose.

Physical Examination
- Unresponsive patient
- Right breast: palpable lump in upper outer quadrant
- Left breast: normal exam

Ultrasound

Frequency
- 10 MHz

Mass (Fig. 29.1)
- Margin: ill defined
- Echogenicity: hypoechoic
- Retrotumoral acoustic appearance: bilateral edge shadowing
- Shape: lobulated

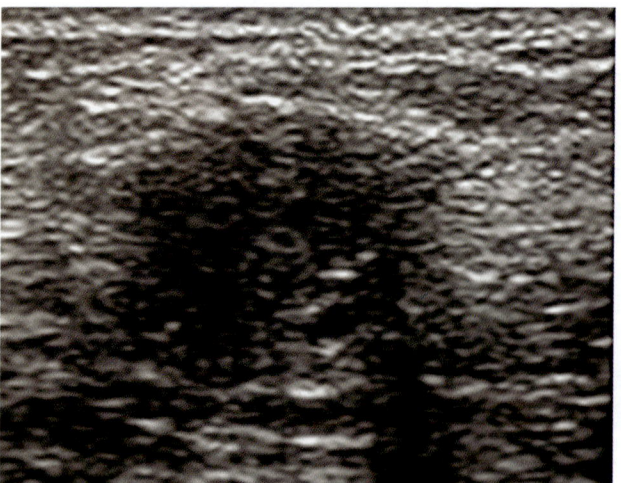
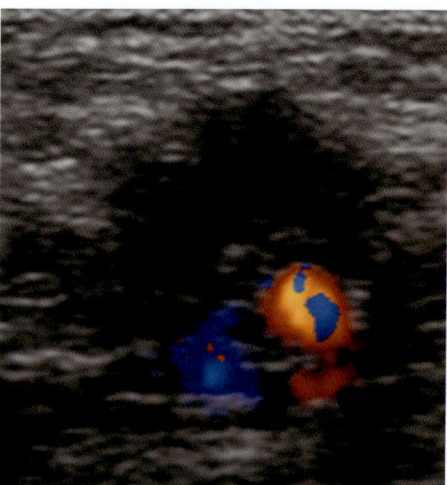

Fig. 29.1 The palpable lump corresponds to a lobulated hypoechoic mass. (**A**) Right radial breast sonogram. (**B**) Right radial color Doppler breast sonogram.

Other Modalities: Brain MRI (Fig. 29.2)

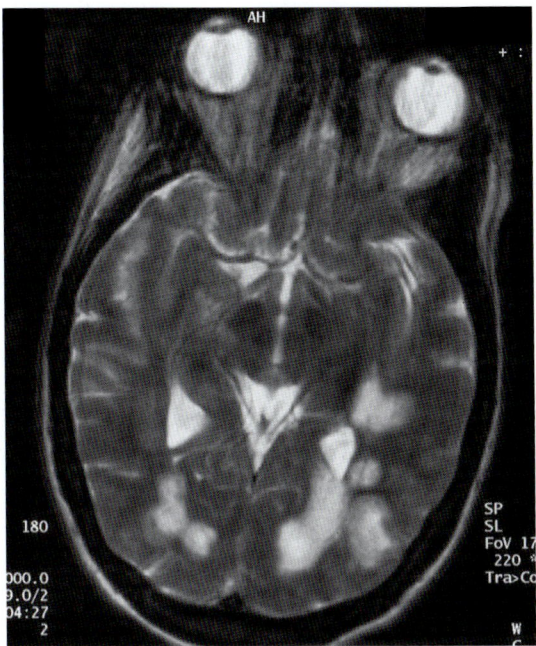

Fig. 29.2 T2-weighted transverse image of the brain. There are numerous high-intensity white matter abnormalities.

Pathology
- Infiltrating ductal carcinoma

Management
- BI-RADS assessment category 4, suspicious; biopsy should be considered.

Pearls and Pitfalls

- In this patient, the encephalomyelitis was a paraneoplastic syndrome caused by the breast cancer. The patient was treated with mastectomy, and her symptoms improved, but she retained chronic left-sided paralysis and contractures.
- When tumors produce symptoms at anatomical locations that are distant from the primary tumor or its metastases, these symptoms are described as paraneoplastic syndromes. Paraneoplastic syndromes may be classified as (1) endocrine (e.g., ectopic adrenocorticotropic hormone, inappropriate antidiuretic hormone), (2) hematologic (e.g., anemia, erythrocytosis, thrombophlebitis), (3) gastrointestinal (e.g., protein-losing enteropathy, anorexia-cachexia), (4) renal (e.g., membranous nephropathy, hemolytic uremic syndrome), (5) cutaneous (e.g., pigmented lesions, keratoses, erythemas, bullae, urticaria), and (6) neurologic (e.g., encephalomyelitis, cerebellar degeneration, Lambert-Eaton myasthenic syndrome, dermatomyositis). Neurologic paraneoplastic syndromes occur in less than 1% of cancer patients. The etiology of encephalomyelitis is unknown. There is no specific treatment, and patients generally suffer chronic severe debilitation.
- In rare situations, patients cannot tolerate or cooperate adequately to produce a mammogram. In a clinically suspicious situation, if a palpable lump is present, sonography is useful for clarifying a specific problem. If no lump is present, then MRI is useful to evaluate the breasts.

Suggested Reading

Arnold SM, Patchell R, Lowy AM, Foon KA. Paraneoplastic syndromes. In: DeVita VT, Hellman S, Rosenberg SA, eds. Cancer Principles and Practice of Oncology. 6th ed. Philadelphia: Lippincott Williams & Wilkins; 2001:2511–2536

Cosmacini P, Veronesi P, Galimberti V, Ferranti C, Viganotti G, Coopmans de Yoldi G. Ultrasonographic evaluation of palpable breast masses: analysis of 134 cases. Tumori 1990;76:495–498

Dalmau JO, Posner JB. Paraneoplastic syndromes affecting the nervous system. Semin Oncol 1997;24:318–328

30 Palpable Masses

Case 30.1: Young Women—Diabetic Mastopathy

Case History

A 74-year-old woman presents with a left breast lump. She was identified with type 1 diabetes 40 years ago and is on an insulin pump.

Physical Examination
- Left breast: firm 2 cm palpable mass at the 6 o'clock position
- Right breast: normal exam

Mammogram (Fig. 30.1)

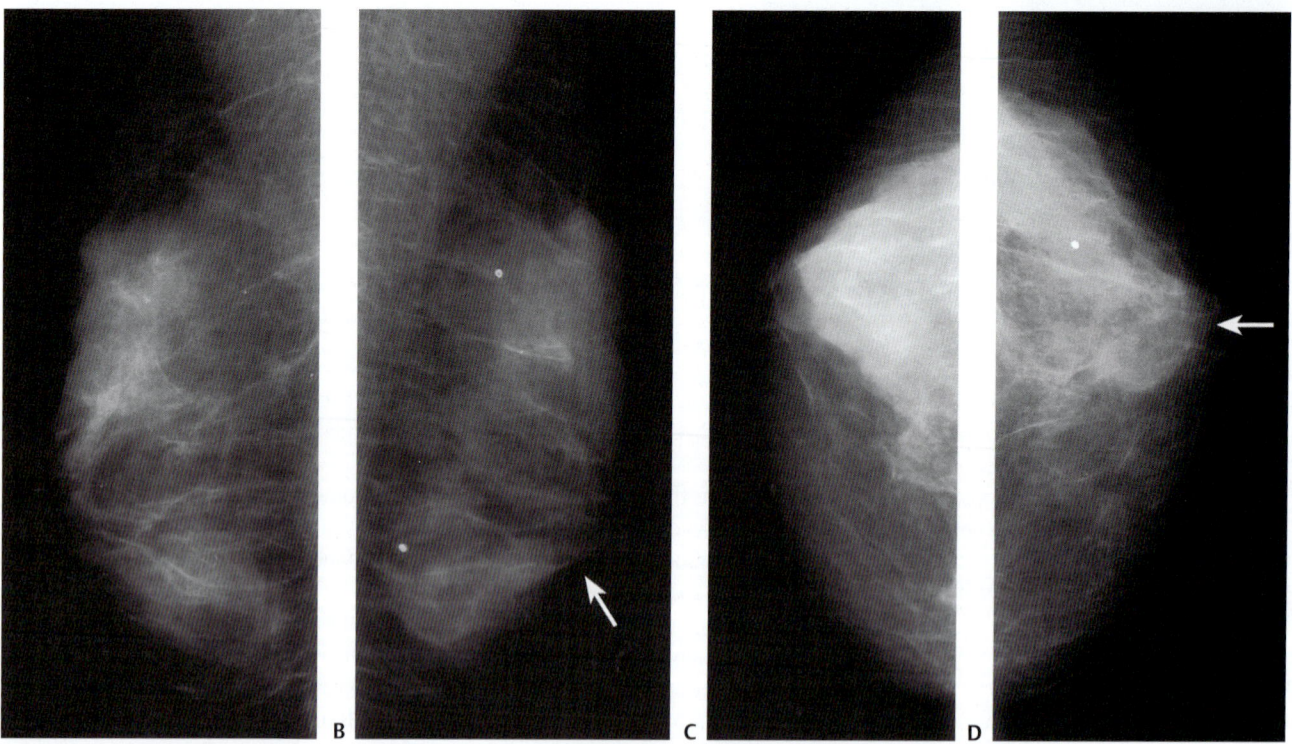

Fig. 30.1 The left palpable mass is marked with an arrow. No focal mass is identified. Bilateral mammograms are normal. (**A**) Right MLO mammogram. (**B**) Left MLO mammogram. (**C**) Right CC mammogram. (**D**) Left CC mammogram.

Ultrasound

Low Frequency

Frequency
- 6 MHz

Mass (Fig. 30.2)
- Margin: ill defined
- Echogenicity: hypoechoic
- Retrotumoral acoustic appearance: severe shadowing, mass completely obscured
- Shape: irregular

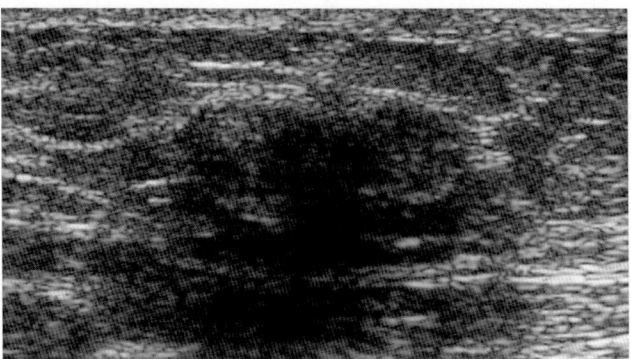

Fig. 30.2 Because the mass is obscured with the high-frequency examination, lower frequencies were applied. With 8 MHz (**A**), the mass is mildly hypoechoic. However, normal parenchymal lines are identified running through the mass. With 6 MHz (**B**), the hypoechogenicity and mass almost disappear. (**A**) Left antiradial breast sonogram (8 MHz). (**B**) Left antiradial breast sonogram (6 MHz).

High Frequency

Frequency
- 11.5 MHz

Associated Findings (Fig. 30.3)

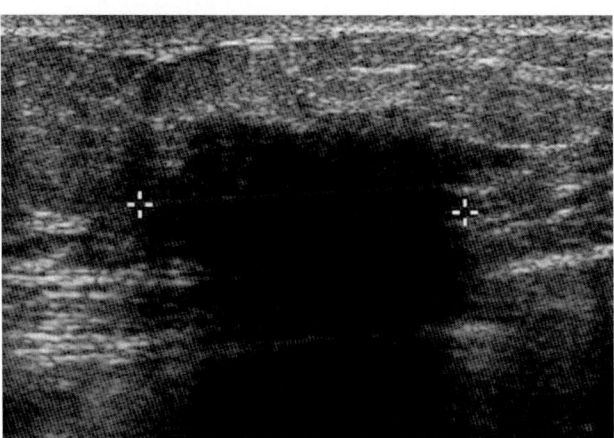

Fig. 30.3 Left antiradial breast sonogram. The palpable mass corresponds to a hypoechoic mass with severe shadowing.

Pathology
- Diabetic mastopathy

Management
- BI-RADS assessment category 4, suspicious; biopsy should be considered.

Pearls and Pitfalls

- Diabetic mastopathy is identified in less than 1% of benign breast biopsies but represents approximately 13% of benign biopsies in women with type 1 diabetes. Clinically, this abnormality affects young women between the ages of 25 and 40 years who have had a long history of diabetes (usually more than 10 years). This patient is much older than most patients who present with this problem. The mastopathy presents as a painless, hard, irregular mass. About 50% of patients will have multiple masses.
- Mammographically, these masses are commonly not identifiable. Sometimes there is an asymmetric focal density or ill-defined mass.
- Sonographically, these masses highly attenuate sound. Therefore, when using a high-frequency transducer, the mass will appear as a focal area of heavy shadowing. With lower frequencies, the shadowing and hypoechogenicity will decrease, and no definite mass is evident. Sonographically, these findings do not prevent a biopsy. However, if the biopsy result is diabetic mastopathy, there is good sonographic and pathologic correlation.

Suggested Reading

Boullu S, Andrac L, Piana L, Darmon P, Dutour A, Oliver C. Diabetic mastopathy, complication of type 1 diabetes mellitus: report of two cases and a review of the literature. Diabetes Metab 1998;24:448–454

Hunfeld KP, Bässler R. Lymphocytic mastitis and fibrosis of the breast in long-standing insulin-dependent diabetics: a histopathologic study on diabetic mastopathy and report of ten cases. Gen Diagn Pathol 1997;143:49–58

Logan WW, Hoffman NY. Diabetic fibrous breast disease. Radiology 1989;172:667–670

Case 30.2: Young Women—Juvenile Fibroadenoma

Case History
A 14-year-old girl presents with new left breast lump.

Physical Examination
- Left breast: 3 cm smooth mass extending from the 10 o'clock to the 2 o'clock positions along the areolar margin
- Right breast: normal exam

Ultrasound

Frequency
- 7 MHz

Mass (Fig. 30.4)
- Margin: well defined
- Echogenicity: hypoechoic
- Retrotumoral acoustic appearance: no shadowing
- Shape: ellipsoid

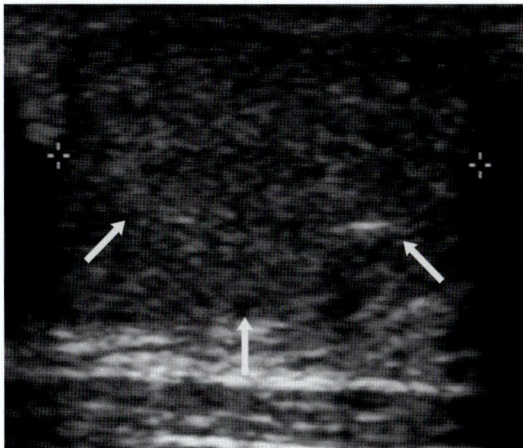

Fig. 30.4 Left radial breast sonogram. The palpable mass corresponds to a well-defined, hypoechoic mass with a thin, lucent rim (*arrows*).

Pathology
- Juvenile fibroadenoma

Management
- BI-RADS assessment category 3, probably benign; short-interval follow-up

Pearls and Pitfalls

- Fibroadenoma is the most common mass in adolescent girls. Most of these fibroadenomas are the adult type of histology. However, some adolescents have juvenile fibroadenomas, which are variants of the adult type. These patients commonly present with a rapidly growing mass. Microscopically, the tumor demonstrates a pericanalicular growth pattern, as opposed to the usual intracanalicular pattern of adult fibroadenomas. Furthermore, the stroma is more cellular than the adult type.
- Because these masses are palpable and occur in young women, they are generally initially identified sonographically. Their appearance is identical to adult fibroadenomas. They are generally well-defined oval or lobulated hypoechoic masses. Because these lesions tend to be large and growing, they are commonly biopsied even though their appearance is sonographically relatively benign (as in this case).

Suggested Reading

Ashikari R, Farrow JH, O'Hara J. Fibroadenomas in the breast of juveniles. Surg Gynecol Obstet 1971;132:259–262

Devitt JE. Juvenile giant fibroadenoma of the breast. Can J Surg 1974;17:205–207

Tavassoli FA, Fattaneh A. Pathology of the Breast. 2nd ed. Stamford: Appleton and Lange; 1999:583–586

Case 30.3: Pregnant or Lactating Women—Lactating Adenoma

Case History
A 37-year-old woman who is 9-months postpartum presents with a new right breast lump. She recently had symptoms of right breast mastitis that have improved on antibiotics. She is still nursing her baby.

Physical Examination
- Right breast: smooth, soft, mobile mass at the 6 o'clock position
- Left breast: normal exam

Ultrasound

Frequency
- 10 MHz

Mass
- Margin: well defined
- Echogenicity: heterogeneous
- Retrotumoral acoustic appearance: no shadowing
- Shape: ellipsoid (**Fig. 30.5**)

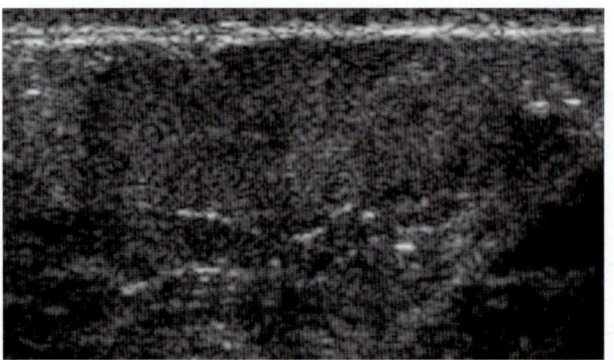
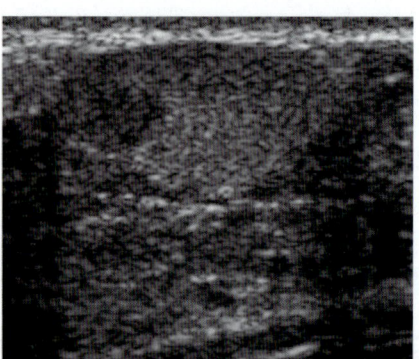
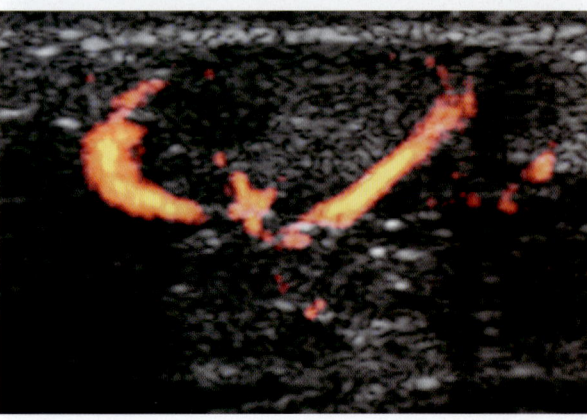

Fig. 30.5 The palpable lump corresponds to a well-defined, oval mass with heterogeneous echogenicity. (**A**) Right radial breast sonogram. (**B**) Right antiradial breast sonogram. (**C**) Right antiradial color power Doppler breast sonogram.

Pathology
- Lactating adenoma

Management
- BI-RADS assessment category 4, suspicious; biopsy should be considered.

Pearls and Pitfalls
- Adenomas are benign tumors consisting of epithelial and myoepithelial lined tubules. Adenomas differ from fibroadenomas because adenomas have little stroma. In fibroadenomas, stromal cells are the dominant feature.
- Lactating adenomas occur in young women who are either pregnant or nursing. Of an Armed Forces Institute of Pathology (AFIP) series of 88 lactating adenomas, the oldest woman was 38 years.
- Because lactating adenomas present as palpable masses in young pregnant or nursing women, these masses are commonly imaged only with sonography. They are generally well-defined, oval or lobulated masses that are hypoechoic or heterogeneous in echogenicity. They are sonographically similar to fibroadenomas.

Suggested Reading
Bassett LW, Ysrael M, Gold RH, Ysrael C. Usefulness of mammography and sonography in women less than 35 years of age. Radiology 1991;180:831–835

Hertel BF, Zaloudek C, Kempson RL. Breast adenomas. Cancer 1976;37:2891–2905

Tavassoli FA, Fattaneh A. Pathology of the Breast. 2nd ed. Stamford: Appleton & Lange; 1999:157–165

Case 30.5: Scattered Heterogeneous or Extremely Dense Mammogram—Angiosarcoma

Case History
A 68-year-old woman had right lumpectomy and radiation therapy 7 years ago for breast cancer. She now presents with new red skin lesions on the incision site.

Physical Examination
- Right breast: three red quarter-sized lesions around the healed lumpectomy scar
- Left breast: normal exam

Mammogram (Fig. 30.8)

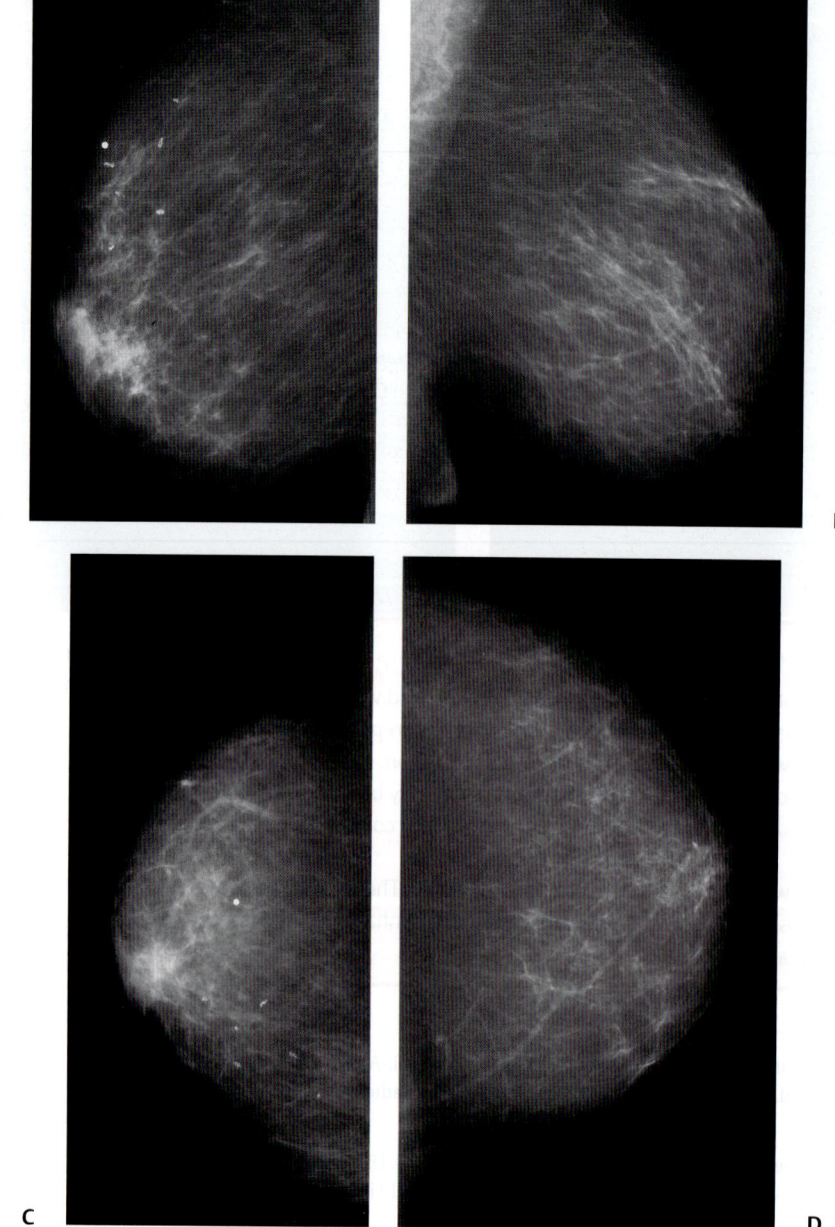

Fig. 30.8 There is ill-defined increased density and coarsening of the trabecular pattern of the right breast consistent with previous radiation therapy. No mass corresponding to the skin abnormalities is identified. Left breast is normal. (**A**) Right MLO mammogram. (**B**) Left MLO mammogram. (**C**) Right CC mammogram. (**D**) Left CC mammogram.

Other Modalities (Fig. 30.9)

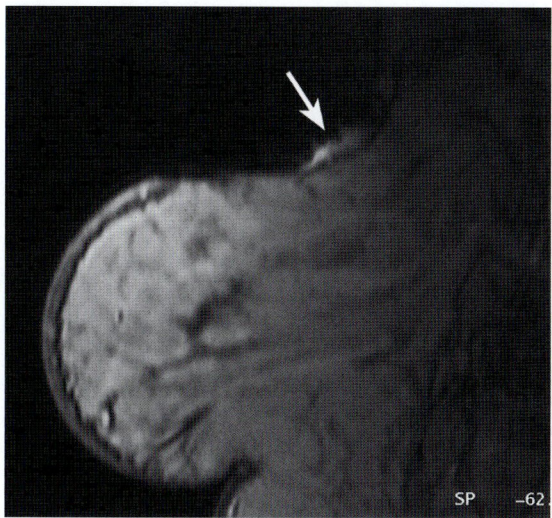

Fig. 30.9 Right longitudinal dynamic bolus three-dimensional (3D) volume-gradient series breast MRI. There is abnormal enhancement of an irregular superficial mass (*arrow*) in the upper outer quadrant.

Pathology
- Angiosarcoma

Management
- BI-RADS assessment category 4, suspicious; biopsy should be considered.

Pearls and Pitfalls

- The breast is a relatively common site for angiosarcoma. In a series of 33 patients from Memorial Sloan-Kettering Cancer Center, breast was fourth (9%) behind head (27%), thigh (18%), and arm (12%). However, compared with other breast malignancies, this tumor is rare. It accounts for less than 0.05% of primary breast cancers. Women who have had breast cancer have an increased risk of developing this tumor. The reason for this association is not clear.
- Angiosarcomas generally present as a palpable mass. A blue-red skin discoloration is commonly present. Generally, nipple discharge, retraction, and axillary adenopathy are absent even with large masses.
- Mammographically, these tumors are lobulated or irregular in shape and have ill-defined margins. Calcifications have been described in 10% of masses and skin thickening in 5% of cases. Many (35%) of these tumors are not visible mammographically.
- Sonographically, these masses appear ellipsoid, lobulated, or irregular with either well-defined or ill-defined margins. The masses are hypoechoic, heterogeneous, or hyperechoic in echogenicity.
- With MRI, these tumors have a low to intermediate signal intensity on T1-weighted studies and high signal intensity on T2-weighted sequences.

Suggested Reading

Cozen W, Bernstein L, Wang F, Press MF, Mack TM. The risk of angiosarcoma following primary breast cancer. Br J Cancer 1999;81:532–536

Grant EG, Holt RW, Chun B, Richardson JD, Orson LW, Cigtay OS. Angiosarcoma of the breast: sonographic, xeromammographic, and pathologic appearance. AJR Am J Roentgenol 1983;141:691–692

Liberman L, Dershaw DD, Kaufman RJ, Rosen PP. Angiosarcoma of the breast. Radiology 1992;183:649–654

Tavassoli FA, Fattaneh A. Pathology of the Breast. 2nd ed. Stamford: Appleton & Lange; 1999:633–673

Case 30.6: Scattered Heterogeneous or Extremely Dense Mammogram—Ductal Carcinoma in Situ

Case History
A 42-year-old woman presents with a new left breast lump.

Physical Examination
- Left breast: ill-defined 5 cm area of thickening in the upper outer quadrant
- Right breast: normal exam

Mammogram (Fig. 30.10)

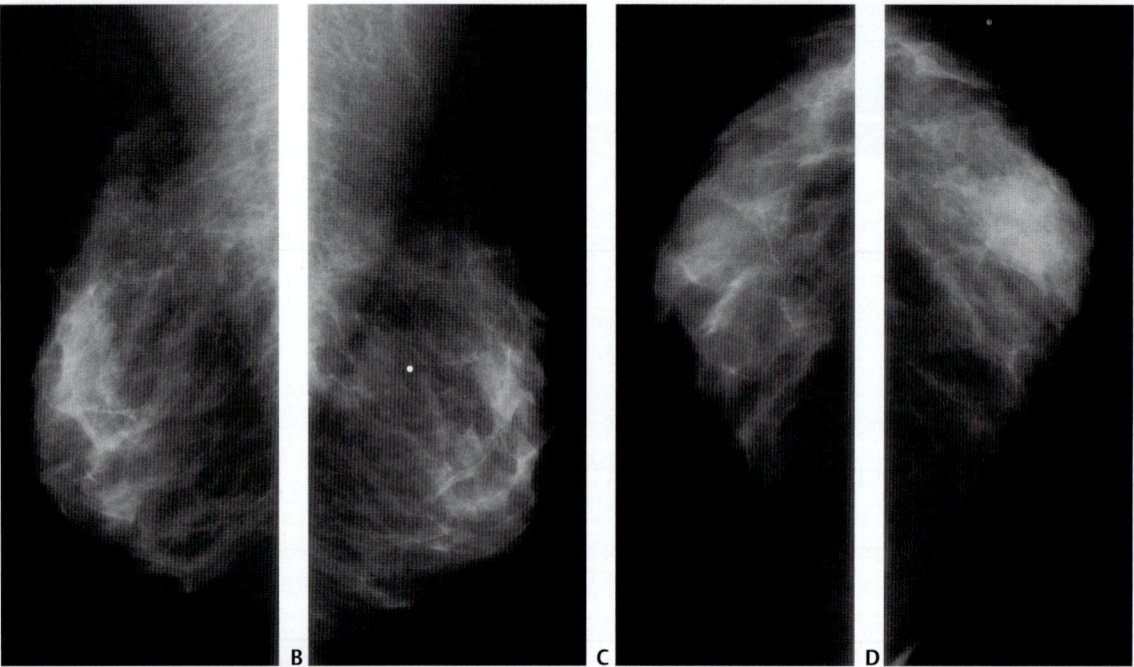

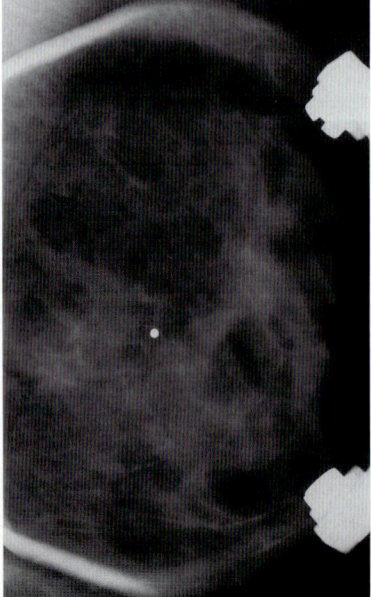

Fig. 30.10 Bilateral mammograms demonstrate scattered fibroglandular densities. The palpable mass (labeled with a radiographic marker) is associated with an area of focal increased density in the left breast visible only on the MLO view (**B,E**). (**A**) Right MLO mammogram. (**B**) Left MLO mammogram. (**C**) Right CC mammogram. (**D**) Left CC mammogram. (**E**) Left MLO spot magnification mammogram of region of palpable mass.

Ultrasound

Frequency
- 11.5 MHz

Mass (Fig. 30.11)
- Margin: ill defined
- Echogenicity: hypoechoic
- Retrotumoral acoustic appearance: no shadowing
- Shape: ellipsoid

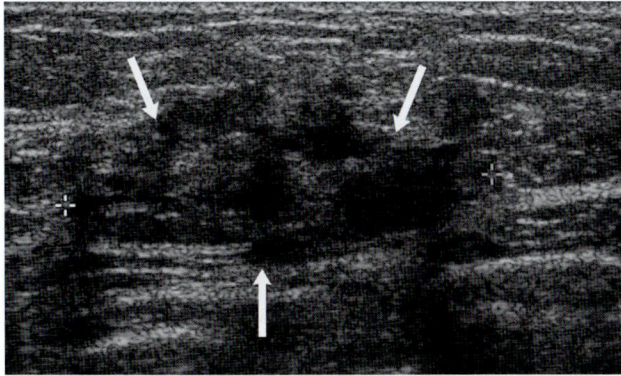

Fig. 30.11 Left radial breast sonogram. The palpable thickening corresponded to an area of ill-defined hypoechogenicity (*arrows*).

Pathology
- Ductal carcinoma in situ (DCIS)
- 4 cm of low-grade DCIS

Management
- BI-RADS assessment category 4, suspicious; biopsy should be considered.

Pearls and Pitfalls

- Occasionally, DCIS presents as a palpable mass. Sonographically, this malignancy is relatively difficult to identify. Sonographic findings include calcifications, irregular hypoechoic mass, focally dilated ducts, and an ill-defined hypoechoic area. This case illustrates the last type of appearance.

Suggested Reading

Rickard MT. Ultrasound of malignant breast microcalcifications: role in evaluation and guided procedures. Australas Radiol 1996;40:26–31

Schoonjans JM, Brem RF. Sonographic appearance of ductal carcinoma in situ diagnosed with ultrasonographically guided large core needle biopsy: correlation with mammographic and pathologic findings. J Ultrasound Med 2000;19:449–457

Case 30.7: Scattered Heterogeneous or Extremely Dense Mammogram—Infiltrating Ductal Carcinoma

Case History
A 35-year-old woman found a right breast lump on breast self-examination.

Physical Examination
- Right breast: irregular movable mass at the 10 o'clock position
- Left breast: normal exam

Mammogram (Fig. 30.12)

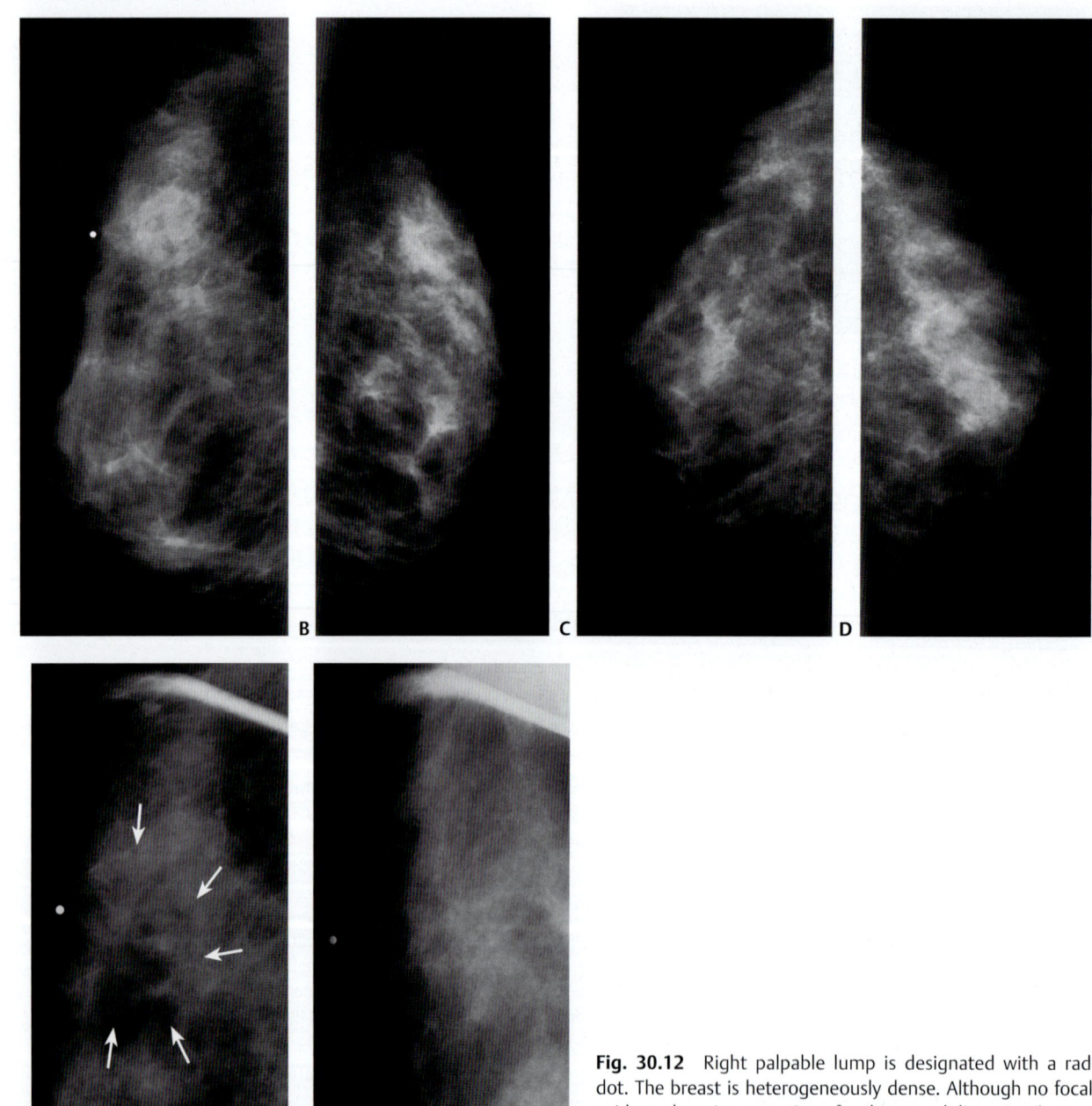

Fig. 30.12 Right palpable lump is designated with a radiopaque dot. The breast is heterogeneously dense. Although no focal mass is evident, there is suggestion of architectural distortion (*arrows*) on the right spot compression view (**E**). (**A**) Right MLO mammogram. (**B**) Left MLO mammogram. (**C**) Right CC mammogram. (**D**) Left CC mammogram. (**E**) Right MLO spot compression mammogram. (**F**) Right XCCL spot compression mammogram.

Ultrasound

Frequency
- 11.5 MHz

Mass (Fig. 30.13)
- Margin: ill defined
- Echogenicity: hypoechoic
- Retrotumoral acoustic appearance: posterior shadowing distal to mass
- Shape: irregular

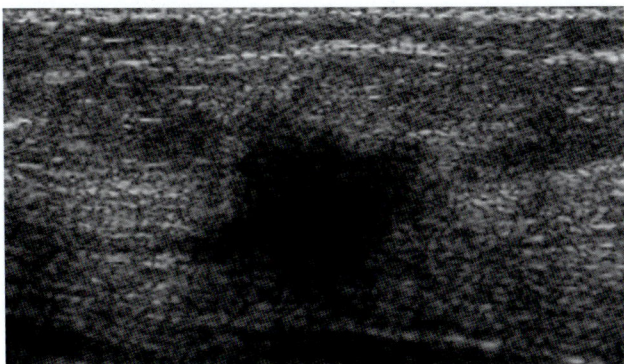

Fig. 30.13 Right radial breast sonogram. An ill-defined irregular mass of heterogeneous echogenicity corresponds to the palpable mass.

Pathology
- Infiltrating ductal carcinoma
- 1.6 cm primary tumor; one of eight axillary nodes positive for metastatic tumor

Management
- BI-RADS assessment category 4, suspicious; biopsy should be considered.

Pearls and Pitfalls

- One of the well-established reasons for breast sonography is examination of a palpable mass that is not mammographically identified. Lack of mammographic identification may be due to a variety of factors, including suboptimal technique, unusual position of mass, and overlap of tumor with fibroglandular tissue.

Suggested Reading

Cosmacini P, Veronesi P, Galimberti V, Ferranti C, Viganotti G, Coopmans de Yoldi G. Ultrasonographic evaluation of palpable breast masses: analysis of 134 cases. Tumori 1990;76:495–498

Dennis MA, Parker SH, Klaus AJ, Stavros AT, Kaske TI, Clark SB. Breast biopsy avoidance: the value of normal mammograms and normal sonograms in the setting of a palpable lump. Radiology 2001;219:186–191

Zonderland HM. The role of ultrasound in the diagnosis of breast cancer. Semin Ultrasound CT MR 2000;21:317–324

Case 30.8: Scattered Heterogeneous or Extremely Dense Mammogram—Fibrous Histiocytoma

Case History
A 45-year-old woman presents with a palpable lump.

Physical Examination
- Right breast: small palpable lump at the 4:30 clock position associated with skin thickening and mild redness
- Left breast: normal exam

Mammogram (Fig. 30.14)

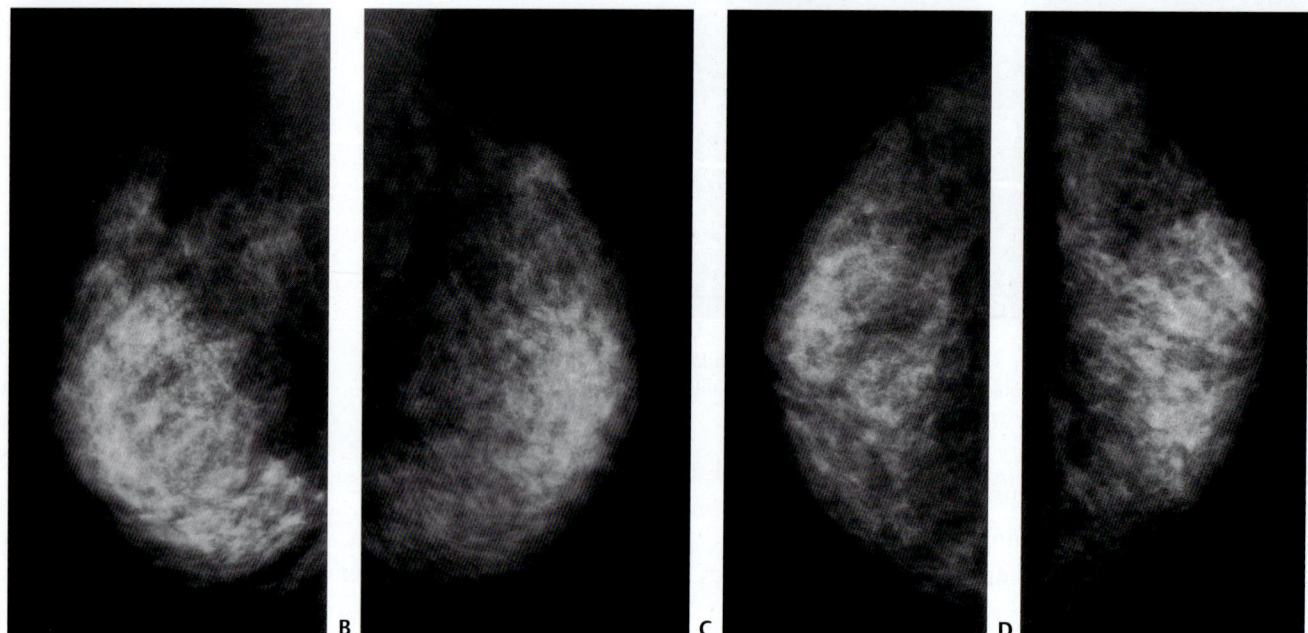

Fig. 30.14 The palpable mass is not evident on the heterogeneously dense mammograms. (**A**) Right MLO mammogram. (**B**) Left MLO mammogram. (**C**) Right CC mammogram. (**D**) Left CC mammogram.

Ultrasound

Frequency
- 13 MHz

Mass (Fig. 30.15)
- Margin: ill defined
- Echogenicity: hypoechoic
- Retrotumoral acoustic appearance: bilateral edge shadowing
- Shape: irregular

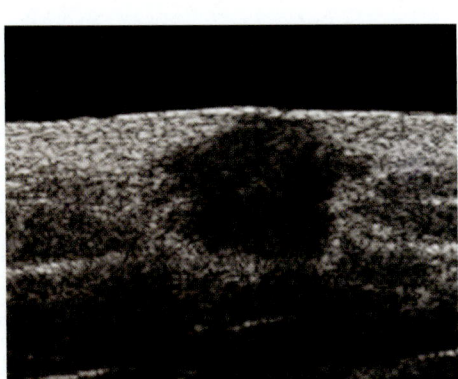
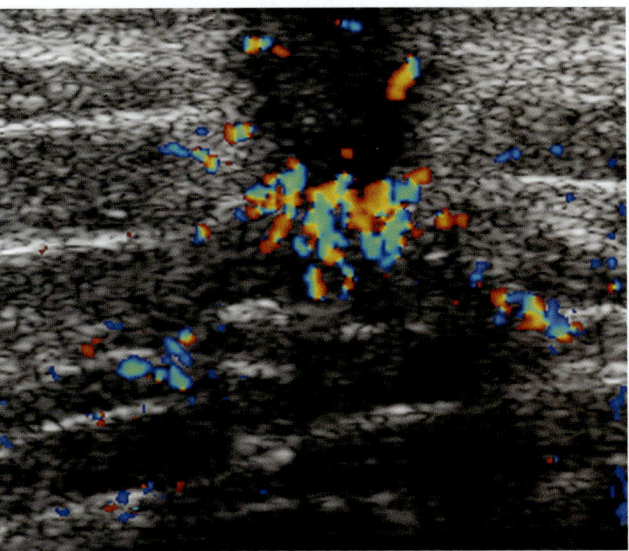

Fig. 30.15 The palpable mass corresponds to an irregular, hypoechoic mass. The mass extends into the hyperechoic skin. (**A**) Right radial breast sonogram. (**B**) Right radial color Doppler breast sonogram.

Pathology
- Malignant fibrous histiocytoma

Management
- BI-RADS assessment category 4, suspicious; biopsy should be considered.

Pearls and Pitfalls

- Malignant fibrous histiocytomas are an unusual breast sarcoma. Most reported cases are idiopathic, but this lesion has been related to previous radiation therapy. In an AFIP series of 24 tumors, 5 tumors were in men. The mean patient age was 58 years.
- In this case, the tumor is an irregular, ill-defined, hypoechoic solid mass that is indistinguishable from other tumors.

Suggested Reading

Horii R, Fukuuchi A, Nishi T, Takanashi R. A case of malignant fibrous histiocytoma after breast conserving therapy for breast cancer. Breast Cancer 2000;7:75–77

Tavassoli FA, Fattaneh A. Pathology of the Breast. 2nd ed. Stamford: Appleton & Lange; 1999:718–729

Case 30.9: Scattered Heterogeneous or Extremely Dense Mammogram—Normal Structures

Case History
A 39-year-old woman presents with a palpable left breast lump.

Physical Examination
- Left breast: 5 mm lump in the upper outer quadrant
- Right breast: normal exam

Mammogram (Fig. 30.16)

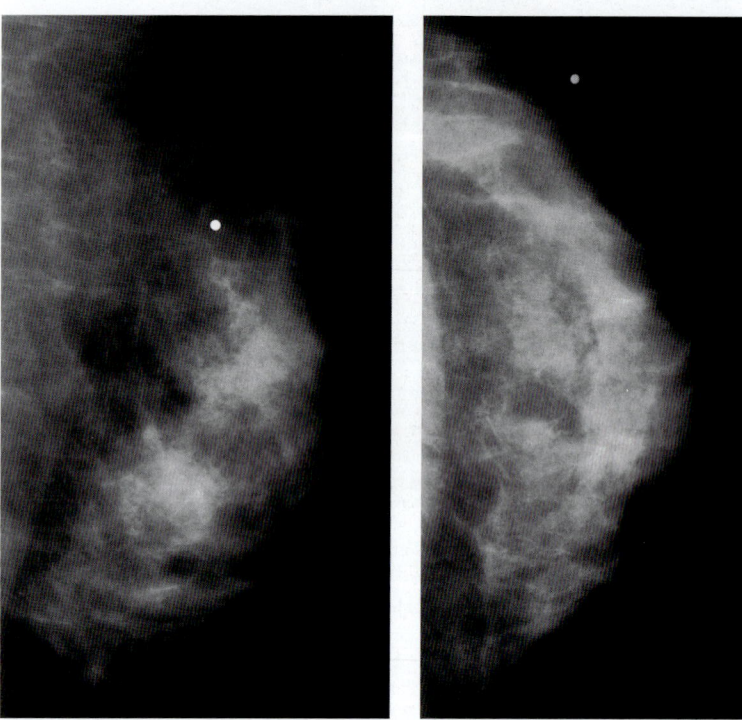

Fig. 30.16 Normal left mammogram. The breast is extremely dense. No mass is associated with the palpable lump, which is marked with a radiopaque dot. (**A**) Left MLO mammogram. (**B**) Left CC mammogram.

Ultrasound

Frequency
- 13 MHz (**Fig. 30.17**)

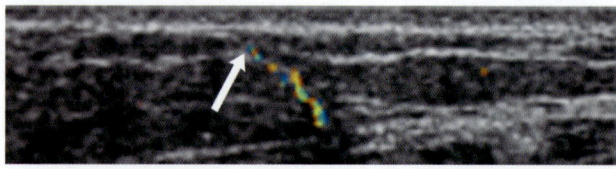

Fig. 30.17 Left oblique breast color Doppler sonogram. The palpable lump corresponds to a Cooper's ligament attachment (*arrow*).

Pathology
- Cooper's ligament attachment

Management
- BI-RADS assessment category 2, benign finding

Pearls and Pitfalls

- With higher-frequency sonography, the normal breast structures are better visualized. Many palpable lumps are due to normal breast structures. Cooper's ligament attachments are commonly palpable, particularly in the upright position. Sometimes one attachment is more prominent, as illustrated in this case. After identifying the attachment as the etiology of the lump, you can generally confirm the presence of similar (but less obvious) lumps throughout the breast that also correspond to these ligaments sonographically. Other common palpable lumps include lobular fibroglandular tissue, fat lobules, and blood vessels. To assign a BI-RADS category 2 (benign) or 3 (probably benign) to a palpable lump, it is critical that the mammogram also be normal.
- The main reasons for missing a neoplasm when "normal" structures are identified are (1) not using high-resolution sonography, (2) not palpating the correct abnormality, (3) not correlating the sonogram to the mammogram, (4) not linking the palpable lump to a specific normal structure, and (5) suboptimal sonographic technique (e.g., inadequate contrast). Some lesions, such as ductal carcinoma in situ, are present with minimal disruption of breast architecture. Therefore, I would not assign a category 2 to a negative breast sonogram for the following situations: (1) The patient has an unusually high risk for cancer (e.g., previous history of cancer, high-risk gene pool). (2) The patient has any other symptoms besides a palpable lump (e.g., nipple discharge). (3) The lump size is discordant with the size of the normal structure. (4) The mammogram has any abnormality or asymmetry. (5) High-frequency sonography is not available.

Suggested Reading

Dennis MA, Parker SH, Klaus AJ, Stavros AT, Kaske TI, Clark SB. Breast biopsy avoidance: the value of normal mammograms and normal sonograms in the setting of a palpable lump. Radiology 2001;219:186–191

Case 30.10: Fatty Mammogram—Fat Necrosis

Case History
A 76-year-old woman presents with a new right palpable lump.

Physical Examination
- Right breast: firm lump associated with a bruise at the 12 o'clock position
- Left breast: normal exam

Mammogram (Fig. 30.18)

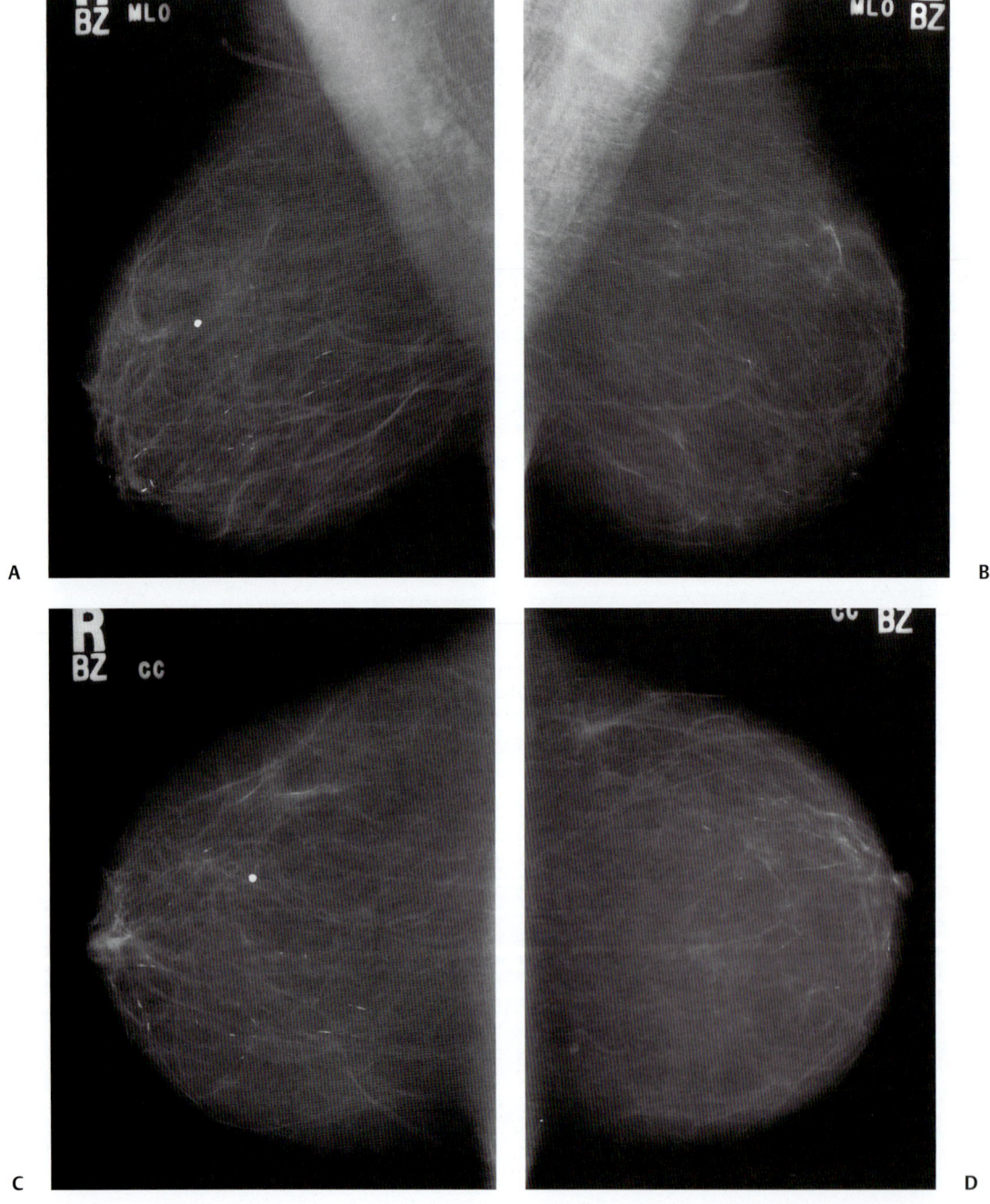

Fig. 30.18 There are benign calcifications in the right breast. Both breasts are predominantly fatty and normal in appearance. (**A**) Right MLO mammogram. (**B**) Left MLO mammogram. (**C**) Right CC mammogram. (**D**) Left CC mammogram.

Ultrasound

Frequency
- 13 MHz

Mass (Fig. 30.19)
- Margin: ill defined
- Echogenicity: hyperechoic
- Retrotumoral acoustic appearance: no shadowing
- Shape: irregular

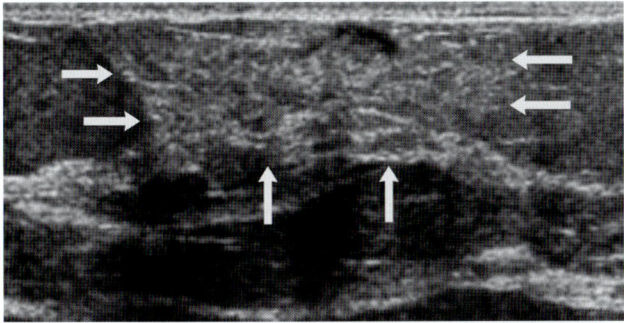

Fig. 30.19 Right antiradial breast sonogram. The palpable lump corresponds to a uniformly hyperechoic area (*arrows*). The superficial linear hypoechogenicity corresponded to a small vessel by color Doppler.

Pathology
- Fat necrosis

Management
- BI-RADS assessment category 3, probably benign; short-interval follow-up

Pearls and Pitfalls

- Homogeneous, circumscribed hyperechoic sonographic masses are generally benign. Differential diagnosis includes fat necrosis, fibrosis, hyalinized fibroadenomas, and angiolipomas. In this clinical setting, fat necrosis is the most likely etiology for the sonographic findings. The patient was not biopsied. She returned 1 month later, and the palpable lump and sonographic findings had decreased greatly in size.

Suggested Reading

Stavros AT, Thickman D, Rapp CL, Dennis MA, Parker SH, Sisney GA. Solid breast nodules: use of sonography to distinguish between benign and malignant lesions. Radiology 1995;196:123–134

Case 30.11: Fatty Mammogram—Infiltrating Ductal Carcinoma

Case History
- A 58-year-old woman presents with a palpable left breast lump.

Physical Examination
- Left breast: 1 cm soft nodule in the upper outer quadrant
- Right breast: normal exam

Mammogram

Mass (Fig. 30.20)
- Architectural distortion

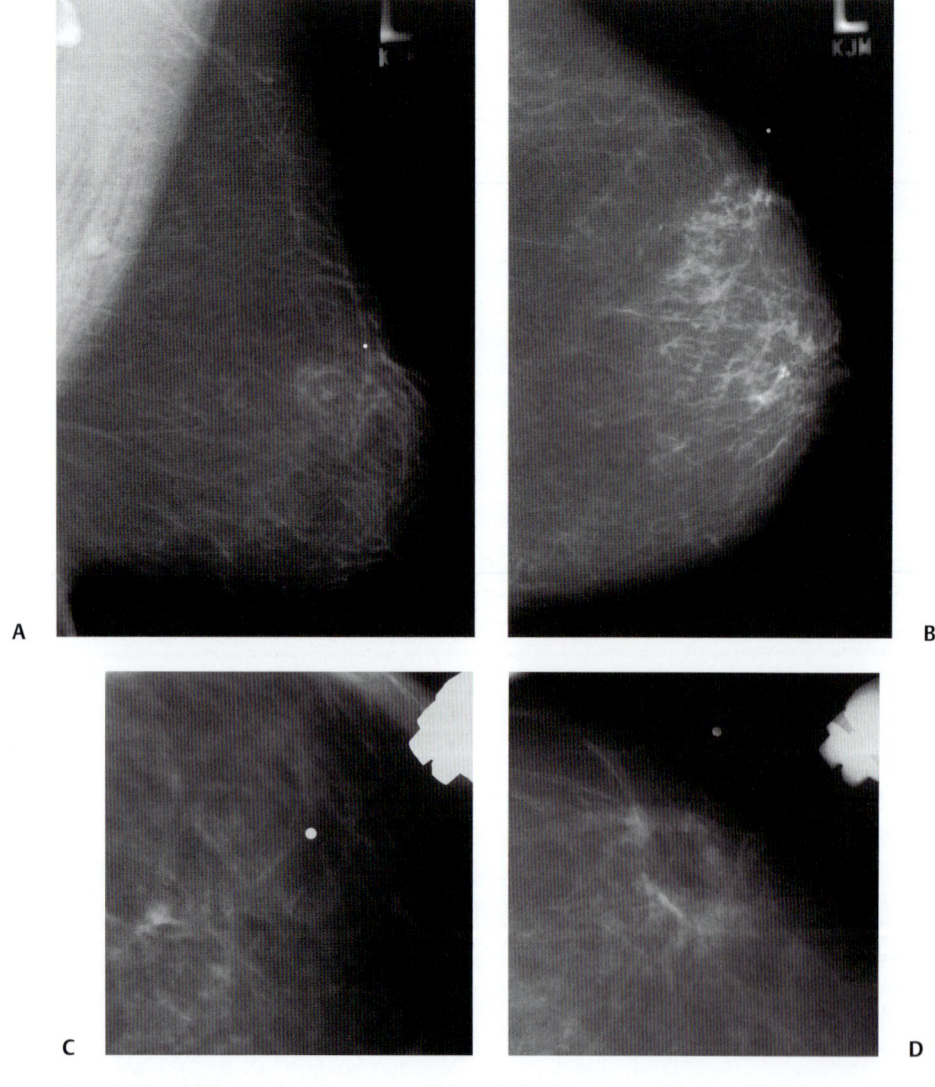

Fig. 30.20 Left breast mammograms. Although the breast is predominantly fatty in composition, no mass is associated with the radiographic marker. The marker identifies the location of a palpable lump. In the CC spot compression view, there is a subtle, small area of architectural distortion associated with the radiographic marker. (**A**) Left MLO mammogram. (**B**) Left CC mammogram. (**C**) Left MLO spot compression mammogram. (**D**) Left CC spot compression mammogram.

Ultrasound

Low Frequency

Frequency
- 7 MHz

Mass (Fig. 30.21)
- Margin: ill defined
- Echogenicity: hypoechoic
- Retrotumoral acoustic appearance: no shadowing
- Shape: oval with large lobulations

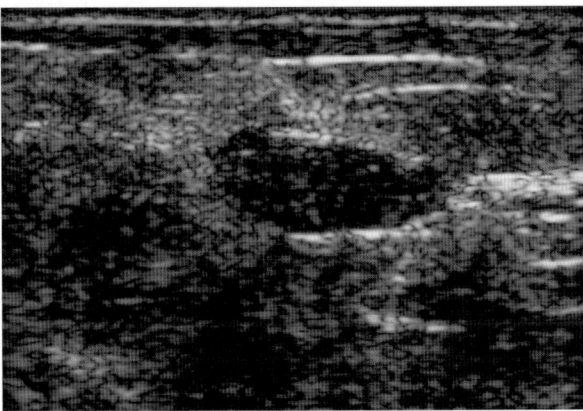

Fig. 30.21 Left breast antiradial sonogram. The palpable lump corresponds to a well-defined oval hypoechoic mass without posterior acoustic shadowing. Increased echogenicity superficial to the mass may be due to architectural distortion.

High Frequency

Frequency
- 11.5 MHz (**Fig. 30.22**)

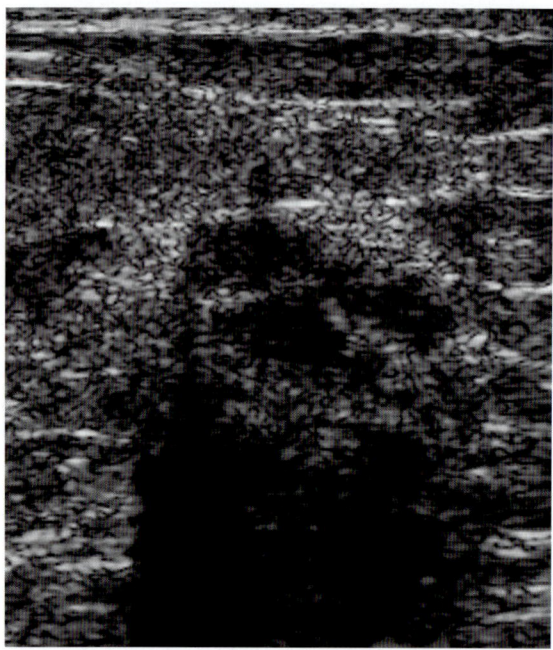

Fig. 30.22 Left breast antiradial sonogram. Higher-frequency sonographic examination of the same mass as in **Fig. 30.21** demonstrates more internal heterogeneous echogenicity compared with the lower-frequency examination. Furthermore, the higher-frequency examination demonstrates that the margin of the mass is ill defined, and there is diffuse posterior acoustic shadowing.

Pathology
- Infiltrating ductal carcinoma

Management
- BI-RADS assessment category 4, suspicious; biopsy should be considered.

Pearls and Pitfalls

- This case demonstrates that sonographic information is useful even in a predominantly fatty breast. The mammographic architectural distortion is subtle, but the sonographic exam clearly identifies a suspicious mass. This case also demonstrates that high-frequency sonography provides additional diagnostic information that improves diagnostic confidence. If one ignores or overlooks the anterior hyperechogenicity on the low-frequency exam, one may erroneously decide to characterize this mass as a probably benign lesion. However, the high-frequency study clearly demonstrates several malignant characteristics (i.e., ill-defined margin, heterogeneous echogenicity).

Suggested Reading
Stavros AT, Thickman D, Rapp CL, Dennis MA, Parker SH, Sisney GA. Solid breast nodules: use of sonography to distinguish between benign and malignant lesions. Radiology 1995;196:123–134

31 Mammogram Underestimates Tumor Size

Case 31.1: Mammogram Underestimates Tumor Size

Case History

A 69-year-old woman presents for screening mammogram.

Physical Examination
- Bilateral breast: multiple lumps

Mammogram

Calcifications (Fig. 31.1)
- Type: pleomorphic/heterogeneous
- Distribution: grouped/clustered

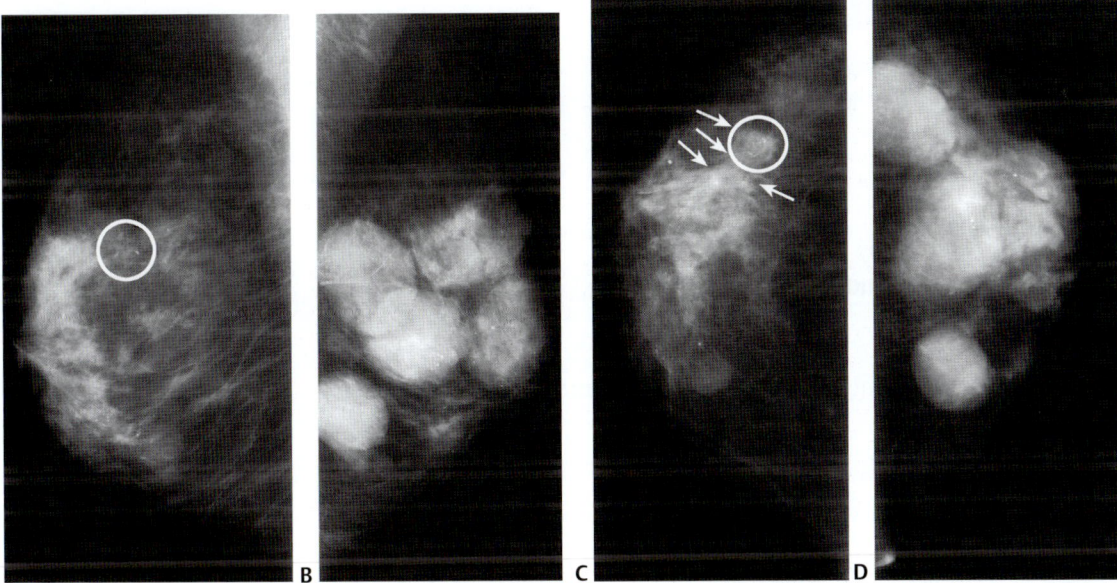
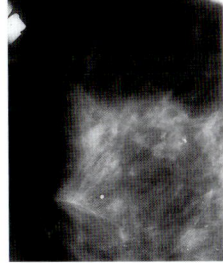

Fig. 31.1 The right breast has a cluster of heterogeneous calcifications (*circle*) in the upper outer breast. These calcifications are associated with architectural distortion in the CC view. The left breast has multiple round and oval masses that have been stable for several years. (**A**) Right MLO mammogram. (**B**) Left MLO mammogram. (**C**) Right CC mammogram. (**D**) Left CC mammogram. (**E**) Right ML spot magnification mammogram.

Ultrasound

Frequency
- 12 MHz

Mass (Fig. 31.2)
- Margin: ill defined
- Echogenicity: hypoechoic
- Retrotumoral acoustic appearance: posterior shadowing distal to mass
- Shape: irregular

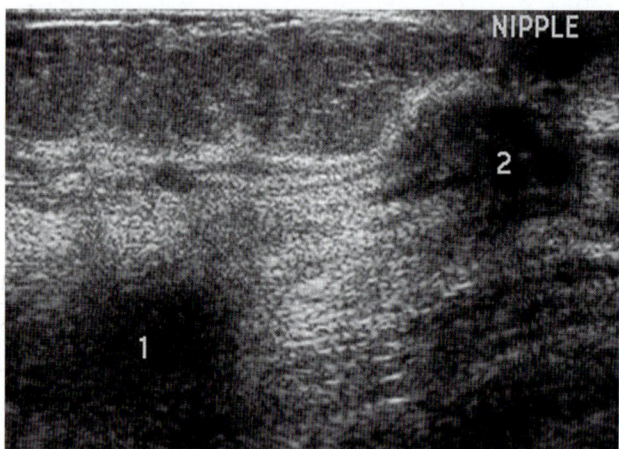

Fig. 31.2 Right radial breast sonogram. Two hypoechoic irregular masses are present. Mass 1 is in the upper outer quadrant, and mass 2 is next to the nipple.

Pathology
- Mixed ductal and lobular carcinoma
- Two separate foci of mixed ductal and lobular carcinoma

Management
- BI-RADS assessment category 5, highly suggestive of malignancy

Pearls and Pitfalls

- In this case, it was not clear if the architectural distortion was associated with the abnormal calcifications, as the distortion was visible in only one view. Furthermore, the architectural distortion appeared much larger than the area of the calcifications. Sonography may be helpful when there is a mammographic imaging discrepancy. In this case, the abnormal mammographic calcifications and architectural distortion correspond to multifocal disease.

Suggested Reading

Baker JA, Soo MS. The evolving role of sonography in evaluating solid breast masses. Semin Ultrasound CT MR 2000;21:286–296

Buchberger W, Niehoff A, Obrist P, DeKoekkoek-Doll P, Dünser M. Clinically and mammographically occult breast lesions: detection and classification with high-resolution sonography. Semin Ultrasound CT MR 2000;21:325–336

Case 31.2: Mammogram Underestimates Tumor Size

Case History
A 45-year-old woman presents with thickening in the right breast, which she thinks might be a pulled muscle.

Physical Examination
- Right breast: large, mildly tender firm area extending from the 9 o'clock to the 12 o'clock positions in the right breast
- Left breast: normal exam

Mammogram

Mass (Fig. 31.3)
- Margin: ill defined
- Shape: oval
- Density: isodense

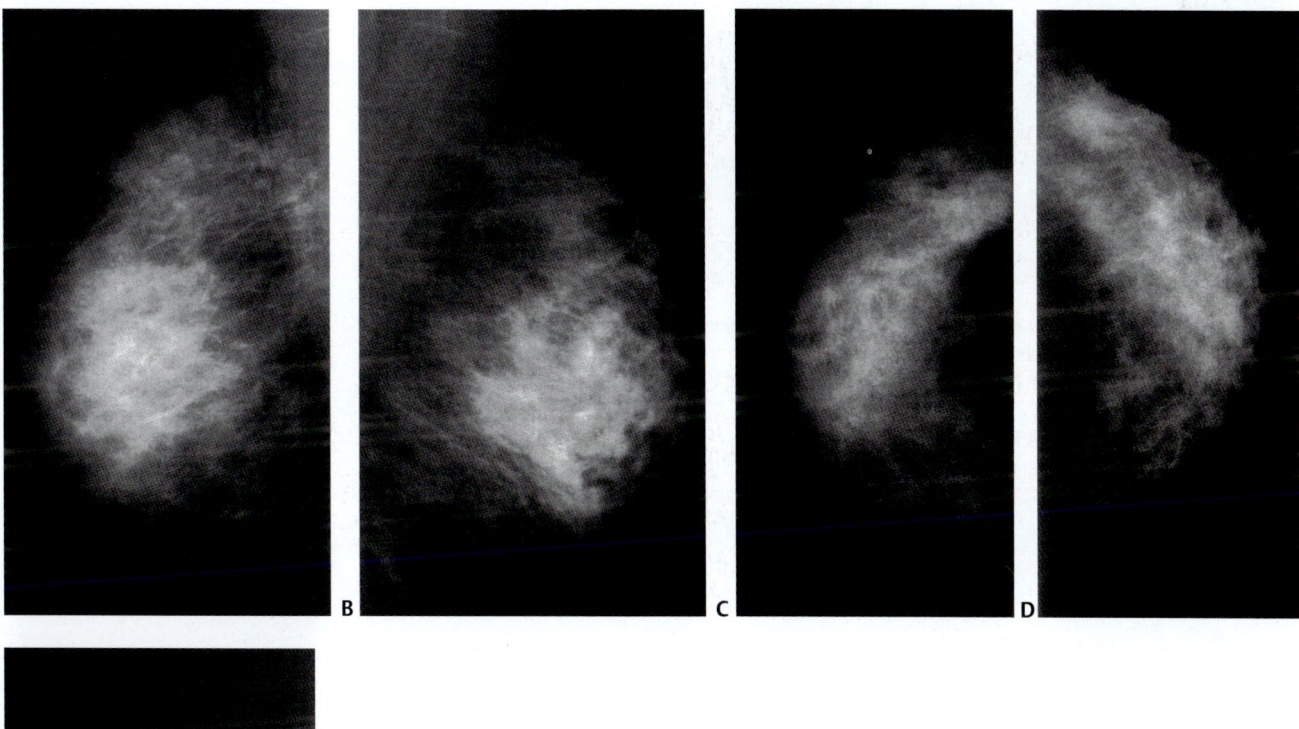

Fig. 31.3 There is an ill-defined mass in the right upper outer quadrant. The size of the mass is difficult to determine because of the surrounding heterogeneous parenchymal density. (**A**) Right MLO mammogram. (**B**) Left MLO mammogram. (**C**) Right CC mammogram. (**D**) Left CC mammogram. (**E**) Right MLO spot compression mammogram.

Ultrasound

Frequency
- 10 MHz

Mass (Fig. 31.4)
- Margin: ill defined
- Echogenicity: hypoechoic
- Retrotumoral acoustic appearance: extensive acoustic shadowing
- Shape: irregular

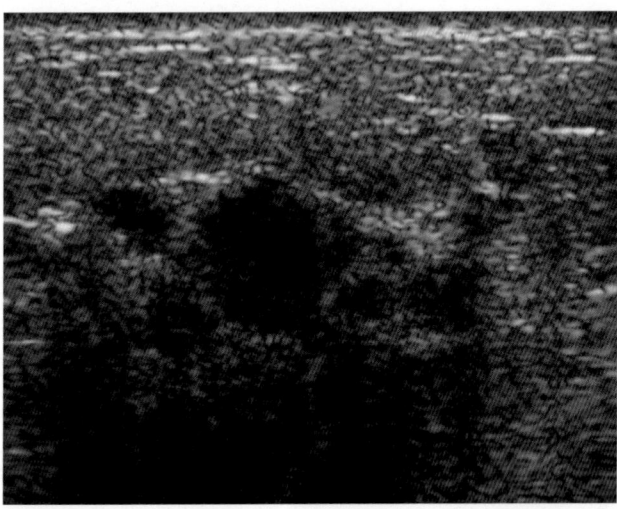

Fig. 31.4 Right radial breast sonogram. In the upper outer quadrant, there are several hypoechoic, ill-defined solid nodules.

Other Modalities (Fig. 31.5)

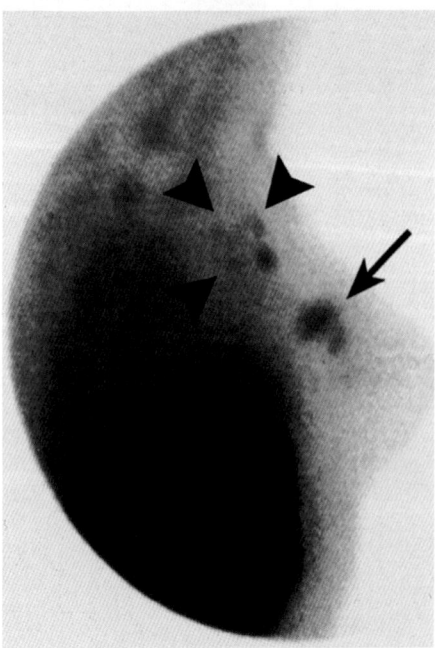

Fig. 31.5 Technetium 99m sestamibi scan. The exam shows abnormal increased uptake within the breast (*arrow*) and in axillary lymph nodes (*arrowheads*).

Pathology
- Infiltrating ductal carcinoma
- Stage IIB infiltrating ductal carcinoma with 9 of 13 nodes positive

Management
- BI-RADS assessment category 4, suspicious; biopsy should be considered.

Pearls and Pitfalls

- When the size or extent of a malignancy is not clear, ultrasound, MRI, and scintimammography can be helpful in determining the extent of tumors. In this case, scintimammography was useful, as it demonstrated malignant extension into the axillary nodes.

Suggested Reading

Klaus AJ, Klingensmith WC III, Parker SH, Stavros AT, Sutherland JD, Aldrete KD. Comparative value of 99mTc-sestamibi scintimammography and sonography in the diagnostic workup of breast masses. AJR Am J Roentgenol 2000;174:1779–1783

Palmedo H, Biersack HJ, Lastoria S, et al. Scintimammography with technetium-99m methoxyisobutylisonitrile: results of a prospective European multicentre trial. Eur J Nucl Med 1998;25:375–385

Waxman AD. The role of (99m)Tc methoxyisobutylisonitrile in imaging breast cancer. Semin Nucl Med 1997;27:40–54

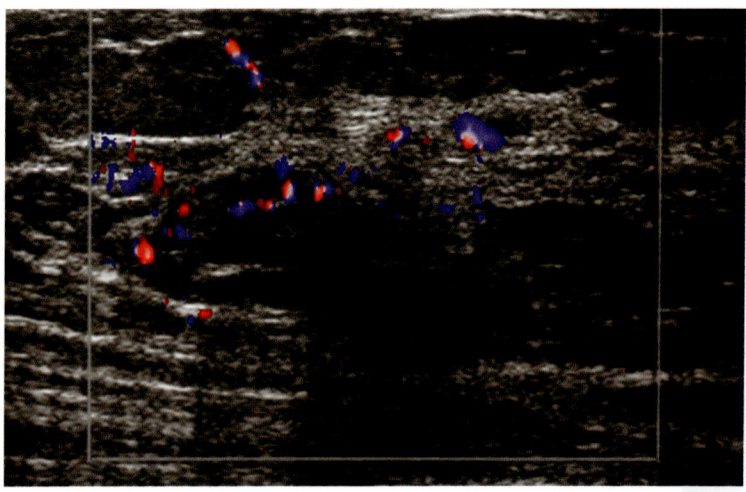

Fig. 31.9 Right upper outer quadrant radial color Doppler breast sonogram. This sonographic exam is performed to identify the right upper outer MRI mass. The segmental non-mass MRI enhancement corresponds to an area of subtly decreased echogenicity with increased color Doppler flow compared with the surrounding tissues. The patient refused sonographic biopsy and chose to have an MRI biopsy of this area.

Pathology
- Right mastectomy: 0.7 mm invasive ductal carcinoma surrounded with a large area of extensive intraductal component

Management
- BI-RADS assessment category 5, highly suggestive of malignancy

Pearls and Pitfalls
- Unlike invasive cancer, ductal carcinoma in situ (DCIS) commonly presents with a non-mass morphology, generally clumped with ductal or segmental distribution. DCIS that appears as a mammographic mass, more often, has a suspicious kinetic curve compared with those that present as mammographic calcifications. However, there is no correlation between kinetic enhancement curves and DCIS nuclear grade.
- This case illustrates that color Doppler may increase diagnostic confidence in cross-correlating subtle sonographic findings with the MRI abnormality.

Suggested Reading

Groves AM, Warren RML, Godward S, Rajan PS. Characterization of pure high-grade DCIS on magnetic resonance imaging using the evolving breast MR lexicon terminology: can it be differentiated from pure invasive disease? Magn Reson Imaging 2005;23:733–738

Jansen SA, Newstead GM, Abe H, Shimauchi A, Schmidt RA, Karczmar GS. Pure ductal carcinoma in situ: kinetic and morphologic MR characteristics compared with mammographic appearance and nuclear grade. Radiology 2007;245:684–691

Menell JH. Ductal carcinoma in situ. In: Morris EA, Liberman L, eds. Breast MRI Diagnosis and Intervention. New York: Springer; 2005:164–172

Raza S. DCIS. In: Berg WA, Birdwell RL, Gombos EC, Wang S-C, Parkinson BT, Raza S, Green GE, Kennedy A, Kettler MD, eds. Diagnostic Imaging Breast. Altona, Manitoba: Friesens; 2006: IV-2-106-121

Raza S. Clumped. In: Berg WA, Birdwell RL, Gombos EC, Wang S-C, Parkinson BT, Raza S, Green GE, Kennedy A, Kettler MD, eds. Diagnostic Imaging Breast. Altona, Manitoba: Friesens; 2006:IV-1-166-167

Rigauts H, Casselman J, Steyaert L, Devlies F, Pattyn G. Contribution of MRI and color Doppler sonography in breast cancer diagnosis. J Belge Radiol 1993;76:226–231

Rosen EL, Smith-Foley SA, DeMartini WB, Eby PR, Peacock S, Lehman CD. BI-RADS MRI enhancement characteristics of ductal carcinoma in situ. Breast J 2007;13:545–550

32 Mass in Unusual Locations

Case 32.1: Mass in Unusual Locations

Case History
A 42-year-old woman presents with a small, superficial left breast lump.

Physical Examination
- Left breast: a soft, superficial lump at the 12 o'clock position
- Right breast: normal exam

Ultrasound

Frequency
- 10 MHz

Mass (Fig. 32.1)
- Margin: ill defined
- Echogenicity: heterogeneous
- Retrotumoral acoustic appearance: posterior shadowing distal to mass
- Shape: ellipsoid

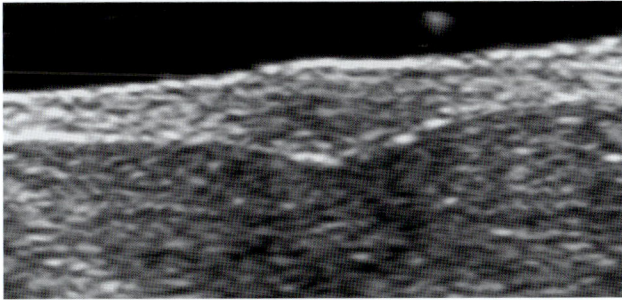

Fig. 32.1 Left antiradial breast sonogram. The palpable lump corresponds to an ill-defined oval mass with heterogeneous echogenicity that is within the skin.

Pathology
- Smooth muscle hamartoma

Management
- BI-RADS assessment category 3, probably benign; short-interval follow-up

Pearls and Pitfalls

- Sonography is useful to identify superficial palpable masses. If additional mammographic imaging is needed, then a radiopaque dot may be placed over the sonographic mass, and tangential mammographic views may be performed.

Suggested Reading
Ragsdale BD. Tumors of fatty, muscular, and osseous tissue. In: Elder D, ed. Histolopathology of the Skin. Philadelphia: Lippincott-Raven, 1997:933–975

Case 32.2: Mass in Unusual Locations

Case History
A 40-year-old woman presents with a palpable right breast lump.

Physical Examination
- Right breast: skin dimpling associated with irregular mass, which is fixed to the chest wall at the 4 o'clock position in the inframammary fold
- Left breast: normal exam

Mammogram

Mass (Fig. 32.2)
- Margin: indistinct
- Shape: focal asymmetric density
- Density: high density

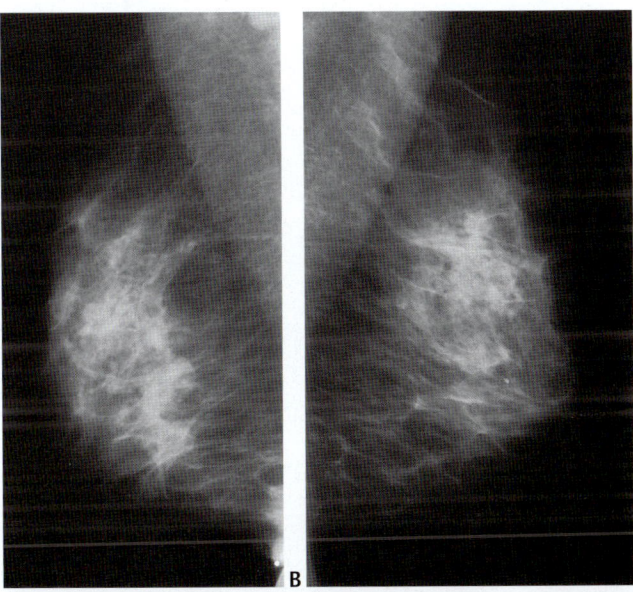
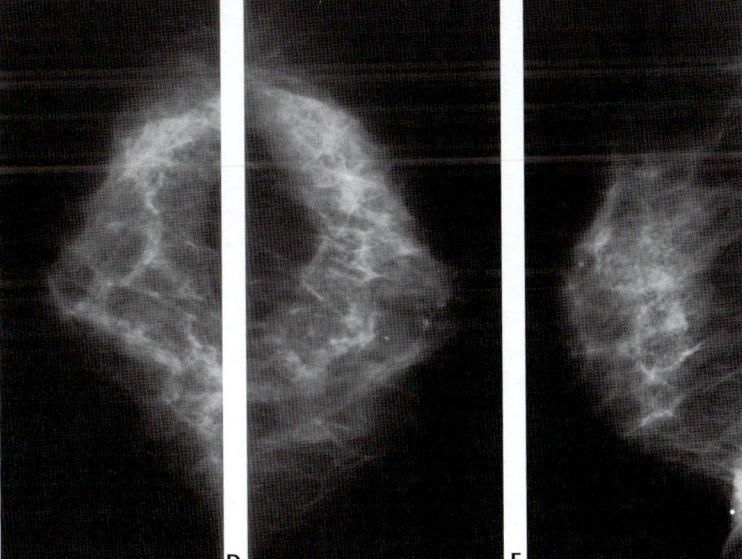

Fig. 32.2 In the right inframammary fold (**A,E**), there is skin thickening and focal ill-defined density. (**A**) Right MLO mammogram. (**B**) Left MLO mammogram. (**C**) Right CC mammogram. (**D**) Left CC mammogram. (**E**) Right ML mammogram.

Ultrasound

Frequency
- 7.5 MHz

Mass (Fig. 32.3)
- Margin: ill defined
- Echogenicity: hypoechoic
- Retrotumoral acoustic appearance: severe shadowing, mass completely obscured
- Shape: irregular

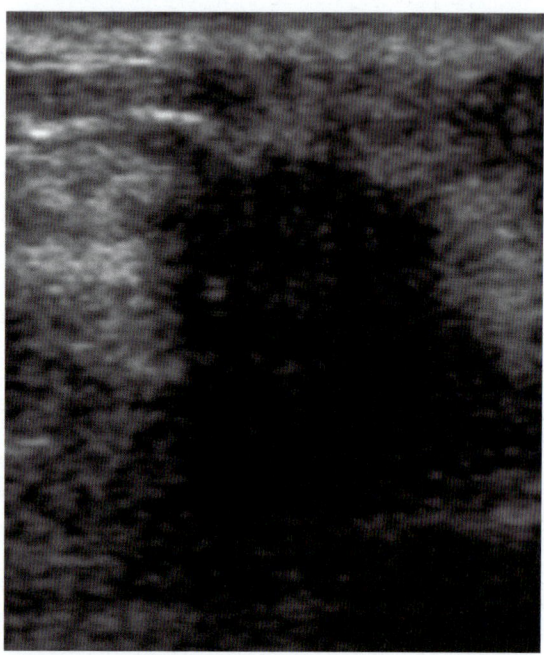

Fig. 32.3 Right antiradial breast sonogram. The palpable mass corresponds to an irregular, hypoechoic, heavily shadowing mass. Superficially, there is extension of the spiculations into the skin.

Pathology
- Infiltrating ductal carcinoma
- Tumor infiltrated into dermis

Management
- BI-RADS assessment category 5, highly suggestive of malignancy

> **Pearls and Pitfalls**
>
> - This is an example of an unusual location for tumor. When masses are in the extreme periphery of the breast (e.g., inframammary fold, peripheral axilla), they are commonly a greater challenge to image mammographically. Optimal imaging is also dependent on the body habitus and flexibility of the patient. In these cases, sonography is useful to assist characterization of the lesion and provide guidance for biopsy.

Suggested Reading

American College of Radiology Committee on Quality Assurance in Mammography. Mammography Quality Control Manual. Reston: ACR; 1999

Jackson VP. Breast sonography. In: Bassett LW, Jackson VP, Jahan R, Fu YS, Gold RH, eds. Diagnosis of the Diseases of the Breast. Philadelphia: WB Saunders; 1997:185–196

33 Ductal Abnormalities

Case 33.1: Intraductal Papilloma

Case History
A 46-year-old woman presents with right nipple discharge.

Physical Examination
- Right breast: clear discharge expressed from nipple
- Left breast: normal exam, no discharge

Mammogram (Fig. 33.1)

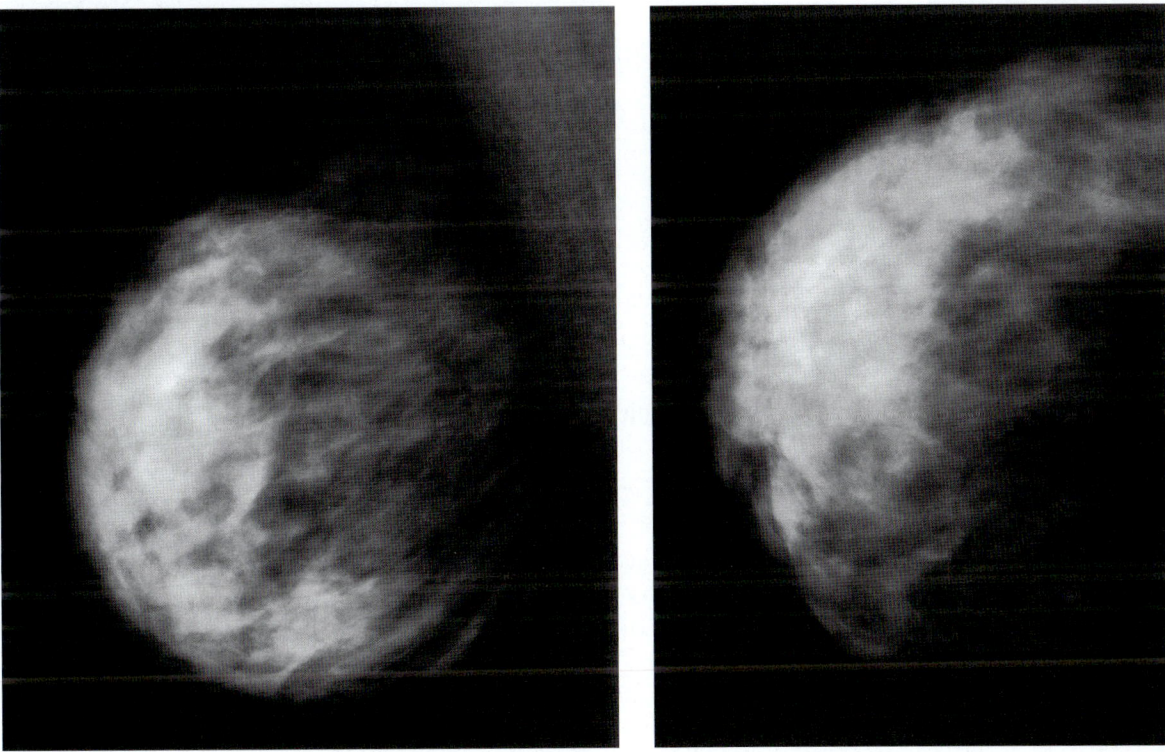

Fig. 33.1 Normal heterogeneously dense right breast. (**A**) Right MLO mammogram. (**B**) Right CC mammogram.

Ultrasound

Frequency
- 13 MHz

Mass (Figs. 33.2 and 33.3)
- Echogenicity: hypoechoic
- Retrotumoral acoustic appearance: no shadowing
- Shape: ellipsoid

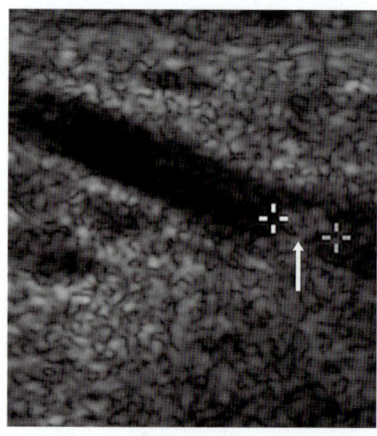

Fig. 33.2 Right radial breast sonogram. At the 6 o'clock position of the nipple, there is a dilated duct. Within the duct is a small, solid, hypoechoic mass (*arrow*).

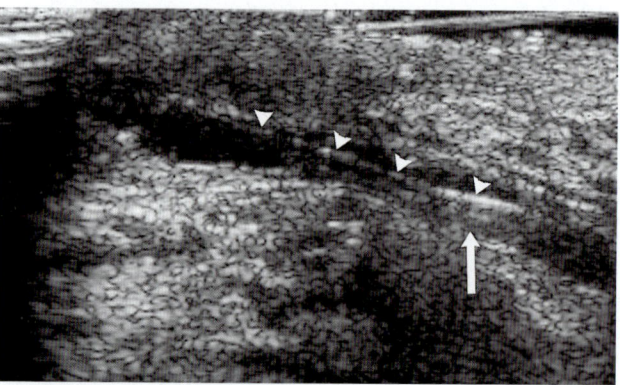

Fig. 33.3 Right radial breast sonogram. Sonography was used intraoperatively to identify the dilated duct demonstrated in **Fig. 33.2**. The surgeon inserted a wire into the nipple. With real-time sonography, the wire (*arrowheads*) was demonstrated within the abnormal duct touching the intraductal mass (*arrow*).

Pathology
- Benign papilloma

Management
- BI-RADS assessment category 4, suspicious; biopsy should be considered.

Pearls and Pitfalls

- Although ductography is the usual method to evaluate ducts, high-frequency sonography may be used to systematically evaluate ducts around the nipple. The operator places one end of the transducer at the nipple and rotates the transducer around the nipple. The ducts are demonstrated in a radial orientation, so they appear as linear anechoic fluid collections. In patients with abnormal nipple discharge, sonographic findings that suggest a focal etiology of the discharge include one or a few dilated ducts within the same quadrant, an intraductal or intracystic solid mass, or a solid mass near the nipple not associated with fluid. If no ducts or masses are identified or if all the ducts are dilated, then ductography is necessary to further evaluate the ducts.

Suggested Reading
Sardanelli F, Imperiale A, Zandrino F, et al. Breast intraductal masses: US-guided fine-needle aspiration after galactography. Radiology 1997;204:143–148

Case 33.2: Intraductal Papilloma

Case History
A 71-year-old woman presents with left bloody nipple discharge.

Physical Examination
- Left breast: small clear, yellow discharge from a duct at the 3 o'clock position; no bloody discharge observed
- Right breast: normal exam

Mammogram (Figs. 33.4 and 33.5)

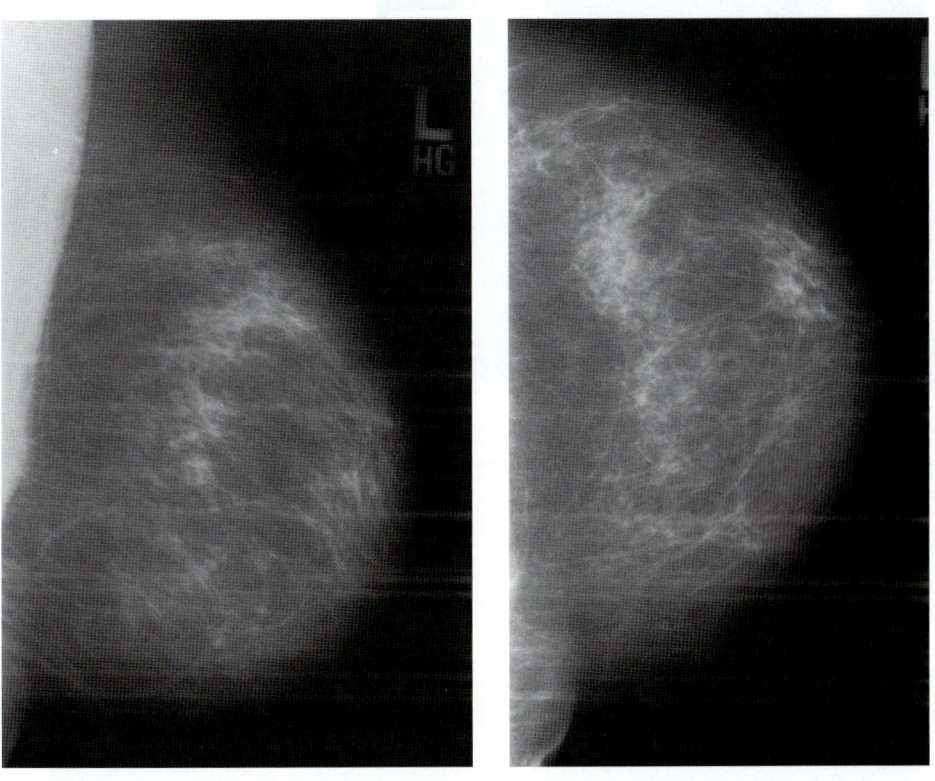

Fig. 33.4 Normal left breast mammogram. (**A**) Left MLO mammogram. (**B**) Left CC mammogram.

Ultrasound

Frequency
- 13 MHz

Mass (Fig. 33.7)
- Margin: well defined
- Echogenicity: hypoechoic
- Retrotumoral acoustic appearance: no shadowing
- Shape: ellipsoid

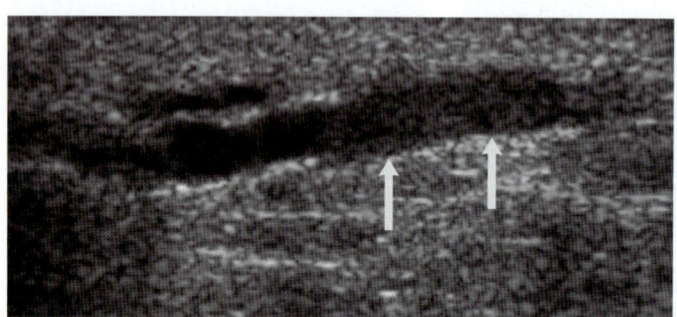
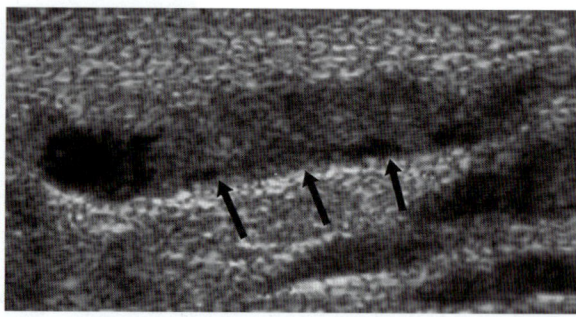
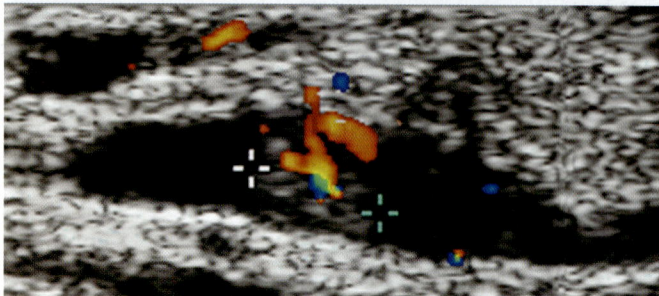

Fig. 33.7 At the 4 o'clock position of the left breast, there is a dilated duct containing a hypoechoic sausage-shaped solid mass (*arrows*). (**A**) Left radial breast sonogram. (**B**) Left radial breast sonogram: close-up image of the mass (*arrows*). (**C**) Left oblique color Doppler breast sonogram. Color Doppler demonstrates vessels within the mass.

Pathology
- Ductal carcinoma in situ

Management
- BI-RADS assessment category 4, suspicious; biopsy should be considered.

Pearls and Pitfalls

- When sonography is performed for bloody discharge, dilatation of one or a few ducts in one quadrant is a serious finding. If no intraductal mass is identified, and the surgeon opts for more imaging, then ductography should be performed. However, if sonographic intraductal or intracystic mass is identified, then biopsy or excision should be recommended.

Suggested Reading

Chung SY, Lee KW, Park KS, Lee Y, Bae SH. Breast tumors associated with nipple discharge: correlation of findings on galactography and sonography. Clin Imaging 1995;19:165–171

Hashimoto BE, Kramer DJ, Picozzi VJ. High detection rate of breast ductal carcinoma in situ calcifications on mammographically directed high-resolution sonography. J Ultrasound Med 2001;20:501–508

Satake H, Shimamoto K, Sawaki A, et al. Role of ultrasonography in the detection of intraductal spread of breast cancer: correlation with pathologic findings, mammography and MR imaging. Eur Radiol 2000;10:1726–1732

Case 33.4: Ductal Carcinoma in Situ—Intraductal Mass

Case History
An 80-year-old woman presents with left bloody discharge.

Physical Examination
- Left breast: bloody discharge from duct at the 5 o'clock position; otherwise normal exam
- Right breast: normal exam

Mammogram (Figs. 33.8 and 33.9)

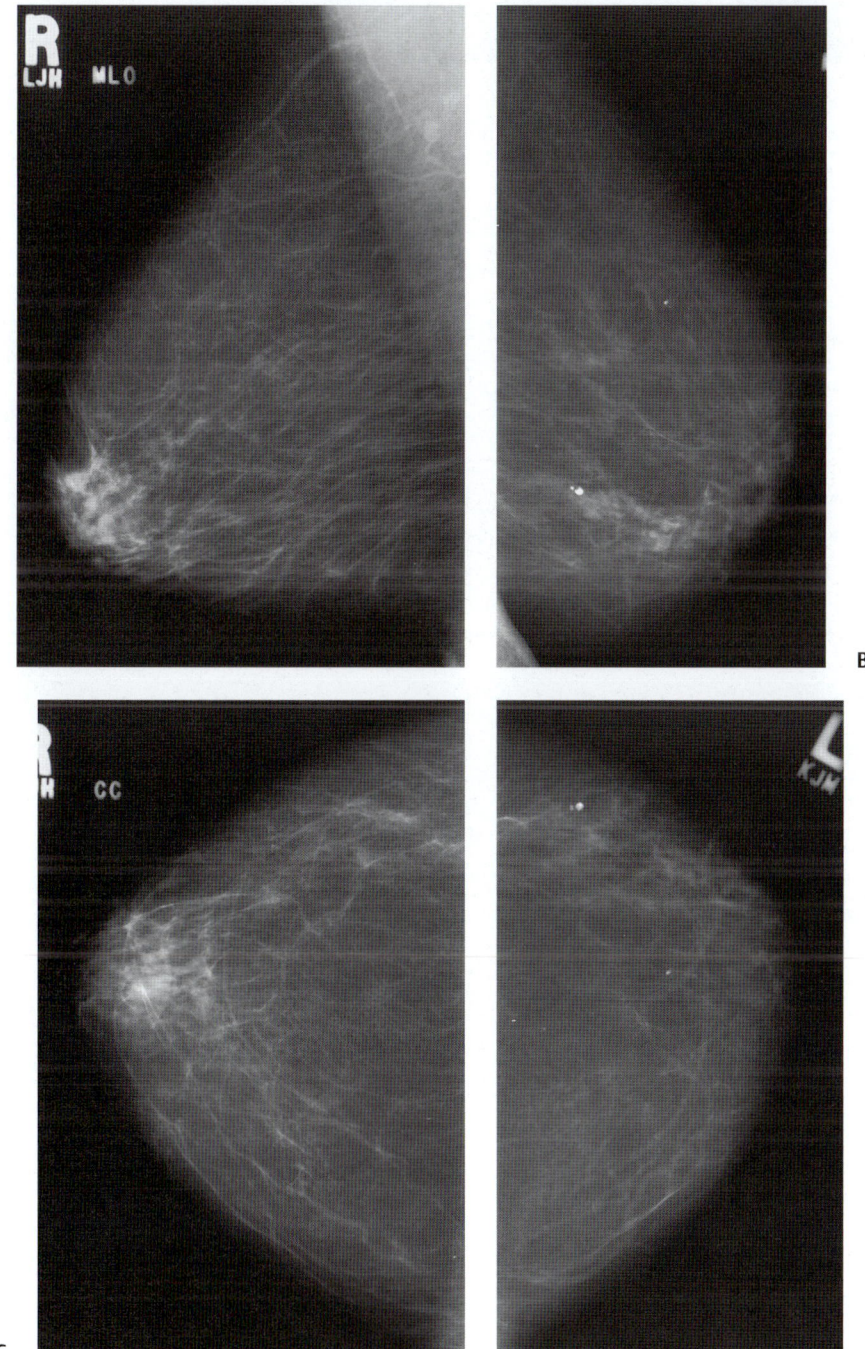

Fig. 33.8 Left breast has prominent ducts in the inferior outer breast. (**A**) Right MLO mammogram. (**B**) Left lateral medial (LM) mammogram. (**C**) Right CC mammogram. (**D**) Left CC mammogram.

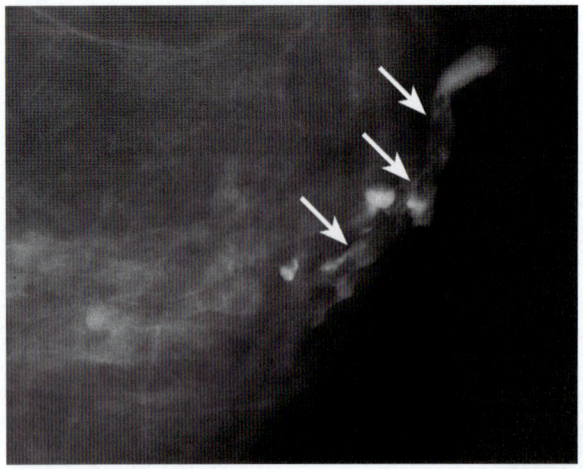 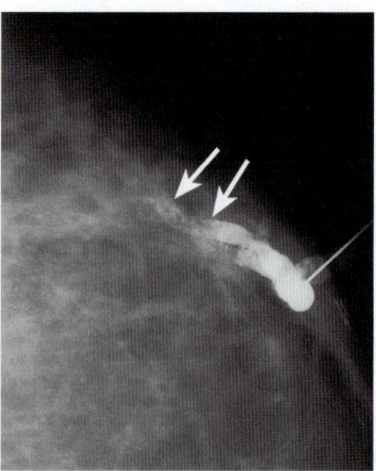

Fig. 33.9 Left breast ductogram. The contrast was injected into the duct at the 5 o'clock position. The duct contains multiple filling defects (*arrows*) associated with contour irregularities. (**A**) Left ML breast ductogram. (**B**) Left CC breast ductogram.

Pathology
- Ductal carcinoma in situ

Management
- BI-RADS assessment category 4, suspicious; biopsy should be considered.

Pearls and Pitfalls

- Between 5 and 15% of intraluminal masses with ductography are due to malignancy.
- Findings of malignancy on ductography include (1) intraluminal filling defects, (2) duct contour irregularity, (3) abrupt duct cutoff, (4) duct displaced or draped around a mass, and (5) duct extravasation. Numerous intraluminal masses and extensive contour irregularity have a higher association with malignancy.

Suggested Reading

Cardenosa G. Ductography. In: Cardenosa G. Breast Imaging Companion. Philadelphia: Lippincott-Raven; 1997:372–383

Dinkel HP, Trusen A, Gassel AM, et al. Predictive value of galactographic patterns for benign and malignant neoplasms of the breast in patients with nipple discharge. Br J Radiol 2000;73:706–714

Van Zee KJ, Ortega Pérez G, Minnard E, Cohen MA. Preoperative galactography increases the diagnostic yield of major duct excision for nipple discharge. Cancer 1998;82:1874–1880

Case 33.5: Ductal Carcinoma in Situ—Thick Wall Ducts

Case History
An 80-year-old woman presents with left milky discharge.

Physical Examination
- Left breast: milky discharge; otherwise normal exam
- Right breast: normal exam

Mammogram (Fig. 33.10)

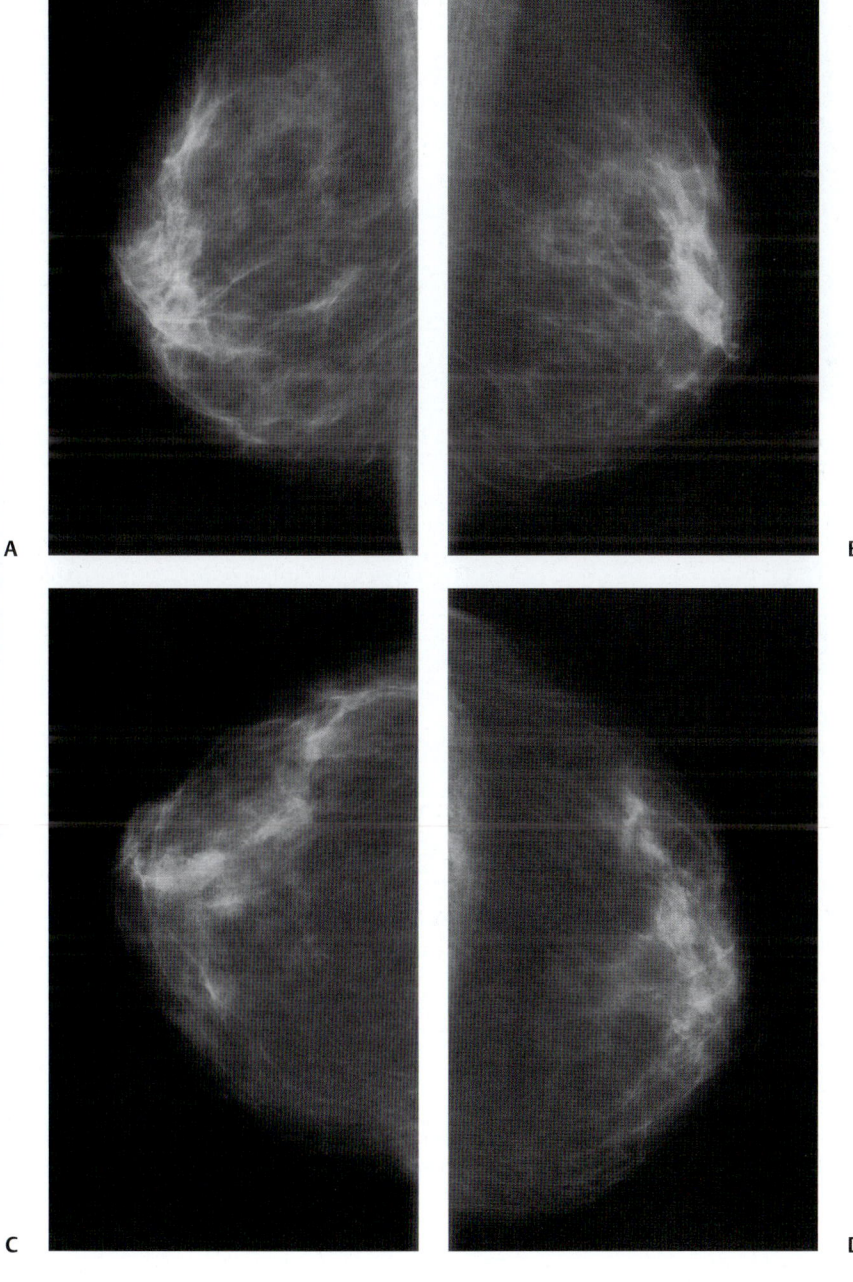

Fig. 33.10 Normal bilateral mammograms with scattered fibroglandular densities. (**A**) Right MLO mammogram. (**B**) Left MLO mammogram. (**C**) Right CC mammogram. (**D**) Left CC mammogram.

Ultrasound

Frequency
- 11.5 MHz (**Figs. 33.11** and **33.12**)

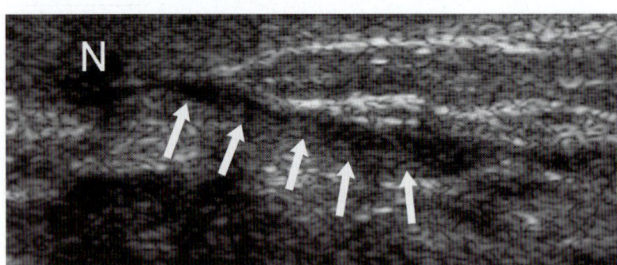
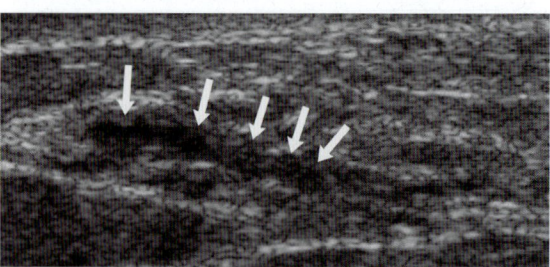

Fig. 33.11 There were multiple thick-walled ducts in the left upper outer quadrant, which were irregular in caliber and contour (*arrows*). Ducts in the other quadrants appeared normal. N, nipple. (**A**) Left radial breast sonogram. (**B**) Left radial breast sonogram.

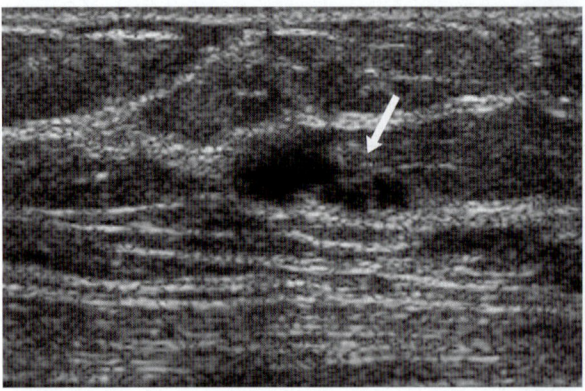

Fig. 33.12 Left antiradial breast sonogram. A cross section of one abnormal duct demonstrates some asymmetric thickening on one wall (*arrow*).

Pathology
- Ductal carcinoma in situ
- 6 cm of high-grade ductal carcinoma in situ in the left upper outer quadrant

Management
- BI-RADS assessment category 4, suspicious; biopsy should be considered.

Pearls and Pitfalls

- Sonographically, ductal carcinoma in situ may appear as (1) isolated calcifications, (2) an irregular hypoechoic mass (with or without calcifications), (3) an ill-defined hypoechoic area, or (4) abnormally focally dilated ducts. The dilated ducts may be single or multiple but are grouped together in a segment or quadrant. The ducts may contain calcifications, hypoechoic debris, or focal masses. In this case, the malignancy appears as an irregular thickening of the ductal walls. Rarely, invasive ductal carcinoma is identified as a dilated duct.

Suggested Reading

Tohno D, Cosgrove DO, Sloane JP, eds. Malignant disease: primary carcinomas. In: Tohno D, Cosgrove DO, Sloane JP, eds. Ultrasound Diagnosis of Breast Diseases. New York: Churchill Livingstone; 1994:157–180

Yang WT, King W, Metreweli C. Clinically and mammographically occult invasive ductal carcinoma diagnosed by ultrasound: the focally dilated duct. Australas Radiol 1997;41:73–75

34 Mammographically Occult MRI Lesions

Case 34.1: Benign MRI Mass

Case History

A 56-year-old woman, status post–left lumpectomy, which was done at another institution, is seeking a second opinion. Microscopic examination suggests that the margins of the invasive malignancy are close to the surgical margins, so breast MRI is performed.

Physical Examination
- Left breast: healing lumpectomy site
- Right breast: normal

Other Modalities: MRI (Fig. 34.1)

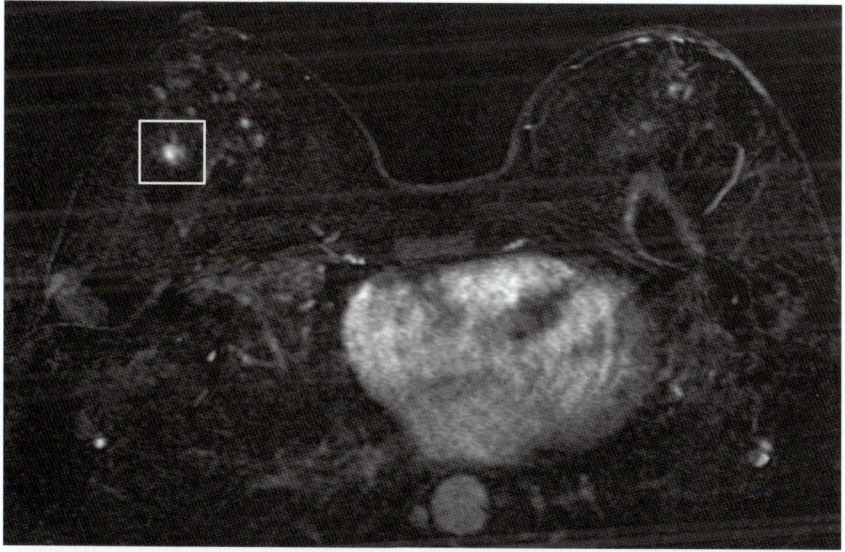

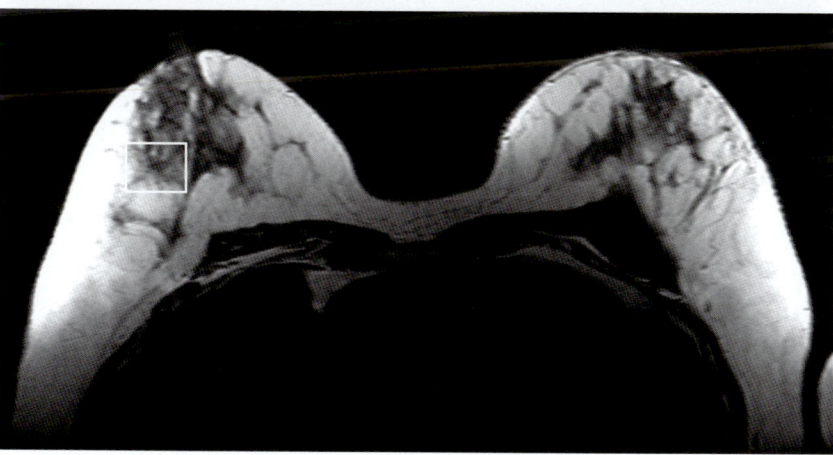

Fig. 34.1 After contrast injection, there is no abnormal enhancement associated with the rim of the left lumpectomy cavity. However, in the right upper outer quadrant, there is a 7 mm irregular, rapidly enhancing mass that appears as a spiculated solid mass on the T1 image, which does not have fat suppression (*square*). (**A**) Dynamic bolus T1-weighted, 2-minute subtraction axial bilateral breast MRI. (**B**) T1-weighted axial bilateral breast MRI.

Pathology
- Left breast: reexcision of the lumpectomy cavity; no residual malignancy
- Right breast: radial scar

Management
- Right MRI enhancing mass: BI-RADS assessment category 4, suspicious; biopsy should be considered.

Pearls and Pitfalls
- Radial scars that are surrounded by fat appear as solid spiculated masses on T1-weighted images that are not fat suppressed. With contrast, radial scars exhibit variable enhancement characteristics; they may or may not enhance. If they enhance, then they appear as highly suspicious spiculated masses on T1 fat-suppressed images. Small series do not appear to identify characteristics that differentiate benign radial scars from those associated with malignancy. Therefore, once identified, these lesions should be completely excised.

Suggested Reading

Berg WA. Radial scar. In: Berg WA, Birdwell RL, Gombos EC, Wang S-C, Parkinson BT, Raza S, Green GE, Kennedy A, Kettler MD, eds. Diagnostic Imaging Breast. Altona, Manitoba: Friesens; 2006:IV-2-84-89

Nunes LW, Schnall MD, Orel SG, et al. Correlation of lesion appearance and histologic findings for the nodes of a breast MR imaging interpretation model. Radiographics 1999;19:79–92

Pediconi F, Occhiato R, Venditti F, et al. Radial scars of the breast: contrast-enhanced magnetic resonance mammography appearance. Breast J 2005;11:23–28

Case 34.2: Malignant MRI Mass

Case History
A 51-year-old woman presents for screening MRI. She has the *BRCA1* gene. She had right breast cancer 14 years prior and left breast cancer 15 years prior. She is status post–bilateral lumpectomy, radiation therapy, and axillary dissections. Her previous breast MRI (1 year prior) and bilateral mammograms (8 months prior) were negative.

Physical Examination
- Normal exam

Mammogram (Fig. 34.2)
- Normal exam

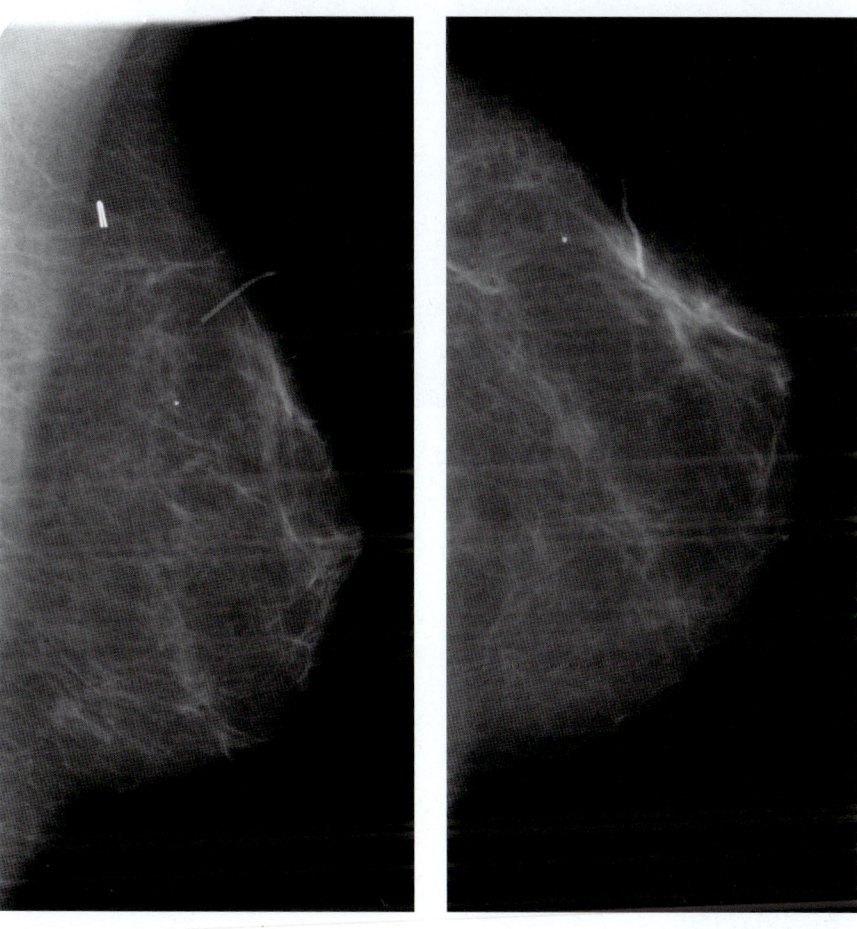

Fig. 34.2 The patient has a lumpectomy scar in the left upper outer quadrant. (**A**) Left MLO mammogram. (**B**) Left CC mammogram.

Other Modalities: MRI and Second Look Sonography (Figs. 34.3 and 34.4)

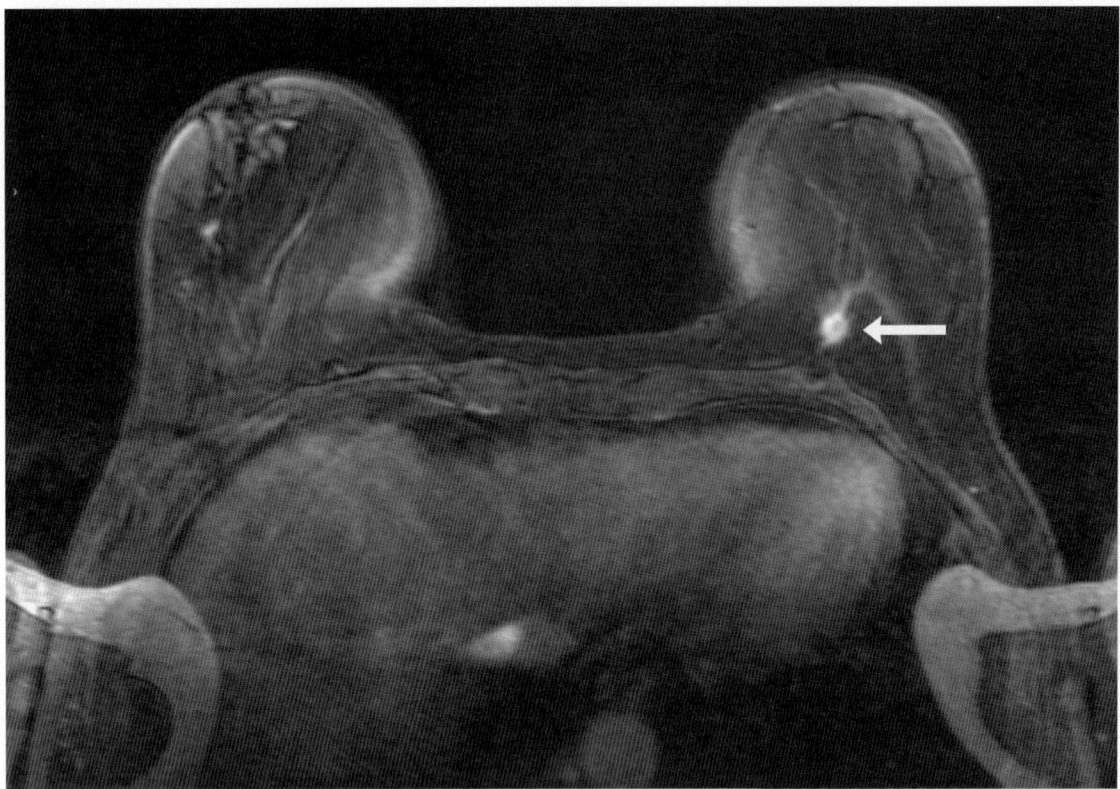

Fig. 34.3 Bilateral contrast-enhanced axial breast high-resolution MRI, delayed image. At the 7 o'clock position of the left breast, there is a new enhancing oval mass (*arrow*).

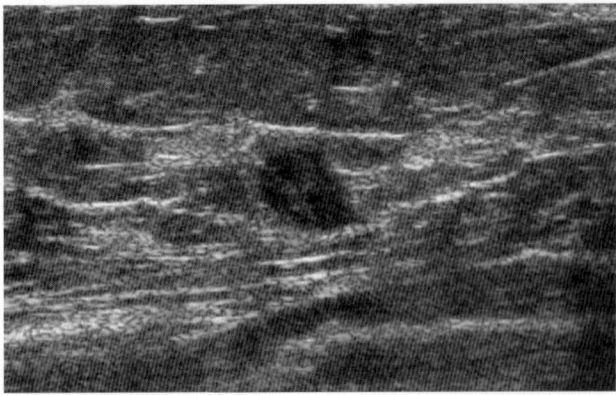

Fig. 34.4 Left radial breast sonogram at the 7 o'clock position. This sonogram was performed as a result of the abnormal screening MRI. There is an oval hypoechoic solid mass, which corresponds to the screening MRI mass.

Pathology
- Infiltrating ductal carcinoma, grade 3

Management
- Left breast MRI enhancing mass: BI-RADS assessment category 4, suspicious; biopsy should be considered.

Pearls and Pitfalls

- *BRCA1* and *BRCA2*, genes that normally suppress cell growth, are on chromosomes 17 and 13, respectively. Patients with mutated *BRCA1* and *BRCA2* genes have a higher risk of breast, ovarian, and prostate cancer. The prevalence of *BRCA1* in women with breast cancer is 5.3% in patients younger than 40 years, 2.2% between ages 40 and 49 years, and 1.1% between ages 50 and 70 years. The lifetime risk of breast cancer in patients with *BRCA1* or *BRCA2* is 85%.
- The American Cancer Society has recommended MRI screening for patients with a lifetime risk greater than 20 to 25%. This recommendation is based on the results of multiple screening studies, which have found that for high-risk women, MRI has a higher sensitivity than mammography (77–100% vs 16–40%). MRI specificities are slightly lower than mammography in this group (81–99% vs 93–99%). Besides women with *BRCA1* and *BRCA2*, women who have received chest radiation therapy treatment for Hodgkin's disease should also be screened by MRI. Other possible screening candidates are women with increased risk due to strong personal and family history.
- Patients with *BRCA1* and *BRCA2* have a greater risk of high-grade carcinoma, which commonly appears as enhancing oval or lobulated masses on MRI and sonographically simulate complex cysts (oval or lobulated, mildly hypoechoic with increased acoustic transmission) or appear similar to fibroadenomas. Therefore, biopsy should not be deferred if a new sonographic benign-appearing mass is detected in a patient with elevated genetic breast cancer risk.

Suggested Reading

Causer PA, Jong RA, Warner E, et al. Breast cancers detected with imaging screening in the *BRCA* population: emphasis on MR imaging with histopathologic correlation. Radiographics 2007;27(Suppl 1):S165–S182

Lee JM, Kopans DB, McMahon PM, et al. Breast cancer screening in *BRCA1* mutation carriers: effectiveness of MR imaging—Markov Monte Carlo decision analysis. Radiology 2008; 246:763–771

Lehman CD, Isaacs C, Schnall MD, et al. Cancer yield of mammography, MR, and US in high-risk women: prospective multi-institution breast cancer screening study. Radiology 2007;244:381–388

Lynch HT, Lemon SJ, Marcus JN, Lehman C, Lynch J, Narod S. Breast cancer genetics: heterogeneity, molecular genetics, syndrome diagnosis, and genetic counseling. In: Bland KI, Copeland EM, eds. The Breast. 2nd ed. Philadelphia: WB Saunders; 1998:370-394

Riedl CC, Ponhold L, Flöry D, et al. Magnetic resonance imaging of the breast improves detection of invasive cancer, preinvasive cancer, and premalignant lesions during surveillance of women at high risk for breast cancer. Clin Cancer Res 2007;13):6144–6152

Saslow D, Boetes C, Burke W, et al. American Cancer Society Breast Cancer Advisory Group. American Cancer Society guidelines for breast screening with MRI as an adjunct to mammography. CA Cancer J Clin 2007;57:75–89

Schrading S, Kuhl CK. Mammographic, US, and MR imaging phenotypes of familial breast cancer. Radiology 2008;246:58–70

Stavros AT. Ultrasound of solid breast nodules: distinguishing benign from malignant. In: Stavros AT, Breast Ultrasound. Philadelphia: Lippincott Williams & Wilkins; 2004:445-527

Willey SC, Cocilovo C. Screening and follow-up of the patient at high risk for breast cancer. Obstet Gynecol 2007;110:1404–1416

Case 34.3: Malignant MRI Mass

Case History
An 81-year-woman presents for screening mammography.

Physical Examination
- Normal examination

Mammogram

Mass (Fig. 34.5)
- Margin: spiculated
- Shape: irregular
- Density: high

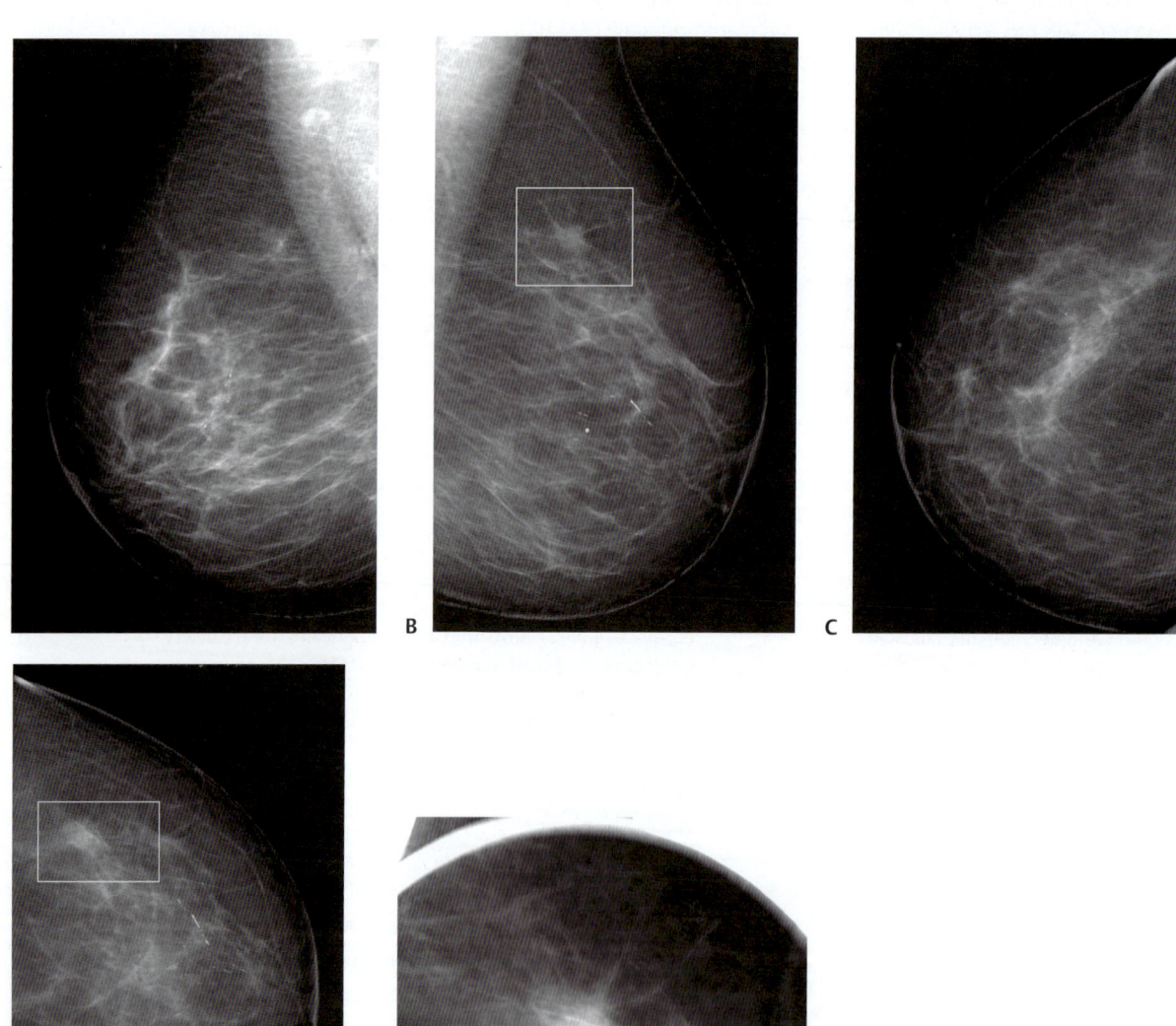

Fig. 34.5 In the left upper outer quadrant, there is a spiculated mass (*square*). (**A**) Right MLO mammogram. (**B**) Left MLO mammogram. (**C**) Right CC mammogram. (**D**) Left CC mammogram. (**E**) Left CC spot compression mammogram.

Ultrasound

Frequency (Fig. 34.6)
- 14 MHz

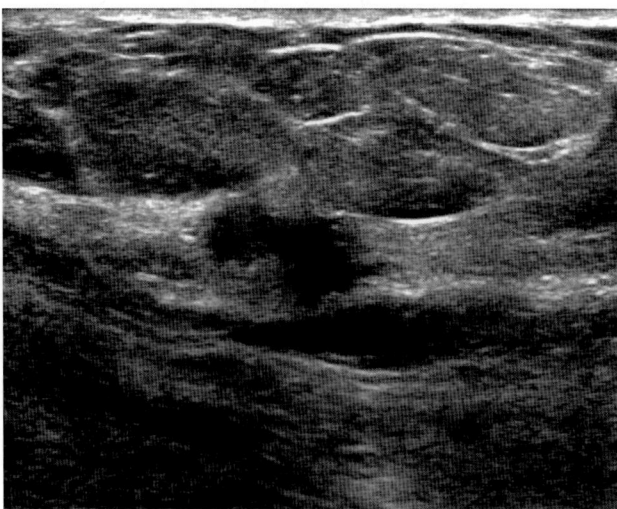

Fig. 34.6 Left radial sonogram. In the upper outer quadrant, there is a solid, hypoechoic, irregular solid mass with a hyperechoic haze and spiculations, which corresponds to the left mammographic spiculated mass.

Other Modalities: MRI and Second Look Sonography (Figs. 34.7, 34.8, and 34.9)

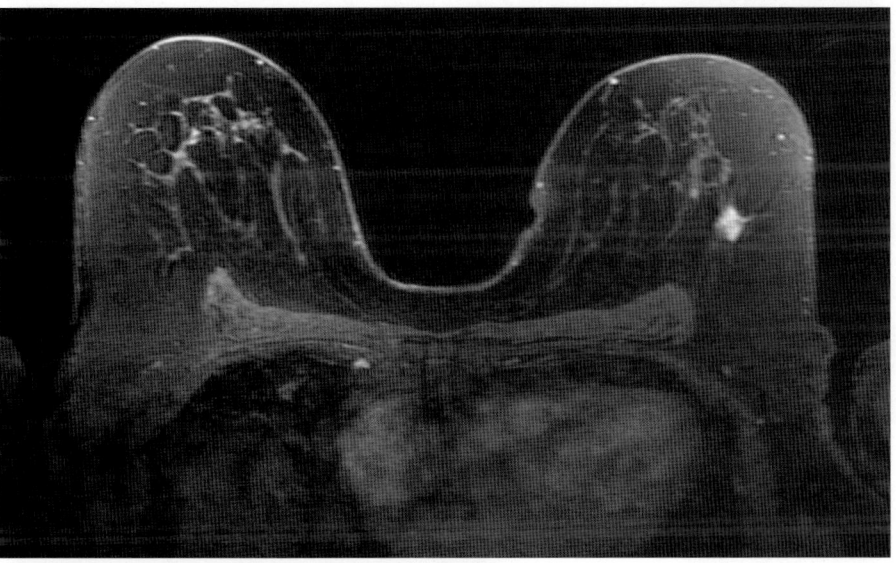

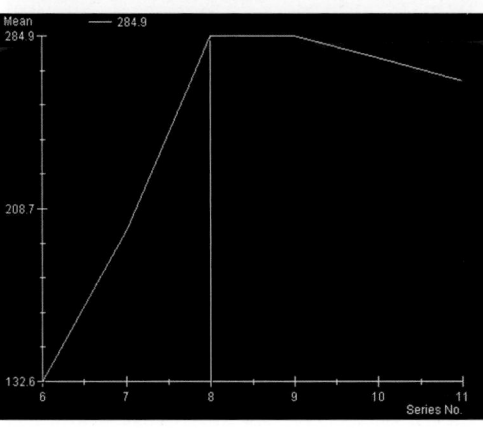

Fig. 34.7 The left mammographic mass corresponds to a homogeneous irregular spiculated mass that exhibits fast initial enhancement that peaks at 2 to 3 minutes, then exhibits washout (type III kinetic curve). (**A**) Bilateral contrast-enhanced axial breast high-resolution MRI. (**B**) Signal-intensity time curve of the left MRI mass.

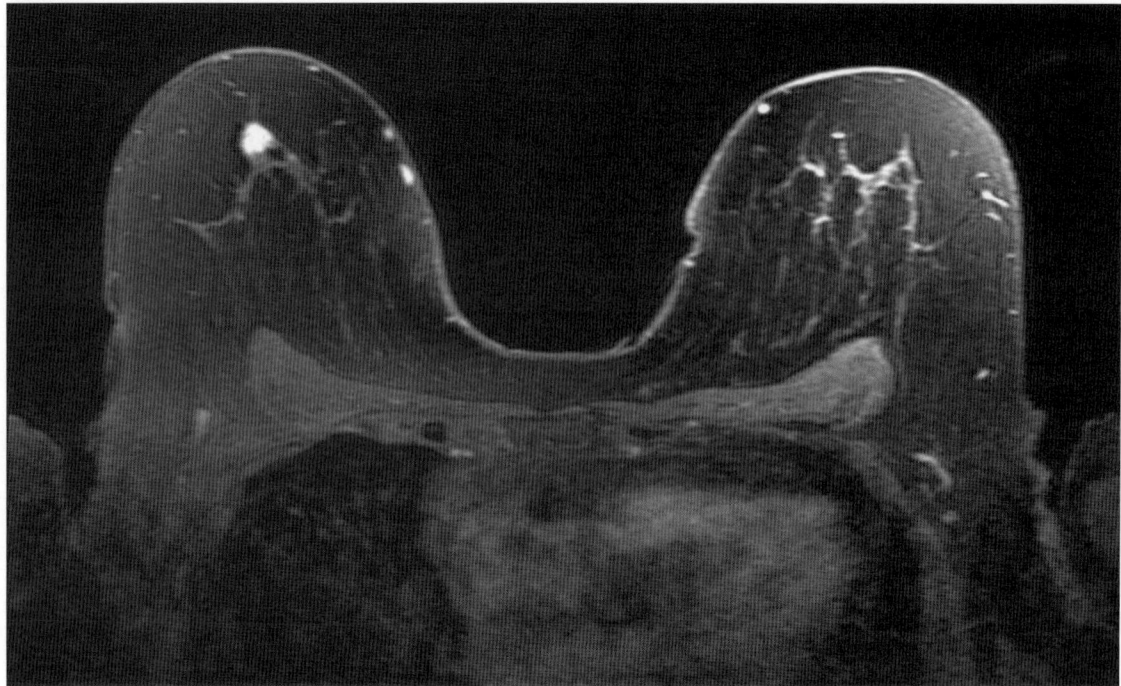

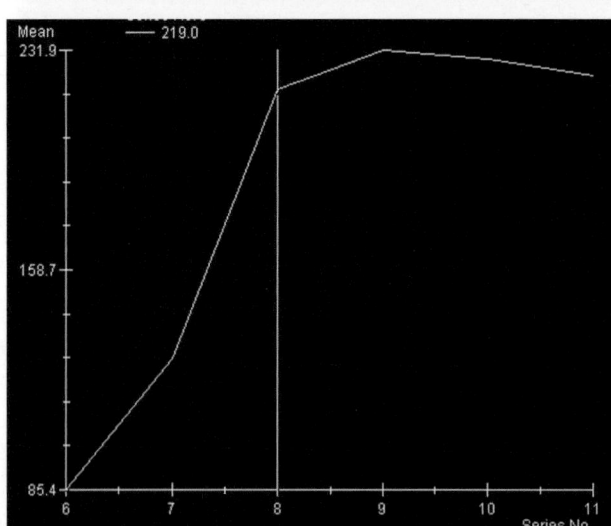

Fig. 34.8 In the right upper outer quadrant, there is an oval mass with irregular margins and homogeneous enhancement. This mass exhibits fast initial enhancement with a plateau curve in the later contrast phases (type II kinetic curve). (**A**) Bilateral contrast-enhanced axial breast high-resolution MRI. (**B**) Signal-intensity time curve of the right MRI mass.

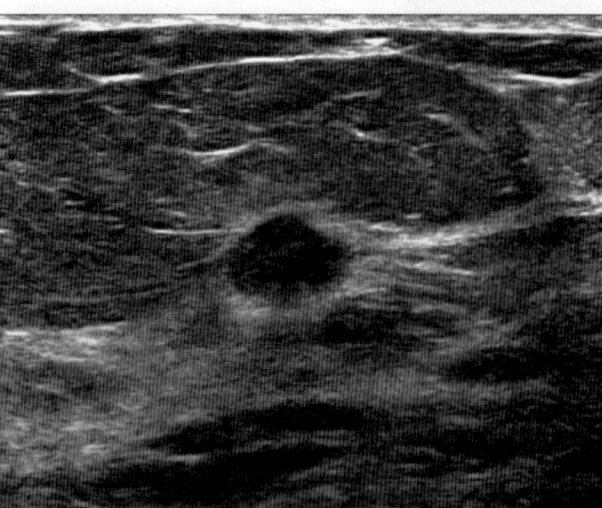

Fig. 34.9 Right radial sonogram. This sonogram is performed to identify the MRI mass for sonographic biopsy. In the upper outer quadrant, there is a hypoechoic oval mass with a hyperechoic haze and spiculations, which corresponds to the right breast MRI mass. This mass was not identified mammographically.

Pathology
- Left breast: invasive lobular carcinoma
- Right breast: invasive ductal carcinoma, grade 1

Management
- Left mammographic and sonographic mass: BI-RADS assessment category 5, highly suggestive of malignancy
- Right MRI and sonographic mass: BI-RADS assessment category 5, highly suggestive of malignancy

Pearls and Pitfalls

- Besides morphology, enhancement kinetics may be helpful in characterizing a mass. There are three types of kinetic curves. Type I curves exhibit continuous increasing enhancement with time. Type II curves reach maximum signal intensity approximately 2 to 3 minutes after injection, then plateau and remain constant. Type III curves reach a maximum enhancement after 2 to 3 minutes, then rapidly decrease in signal. This decrease in signal is called "washout." In general, type I curves are associated with benign lesions. Malignant lesions are associated with type II and type III curves.
- When assessing an MRI lesion, one should first characterize the morphology of the lesion. If the morphology is clearly suspicious, such as a spiculated mass, then biopsy should be recommended, regardless of the appearance of the kinetic curve. The kinetic curve of a morphologically suspicious mass should not downgrade the assessment of the mass. If the mass is morphologically probably benign, such as an oval, circumscribed mass, then a suspicious kinetic curve (type III) should result in a final recommendation of a biopsy. If the mass is morphologically probably benign and has a benign (type I) curve, then a final assessment of probably benign is appropriate.

Suggested Reading

Kuhl CK. MRI of breast tumors. Eur Radiol 2000;10:46–58

Kuhl CK. Dynamic breast magnetic resonance imaging. In: Morris EA, Liberman L, eds. Breast MRI Diagnosis and Intervention. New York: Springer; 2005:79-139

Case 34.4: Malignant MRI Mass

Case History
A 43-year-old woman presents with a palpable left breast lump at the 6 o'clock position.

Physical Examination
- Left breast mass at the 6 o'clock position approximately 1 cm from the nipple

Mammogram (Fig. 34.10)
- Normal exam

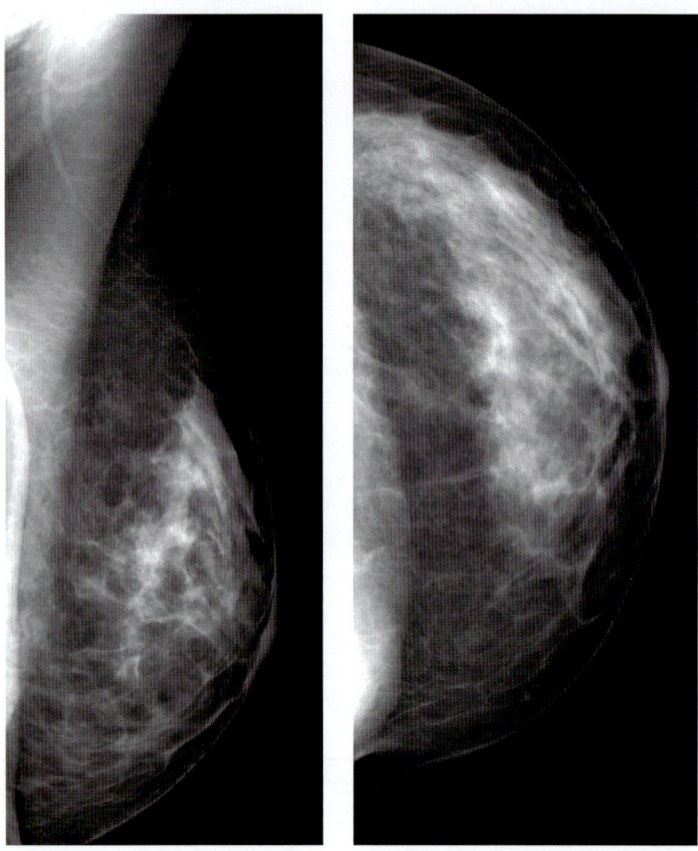

Fig. 34.10 Left breast mammograms are normal. (**A**) Left MLO mammogram. (**B**) Left CC mammogram.

Ultrasound

Frequency (Fig. 34.11)
- 14 MHz

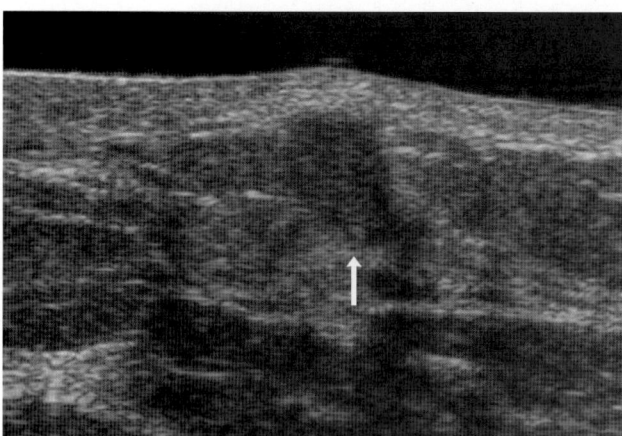

Fig. 34.11 Left breast radial sonogram. The palpable lump at the 6 o'clock position corresponds to a superficial irregular hypoechoic mass (*arrow*).

Other Modalities: MRI and Second Look Sonography (Figs. 34.12, 34.13, and 34.14)

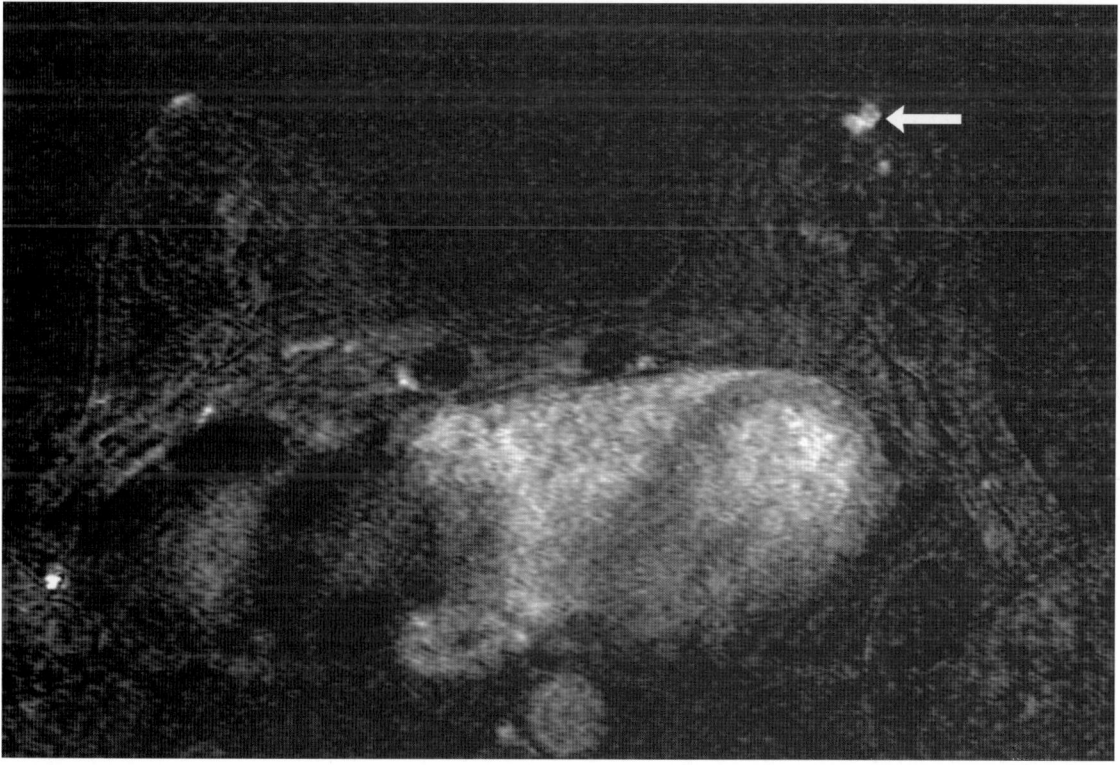

Fig. 34.12 Dynamic bolus T1-weighted, 2-minute subtraction axial bilateral breast MRI. The palpable lump corresponds to a lobulated mass (*arrow*) at the 6 o'clock position. This mass exhibits rapid initial enhancement with later plateau kinetics.

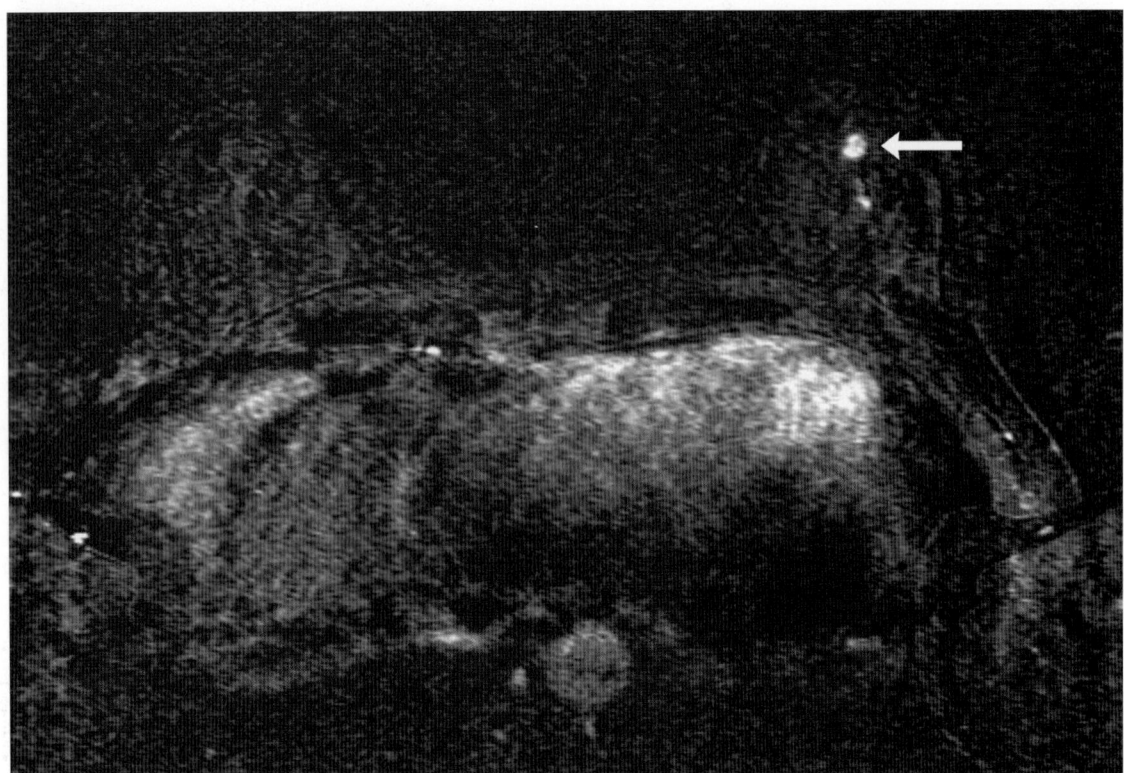

Fig. 34.13 Dynamic bolus T1-weighted, 2-minute subtraction axial bilateral breast MRI inferior to the left palpable lump (**Fig. 34.12**). There is a second left oval mass at the 6 o'clock position (*arrow*). This mass exhibits rapid initial enhancement and late-phase plateau kinetics.

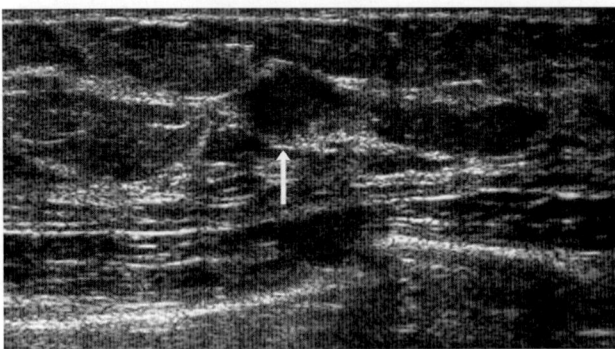

Fig. 34.14 Left breast radial sonogram. This exam was performed after the MRI. The second left breast MRI mass at the 6 o'clock position corresponds to this oval solid mass (*arrow*).

Pathology
- Left palpable mass at the 6 o'clock position: infiltrating ductal carcinoma
- Left nonpalpable mass at the 6 o'clock position: infiltrating ductal carcinoma. At mastectomy, these masses were 3.5 cm apart.

Management
- Left breast sonographic palpable mass at the 6 o'clock position: BI-RADS assessment category 4, suspicious; biopsy should be considered.
- Left breast MRI/sonographic nonpalpable mass at the 6 o'clock position: BI-RADS assessment category 4, suspicious; biopsy should be considered.

Pearls and Pitfalls

- Although masses that are round, oval, and lobulated in shape are generally benign, when these masses have a suspicious kinetic curve, they should be considered suspicious, and biopsy should be recommended.

Suggested Reading

Kuhl CK. Dynamic breast magnetic resonance imaging. In: Morris EA, Liberman L, eds. Breast MRI Diagnosis and Intervention. New York: Springer; 2005:79-139

Tozaki M, Igarashi T, Matsushima S, Fukuda K. High-spatial-resolution MR imaging of focal breast masses: interpretation model based on kinetic and morphological parameters. Radiat Med 2005;23:43–50

Case 34.5: MRI Focus

Case History
A 78-year-old woman presents for screening mammogram.

Physical Examination
- Normal exam

Mammogram

Mass (Fig. 34.15)
- Margin: indistinct
- Shape: irregular
- Density: equal density

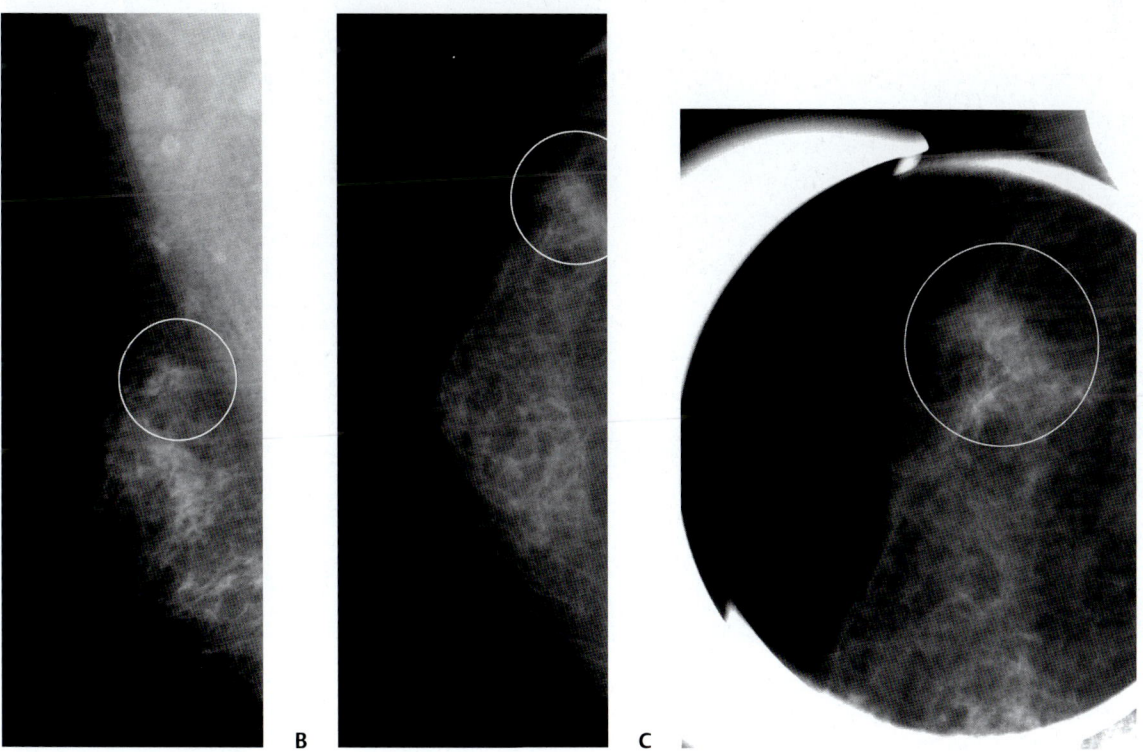

Fig. 34.15 In the right upper outer quadrant (*circle*), there is an irregular mass with indistinct margins. (**A**) Right MLO mammogram. (**B**) Right CC mammogram. (**C**) Right CC spot compression mammogram.

Ultrasound

Frequency (Fig. 34.16)
- 14 MHz

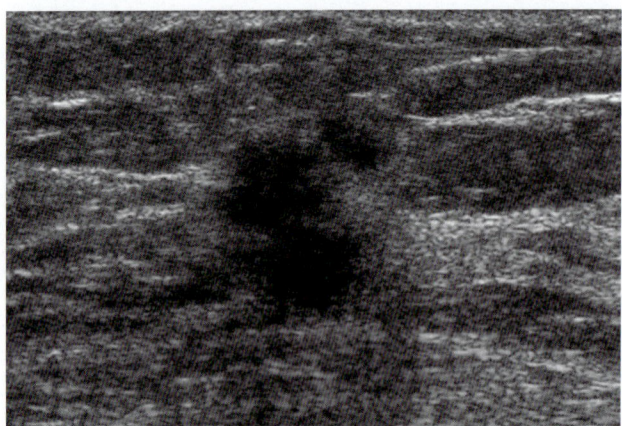

Fig. 34.16 Right radial breast sonogram. In the right upper outer quadrant, there is an irregular hypoechoic solid mass that corresponds to the mammographic mass.

Other Modalities: MRI (Figs. 34.17 and 34.18)

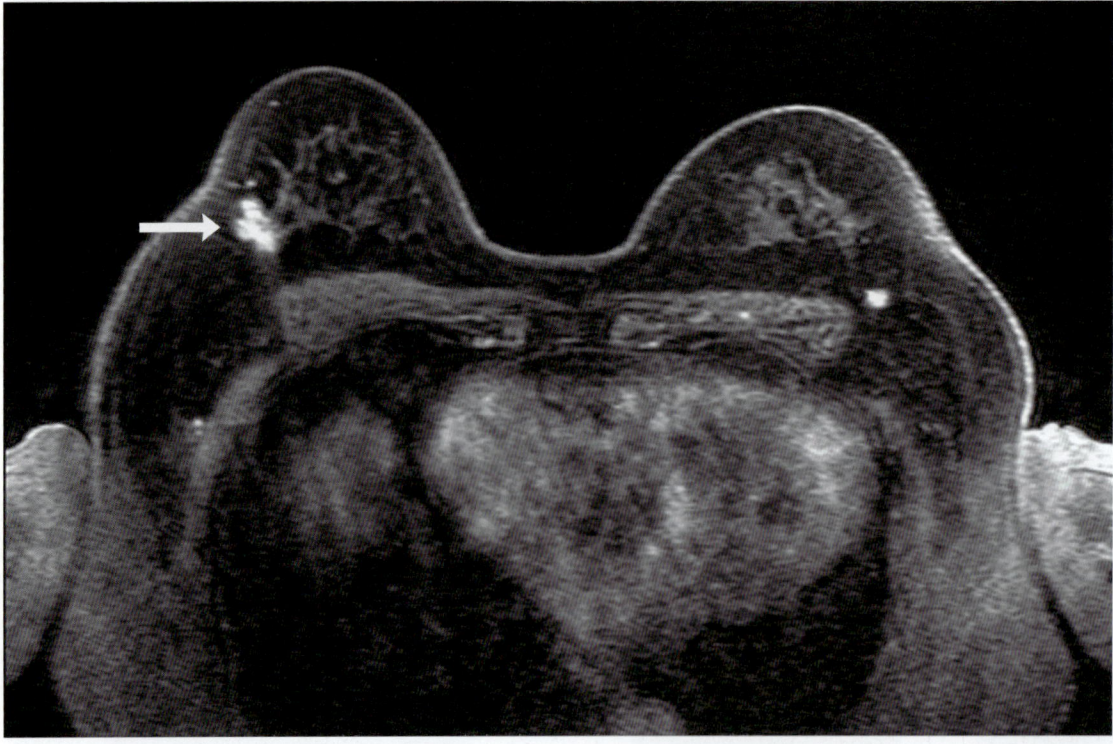

Fig. 34.17 Bilateral contrast-enhanced axial breast high-resolution MRI, delayed image. The known mammographic mass corresponds to an irregular, rapidly enhancing mass in the right upper outer quadrant (*arrow*). A left enhancing axillary lymph node is also evident. This lymph node was later sonographically examined and appeared normal.

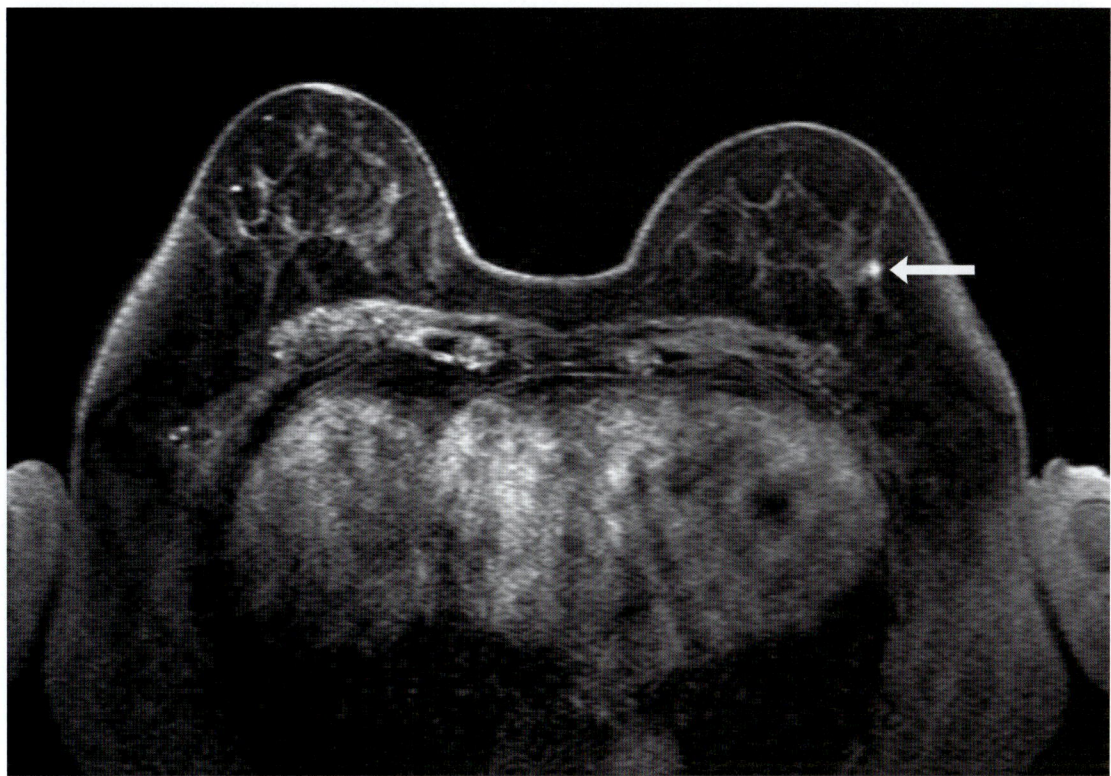

Fig. 34.18 Bilateral contrast-enhanced axial breast high-resolution MRI, delayed image. In the left upper outer breast, there was an enhancing focus (*arrow*). This focus was biopsied with MRI guidance.

Pathology
- Right breast mass: 1.3 cm invasive carcinoma with ductal and lobular features
- Left breast MRI enhancing focus: 0.4 cm ductal carcinoma in situ (DCIS)
- Bilateral sentinel nodes were normal without metastatic disease.

Management
- Right breast mammographic and sonographic mass: BI-RADS assessment category 5, highly suggestive of malignancy
- Left breast MRI enhancing focus: BI-RADS assessment category 4, suspicious; biopsy should be considered

Pearls and Pitfalls

- The most common morphologic MRI features of invasive ductal carcinoma include irregular shape (56%), irregular (33%) or spiculated margin (49%), and heterogeneous internal enhancement (60%). Rim and central enhancement are also considered suspicious MRI findings for malignancy. Finally, if the mass has rapid initial enhancement and washout, the likelihood of malignancy is 87%. For discussion on MRI focus see Case 22.5.

Suggested Reading

Kim SJ, Morris EA, Liberman L, et al. Observer variability and applicability of BI-RADS terminology for breast MR imaging: invasive carcinomas as focal masses. AJR Am J Roentgenol 2001;177:551–557

Kuhl CK, Mielcareck P, Klaschik S, et al. Dynamic breast MR imaging: are signal intensity time course data useful for differential diagnosis of enhancing lesions? Radiology 1999;211:101–110

Liberman L, Morris EA, Lee MJ-Y, et al. Breast lesions detected on MR imaging: features and positive predictive value. AJR Am J Roentgenol 2002;179:171–178

Nunes LW, Schnall MD, Orel SG, et al. Breast MR imaging: interpretation model. Radiology 1997;202:833–841

Nunes LW, Schnall MD, Siegelman ES, et al. Diagnostic performance characteristics of architectural features revealed by high spatial-resolution MR imaging of the breast. AJR Am J Roentgenol 1997;169:409–415

Sherif H, Mahfouz A-E, Oellinger H, et al. Peripheral washout sign on contrast-enhanced MR images of the breast. Radiology 1997;205:209–213

Tozaki M, Igarashi T, Matsushima S, Fukuda K. High-spatial-resolution MR imaging of focal breast masses: interpretation model based on kinetic and morphological parameters. Radiat Med 2005;23:43–50

Masses Poorly Identified Mammographically

Case 34.6: MRI Duct

Case History

A 62-year-old woman presents with a palpable right breast mass. Because both the mammograms and the right breast sonogram are interpreted as normal, breast MRI is performed.

Physical Examination

- Ill-defined thickening or firmness in the right upper outer quadrant

Mammogram (Fig. 34.19)

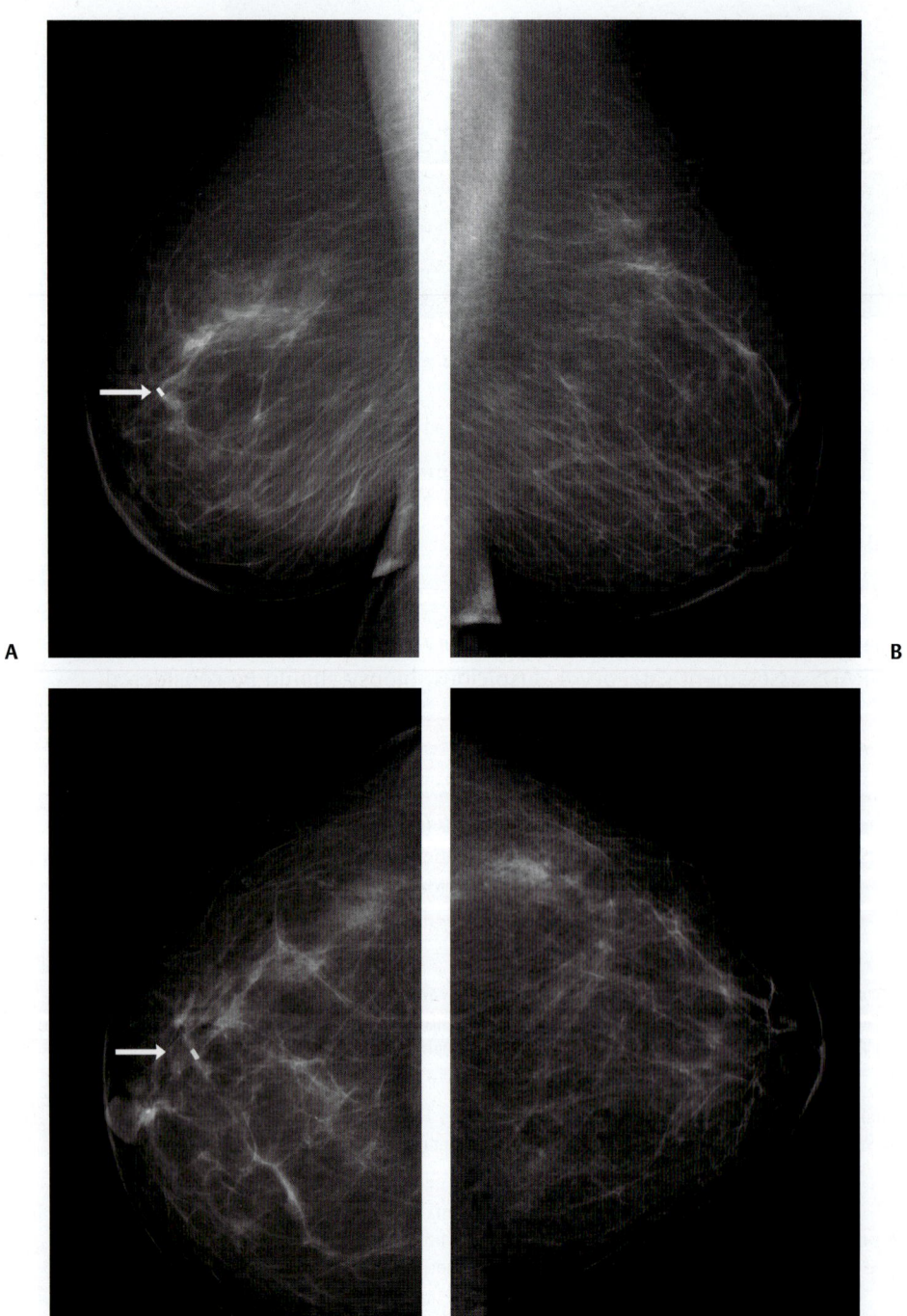

Fig. 34.19 The mammograms are normal. There is mild asymmetry in the right upper outer quadrant, but this asymmetry has been stable for 8 years. The clip (*arrow*) denotes the location of the ultrasound-guided biopsy, which will be subsequently described. (**A**) Right MLO mammogram. (**B**) Left MLO mammogram. (**C**) Right CC mammogram. (**D**) Left CC mammogram.

Ultrasound

Frequency (Fig. 34.20)
- 14 MHz

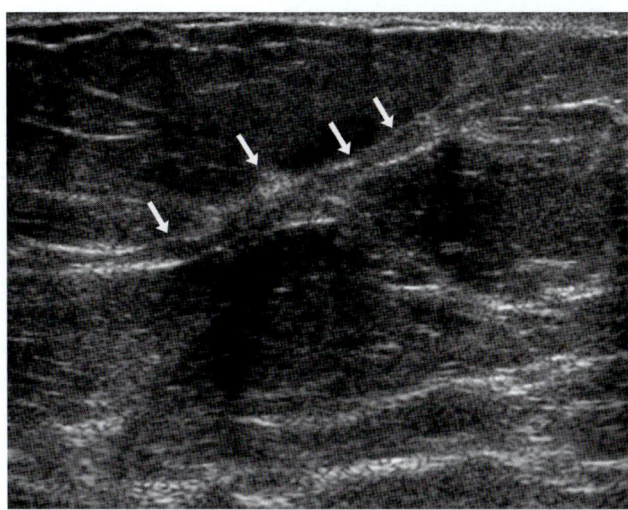
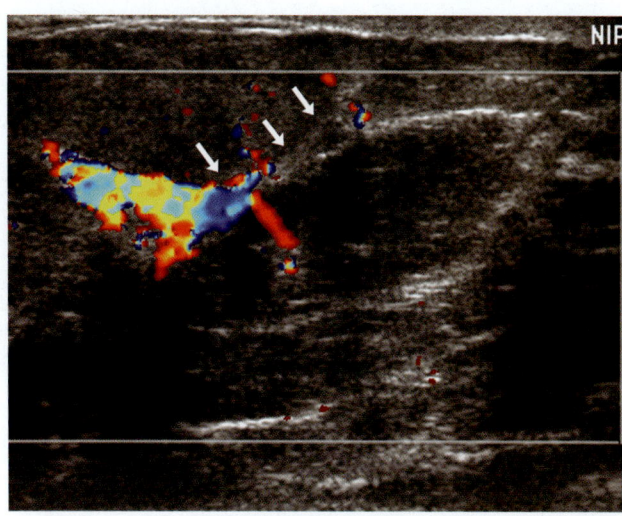

Fig. 34.20 Right radial breast sonogram. The first sonogram is performed to examine the palpable mass and is interpreted as normal. Later, a second sonogram is performed to examine the MRI abnormality that is in the same location as the previously identified palpable lump. The MRI lesion corresponded to this dilated duct (*arrows*), which appears to be filled with material. This duct exhibits increased color flow Doppler and is sonographically biopsied. The clip from this biopsy is present on previously shown right breast mammograms. (**A**) Right radial breast sonogram. (**B**) Right radial breast sonogram in the same location as **A** with color flow Doppler.

Other Modalities: MRI (Fig. 34.21)

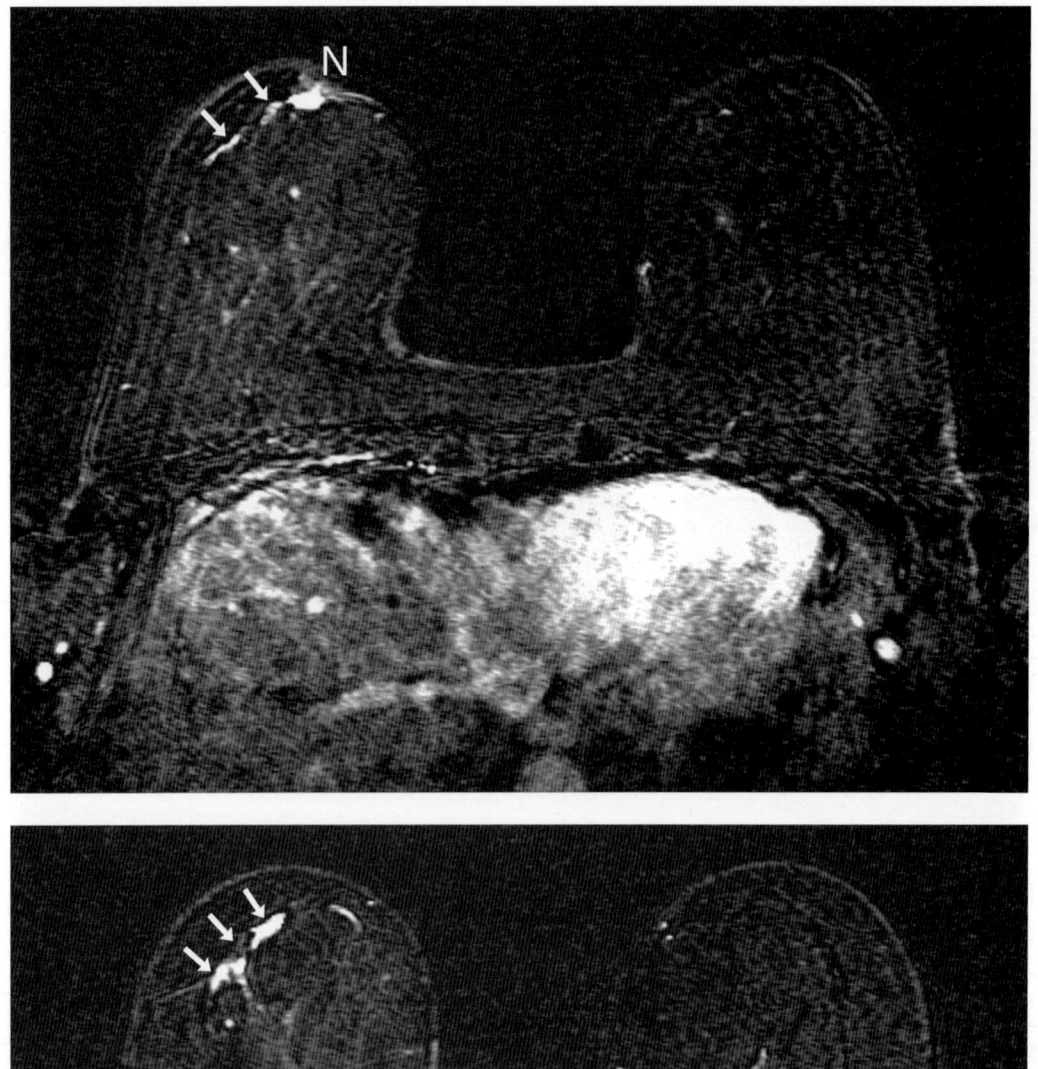

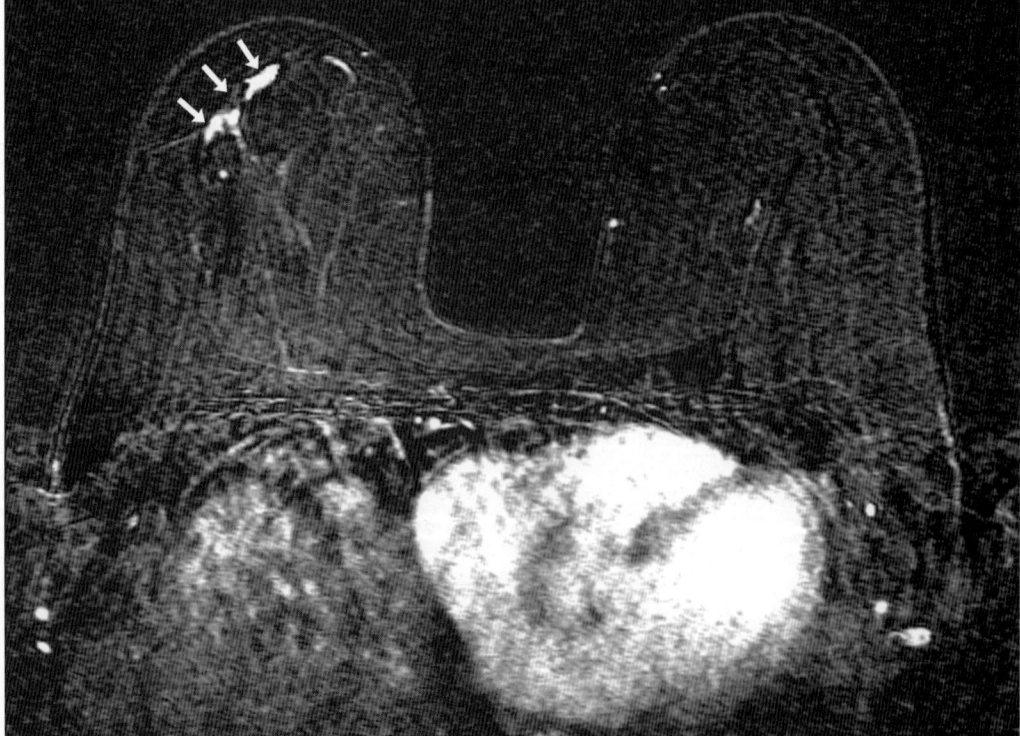

Fig. 34.21 Bilateral contrast-enhanced breast MRI. In the outer right breast near the 3 o'clock position, there is a rapidly enhancing dilated duct (*arrows*). The duct starts at the nipple (N) and branches in the outer breast. (**A**) Dynamic bolus T1-weighted, 3-minute subtraction axial bilateral breast MRI. (**B**) Dynamic bolus T1-weighted, 3-minute subtraction axial bilateral breast MRI.

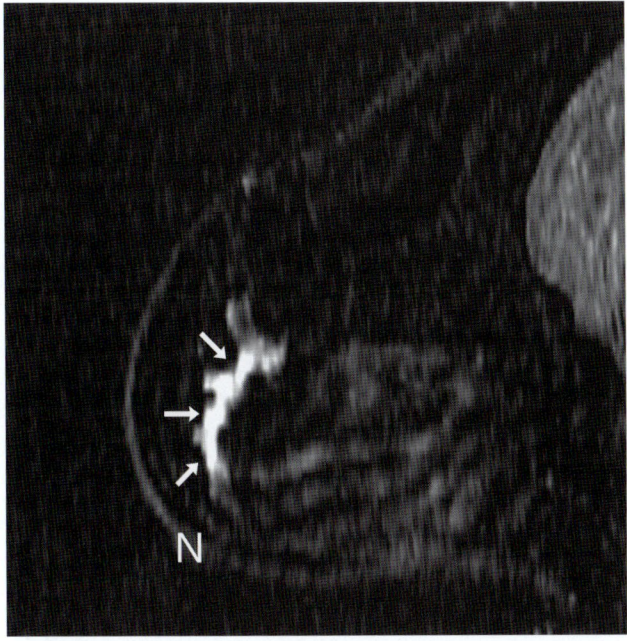

Fig. 34.21 *(Continued)* **(C)** Sagittal reconstructed dynamic bolus T1-weighted, 3-minute subtraction right breast MRI.

Pathology
- Invasive lobular carcinoma

Management
- Breast MRI enhancing duct: BI-RADS assessment category 5, highly suggestive of malignancy

Pearls and Pitfalls
- When the MRI finding is suspicious, sonographic examination may be used to localize for biopsy. In these situations, the sonographic findings commonly do not correspond to the classic sonographic mass. In this case, because the MRI abnormality appears to be an abnormally dilated duct, the imager should sonographically identify a dilated duct. The presence of increased color Doppler (compared with normal surrounding tissue) provides further evidence that this duct corresponds to the MRI lesion.
- Invasive lobular carcinoma most commonly appears as an enhancing irregular mass with irregular or spiculated margins, either with or without rim enhancement. However, compared with invasive ductal carcinoma, invasive lobular cancer appears to have a wider variety of appearances, including homogeneous and heterogeneous regional and segmental enhancement.
- MRI has been found to be particularly useful in presurgical staging of lobular cancer. Rodenko and colleagues[1] found that MRI has been found to correlate more closely with pathologic results compared with mammography (85% vs 32%). Furthermore, in multiple studies, the additional MRI information has been found to change treatment management in between 14 and 50% of cases. Bedrosian et al[2] found that MRI was twice as likely to change management in patients with invasive lobular compared with other breast tumor histologies.

References

1. Rodenko GN, Harms SE, Pruneda JM, et al. MR imaging in the management before surgery of lobular carcinoma of the breast: correlation with pathology. AJR Am J Roentgenol 1996;167:1415–1419

2. Bedrosian I, Mick R, Orel SG, et al. Changes in the surgical management of patients with breast carcinoma based on preoperative magnetic resonance imaging. Cancer 2003;98:468–473

Suggested Reading

Biglia N, Mariani L, Sgro L, Mininanni P, Moggio G, Sismondi P. Increased incidence of lobular breast cancer in women treated with hormone replacement therapy: implications for diagnosis, surgical and medical treatment. Endocr Relat Cancer 2007;14:549–567

Munot K, Dall B, Achuthan R, Parkin G, Lane S, Horgan K. Role of magnetic resonance imaging in the diagnosis and single-stage surgical resection of invasive lobular carcinoma of the breast. Br J Surg 2002;89:1296–1301

Rigauts H, Casselman J, Steyaert L, Devlies F, Pattyn G. Contribution of MRI and color Doppler sonography in breast cancer diagnosis. J Belge Radiol 1993;76:226–231

Weinstein SP, Orel SG, Heller R, et al. MR imaging of the breast in patients with invasive lobular carcinoma. AJR Am J Roentgenol 2001;176:399–406

Yeh ED, Slanetz PJ, Edmister WB, Talele A, Monticciolo D, Kopans DB. Invasive lobular carcinoma: spectrum of enhancement and morphology on magnetic resonance imaging. Breast J 2003;9:13–18

Case 34.7: MRI-Associated Findings

Case History
A 47-year-old woman presents with 4 months of right breast pain and bloody nipple discharge.

Physical Examination
The right nipple exhibits signs of excoriation and is swollen and tender. No breast or axillary mass is palpable.

Mammogram (Fig. 34.22)
- Normal exam

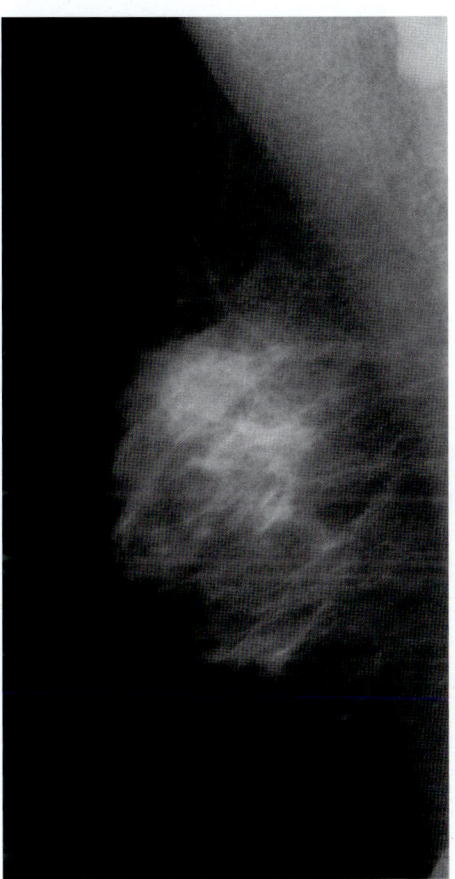
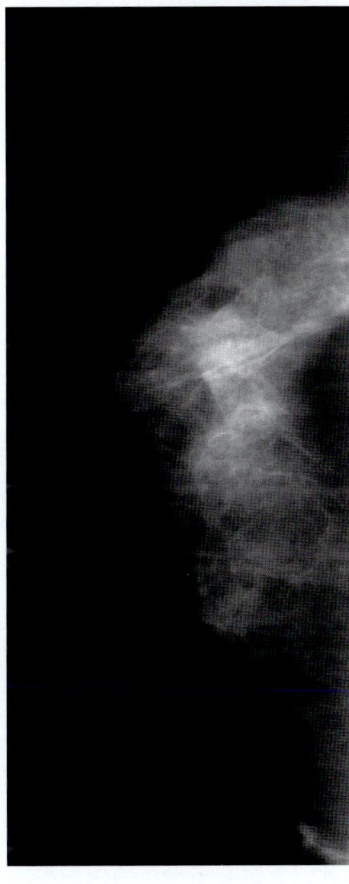

Fig. 34.22 Right breast mammograms are normal. (**A**) Right MLO mammogram. (**B**) Right CC mammogram.

Ultrasound

Frequency (Fig. 34.23)
- 14 MHz

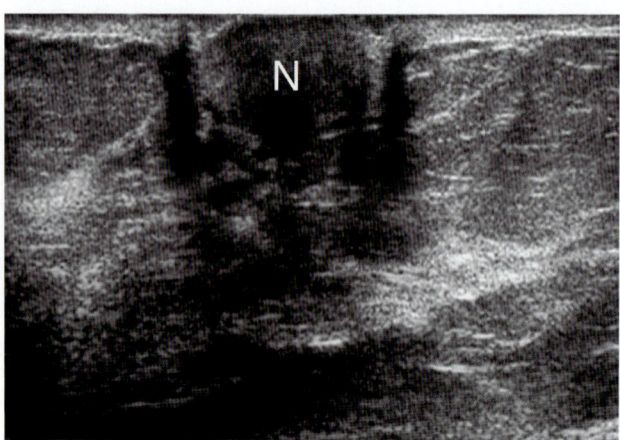

Fig. 34.23 Right radial breast sonogram. The sonographic appearance of the nipple (N) is normal. No masses are identified.

Other Modalities: MRI and Second Look Sonography (Figs. 34.24, 34.25, and 34.26)

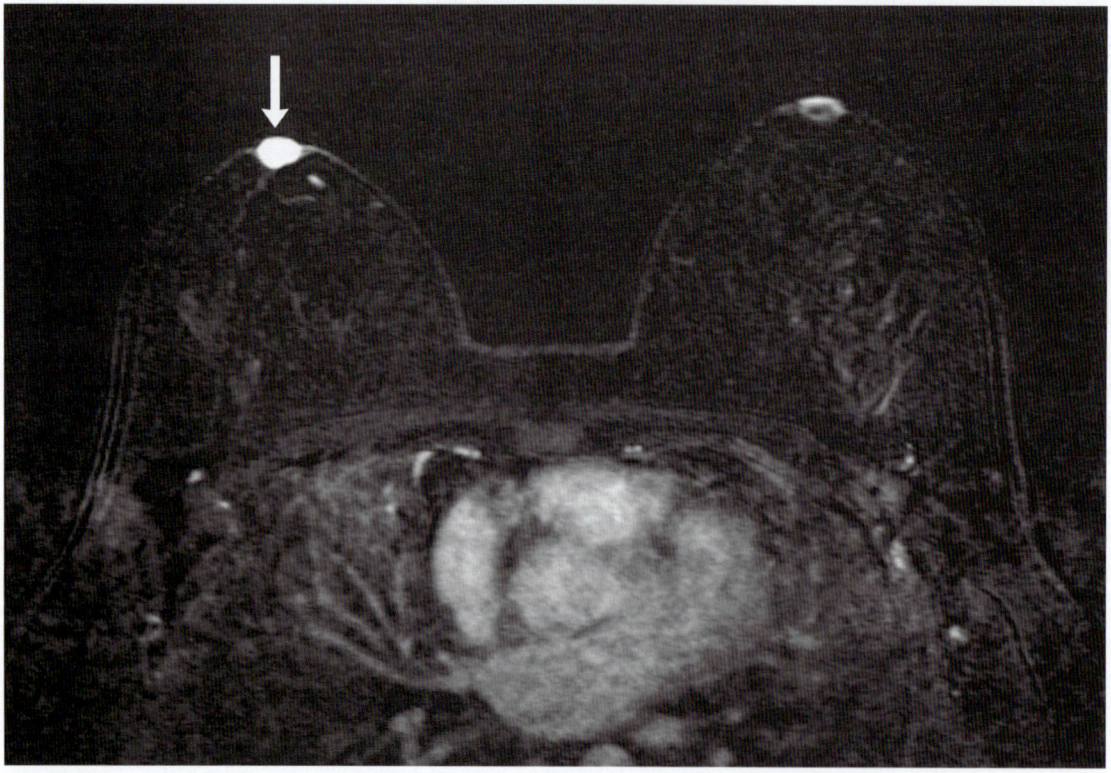

Fig. 34.24 Dynamic bolus T1-weighted, 2-minute subtraction axial bilateral breast MRI. The enhancement of the right nipple (*arrow*) is rapid and is much greater than the left.

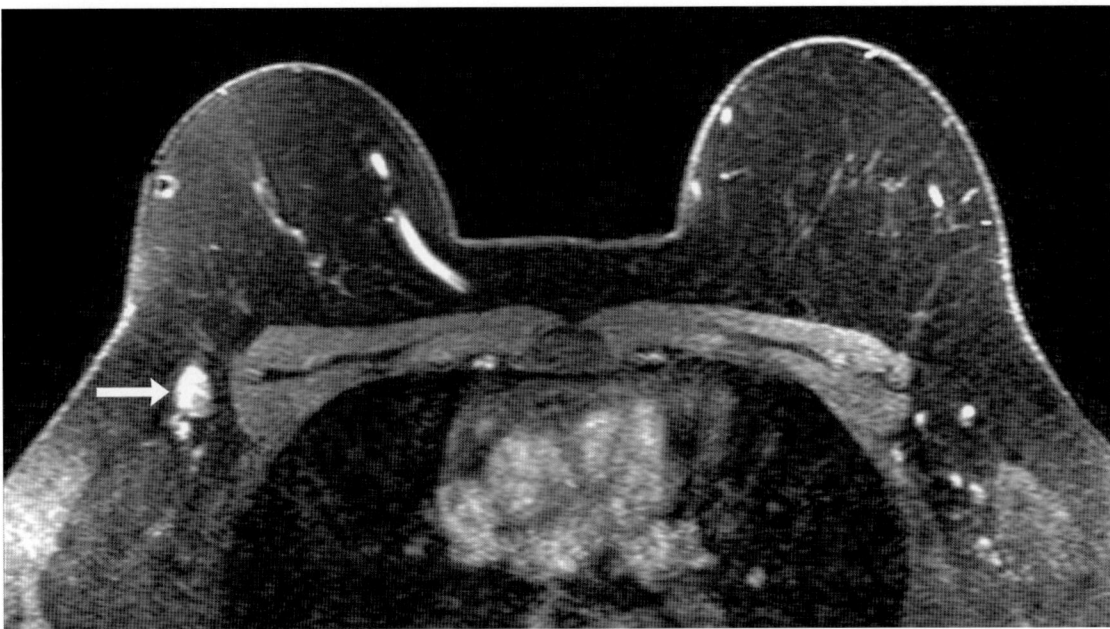

Fig. 34.25 Bilateral contrast-enhanced axial breast high-resolution MRI, delayed image. In the axilla, there is an enhancing axillary lymph node (*arrow*). This lymph node exhibits rapid enhancement and moderate asymmetric thickening of the cortex.

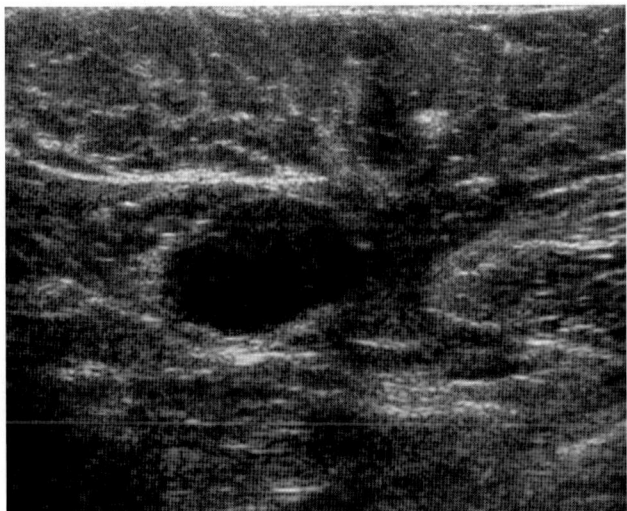

Fig. 34.26 Right radial breast sonogram. This sonographic exam is done to characterize the abnormal axillary lymph node originally identified by MRI. The lymph node is hypoechoic and has lost its normal hyperechoic hilum.

Pathology
- Punch biopsy of nipple and later partial mastectomy: 1.5 cm invasive ductal carcinoma, high grade. Malignancy involved epidermis of nipple in conjunction with Paget cells.
- Sonographic biopsy lymph node: metastatic invasive ductal. Axillary dissection: 6 of 11 lymph nodes were positive for metastatic malignancy.

Management
- Right MRI enhancing nipple and axillary lymph nodes: BI-RADS assessment category 5, highly suggestive of malignancy

> **Pearls and Pitfalls**
>
> - The most common MRI finding of Paget's disease is enhancement and thickening of the nipple-areolar complex. In three small studies involving 13 patients, all patients with Paget's disease had this finding. Associated findings are enhancement of dilated subareolar ducts, ductal enhancement separate from the nipple, and segmental clumped enhancement. These latter findings are generally associated with ductal carcinoma in situ (DCIS).
> - Although MRI may be excellent in identifying Paget's disease, it may not be as sensitive to malignancy in patients with Paget's disease compared with other clinical situations. In a separate study, in 13 patients with Paget's disease, MRI identified only 7 (58%) of 12 malignancies, missing 5 neoplasms (1 invasive and 4 DCIS).
> - This case illustrates that sonography may be useful when Paget's disease is associated with a malignant mass such as adenopathy. Signs of metastatic axillary lymph node disease include (1) eccentric cortical thickening, (2) convex cortical bulge into the hilum, (3) severe reduction or obliteration of the hilum, (4) loss of smooth oval contour with development of angular margins, (5) severe hypoechogenicity of the cortex, and (6) loss of ellipsoid shape with abnormal "rounding" of the lymph node.

Suggested Reading

Capobianco G, Spaliviero B, Dessole S, et al. Paget's disease of the nipple diagnosed by MRI. Arch Gynecol Obstet 2006;274:316–318

Echevarria JJ, Lopez-Ruiz JA, Martin D, Imaz I, Martin M. Usefulness of MRI in detecting occult breast cancer associated with Paget's disease of the nipple-areolar complex. Br J Radiol 2004;77:1036–1039

Frei KA, Bonel HM, Pelte M-F, Hylton NM, Kinkel K. Paget disease of the breast: findings at magnetic resonance imaging and histopathologic correlation. Invest Radiol 2005;40:363–367

Morrogh M, Morris EA, Liberman L, Van Zee K, Cody HS III, King TA. MRI identifies otherwise occult disease in select patients with Paget disease of the nipple. J Am Coll Surg 2008;206:316–321

Stavros TA. Evaluation of regional lymph nodes in breast cancer patients. In: Stavros TA. Breast Ultrasound. Philadelphia: Lippincott Williams & Wilkins; 2004:834-876

Case 34.8: MRI-Associated Findings

Case History
An 85-year-old woman presents with a 6-month history of right breast nipple depigmentation and scaliness.

Physical Examination
- Right breast: mildly decreased pigmentation of the areola with dry, excoriated skin around the nipple

Mammogram (Fig. 34.27)

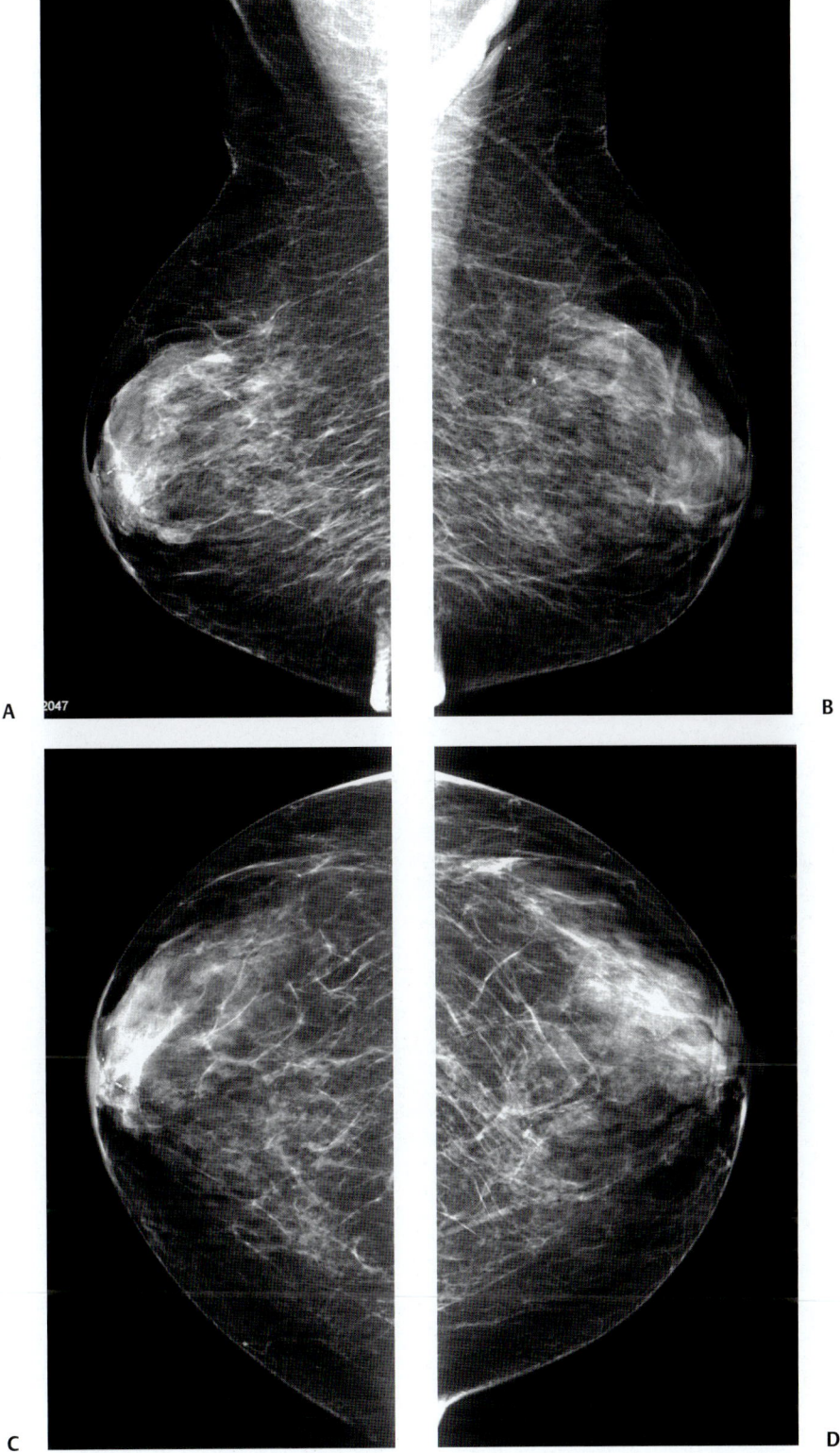

Fig. 34.27 The right mammograms demonstrate flattening of the nipple but are otherwise normal. (**A**) Right MLO mammogram. (**B**) Left MLO mammogram (**C**) Right CC mammogram. (**D**) Left CC mammogram.

Ultrasound

Frequency (Fig. 34.28)
- 14 MHz

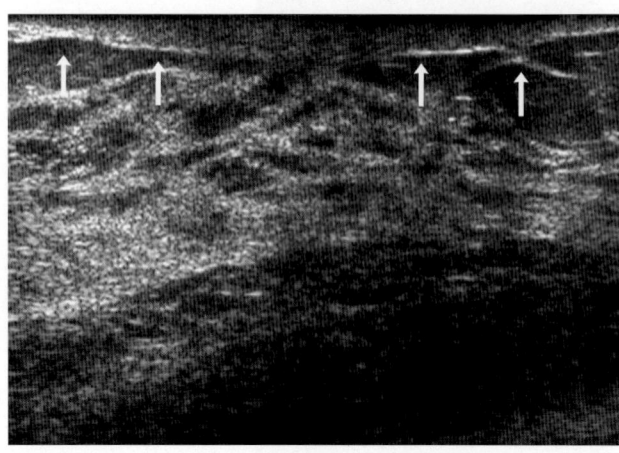

Fig. 34.28 Right radial subareolar sonogram. There is mild skin thickening (*arrows*). Otherwise, the exam is normal. No masses are present.

Other Modalities (Figs. 34.29 and 34.30)

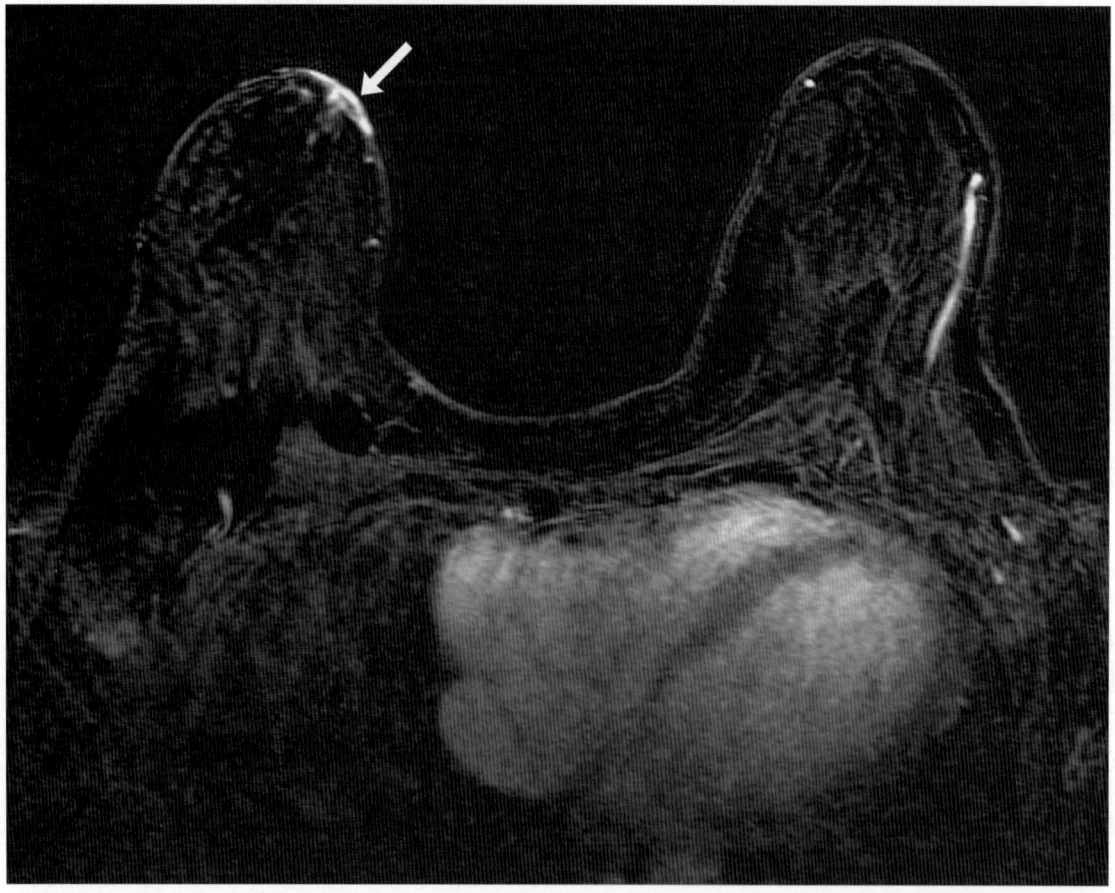

Fig. 34.29 Dynamic bolus T1-weighted, 5-minute subtraction axial bilateral breast MRI. MRI is performed because the mammograms and ultrasound are negative. MRI shows asymmetric enhancement of the right nipple (*arrow*).

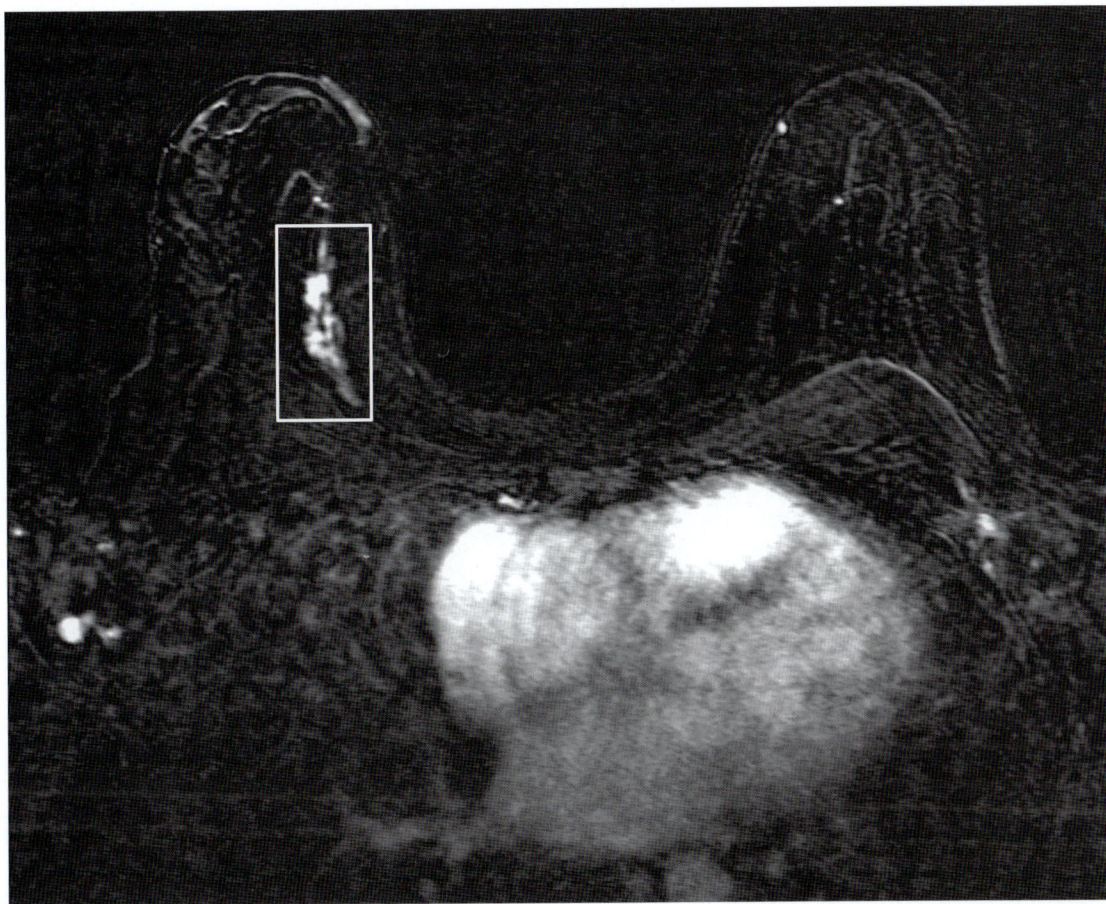

Fig. 34.30 Dynamic bolus T1-weighted, 2-minute subtraction axial bilateral breast MRI. In the upper inner right breast, there is clumped enhancement in a linear distribution (*square*). This area was biopsied by MRI.

Pathology
- Mastectomy specimen showed that the area of MRI enhancement was DCIS. The nipple was also involved with ductal carcinoma in situ (DCIS) and Paget cells.

Management
- MRI findings: BI-RADS assessment category 4, suspicious; biopsy should be considered.

Pearls and Pitfalls

- Paget's disease, described in 1874 by Sir James Paget, represents 1 to 5% of all breast malignancies. Clinically, the nipple is red and pruritic initially. These symptoms progress to eczema, scaling, erosion, and ulceration. About 50% of patients have a palpable mass. Microscopically, Paget cells, identified within the epidermis, are commonly associated with underlying DCIS. In about one third of patients without a palpable mass and in 90% of those with a palpable mass, there is an associated invasive carcinoma. When only DCIS is present and the tumor is completely excised, the 10-year survival rate is 100%.
- Mammographically, the epidermal involvement is generally not visible, so Paget's disease commonly is mammographically occult. Rarely, the intense neoplasia may produce a hazy periareolar density or subareolar dilated ducts. More commonly, the main mammographic features will be malignant calcifications extending from the nipple due to DCIS.
- Unless there is an associated invasive malignancy, sonography may demonstrate periareolar skin thickening but is otherwise usually negative.
- In Paget's disease, MRI demonstrates skin thickening and abnormal skin enhancement.

Suggested Reading

De Paredes ES. Prominent ductal patterns. In: De Paredes ES, Atlas of Mammography. 3rd ed. Philadelphia: Lippincott Williams & Wilkins; 2007:339-362

Eusebi V, Mai KT, Taranger-Charpin A. Tumours of the nipple. In: Tavassoli FA, Deville P, eds. Pathology and Genetics of Tumours of the Breast and Female Genital Organs. Lyon: International Agency for Research on Cancer; 2003:104-106

Kopans DB. Histologic, pathologic, and imaging correlation. In: Kopans DB. Breast Imaging. 3rd ed. Philadelphia: Lippincott Williams & Wilkins; 2007:783-888

Parkinson BT. Paget disease of the nipple. In: Berg WA, Birdwell RL, Gombos EC, Wang SC, Parkinson BT, Raza S, Green GE, Kennedy A, Kettler MD, eds. Diagnostic Imaging Breast. Manitoba, Canada: Friesens, Altona; 2006:IV:3:10-13

Applications of PET-CT

35 Staging

Case 35.1: Staging Locoregional Disease

Case History
A 63-year-old woman presents with a palpable left breast lump.

Physical Examination
- Firm lump in outer left breast near the 3 o'clock position

Mammogram

Mass (Fig. 35.1)
- Margin: ill defined
- Shape: oval
- Density: high

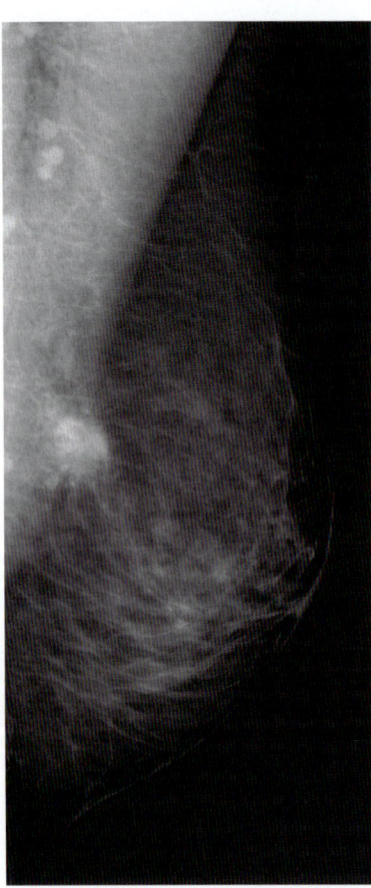 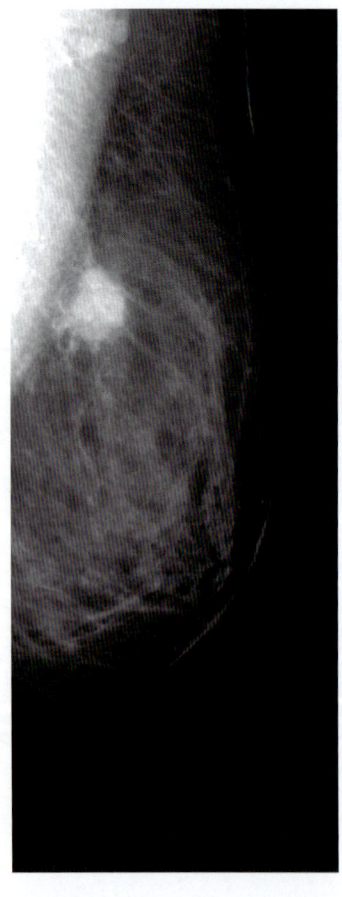

A B

Fig. 35.1 In the outer quadrant, there is an ill-defined oval mass. (**A**) Left MLO mammogram. (**B**) Left exaggerated craniocaudal (XCC) mammogram.

Ultrasound

Frequency (Fig. 35.2)
- 14 MHz

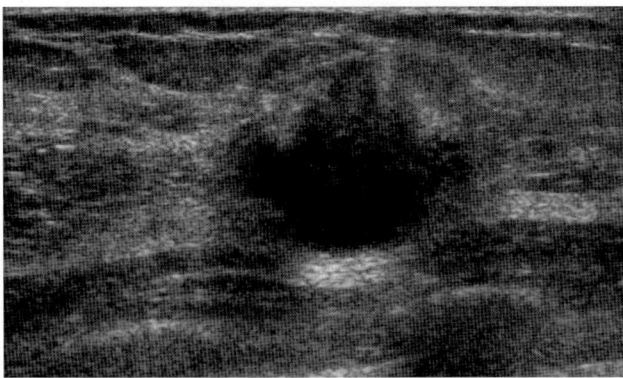

Fig. 35.2 Left breast antiradial sonogram. The mammographic mass and palpable lump correspond to an irregular hypoechoic solid mass near the 3 o'clock position that is associated with spiculations. The mass also distorts the Cooper's ligament and surrounding glandular architecture.

Other Modalities: MRI and PET (Figs. 35.3, 35.4, 35.5, and 35.6)

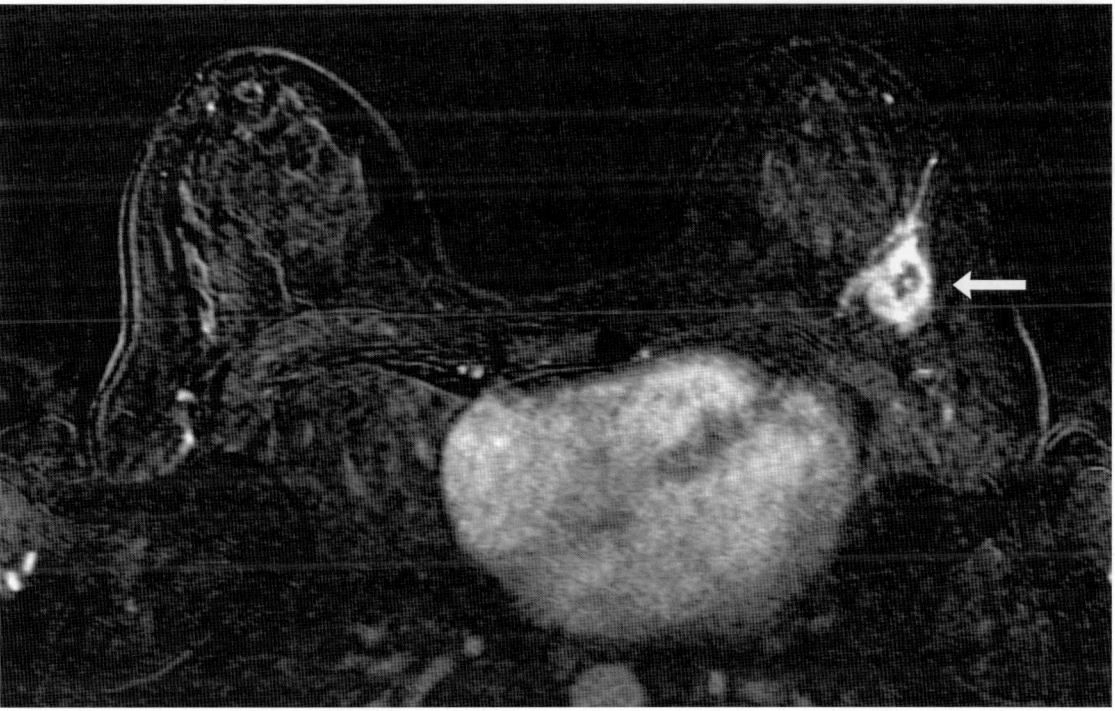

Fig. 35.3 Dynamic bolus T1-weighted, 2-minute subtraction axial bilateral breast MRI. The MRI is performed to further stage the tumor. The primary malignancy is a rapidly enhancing irregular mass in the left 3 o'clock position (*arrow*).

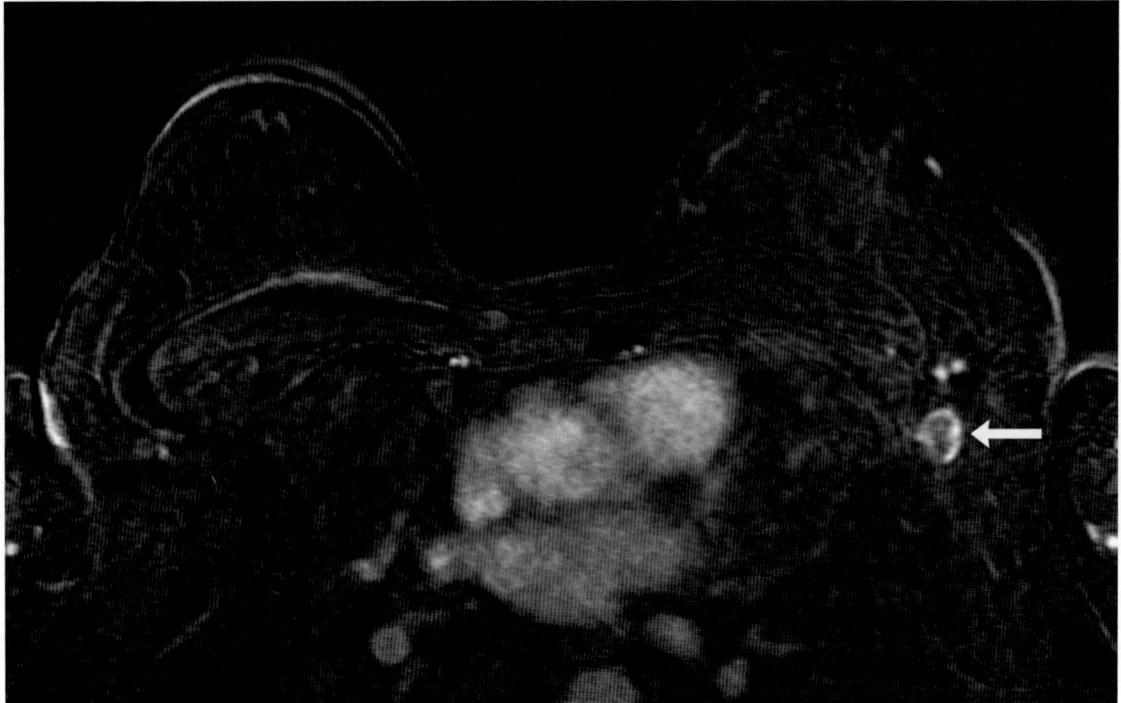

Fig. 35.4 Dynamic bolus T1-weighted, 2-minute subtraction axial bilateral breast MRI. The MRI identifies an abnormal enhancing left axilla (*arrow*).

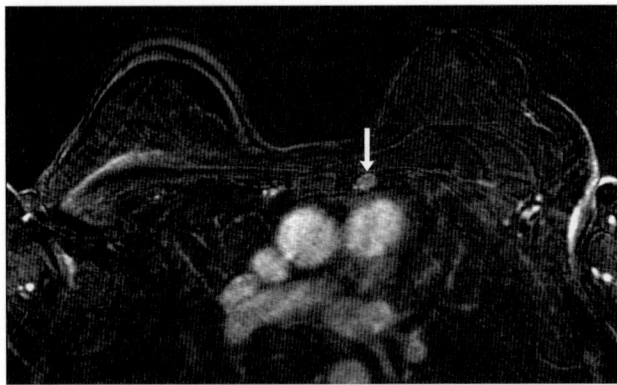

Fig. 35.5 Dynamic bolus T1-weighted, 2-minute subtraction axial bilateral breast MRI. An abnormally enlarged internal mammary lymph node is evident (*arrow*).

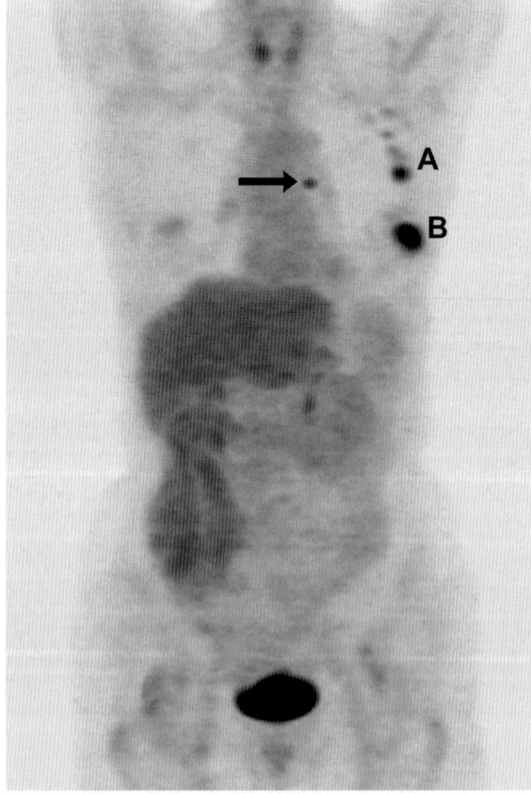

Fig. 35.6 Maximum projection intensity (MIP) positron emission tomography (PET) image. The PET exam demonstrates the primary malignancy (B) and confirms the presence of abnormal axillary nodes (A) and an internal mammary node (*arrow*).

Pathology
- Invasive ductal carcinoma

Management
- Left mammographic and sonographic mass: BI-RADS assessment category 5, highly suggestive of malignancy

Pearls and Pitfalls

- Positron emission tomography (PET) is not recommended for routine staging for patients with early-stage breast cancer because in these patients PET is not as sensitive as sentinel lymph node biopsy for staging axillary metastases. A multicenter trial found that the sensitivity was 61%, and specificity was 80%. Because of a relatively high false-negative rate, sentinel lymph node biopsy or axillary dissection cannot be avoided if the PET scan is negative. PET has a higher sensitivity when the primary breast tumor is large (i.e., > 2 cm) and when the ^{18}F-fluorodeoxyglucose (FDG) uptake of the tumor is high.
- PET has been found to be more accurate than computed tomography (CT) for the identification of internal mammary and mediastinal metastases.

Suggested Reading

Eubank WB, Mankoff DA, Takasugi J, et al. ^{18}Fluorodeoxyglucose positron emission tomography to detect mediastinal or internal mammary metastases in breast cancer. J Clin Oncol 2001;19(15):3516–3523

Greco M, Crippa F, Agresti R, et al. Axillary lymph node staging in breast cancer by 2-fluoro-2-deoxy-D-glucose-positron emission tomography: clinical evaluation and alternative management. J Natl Cancer Inst 2001;93(8):630–635

van der Hoeven JJM, Krak NC, Hoekstra OS, et al. ^{18}F-2-fluoro-2-deoxy-D-glucose positron emission tomography in staging of locally advanced breast cancer. J Clin Oncol 2004;22(7):1253–1259

Wahl RL, Siegel BA, Coleman RE, Gatsonis CG; PET Study Group. Prospective multicenter study of axillary nodal staging by positron emission tomography in breast cancer: a report of the staging breast cancer with PET Study Group. J Clin Oncol 2004;22(2):277–285

Case 35.2: Staging Advanced Disease

Case History
A 73-year-old woman presents for screening mammography.

Physical Examination
- Normal exam

Mammogram

Mass (Fig. 35.7)
- Margin: ill defined and irregular
- Shape: oval
- Density: high

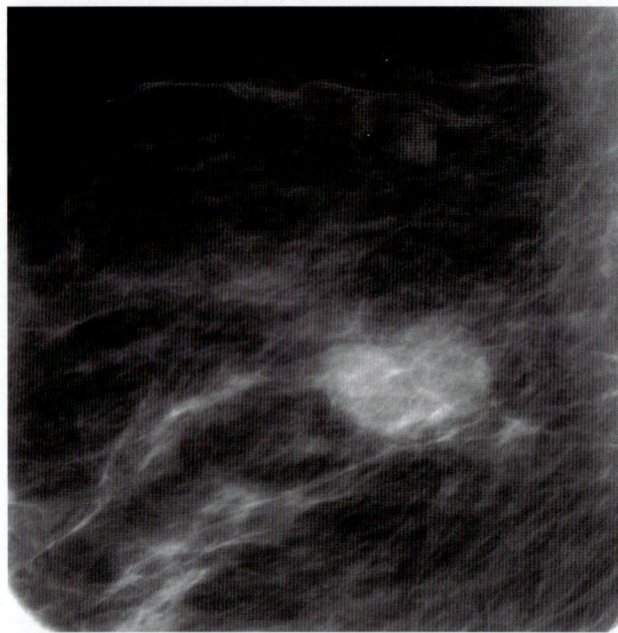

Fig. 35.7 Right MLO spot compression mammogram. There is an oval mass with ill-defined, irregular margins in the upper outer quadrant of the right breast.

Ultrasound

Frequency (Fig. 35.8)
- 14 MHz

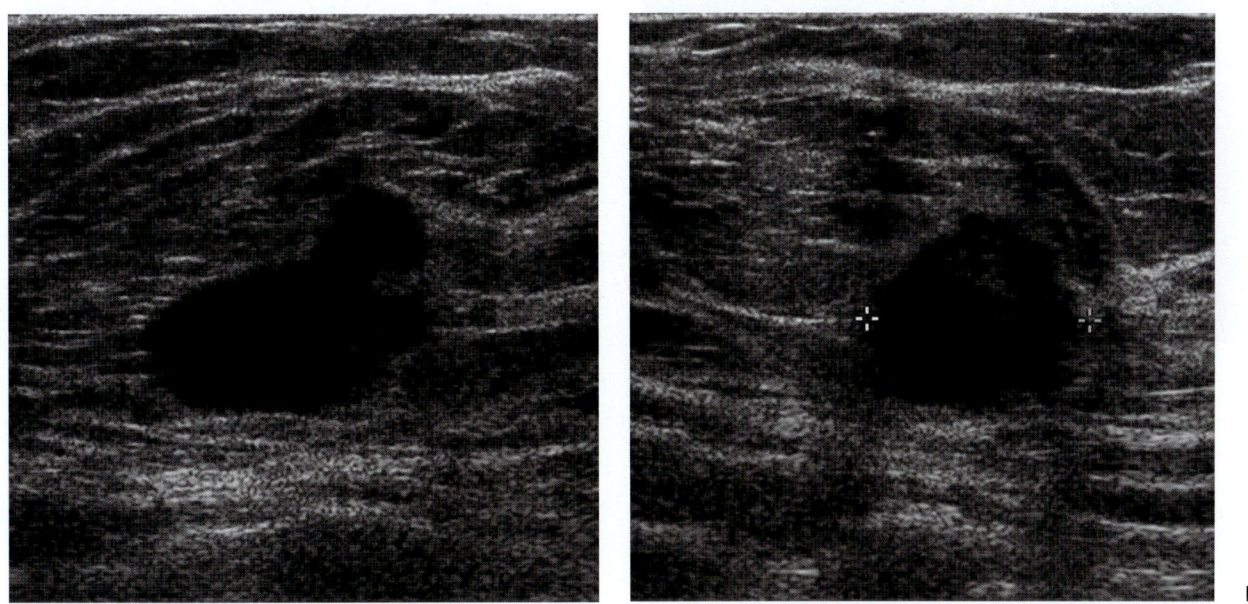

Fig. 35.8 The mammographic mass corresponds to a sonographically solid, hypoechoic, mildly lobulated mass. The margins are mildly irregular on the antiradial image. (**A**) Right radial breast sonogram. (**B**) Right antiradial breast sonogram.

Other Modalities: PET-CT (Fig. 35.9)

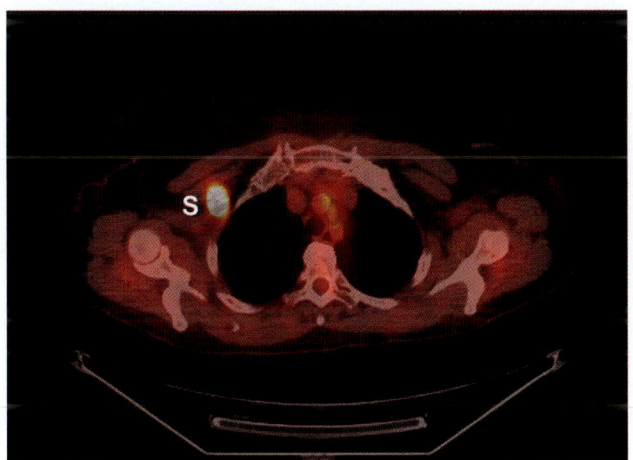
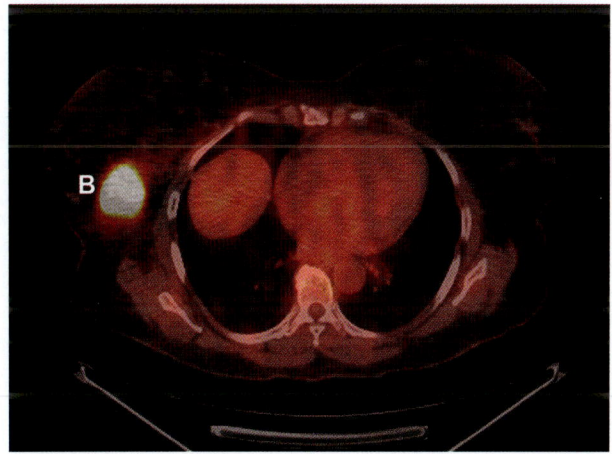

Fig. 35.9 Because the patient's tumor histologically is aggressive, a PET scan is performed, which demonstrates abnormal uptake in the liver (L), right supraclavicular lymph node (S), and right breast (B). The liver and nodal appearance is consistent with metastatic disease. (**A**) Axial positron emission tomography–computed tomography (PET-CT) of upper chest. (**B**) Axial PET-CT of lower chest.

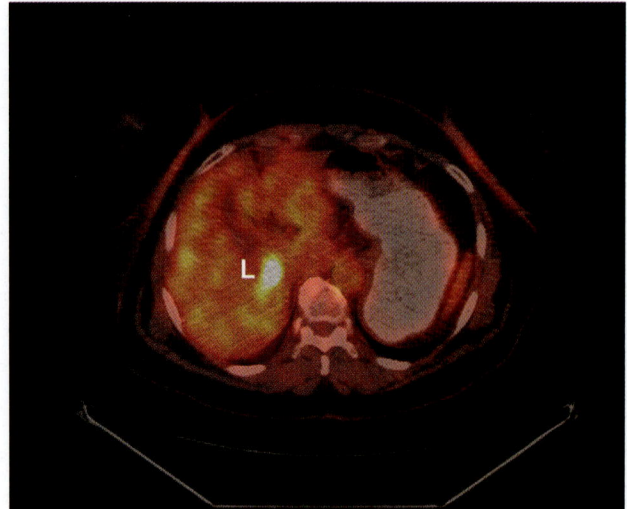
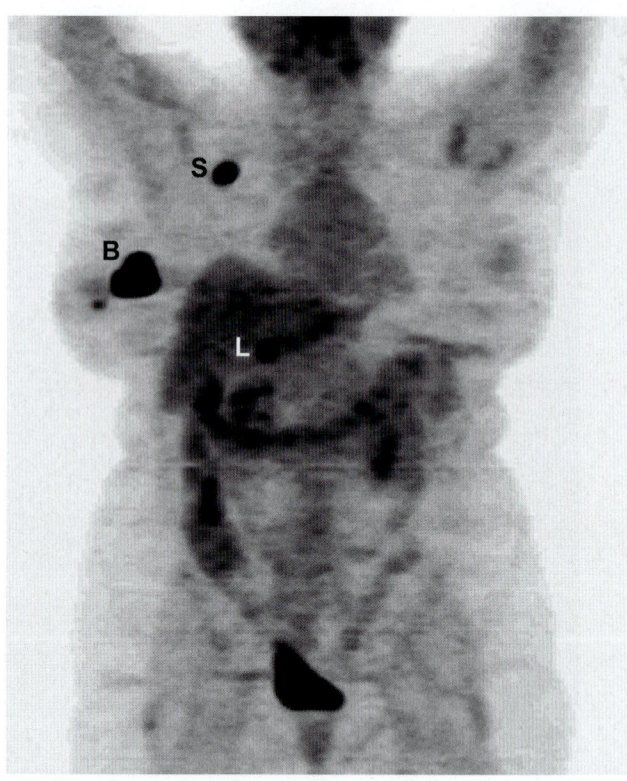

Fig. 35.9 *(continued)* (**C**) Axial PET-CT of the abdomen. (**D**) Maximum intensity projection (MIP) PET image.

Pathology
- A 3.6 cm, high-grade infiltrating ductal carcinoma, estrogen and progesterone receptor negative, with overexpression of HER-2/neu (c-erb-B2)

Management (Mammography and Ultrasound Findings)
- Right mammographic and sonographic mass: BI-RADS assessment category 4, suspicious; biopsy should be considered.

Pearls and Pitfalls
- PET is not recommended as a routine method to stage patients with early-stage breast cancer because they have a low probability of metastatic disease. However, PET has been found to be an excellent method to identify metastatic or recurrent disease. It has been shown to have slightly less than 95% sensitivity and 80 to 90% specificity for recurrent or metastatic disease.
- When researchers have retrospectively examined PET scans of patients with more advanced disease, those patients with tumors in the inner breast are more likely to present with isolated extra-axillary disease and experience progressive disease compared with those with tumors in the outer breast. These extra-axillary sites include the brain, supraclavicular region, mediastinal or internal mammary nodes, bone, liver, lung, and pleura.

Suggested Reading
Eubank WB, Mankoff D, Bhattacharya M, et al. Impact of FDG PET on defining the extent of disease and on the treatment of patients with recurrent or metastatic breast cancer. AJR Am J Roentgenol 2004;183(2):479–486

Moon DH, Maddahi J, Silverman DHS, Glaspy JA, Phelps ME, Hoh CK. Accuracy of whole-body fluorine-18-FDG PET for the detection of recurrent or metastatic breast carcinoma. J Nucl Med 1998;39(3):431–435

Tran A, Pio BS, Khatibi B, Czernin J, Phelps ME, Silverman DHS. ^{18}F-FDG PET for staging breast cancer in patients with inner-quadrant versus outer-quadrant tumors: comparison with long-term clinical outcome. J Nucl Med 2005;46(9):1455–1459

Case 35.3: Staging Advanced Disease

Case History
A 66-year-old woman presents with palpable left breast lump.

Physical Examination
- Palpable firmness in the left inferior outer breast

Mammogram

Mass (Fig. 35.10)
- Margin: spiculated
- Shape: irregular
- Density: high
- Associated calcifications: heterogeneous

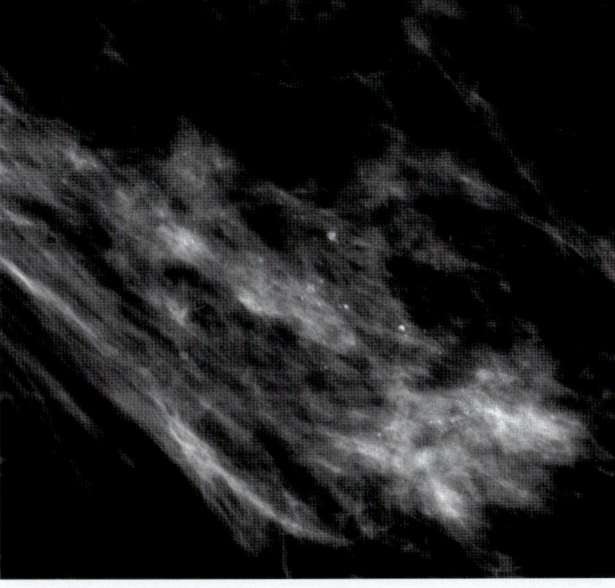

Fig. 35.10 Left ML magnification mammogram. There is an ill-defined, irregular, spiculated mass in the left inferior outer breast that is associated with heterogeneous calcifications that are scattered throughout the quadrant.

Other Modalities: PET-CT (Figs. 35.11, 35.12, and 35.13)

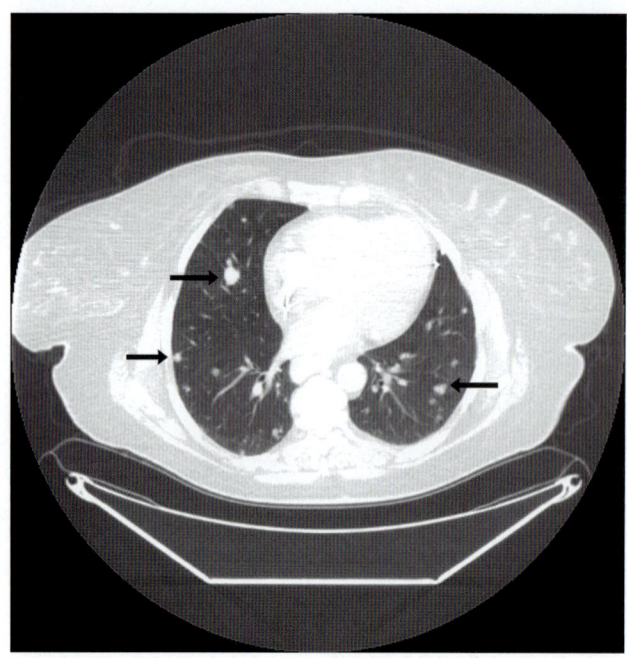

Fig. 35.11 Axial CT of the chest. There are numerous 1 to 2 cm pulmonary nodules (*arrows*) consistent with pulmonary metastases.

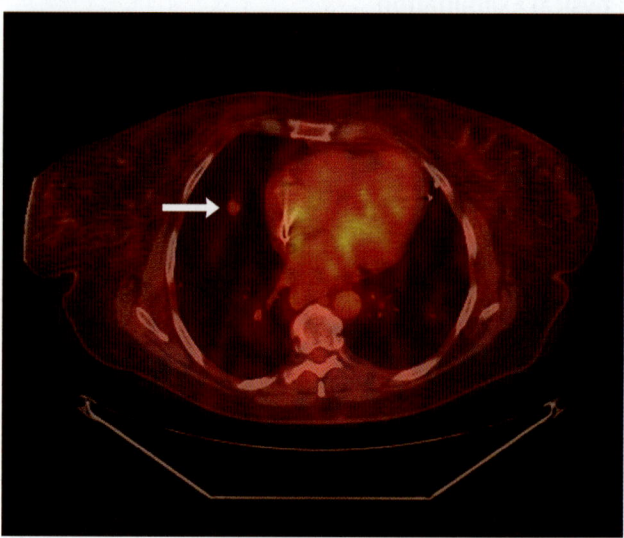

Fig. 35.12 Axial PET-CT image. The pulmonary nodules (*arrow*) do not exhibit significant uptake on the PET-CT images.

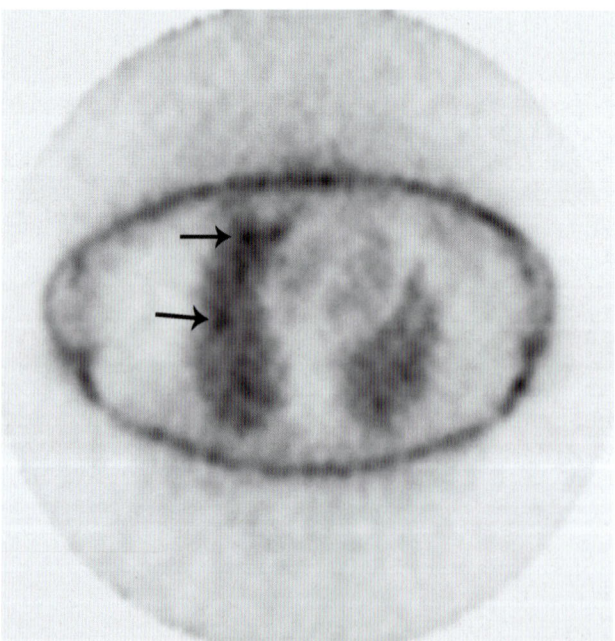

Fig. 35.13 Non-attenuation-corrected axial PET. This image demonstrates focal uptake corresponding to pulmonary nodules (*arrows*), consistent with metastases to the lung.

Pathology
- Invasive ductal carcinoma, grade II (intermediate grade)

Management
- Left mammographic mass: BI-RADS assessment category 5, highly suggestive of malignancy

Pearls and Pitfalls
- PET is useful in identifying metastatic disease in patients who present with advanced-stage breast cancer. Slightly less than 10% of these patients are found to have distant metastases with PET. In a small series, PET identified between 80 and 100% of pulmonary nodules compared with chest radiographs.
- Small pulmonary metastases are often difficult to identify on PET-CT because small nodules challenge the spatial resolution capabilities of PET. However, as this case demonstrates, metastasis can be identified on non-attenuation-corrected images, which often demonstrate uptake in small nodules that are not evident on attenuation-corrected PET-CT images.
- Causes of false-positive PET uptake in the lung or mediastinum include trauma, infection, and inflammatory or granulomatous diseases such as sarcoid.

Suggested Reading

Cermik TF, Mavi A, Basu S, Alavi A. Impact of FDG PET on the preoperative staging of newly diagnosed breast cancer. Eur J Nucl Med Mol Imaging 2008;35(3):475–483

Lind P, Igerc I, Beyer T, Reinprecht P, Hausegger K. Advantages and limitations of FDG PET in the follow-up of breast cancer. Eur J Nucl Med Mol Imaging 2004;31(Suppl 1):S125–S134

Schirrmeister H, Kühn T, Guhlmann A, et al. Fluorine-18 2-deoxy-2-fluoro-D-glucose PET in the preoperative staging of breast cancer: comparison with the standard staging procedures. Eur J Nucl Med 2001;28(3):351–358

van der Hoeven JJM, Krak NC, Hoekstra OS, et al. ^{18}F-2-fluoro-2-deoxy-D-glucose positron emission tomography in staging of locally advanced breast cancer. J Clin Oncol 2004;22(7):1253–1259

Case 35.4: Staging Advanced Disease

Case History
A 46-year-old woman presents with a 3-week history of right breast swelling, redness, and mild tenderness. She has started antibiotics, but her symptoms have not changed.

Physical Examination
- Right breast: warm, indurated, red, and tender
- Left breast: normal exam

Mammogram (Fig. 35.14)
- Right breast: global asymmetry

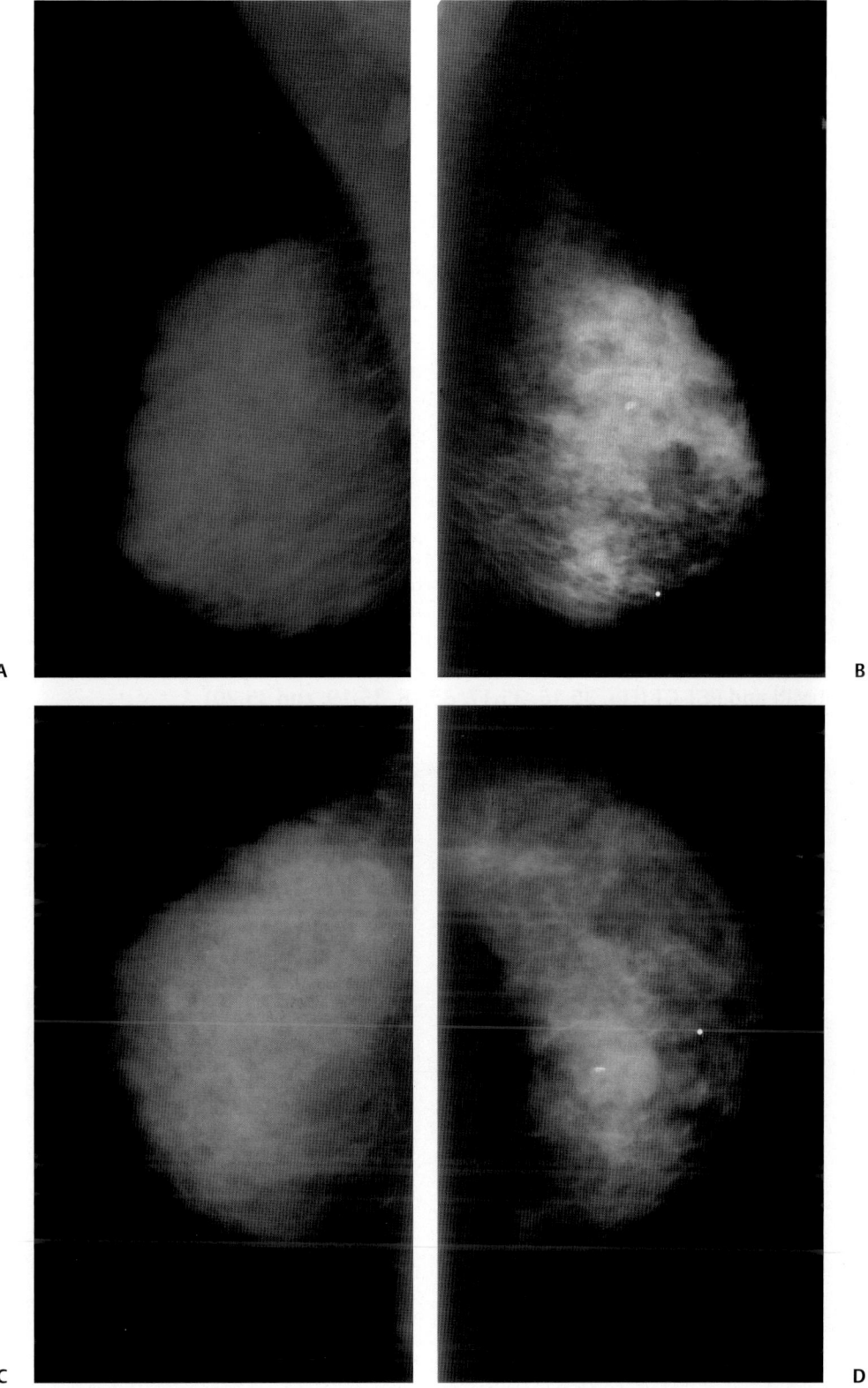

Fig. 35.14 Both breasts exhibit extremely dense composition, but the right breast is denser than the left breast. There are also some enlarged right axillary lymph nodes. (**A**) Right MLO mammogram. (**B**) Left MLO mammogram. (**C**) Right CC mammogram. (**D**) Left CC mammogram.

Ultrasound

Frequency (Fig. 35.15)
- 14 MHz

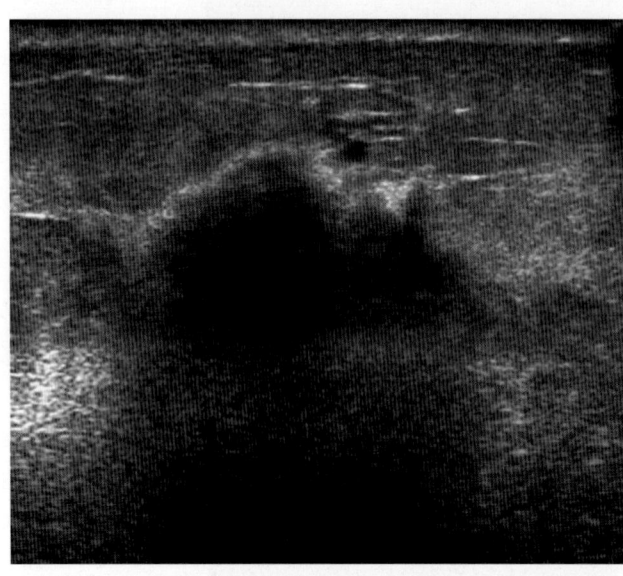

Fig. 35.15 Right radial breast sonogram. There is diffuse edematous change in the breast. The normal landmarks such as Cooper's ligaments are obscured by the edema. In the upper outer quadrant, there is a hypoechoic irregular mass with severe shadowing.

Other Modalities: MRI and PET-CT (Fig. 35.16, 35.17, 35.18, 35.19, and 35.20)

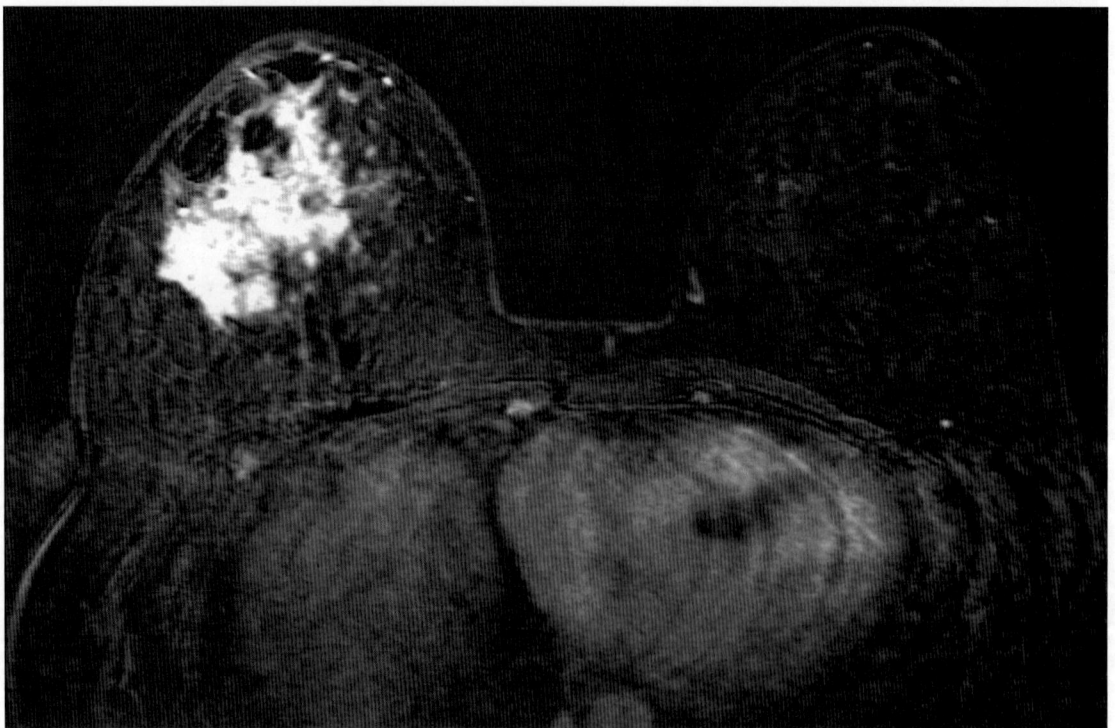

Fig. 35.16 Dynamic bolus T1-weighted, 2-minute subtraction axial bilateral breast MRI demonstrates homogeneous enhancement of the right upper outer quadrant and central breast.

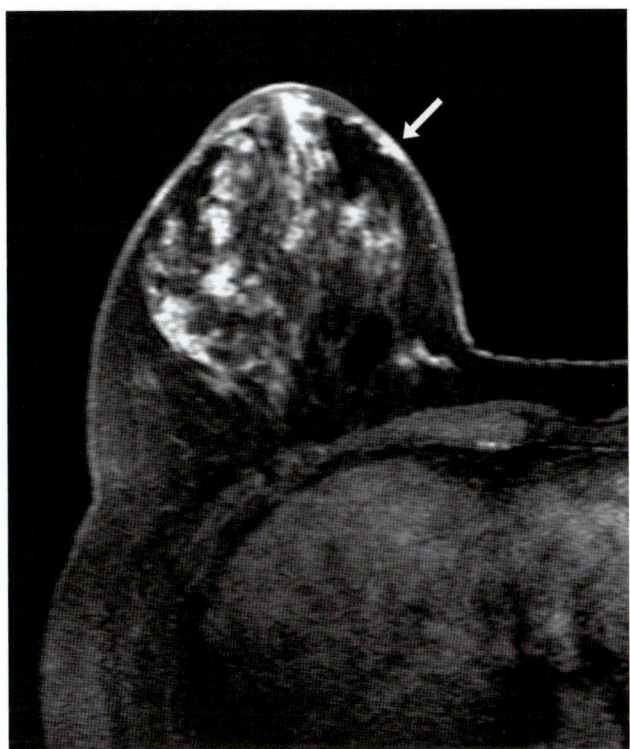

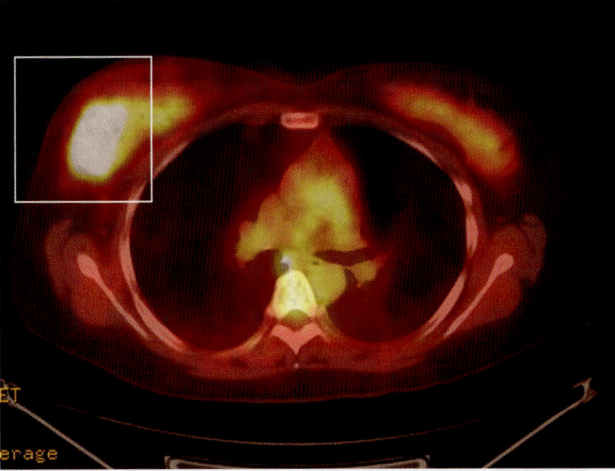

Fig. 35.19 Axial PET-CT. There is high ^{18}F-fluorodeoxyglucose (FDG) uptake in the right breast, consistent with breast malignancy (*square*). The maximum standardized uptake value (SUV) of the breast is 18. On a different axial image (not shown), there is abnormal uptake in a right axillary node.

Fig. 35.17 Dynamic bolus T1-weighted, 2-minute subtraction axial right breast MRI. In the inferior breast, there is clumped enhancement with focal skin thickening distant from the dominant parenchymal enhancement (*arrow*).

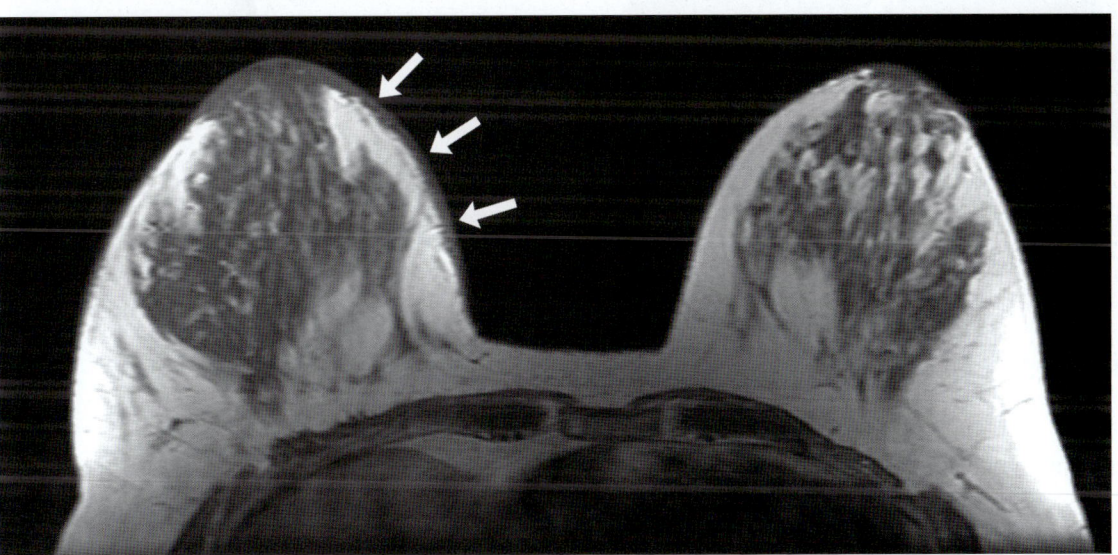

Fig. 35.18 T1-weighted noncontrast axial bilateral breast MRI. Without fat saturation, the diffuse medial skin thickening is evident (*arrows*).

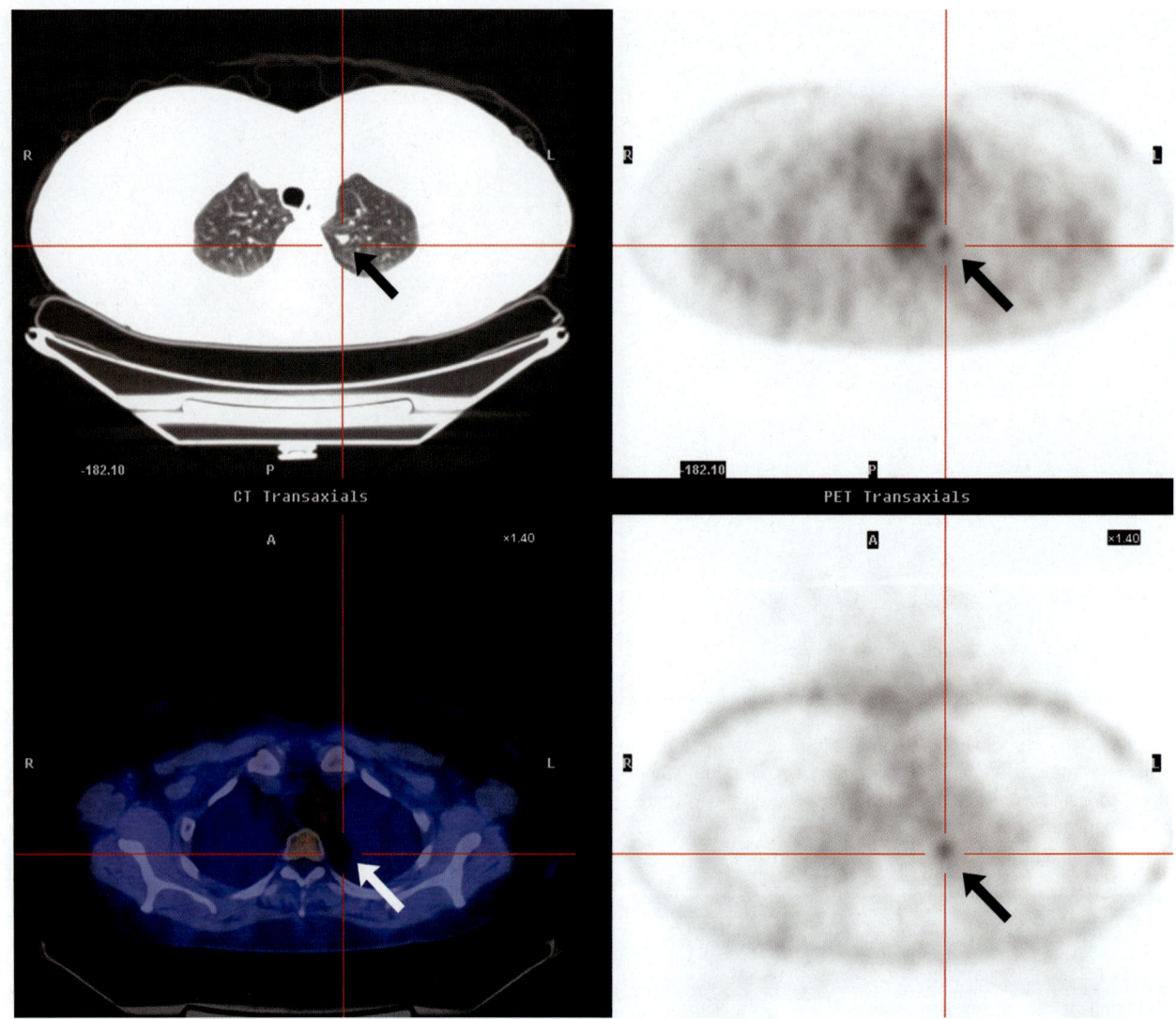

Fig. 35.20 Axial PET-CT with non-attenuation-corrected axial PET images. Right pulmonary nodule (*arrow*) also exhibits abnormal uptake, as shown by the non-attenuation-corrected axial PET images. The cross-hairs cross-correlate the location of the pulmonary nodule on the PET-CT fused image with the separated CT and PET images.

Pathology
- High-grade infiltrating ductal carcinoma

Management
- BI-RADS assessment category 5, highly suggestive of malignancy

Pearls and Pitfalls

- Inflammatory breast cancer accounts for approximately 1 to 5% of all breast cancer cases in the United States. Clinically, the patient presents with inflammatory skin changes, and histologically, the clinical findings are due to lymphatic obstruction from an underlying invasive adenocarcinoma, not to inflammatory cell infiltration. Dermal invasion without the clinical presentation is not sufficient to be considered inflammatory carcinoma.
- Three retrospective studies since 2000 reported the most common mammographic abnormalities of inflammatory breast cancer include skin thickening (83–92%), trabecular thickening (62–81%), microcalcifications (23–56%), mass (15–32%), and axillary adenopathy (24–58%). Two of these studies also recorded sonographic findings, including mass (71–80%), skin thickening (95–96%), and axillary adenopathy (73–93%).
- With contrast-enhanced, T1-weighted, fat-saturated MRI, inflammatory breast cancer may have any of the following findings: irregular rapidly enhancing mass generally with washout, poorly defined regional or diffuse enhancement, reticular/dendritic enhancement, and skin enhancement. The skin enhancement is commonly focal and not necessarily contiguous with the enhancing mass.
- Yang and coworkers[1] noted that in 23/24 (96%) patients with inflammatory breast cancer, PET-CT identified diffuse increased uptake of FDG in the symptomatic breast with skin thickening. Other findings included axillary adenopathy (88%), internal mammary adenopathy (25%), supraclavicular adenopathy (8%), and distant metastases (38%).

Reference

1. Yang WT, Le-Petross HT, Macapinlac H, et al. Inflammatory breast cancer: PET/CT, MRI, mammography, and sonography findings. Breast Cancer Res Treat 2008;109(3):417–426

Suggested Reading

Berg WA. Inflammatory breast cancer. In: Berg WA, Birdwell RL, Gombos EC, Wang S-C, Parkinson BT, Raza S, Green GE, Kennedy A, Kettler MD, eds. Diagnostic Imaging Breast. Altona, Manitoba: Friesens; 2006, IV-2-134-139

de Paredes ES. The thickened skin pattern. In: de Paredes ES. Atlas of Mammography. Philadelphia: Lippincott Williams & Wilkins; 2007:418-444

Ellis IO, Schnitt SJ, Sastre-Garau X, et al. Invasive breast carcinoma. In: Tavassoli FA, Devilee P, eds. Tumours of the Breast and Female Genital Organs. Lyon: IARC Press; 2003:13-59

Günhan-Bilgen I, Ustün EE, Memiş A. Inflammatory breast carcinoma: mammographic, ultrasonographic, clinical, and pathologic findings in 142 cases. Radiology 2002;223(3):829–838

Kushwaha AC, Whitman GJ, Stelling CB, Cristofanilli M, Buzdar AU. Primary inflammatory carcinoma of the breast: retrospective review of mammographic findings. AJR Am J Roentgenol 2000;174(2):535–538

Merajver SD, Sabel MS. Inflammatory breast cancer. In: Harris JR, Lippman ME, Morrow M, Osborne CK, eds. Diseases of the Breast. 3rd ed. Philadelphia: Lippincott Williams & Wilkins; 2004:971-982

Case 35.5: Staging Advanced Disease

Case History
A 73-year-old woman presents with a left breast mass.

Physical Examination
- Palpable left breast mass in the upper outer quadrant

Mammogram

Mass (Fig. 35.21)
- Margin: ill defined
- Shape: irregular
- Density: high density

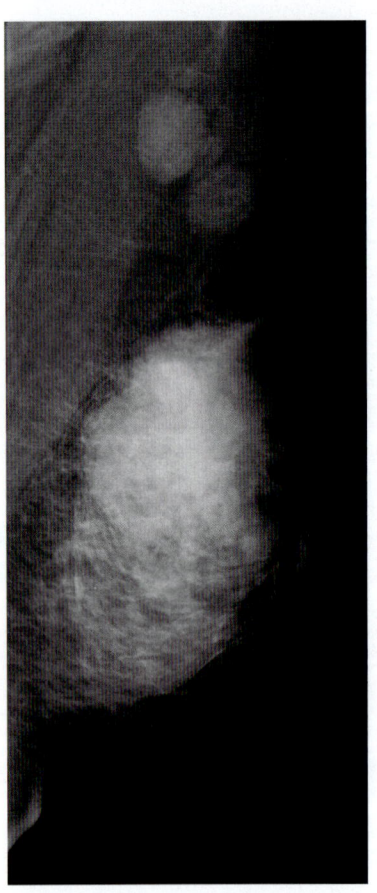
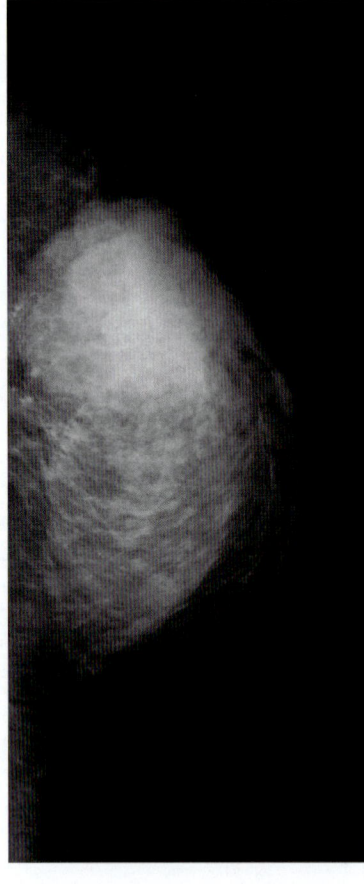

Fig. 35.21 In the left upper outer quadrant, there is a large, ill-defined, irregular, high-density mass that involves the entire quadrant. (**A**) Left MLO mammogram. (**B**) Left exaggerated craniocaudal mammogram.

Staging 587

Ultrasound

High Frequency
- 15 MHz

Mass (Figs. 35.22 and 35.23)
- Retrotumoral acoustic appearance: severe; appearance of mass obscured by shadowing

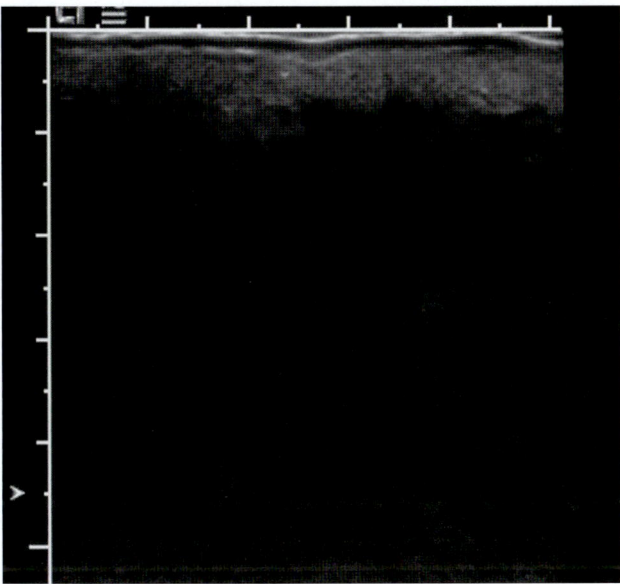

Fig. 35.22 Left antiradial breast sonogram. The mammographic mass corresponds to a heavily shadowing solid mass.

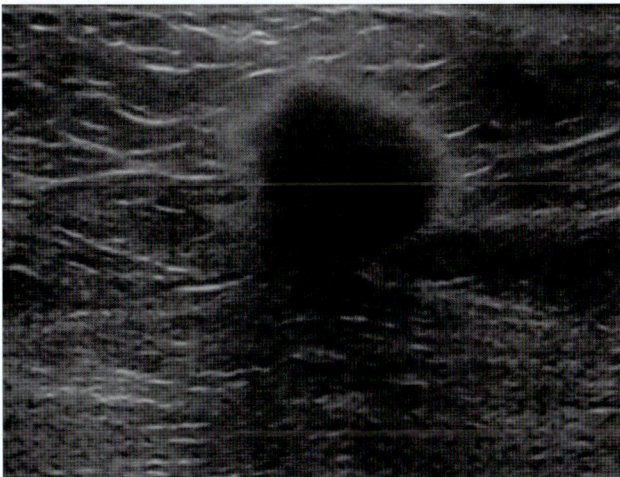

Fig. 35.23 Left axillary breast sonogram. Multiple abnormally enlarged hypoechoic axillary lymph nodes are present. These lymph nodes do not demonstrate a hyperechoic hilum, are angular in shape, and have hyperechoic halos. This combination of signs is highly suggestive of malignancy.

Low Frequency
- 8 MHz

Mass (Fig. 35.24)
- Margins: ill defined
- Echogenicity: hypoechoic
- Retrotumoral acoustic appearance: severe shadowing, but less than high-frequency exam
- Shape: irregular

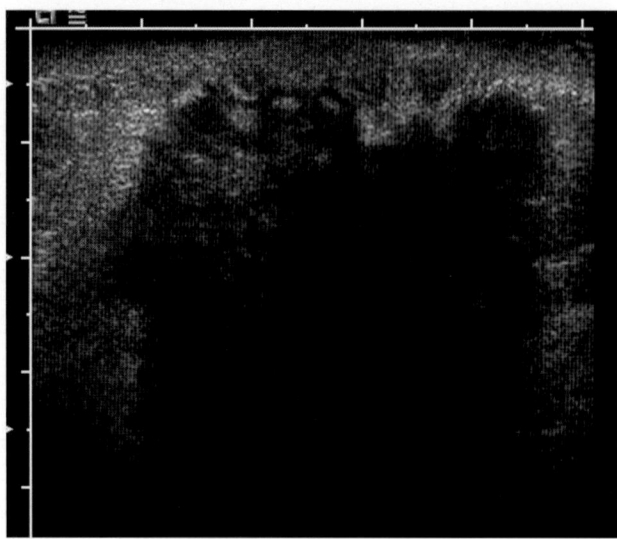

Fig. 35.24 Left antiradial breast sonogram. The shadowing decreases when the frequency is lowered from 15 MHz (**Fig. 35.22**) to 8 MHz. With this technique, the margins are better identified, so the mass may be measured.

Other Modalities: MRI and PET-CT (Figs. 35.25 and 35.26)

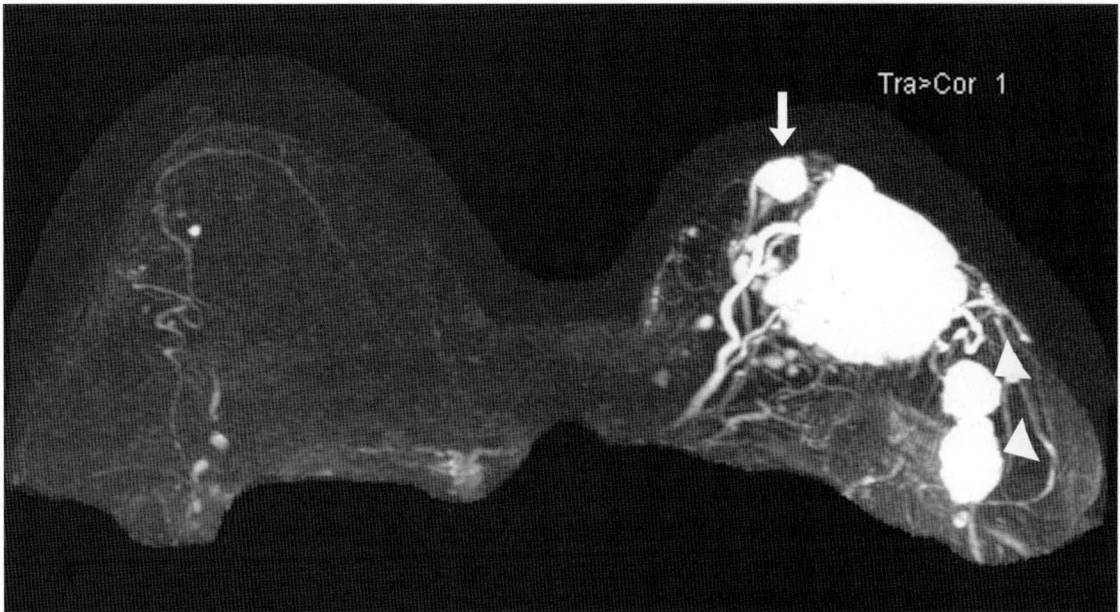

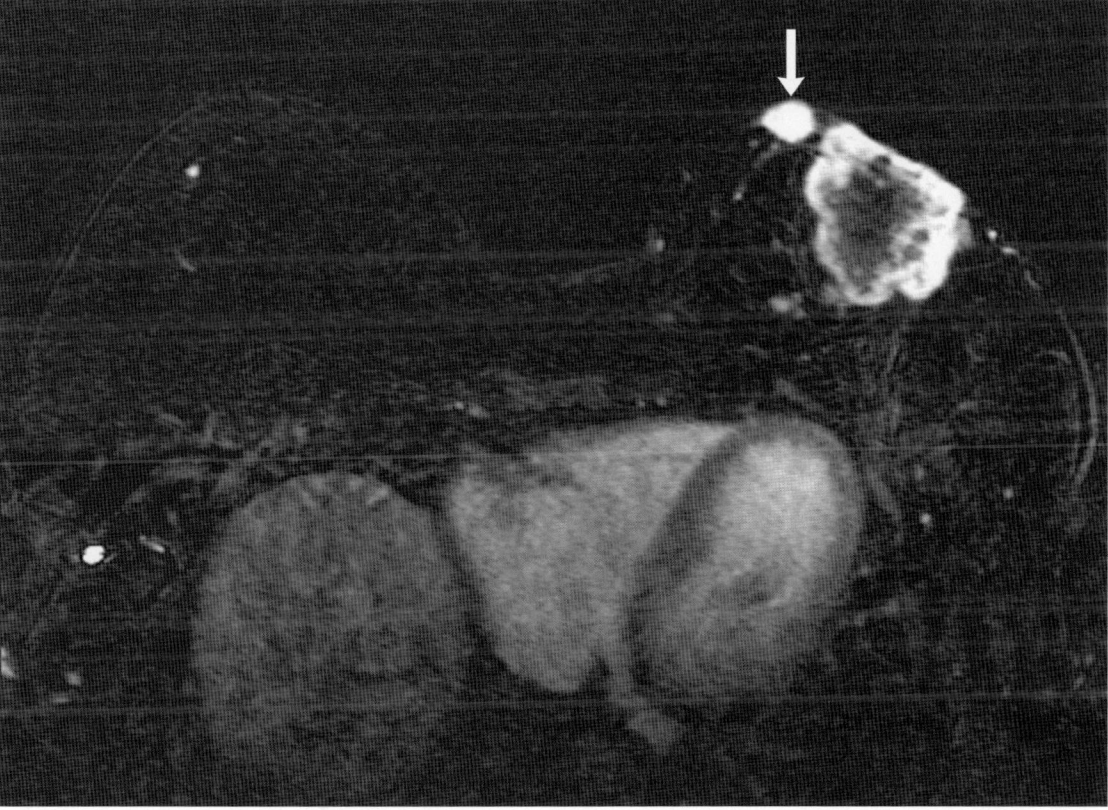

Fig. 35.25 The mammographic and sonographic mass corresponds to a rim-enhancing mass in the left upper outer quadrant. The mass invades the skin. There is a second smaller oval subareolar satellite mass (*arrow*) not previously identified on the other modalities. Large enhancing axillary nodes (*arrowheads*) are also present. (**A**) Contrast-enhanced bilateral breast MRI maximum projection intensity (MIP) image with T1 technique using 2-minute subtraction series. (**B**) Dynamic bolus T1-weighted, 2-minute subtraction axial bilateral breast MRI. *(Continued on page 591)*

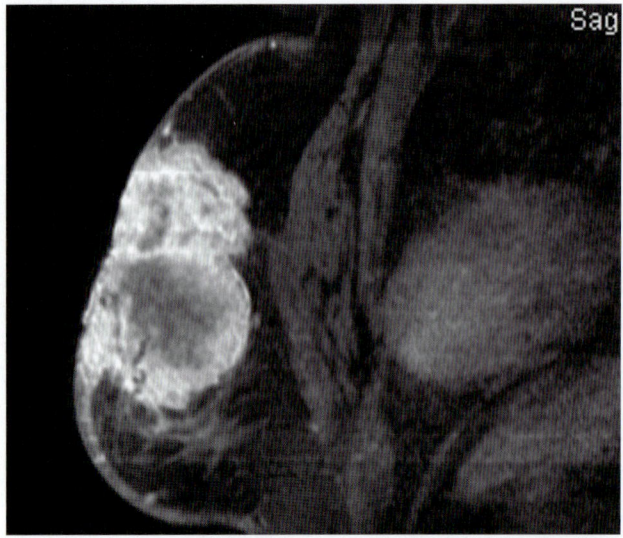

Figure 35.25 *(continued)* (**C**) T1-weighted, fat-suppressed sagittal multiplanar reconstruction (MPR).

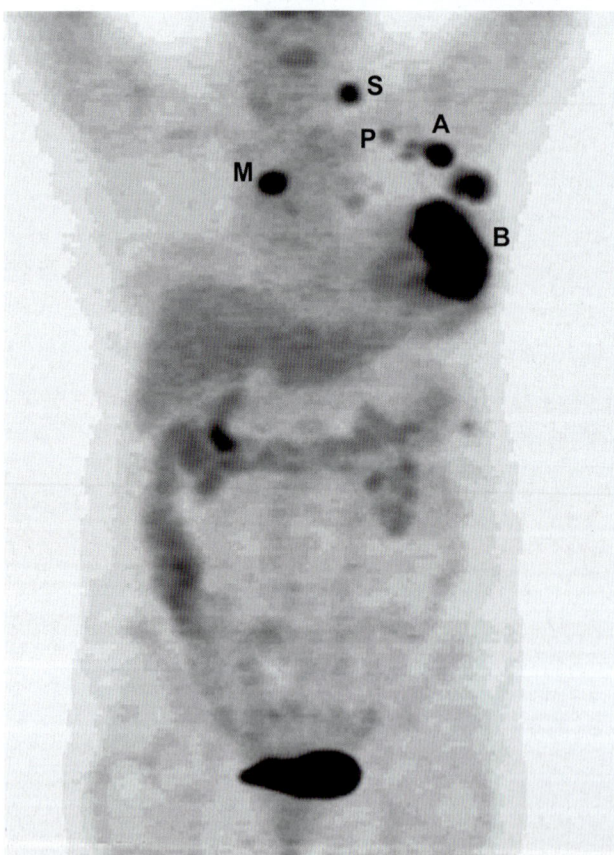

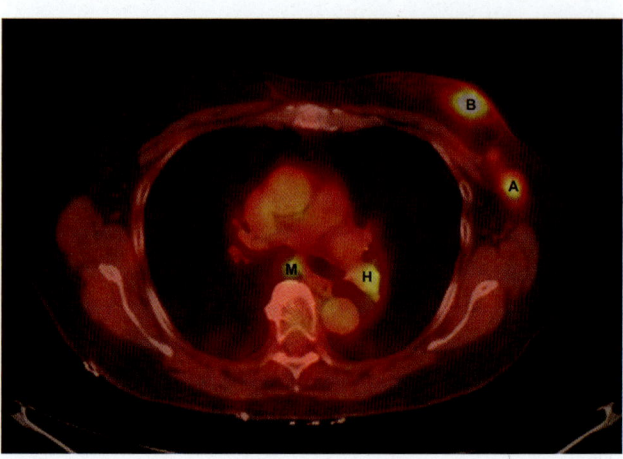

Fig. 35.26 Besides abnormal uptake in the left breast mass (B), the PET scan shows abnormal uptake in mediastinal (M), hilar (H), supraclavicular (S), and axillary (A) lymph nodes, as well as pulmonary nodules (P). (**A**) Maximum projection intensity PET image. (**B**) Axial PET-CT.

Pathology
- Infiltrating ductal carcinoma

Management
- BI-RADS assessment category 5, highly suggestive of malignancy

Pearls and Pitfalls

- This case is an example of a large malignancy presenting as heavy sonographic shadowing. An inexperienced imager may miss the malignancy by confusing the shadowing with hyperechoic benign breast tissue. However, in this case, by lowering the frequency, the observer can identify the margins of the mass.
- Peripheral rim enhancement in a rapidly enhancing irregular MRI mass is highly suggestive of malignancy. The most common benign entities that may produce rim enhancement are inflamed cysts and fat necrosis. Inflamed cysts can be differentiated from malignancies because the rim is thin and circumscribed, and the cyst does not enhance. T2-weighted images further characterize the cystic nature of the mass. Fat necrosis may present as an irregular mass with rim enhancement on T1-weighted images with low central signal on fat-suppressed images. T1-weighted nonsuppressed images are also helpful in this situation, because they demonstrate high central fat signal.
- This case illustrates the utility of PET-CT in staging breast cancer. When CT is added to the PET technique, the diagnostic confidence may be increased by as much as 50% compared with using PET alone due to identification of more malignancies and improved anatomical localization.

Suggested Reading

Abramson AF. Benign lesions. In: Morris EA, Liberman L, eds. Breast MRI Diagnosis and Intervention. New York: Springer; 2005:140-163

Hashimoto BE, Morgan GN, Kramer DJ, Lee ME. Systematic approach to difficult problems in breast sonography. Ultrasound Q 2008;24(1):31–38

Kim SJ, Morris EA, Liberman L, et al. Observer variability and applicability of BI-RADS terminology for breast MR imaging: invasive carcinomas as focal masses. AJR Am J Roentgenol 2001;177(3):551–557

Tatsumi M, Cohade C, Mourtzikos KA, Fishman EK, Wahl RL. Initial experience with FDG-PET/CT in the evaluation of breast cancer. Eur J Nucl Med Mol Imaging 2006;33(3):254–262

36 Assessing Response to Therapy

Case 36.1: Assessing Response to Therapy

Case History
A 47-year-old woman presents with a palpable left breast mass.

Physical Examination
- Palpable lump in the left 4 o'clock position

Mammogram

Mass (Fig. 36.1)
- Two masses have the same characteristics.
- Margin: ill defined
- Shape: irregular
- Density: equal density

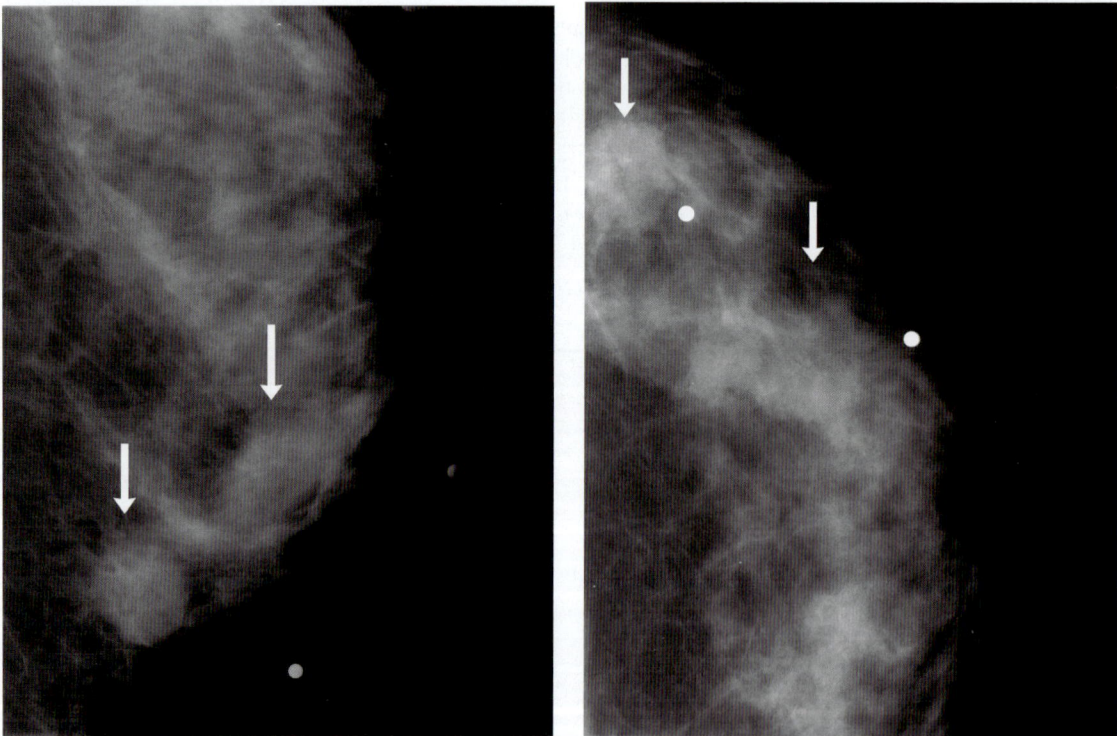

Fig. 36.1 In the left outer inner quadrant, there are two irregular masses (*arrows*). (**A**) Left ML spot compression. (**B**) Left CC spot compression.

Ultrasound (Fig. 36.2)

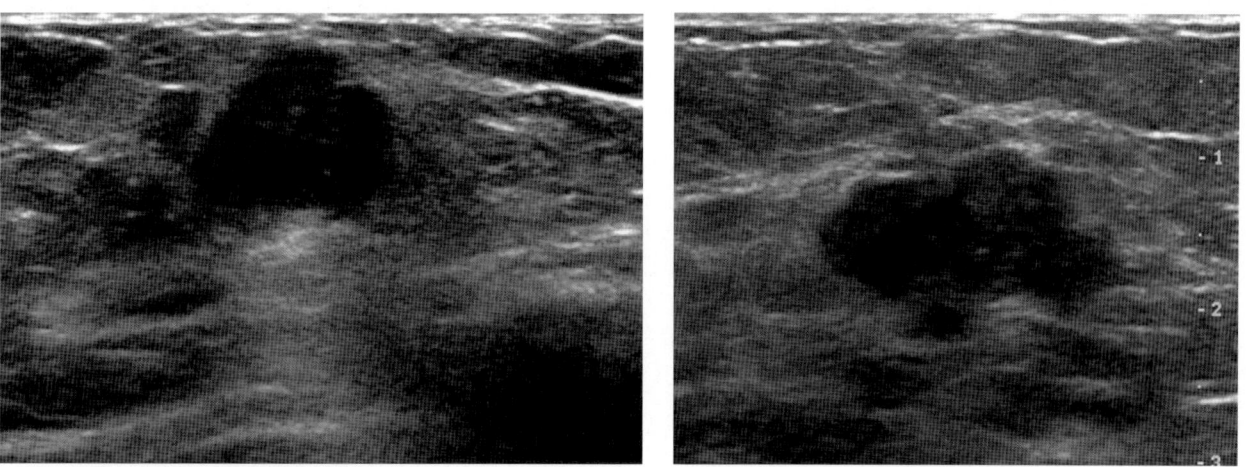

Fig. 36.2 The left breast palpable masses and the mammographic masses correspond to two solid irregular masses at the 4 o'clock and 5 o'clock positions. (**A**) Left transverse breast sonogram of the mass at the 4 o'clock position. (**B**) Left transverse breast sonogram of the mass at the 5 o'clock position.

Other Modalities: MRI and PET-CT (Figs. 36.3, 36.4, and 36.5)

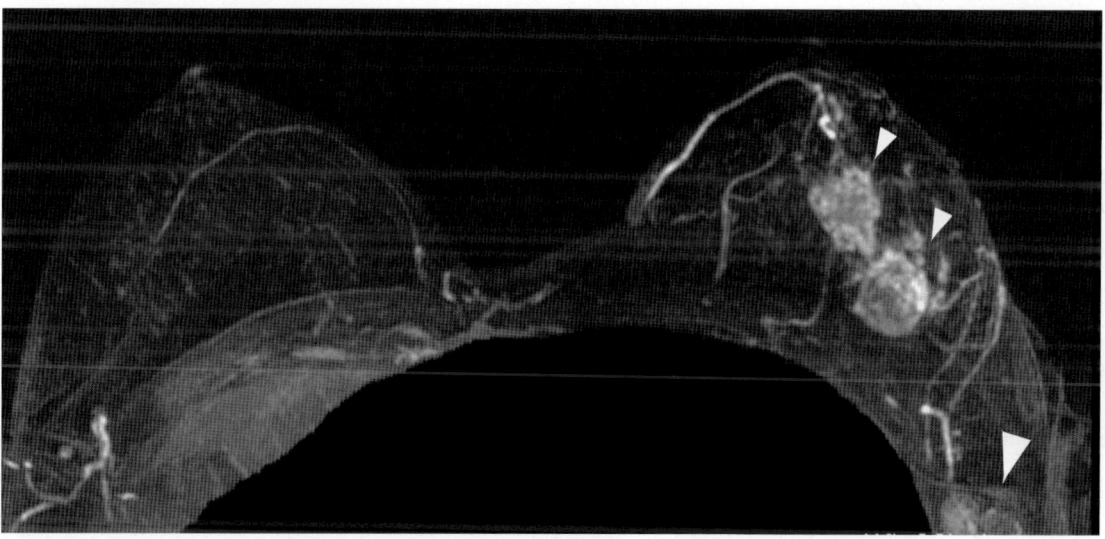

Fig. 36.3 Contrast-enhanced bilateral breast MRI maximum projection intensity (MIP) image. There are two highly enhancing suspicious irregular masses that correspond to the sonographic masses (*small arrowheads*). Suspicious enhancing axillary adenopathy is also evident (*large arrowhead*).

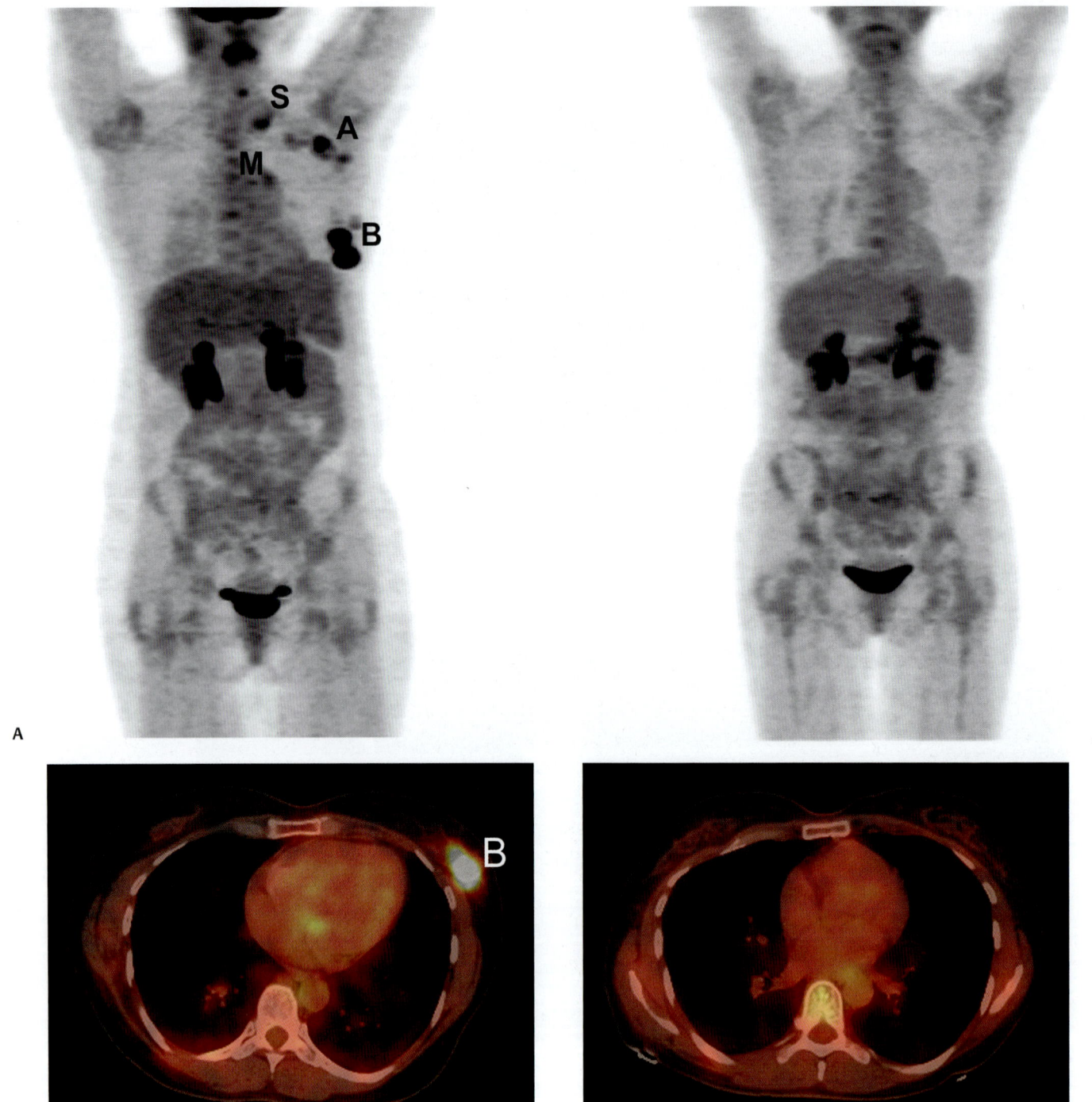

Fig. 36.4 The positron emission tomography–computed tomography (PET-CT) scan performed after the MRI demonstrates extensive ^{18}F-fluorodeoxyglucose (FDG) uptake in the left breast (B), axillary (A), supraclavicular (S), and mediastinal (M) region. (**A**) Maximum intensity projection (MIP) PET image prior to chemotherapy. (**B**) Axial PET-CT prior to chemotherapy.

Fig. 36.5 After 4 months of chemotherapy, PET-CT demonstrates resolution of the uptake in the left breast and previously abnormal lymph nodes. (**A**) MIP PET image after 4 months of chemotherapy. (**B**) Axial PET-CT image after 4 months of chemotherapy.

Pathology
- Left mastectomy and axillary dissection (performed 2 weeks after the second positron emission tomography [PET] scan) demonstrates a residual invasive ductal cancer 0.8 cm in size. Six of eight axillary nodes exhibit metastatic disease. The largest metastatic axillary nodal involvement is < 2 mm.

Management
- Left mammographic and sonographic mass: BI-RADS assessment category 5, highly suggestive of malignancy

Pearls and Pitfalls
- This case illustrates the usefulness of PET in following a patient's response to preoperative neoadjuvant systemic therapy. Multiple investigators have shown that PET is an important method to monitor the effect of these drug regimens. A 55 to 60% serial reduction in the tumor ^{18}F-fluorodeoxyglucose (FDG) uptake has been found to indicate a positive response, with an accuracy of 90% after the second round of chemotherapy. Furthermore, decrease in FDG metabolism often precedes morphologic tumor reduction. However, although this patient shows a dramatic response to treatment, the lack of FDG uptake does not mean that the malignancy has completely resolved because residual tumor is commonly still present, as demonstrated in this case.
- PET and MRI have been shown to be complementary in evaluating tumor response to therapy. Whereas PET is better for predicting poor response to therapy, MRI is better correlated with indicating complete response. Lack of tumor by MRI is strongly correlated with lack of pathologically visible tumor.

Suggested Reading

Chen X, Moore MO, Lehman CD, et al. Combined use of MRI and PET to monitor response and assess residual disease for locally advanced breast cancer treated with neoadjuvant chemotherapy. Acad Radiol 2004;11(10):1115–1124

Mankoff DA, Dunnwald LK, Gralow JR, et al. Changes in blood flow and metabolism in locally advanced breast cancer treated with neoadjuvant chemotherapy. J Nucl Med 2003;44(11):1806–1814

Rousseau C, Devillers A, Sagan C, et al. Monitoring of early response to neoadjuvant chemotherapy in stage II and III breast cancer by [18F]fluorodeoxyglucose positron emission tomography. J Clin Oncol 2006;24(34):5366–5372

Schelling M, Avril N, Nährig J, et al. Positron emission tomography using [(18)F]Fluorodeoxyglucose for monitoring primary chemotherapy in breast cancer. J Clin Oncol 2000;18(8):1689–1695

Wahl RL, Zasadny K, Helvie M, Hutchins GD, Weber B, Cody R. Metabolic monitoring of breast cancer chemohormonotherapy using positron emission tomography: initial evaluation. J Clin Oncol 1993;11(11):2101–2111

Case 36.2: Assessing Response to Therapy

Case History

A 68-year-old woman presents with a left breast 3 cm painful lump at the 2 o'clock position. The patient's mammograms and left breast sonogram were normal. Because the lump persisted, the patient had a breast MRI.

Physical Examination
- Left breast: 3 cm tender lump at the 2 o'clock position approximately 1 cm from the nipple

Mammogram (Fig. 36.6)
- Normal

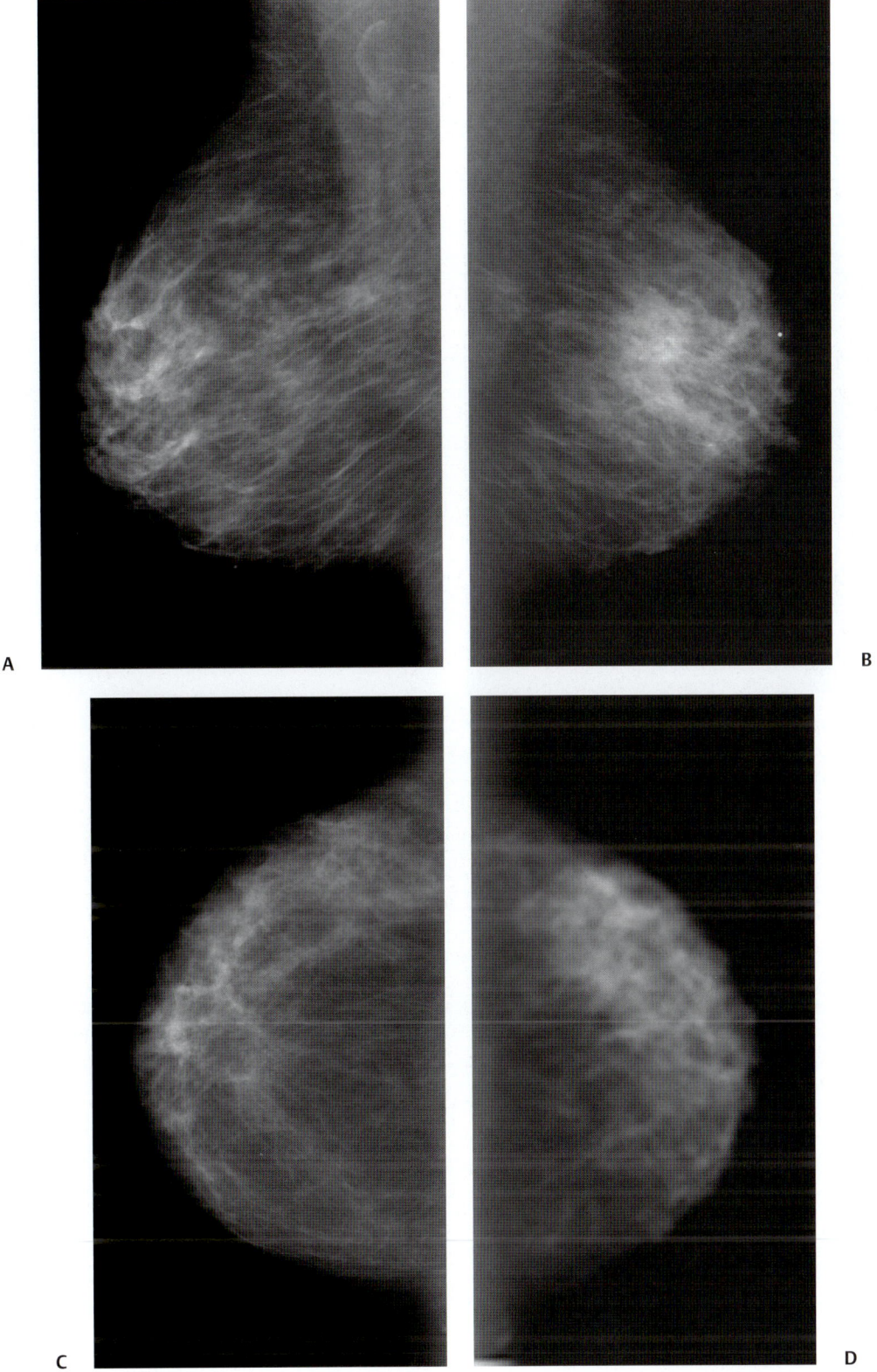

Fig. 36.6 The mammograms were interpreted as negative. In retrospect, there may be slight asymmetry in the left upper outer quadrant, but this asymmetry had been stable for at least 2 years. (**A**) Right MLO mammogram. (**B**) Left MLO mammogram. (**C**) Right CC mammogram. (**D**) Left CC mammogram.

Ultrasound

Frequency (Fig. 36.7)

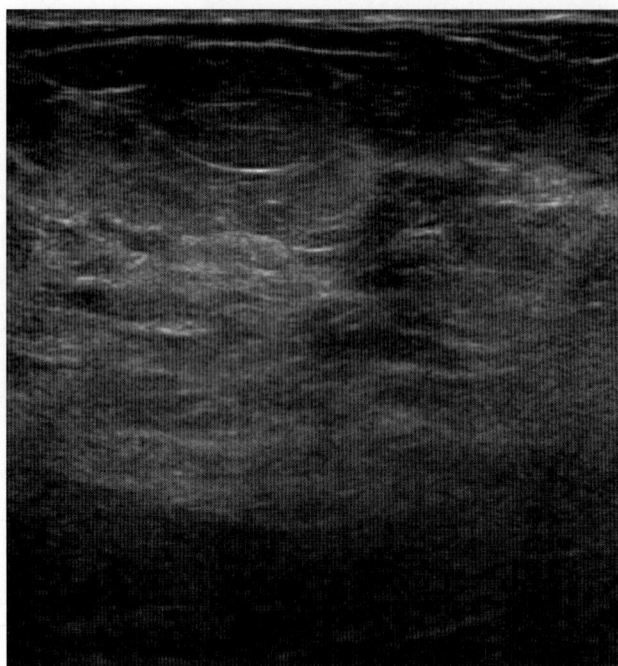

Fig. 36.7 Left breast radial sonogram at the 2 o'clock position. The initial sonographic study examines the left 2 o'clock position, which corresponded to the clinically described mass. This sonogram is normal.

Other Modalities: MRI, Second Look Sonography, and PET-CT (Figs. 36.8, 36.9, 36.10, and 36.11)

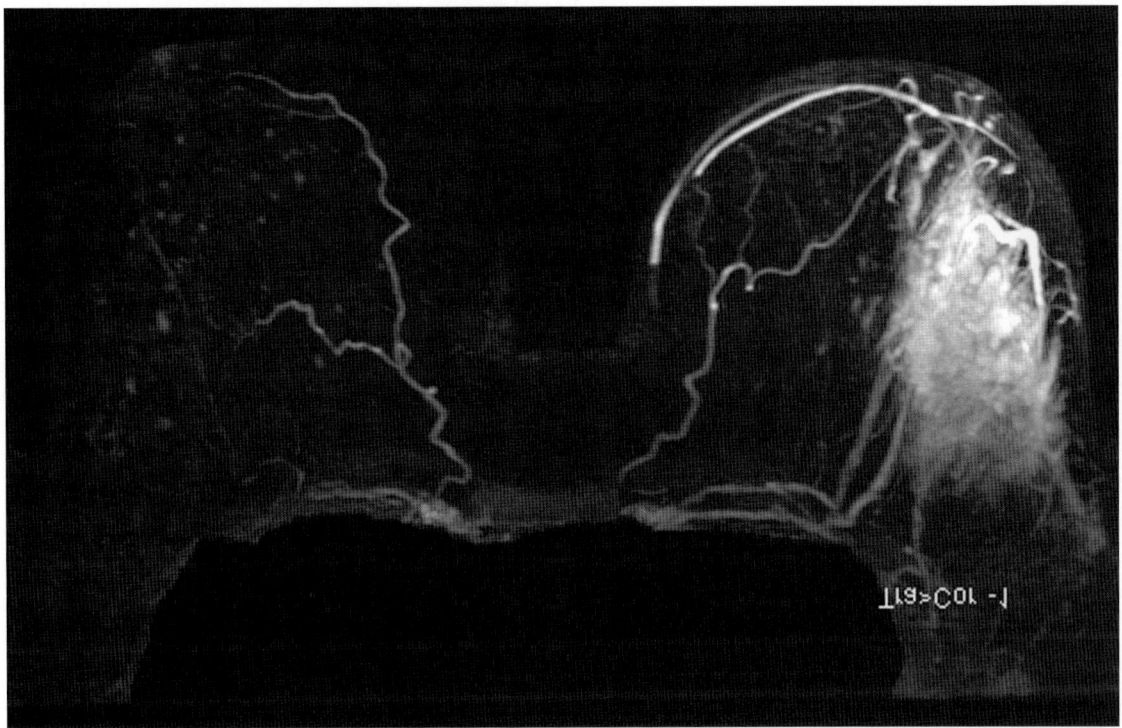

Fig. 36.8 Contrast-enhanced bilateral breast MRI MIP image. MRI demonstrates an enhancing irregular, highly suspicious mass.

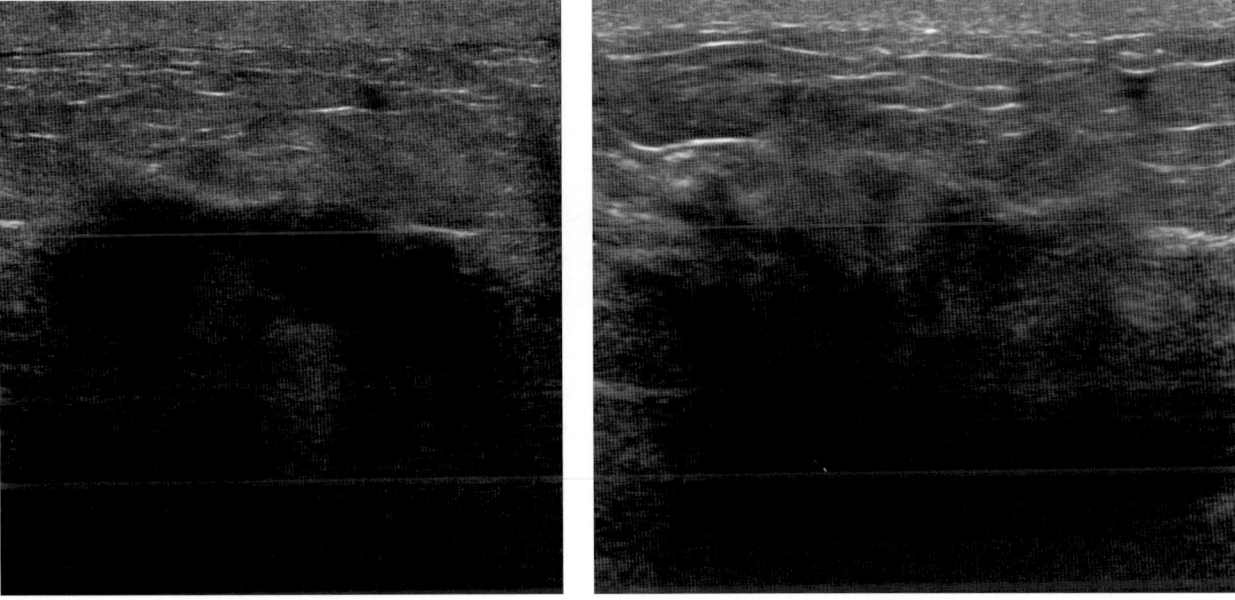

Fig. 36.9 One month after **Fig. 36.7**, the patient returns for a repeat left sonogram to characterize the MRI mass at the 4 o'clock position. The MRI mass corresponds to a large irregular, hypoechoic solid mass. **(A)** Left breast radial sonogram at the 4 o'clock position. **(B)** Left breast antiradial sonogram at the 4 o'clock position.

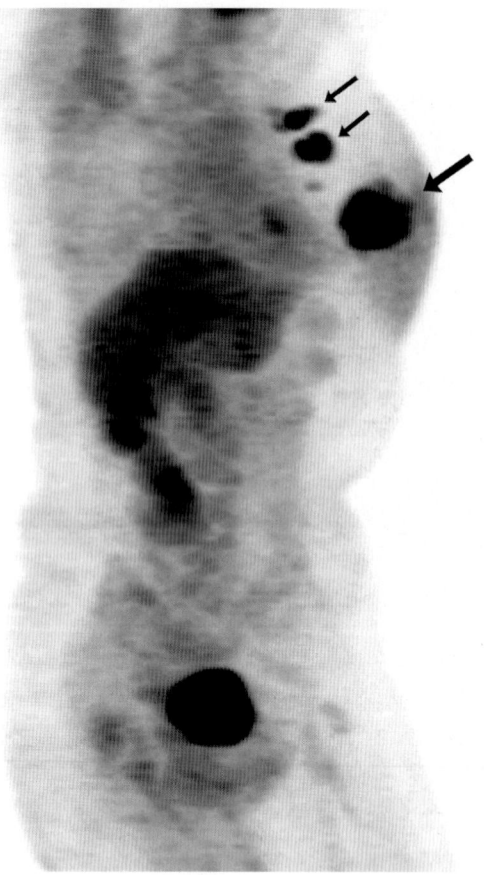 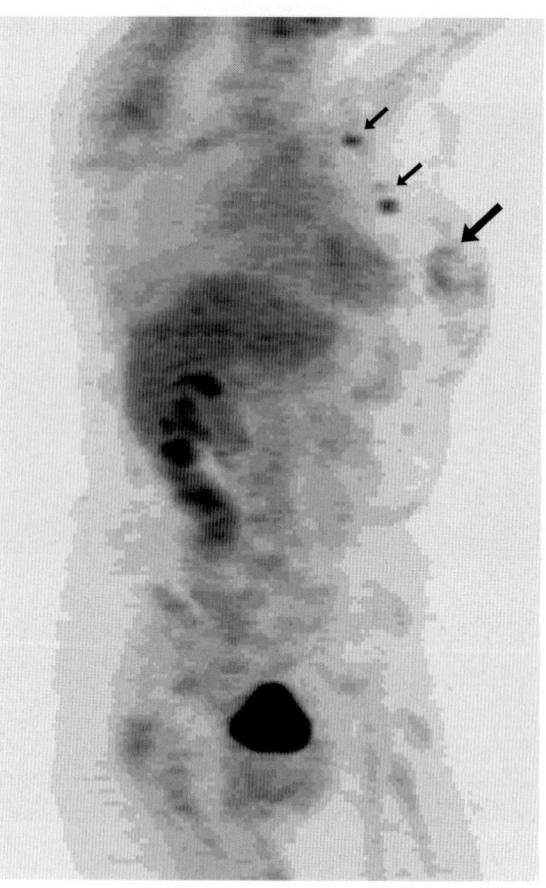

Fig. 36.10 Positron emission tomography (PET) MIP image performed after MRI and prior to chemotherapy. The PET scan demonstrates increased left breast uptake (*large arrow*) in the area of MRI enhancement with a maximum standardized uptake value (SUV) of 17. There are multiple enhancing axillary lymph nodes that have maximum SUVs of 18 (*small arrows*).

Fig. 36.11 PET MIP image performed after 6 months of neoadjuvant chemotherapy. PET scan shows that both the primary breast cancer (*large arrow*) and the axillary disease (*small arrows*) have decreased.

Pathology
- Patient received preoperative neoadjuvant chemotherapy and had a mastectomy and axillary dissection 7 months after discovery of her left breast cancer. Her surgical histology confirmed the initial sonographic biopsy of high-grade invasive ductal carcinoma. Her tumor was 7 cm in size; 26 of 26 axillary nodes were positive for metastatic disease.

Management
- Left MRI breast mass: BI-RADS assessment category 5, highly suggestive of malignancy

Pearls and Pitfalls

- Because the negative predictive value of mammography and ultrasound for identifying malignancy presenting as a palpable mass is > 97%, the American College of Radiology Appropriateness Criteria do not recommend any other imaging. In this case, the initial lack of sonographic identification is due to this modality's small field of view. MRI has been investigated as a possible method to identify malignancy when both mammography and ultrasound are negative. Although investigators have found that MRI complements mammography and ultrasound, there are still not enough data to establish the routine use of MRI in this clinical situation. MRI has been found to have excellent sensitivity (> 90%), but reported specificities have been lower (37–100%). In this case, MRI was useful because the patient and her primary care provider preferred to pursue noninvasive imaging rather than palpation-guided, fine-needle aspiration or core biopsy.
- PET is helpful to follow the effect of neoadjuvant therapy. Studies indicate that the serial change in uptake of FDG during therapy can differentiate responders from nonresponders. Furthermore, multiple studies have found that measurement of FDG after the early cycles (first and second) are particularly predictive of the final response. Rousseau and colleagues[1] found that PET was 61% sensitive and 96% specific after the first cycle, 89% sensitive and 95% specific after the second cycle, and 88% sensitive and 73% specific after the third cycle.

Reference

1. Rousseau C, Devillers A, Sagan C, et al. Monitoring of early response to neoadjuvant chemotherapy in stage II and III breast cancer by [18F]fluorodeoxyglucose positron emission tomography. J Clin Oncol 2006;24(34):5366–5372

Suggested Reading

American College of Radiology. ACR appropriateness criteria (origin 1996; reviewed 2006). (http://acsearch. Acr.org/). Accessed 11/10/08

Moy L, Slanetz PJ, Moore R, et al. Specificity of mammography and US in the evaluation of a palpable abnormality: retrospective review. Radiology 2002;225(1):176–181

Orel SG, Schnall MD. MR imaging of the breast for the detection, diagnosis, and staging of breast cancer. Radiology 2001;220(1):13–30

Rosen EL, Eubank WB, Mankoff DA. FDG PET, PET/CT, and breast cancer imaging. Radiographics 2007;27(Suppl 1):S215–S229

Shetty MK, Shah YP. Prospective evaluation of the value of negative sonographic and mammographic findings in patients with palpable abnormalities of the breast. J Ultrasound Med 2002;21(11):1211–1216, quiz 1217–1219

Soo MS, Rosen EL, Baker JA, Vo TT, Boyd BA. Negative predictive value of sonography with mammography in patients with palpable breast lesions. AJR Am J Roentgenol 2001;177(5):1167–1170

37 Identifications of Recurrent Disease

Case 37.1: Identification of Recurrent Disease

Case History
A 65-year-old woman presents for MRI with a new palpable right chest wall mass and shoulder pain for 4 months. She has had a right modified mastectomy for breast cancer 17 years prior to this examination. Her axillary dissection revealed 3 of 17 nodes with metastatic tumor. She is also status post–right total shoulder arthroplasty 4 years prior to exam. MRI demonstrates a chest wall mass, so mammograms, right breast sonogram, and positron emission tomography–computed tomography (PET-CT) are performed.

Physical Examination
- Patient has a hard right chest wall mass.

Mammogram (Fig. 37.1)

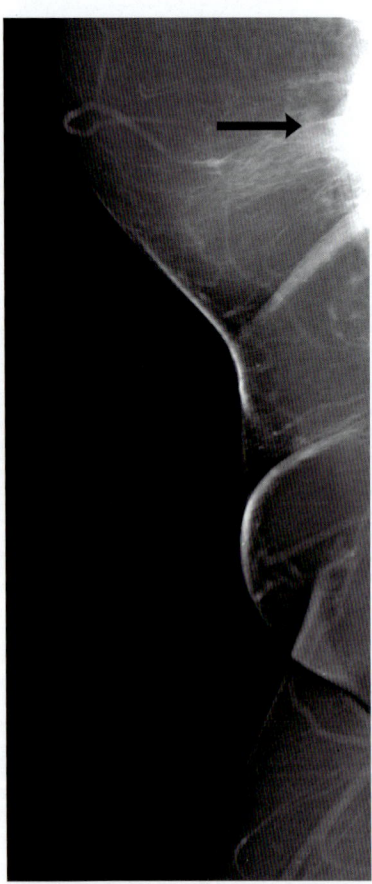

Fig. 37.1 Right axillary mammogram. There is an ill-defined, irregular mass (*arrow*) in the axilla.

Ultrasound

Frequency (Fig. 37.2)
- 14 MHz

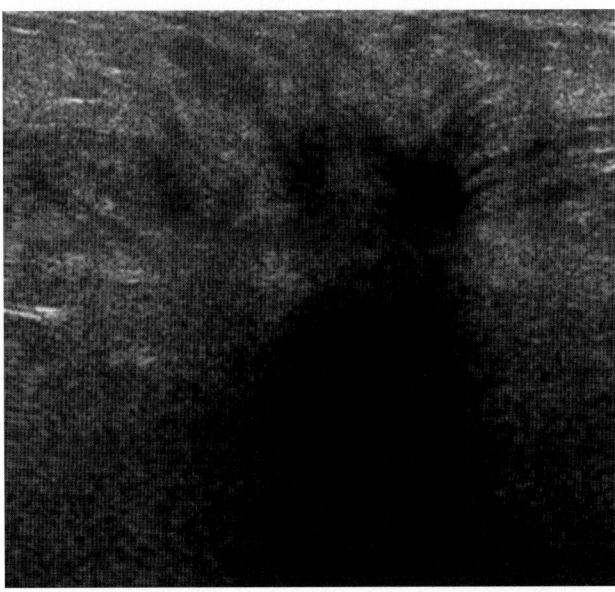

Fig. 37.2 Right chest sonogram. The palpable chest wall mass corresponds to a heavily shadowing, spiculated, hypoechoic solid mass.

Other Modalities: MRI and PET-CT (Figs. 37.3, 37.4, and 37.5)

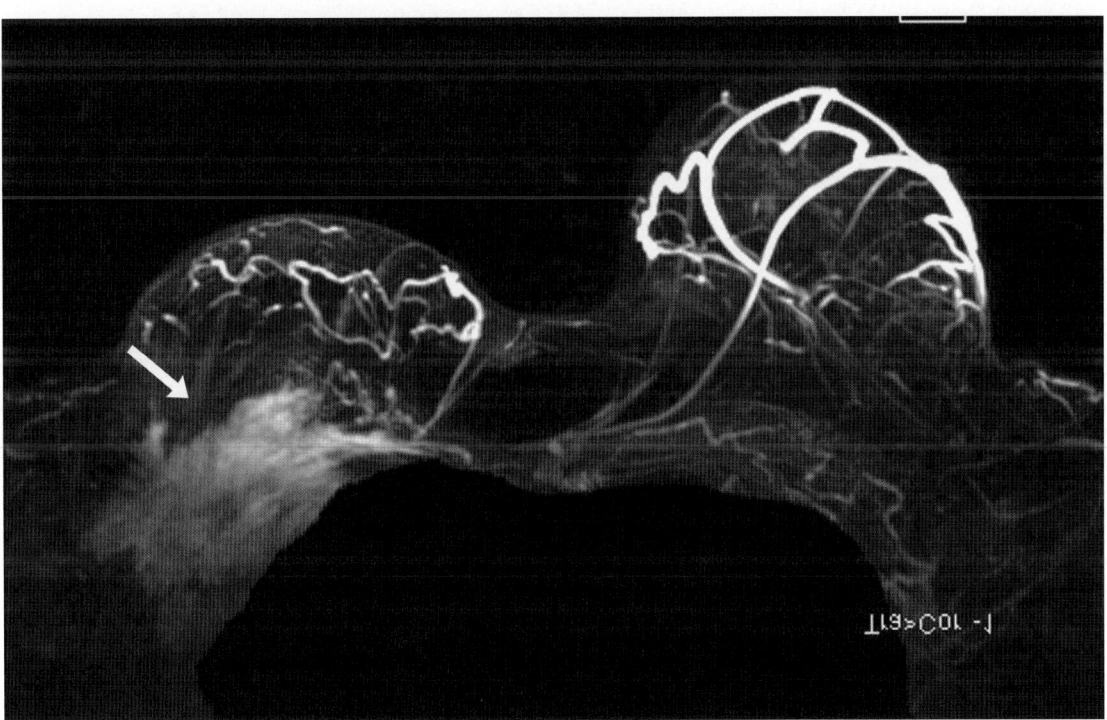

Fig. 37.3 Contrast-enhanced bilateral breast MRI maximum projection intensity (MIP) image. There is an irregular right chest wall mass (*arrow*) that exhibits rapid enhancement and washout.

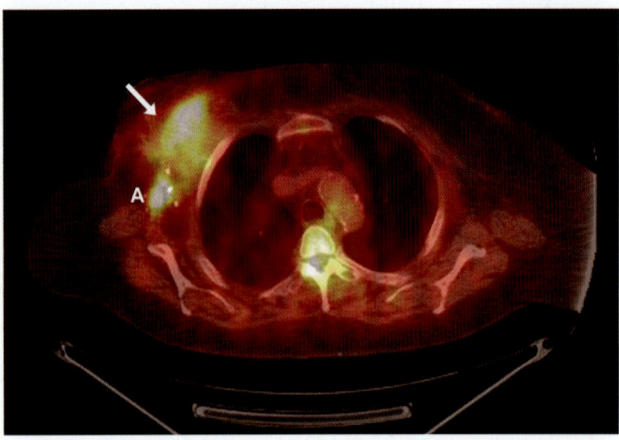 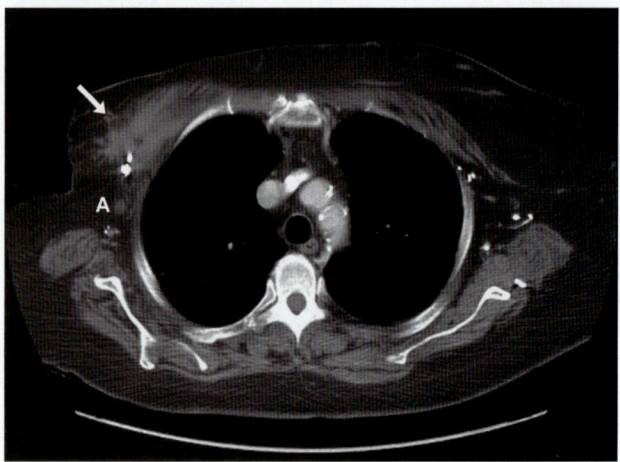

Fig. 37.4 Axial positron emission tomography–computed tomography (PET-CT). There is ¹⁸F-fluorodeoxyglucose (FDG) uptake in the chest wall mass (*arrow*) that invades the pectoralis muscle. This exam also shows abnormal uptake in the right axillary nodes (A).

Fig. 37.5 Axial computed tomography (CT) of the chest. The CT also demonstrates the chest wall mass (*arrow*) and right axillary adenopathy (A) but does not exhibit the physiologic information demonstrated by the PET-CT.

Pathology
- Infiltrating lobular carcinoma

Management
- BI-RADS assessment category 5, highly suggestive of malignancy

Pearls and Pitfalls
- Positron emission tomography (PET) is an excellent method to stage patients for recurrent breast cancer. A meta-analysis of 18 studies found that PET had a median sensitivity of 93% and specificity of 82% for identifying recurrent or metastatic disease.
- PET may have a significant impact on the treatment of patients suspected of having a recurrence. Investigators have found that PET results alter the therapeutic plan in about one third of these patients. PET is particularly useful in asymptomatic patients with elevated tumor markers and negative conventional imaging. It appears to have the least impact when used for staging patients with known metastatic disease. Although PET commonly demonstrates more extensive disease compared with conventional imaging, these findings generally do not change treatment.

Reference
1. Rousseau C, Devillers A, Sagan C, et al. Monitoring of early response to neoadjuvant chemitherapy in stage II and III breast cancer by [18F]fluorodeoxyglucose positron emission tomography. J Clin Oncol 2006;24(34):5366–5372

Suggested Reading
Eubank WB, Mankoff D, Bhattacharya M, et al. Impact of FDG PET on defining the extent of disease and on the treatment of patients with recurrent or metastatic breast cancer. AJR Am J Roentgenol 2004;183:479–486

Hodgson NC, Gulenchyn KY. Is there a role for positron emission tomography in breast cancer staging? J Clin Oncol 2008;26:712–720

Isasi CR, Moadel RM, Blaufox MD. A meta-analysis of FDG-PET for the evaluation of breast cancer recurrence and metastases. Breast Cancer Res Treat 2005;90:105–112

Case 37.2: Identification of Recurrent Disease

Case History
A 46-year-old woman with advanced-stage breast cancer develops right shoulder pain and right proptosis.

Physical Examination
- Patient has weakness of right upper extremity, myosis, and right-sided Horner's syndrome.

Other Modalities: PET (Figs. 37.6 and 37.7)

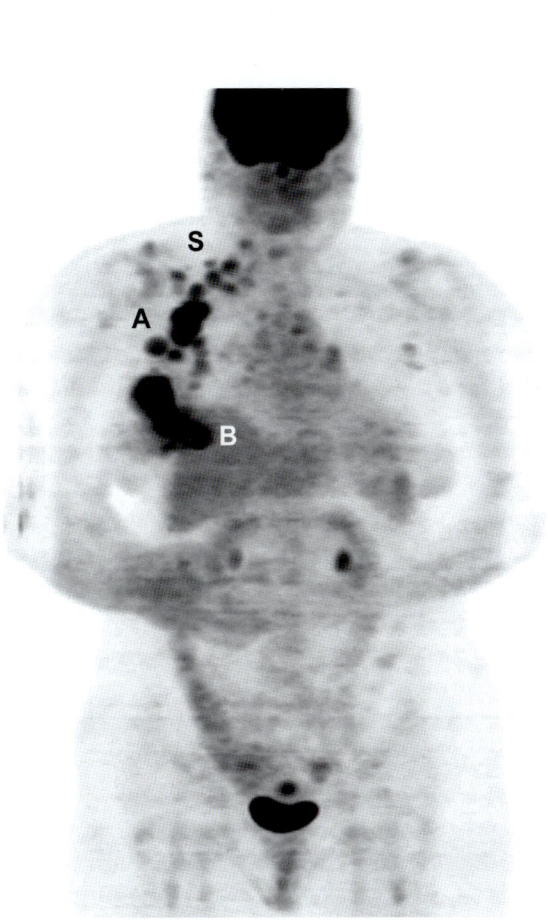

Fig. 37.6 Maximum projection intensity PET image. This image demonstrates extensive FDG uptake in the right breast (B), axilla (A), and supraclavicular (S) region consistent with advanced-stage breast carcinoma.

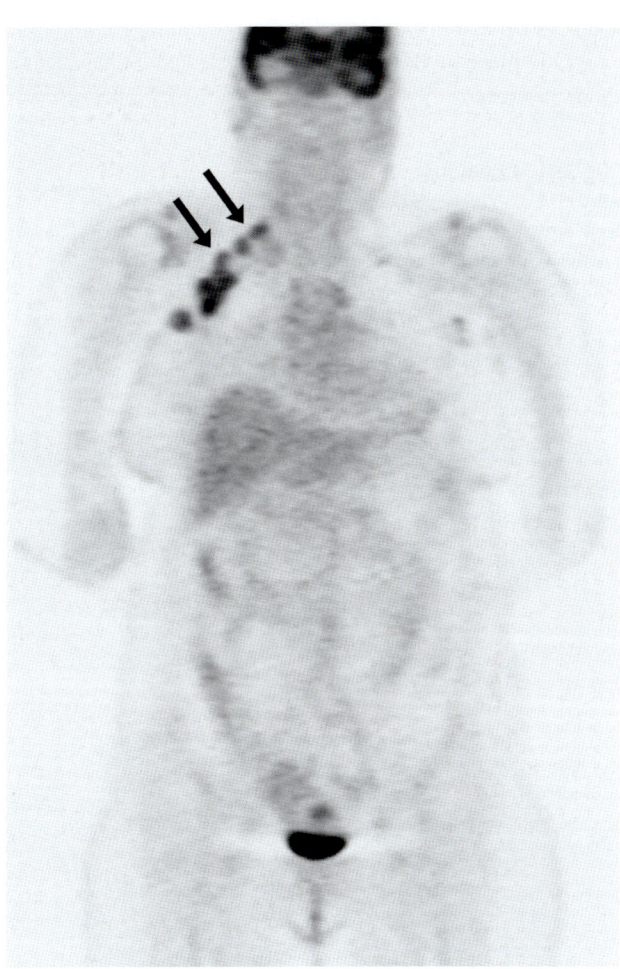

Fig. 37.7 Coronal PET image. This view shows prominent FDG uptake in the right supraclavicular and neck base region (*arrows*) consistent with brachial plexus involvement.

Pathology
- Original breast histology was invasive carcinoma with ductal and lobular features.

Management
- PET findings: BI-RADS assessment category 5, highly suggestive of malignancy

Pearls and Pitfalls

- In this case, PET demonstrates an unusual pattern of metastatic disease that explains all of the patient's symptoms. The distribution of the disease and the patient's symptoms suggest that the metastases have compromised the sympathetic nervous system and the brachial plexus. Damage to the sympathetic nerves may produce a combination of symptoms known as Horner's syndrome: ptosis (drooping upper eyelid), upside-down ptosis (slight elevation of the lower lid), miosis, enophthalmos, and anhidrosis on the affected side of the face. Involvement of the brachial plexus results in a weakness in the arm, diminished reflexes, and associated sensory deficits.
- PET has been found to be useful for breast cancer patients who present with brachial plexus symptoms. PET is more sensitive than computed tomography (CT) in identifying metastatic brachial plexus involvement. MRI is commonly used to examine the brachial plexus because malignancies exhibit higher signal on T1-weighted images compared with radiation fibrosis. Similar to MRI, PET also differentiates fibrosis from neoplasia: increased FDG uptake suggests malignant involvement rather than radiation fibrosis.

Suggested Reading

Ahmad A, Barrington S, Maisey M, Rubens RD. Use of positron emission tomography in evaluation of brachial plexopathy in breast cancer patients. Br J Cancer 1999;79:478–482

Luthra K, Shah S, Purandare N, Medhi S, Rangarajan V, Samuel AM. F-18 FDG PET-CT appearance of metastatic brachial plexopathy in a case of carcinoma of the breast. Clin Nucl Med 2006;31:432–434

38 Additional Malignancies

Case 38.1: Additional Malignancies

Case History
A 78-year-old woman status post–right lumpectomy and radiation therapy 1 year prior to exam presents with right chest wall pain and cough.

Physical Examination
- Right breast: normal lumpectomy scar
- Left breast: normal exam
- Chest: right chest reduced breath sounds at base

Mammogram (Fig. 38.1)
- Right architectural distortion consistent with scar

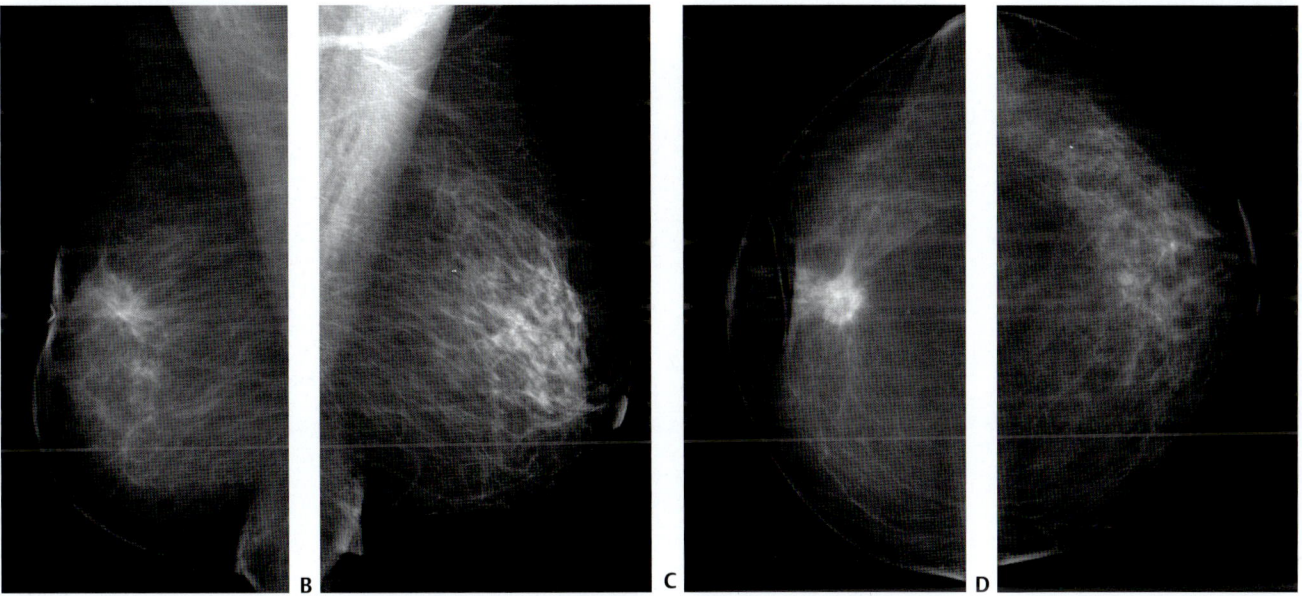

Fig. 38.1 The right breast has architectural distortion consistent with scar. The scar has decreased in size since the previous exam. The left breast is normal. (**A**) Right MLO mammogram. (**B**) Left MLO mammogram. (**C**) Right CC mammogram. (**D**) Left CC mammogram.

Other Modalities: Chest Radiograph and PET-CT (Figs. 38.2 and 38.3)

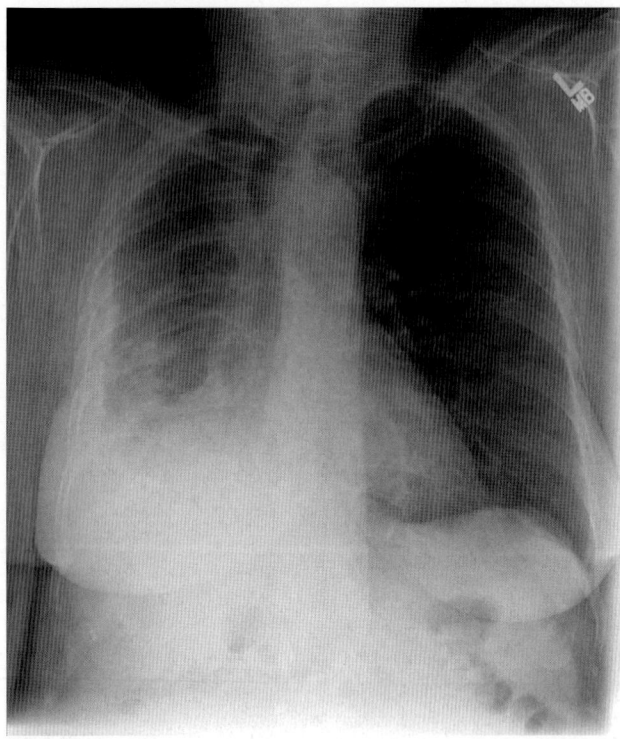

Fig. 38.2 Posteroanterior (PA) chest radiograph. There is a right pleural effusion.

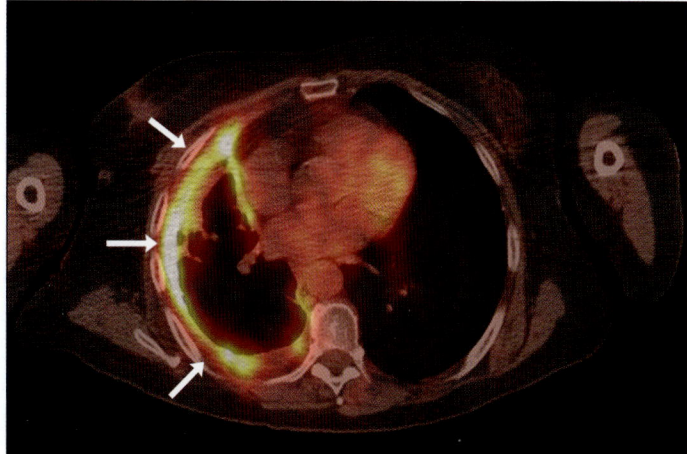
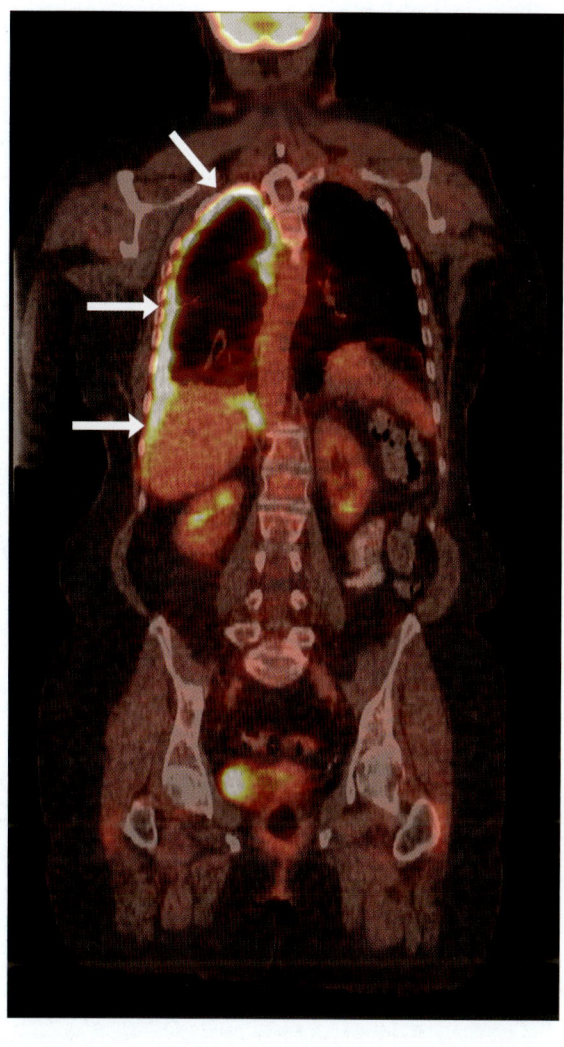

Fig. 38.3 Positron emission tomography–computed tomography (PET-CT) demonstrates extensive ^{18}F-fluorodeoxyglucose (FDG) uptake involving the right pleural surface (*arrows*). There is no significant uptake in the right breast. (**A**) Axial PET-CT. (**B**) Coronal PET/CT.

Pathology
- Pleural biopsy demonstrates mesothelioma.

Management
- Pleural malignancy
- Right breast scar: BI-RADS assessment category 2, benign finding

Pearls and Pitfalls

- This case illustrates an incidental cancer identified by PET-CT. Studies have found that between 1 and 2% of patients with known or suspected neoplasms were found to have unexpected incidental malignant or premalignant lesions that were unrelated to the primary tumor. In the previously described clinical case, the lack of ^{18}F-fluorodeoxyglucose (FDG) uptake in the right breast or in other more common metastatic breast locations strongly suggests that the right chest abnormality is not due to breast carcinoma.

Suggested Reading

Agress H Jr, Cooper BZ. Detection of clinically unexpected malignant and premalignant tumors with whole-body FDG PET: histopathologic comparison. Radiology 2004;230:417–422

Even-Sapir E, Lerman H, Gutman M, et al. The presentation of malignant tumours and pre-malignant lesions incidentally found on PET-CT. Eur J Nucl Med Mol Imaging 2006;33:541–552

Ishimori T, Patel PV, Wahl RL. Detection of unexpected additional primary malignancies with PET/CT. J Nucl Med 2005;46:752–757

39 Unknown Primary

Case 39.1: Unknown Primary

Case History
A 60-year-old woman presents with right chin numbness. Brain MRI identifies a cerebellar mass. Because her physician suspects that the mass is a metastasis, a positron emission tomography–computed tomography (PET-CT) scan is performed, which demonstrates abnormal uptake in the left breast and thyroid. After the PET-CT scan, bilateral mammograms and left breast sonogram are performed. The sonogram identifies a cystic mass that is biopsied and found to be ductal carcinoma in situ. Bilateral breast MRI is then performed demonstrating extensive abnormal left breast enhancement. Because mastectomy is being considered, a second left breast sonogram is performed to identify lesions to biopsy that would be distant from the primary mass.

The PET-CT thyroid abnormalities are also followed up with a thyroid sonogram, which identifies a suspicious right thyroid nodule.

Physical Examination (Figs. 39.1 and 39.2)
- Right chin decreased sensation
- Normal breast examination
- Multiple nodules in both thyroid glands

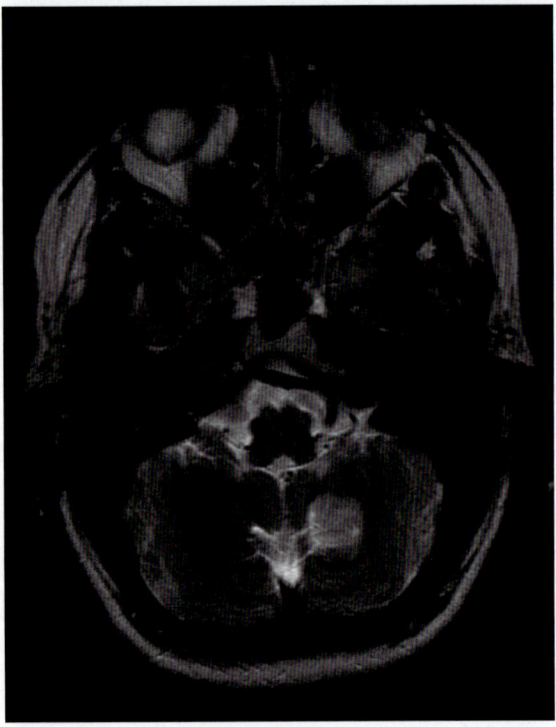

Fig. 39.1 Axial T2-weighted MRI of the brain. There is a high-intensity mass in the left cerebellum. The differential diagnosis is a metastasis versus a slow-growing glioma.

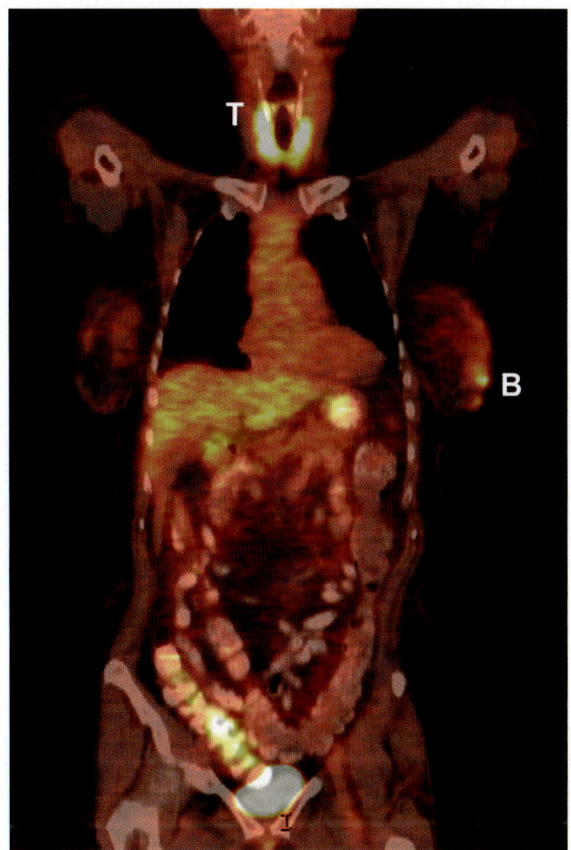

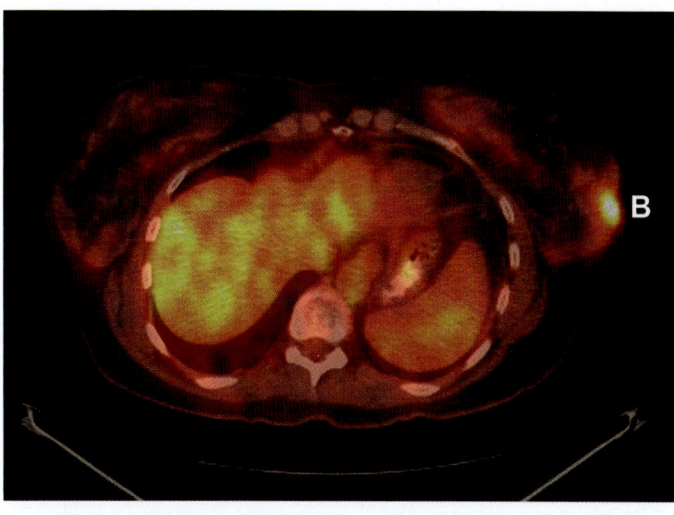

Fig. 39.2 After the cerebellar mass is discovered, positron emission PET-CT scan is performed to identify a primary malignancy. The PET-CT demonstrates increased uptake in the thyroid (T) and the left breast (B). (A) Coronal PET-CT. (B) Axial PET-CT of chest.

Mammogram (Fig. 39.3)
- Normal

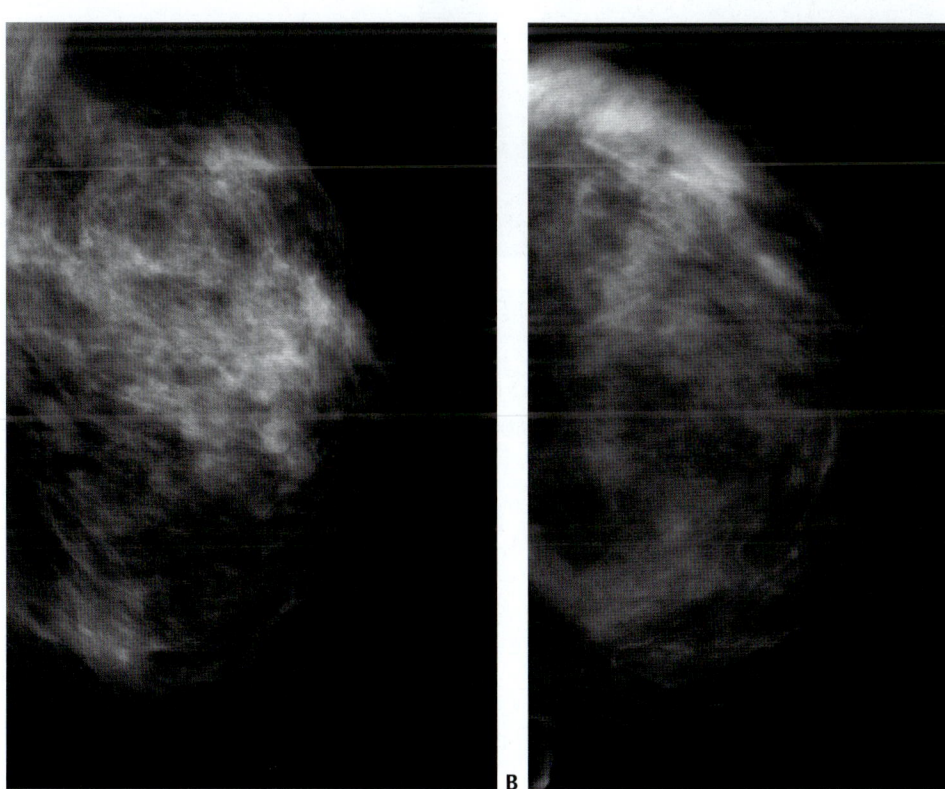

Fig. 39.3 Mammograms are performed as a result of the abnormal PET-CT scan. Left breast has heterogeneous breast composition without suspicious mass or calcifications. (A) Left MLO mammogram. (B) Left CC mammogram.

Applications of PET-CT

Ultrasound

Frequency (Figs. 39.4, 39.5, 39.6, and 39.7)
- 14 MHz

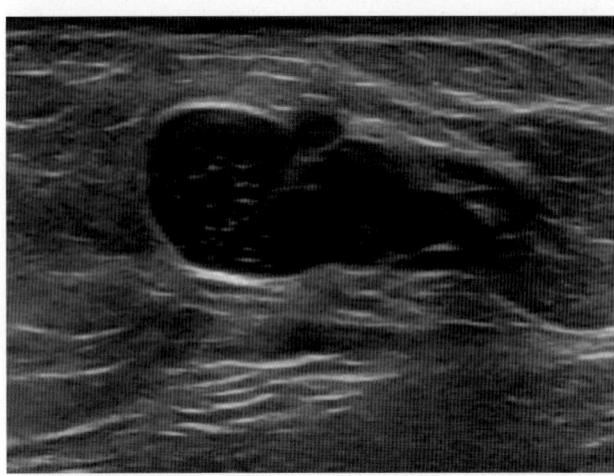

Fig. 39.4 Initial left breast sonogram. Breast sonogram is performed as a result of the abnormal PET-CT scan. A 1.5 cm complex cyst is identified 12 cm from the nipple at the 4 o'clock position. This mass is biopsied and found to be ductal carcinoma in situ (DCIS). It is considered to be the primary malignancy.

Other Modalities: MRI and Second Look Sonography (Figs. 39.5 and 39.6), Thyroid Sonogram (Figs. 39.7)

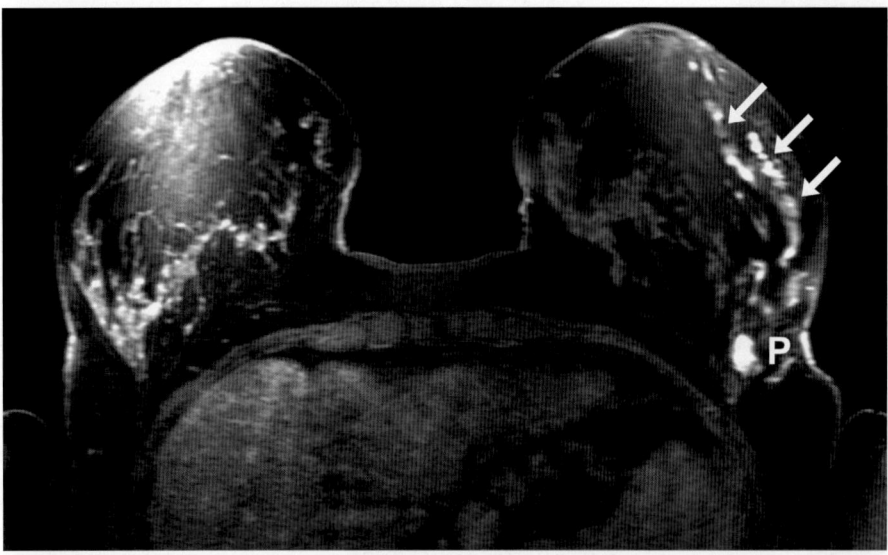

A

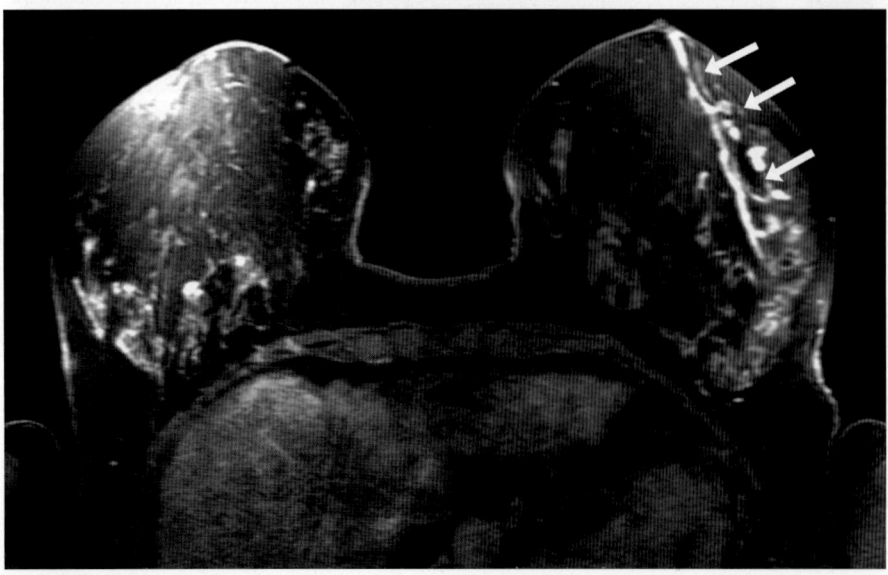

B

Fig. 39.5 After the left breast sonographic mass is found to be DCIS, breast MRI is performed to stage the breast. The MRI demonstrates enhancement of the known primary malignancy (P), as well as the ducts extending from the primary mass to the nipple (*arrows*). (**A**) Bilateral contrast-enhanced, T1-weighted axial breast high-resolution MRI. (**B**) Bilateral contrast-enhanced, T1-weighted axial breast high-resolution MRI, inferior to that in **A**.

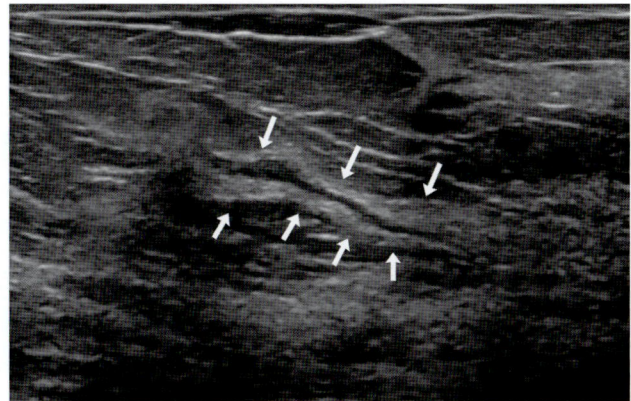
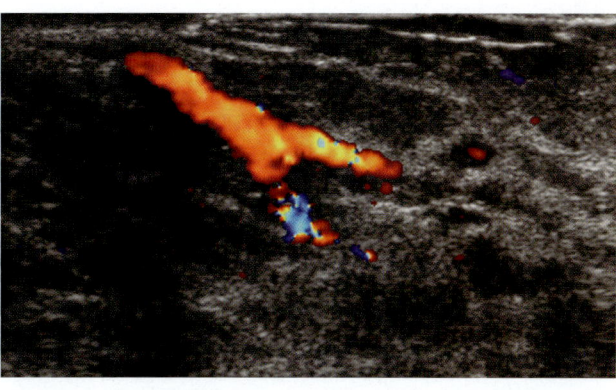

Fig. 39.6 Second left breast sonogram performed after the breast MRI. No suspicious solid or cystic masses are identified close to the nipple. However, the ducts adjacent to the nipple at the 3 o'clock position exhibit a hyperechoic haze (*arrows*) and increased color flow Doppler. (**A**) Left radial breast sonogram at the 3 o'clock position, 2 cm from the nipple. (**B**) Left radial color Doppler breast sonogram at the same location as in **A**.

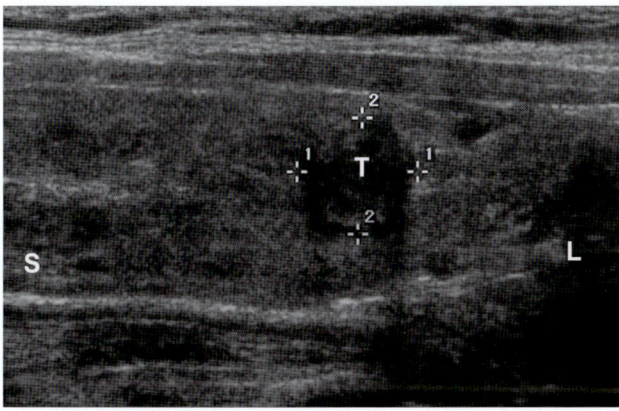

Fig. 39.7 Right longitudinal thyroid sonogram. This exam was performed as a result of the abnormal PET-CT scan. A suspicious solid thyroid nodule (T) is present in the middle right thyroid gland. Fine-needle aspiration of this nodule is papillary cancer. S, superior pole of thyroid; L, lower pole of thyroid.

Pathology
- Left breast primary mass at the 4 o'clock position, 12 cm from nipple; sonographic biopsy: ductal carcinoma in situ (DCIS)
- Left breast duct sonographic biopsy at the 3 o'clock position, 2 cm from the nipple: DCIS
- Left mastectomy specimen demonstrated > 7 cm of ductal carcinoma in situ in the left outer breast.
- Total thyroidectomy demonstrated papillary carcinoma in bilateral glands. Right gland had three foci (largest was 1.2 cm). Left gland had one 0.2 cm cancer.
- No biopsy of cerebellar mass has been performed. The mass did not change in size for 9 months.

Management (Left Breast MRI Findings)
- Sonographic left mass at the 4 o'clock position. BI-RADS assessment category 4, suspicious; biopsy should be considered.

Pearls and Pitfalls

- About 2 to 5% of all new patients with cancer present with malignancy that cannot be attributed to a specific origin and are classified as having occult primary malignancy. In these patients, PET has been found to identify approximately 40% of primary tumors not detected by conventional imaging such as CT.
- Korn et al[1] reported that 6 (1.1%) of 533 women who had PET-CT were found to have incidental focal increased ^{18}F-fluorodeoxyglucose (FDG) uptake in the breast. Five of the six women subsequently were found to have invasive ductal carcinoma. Therefore, women with focally increased FDG in the breast should be worked up for breast cancer.
- DCIS is sometimes difficult to identify on MRI. However, this case illustrates that this malignancy may appear as a mass or as ductal enhancement.
- To biopsy suspicious MRI lesions sonographically, the imager needs to be familiar with the sonographic signs of DCIS. These findings include solid masses, cystic masses, abnormal ducts (duct ectasia—focal or diffuse, intraductal mass or calcifications, thick walled ducts, or ducts affecting the surrounding tissues such as hyperechoic haze), and normal ducts with increased color flow Doppler. When these findings are anatomically matched with the MRI lesion, then biopsy should be performed.

Reference

1. Korn RL, Yost AM, May CC, et al. Unexpected focal hypermetabolic activity in the breast: significance in patients undergoing 18F-FDG PET/CT. AJR Am J Roentgenol 2006;187:81–85

Suggested Reading

Levi F, Te VC, Erler G, Randimbison L, La Vecchia C. Epidemiology of unknown primary tumours. Eur J Cancer 2002; 38:1810–1812

Pelosi E, Pennone M, Deandreis D, Douroukas A, Mancini M, Bisi G. Role of whole body positron emission tomography/computed tomography scan with ^{18}F-fluorodeoxyglucose in patients with biopsy proven tumor metastases from unknown primary site. Q J Nucl Med Mol Imaging 2006;50:15–22

Sève P, Billotey C, Broussolle C, Dumontet C, Mackey JR. The role of 2-deoxy-2-[F-18]fluoro-D-glucose positron emission tomography in disseminated carcinoma of unknown primary site. Cancer 2007;109:292–299

40 Pitfalls of PET

Case 40.1: Low Standardized Uptake Value (SUV)

Case History
A 54-year-old woman presents with left breast pain.

Physical Examination
- Left upper inner quadrant is diffusely tender.

Mammogram (Fig. 40.1)
- Asymmetry in the upper inner quadrant
- Abnormally dense lymph nodes

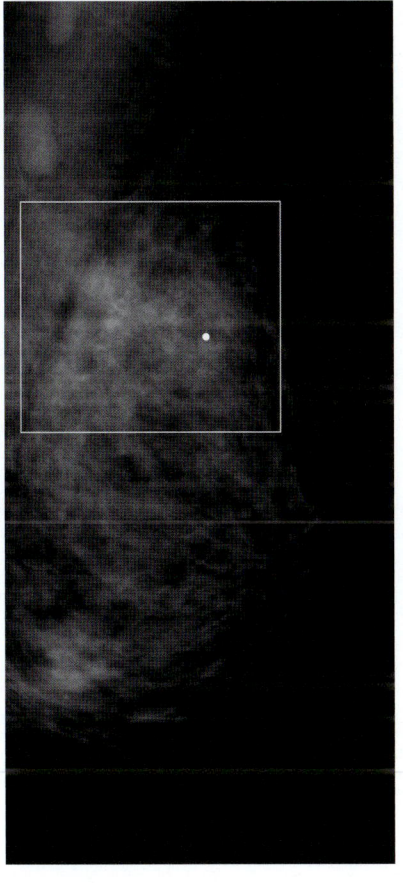
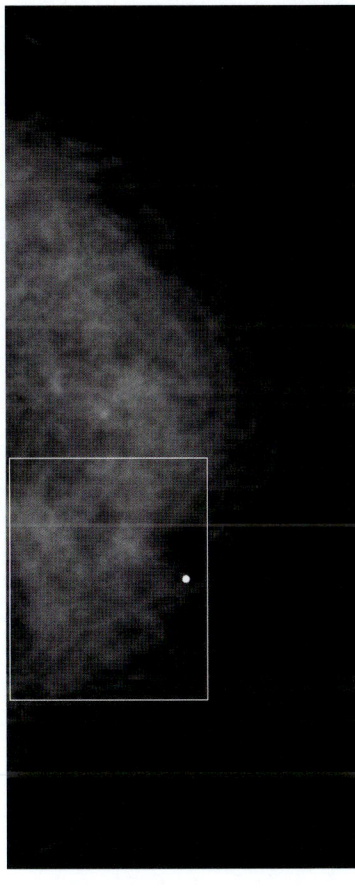

Fig. 40.1 There is asymmetry in the left upper inner quadrant (*square*) associated with abnormal lymph nodes. (**A**) Left ML mammogram. (**B**) Left CC mammogram.

Ultrasound

Frequency (Fig. 40.2)
- 15 MHz

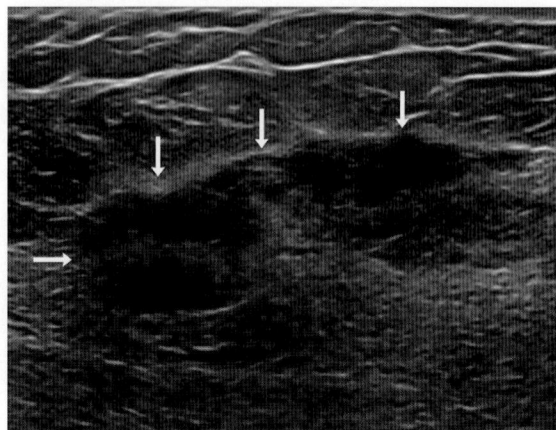
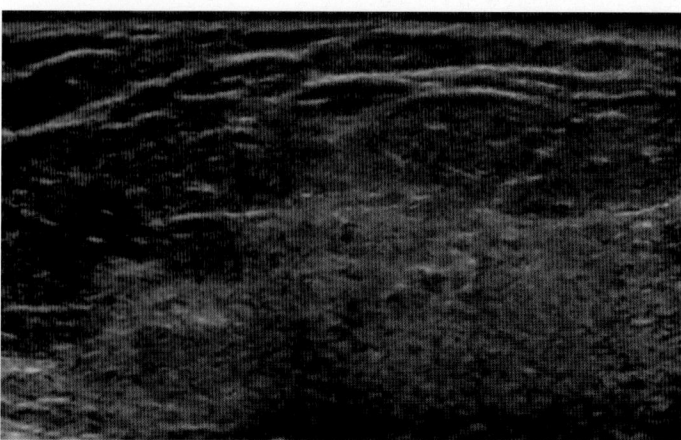
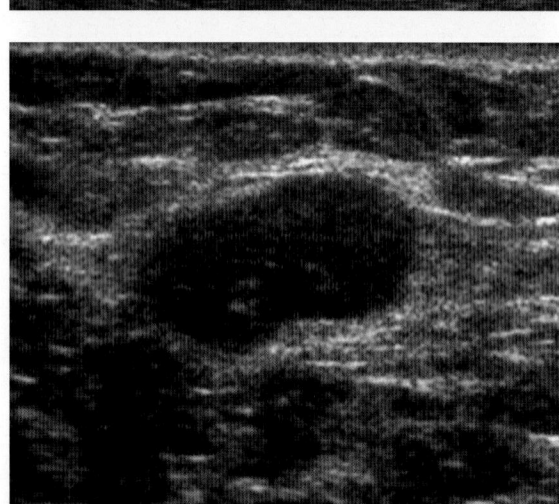

Fig. 40.2 The patient's tenderness and mammographic asymmetry sonographically correspond to a left irregular hypoechoic mass (*arrows*) (**A**). Because the mass is large and ill-defined, the imager may easily miss the mass unless the hyperechoic normal adjacent glandular tissue (**B**) is compared with the hypoechoic mass. Sonography also demonstrates abnormal lymph nodes that lack a central hilum (**C**). (**A**) Left breast sonogram upper outer quadrant. (**B**) Left breast sonogram normal glandular tissue adjacent to mass. (**C**) Left axillary sonogram.

Other Modalities (Figs. 40.3 and 40.4)

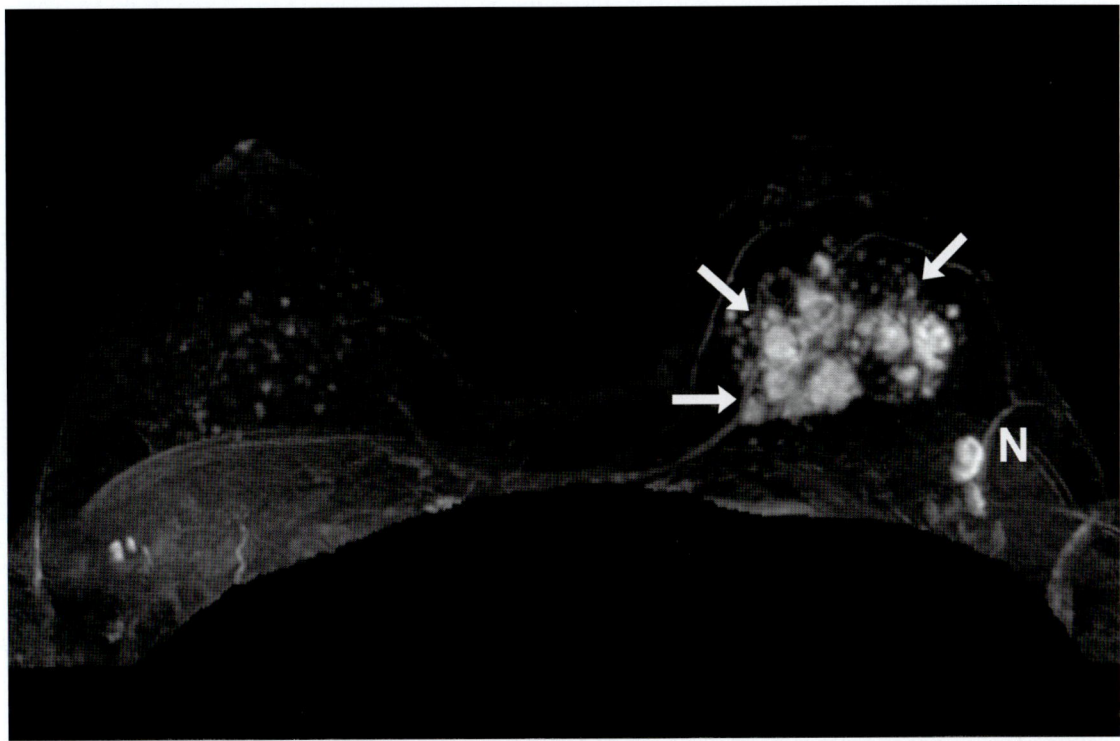

Fig. 40.3 Contrast-enhanced bilateral breast maximum projection intensity (MIP) MRI demonstrates an enhancing, irregular, highly suspicious mass (*arrows*) and a lymph node (N) suspicious for metastatic disease.

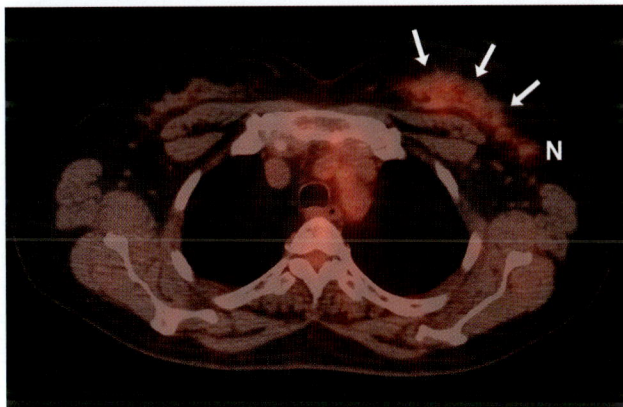

Fig. 40.4 Axial positron emission tomography–computed tomography (PET-CT). The area of MRI enhancement demonstrates only mild diffuse uptake (*arrows*) with maximum standardized uptake value (SUV) of 1.8. The enhancing lymph node (N) at the tail of the mass has a maximum SUV of 1.6.

Pathology
- Primarily invasive lobular carcinoma with a smaller proportion of invasive ductal carcinoma and ductal carcinoma in situ (DCIS). Axillary nodes were positive for metastatic disease.

Management
- Left breast mammographic and sonographic mass: BI-RADS assessment category 5, highly suggestive of malignancy

Pearls and Pitfalls
- Investigators have found that SUVs or tumor-to-background ratios of 2.0 to 2.5 are useful standards for identifying breast malignancies. However, certain malignancies such as invasive lobular, low-grade infiltrating ductal, and DCIS may exhibit SUVs lower than these values. False-negative PET axillary nodal results are due to low tumor burden and relatively poor size resolution (< 1 cm). Furthermore, when the primary tumor has a low SUV, its metastases tend to demonstrate low SUVs. For this reason, PET may not be sensitive for determining the extent of disease in this case, as illustrated by the relatively low SUV in the involved lymph node.

Suggested Reading

Gil-Rendo A, Zornoza G, García-Velloso MJ, Regueira FM, Beorlegui C, Cervera M. Fluorodeoxyglucose positron emission tomography with sentinel lymph node biopsy for evaluation of axillary involvement in breast cancer. Br J Surg 2006;93:707–712

Lovrics PJ, Chen V, Coates G, et al. A prospective evaluation of positron emission tomography scanning, sentinel lymph node biopsy, and standard axillary dissection for axillary staging in patients with early stage breast cancer. Ann Surg Oncol 2004;11:846–853

Zornoza G, Garcia-Velloso MJ, Sola J, Regueira FM, Pina L, Beorlegui C. 18F-FDG PET complemented with sentinel lymph node biopsy in the detection of axillary involvement in breast cancer. Eur J Surg Oncol 2004;30:15–19

Case 40.2: Bone Metastases

Case History
A 76-year-old woman diagnosed with bilateral breast cancer was treated with bilateral mastectomy, axillary node removal, and chemotherapy 9 years prior to examination. She now has lower extremity pain and has been found on axial computed tomography (CT) to have bone metastases.

Physical Examination
- Well-healed mastectomy scars

Other Modalities (Figs. 40.5, 40.6, and 40.7)

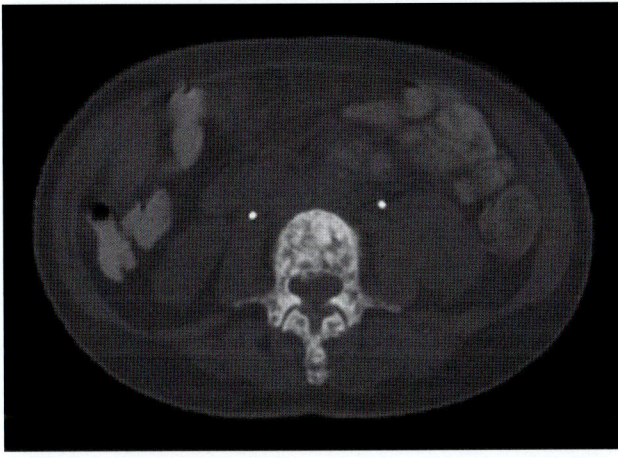

Fig. 40.5 CT of the abdomen. There is a sclerotic destructive process of the third lumbar (L3) vertebral body.

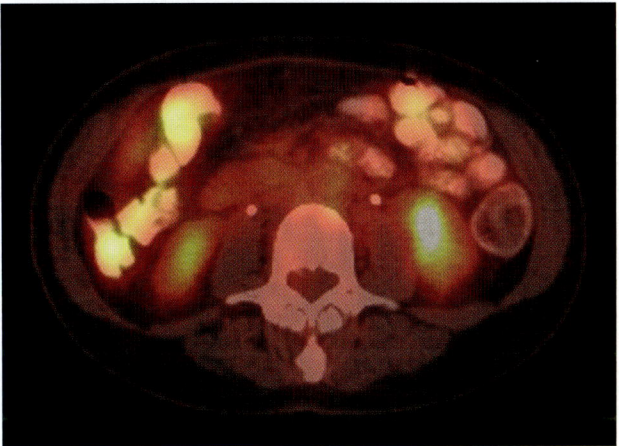

Fig. 40.6 Axial PET-CT of abdomen at same level as **Fig. 40.50**. The L3 sclerotic process does not demonstrate significant ^{18}F-fluorodeoxyglucose (FDG) uptake.

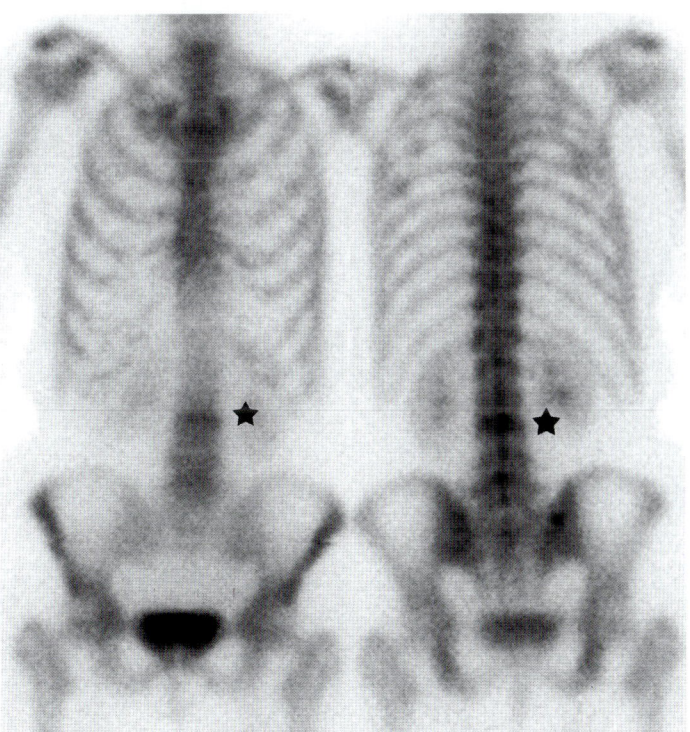

Fig. 40.7 Anteroposterior (AP) technetium 99m (Tc 99m) whole-body bone scan. There is moderate uptake of the Tc 99m at the L3 level (star) in the medial pelvis.

Pathology
- Iliac crest bone biopsy: metastatic breast cancer

Management
- CT and bone scan findings are highly suggestive of metastatic malignancy

Pearls and Pitfalls

- Bone is one of the most common metastatic locations for breast cancer. Although the incidence of bone metastases is only 1 to 2% at the time of initial diagnosis, bone metastases are present in one third of all patients with recurrent disease and in 69% of patients at death.
- This case illustrates that PET-CT often does not demonstrate avid ^{18}F-fluorodeoxyglucose (FDG) uptake in osteoblastic or sclerotic metastases. Bone scan is more sensitive than PET for detection of osteoblastic metastases. Analysis of six combined studies suggests that PET and bone scan are similar when evaluating patient-based sensitivity and specificity of bone metastases (PET: 81% sensitivity, 93% specificity; bone scan: 78% sensitivity, 79% specificity). However, PET is less sensitive than bone scan (69% vs 88%) for individual lesion-based detection, probably due to its relative insensitivity to blastic metastases and to differences in field of view.

Suggested Reading

Cook GJ, Houston S, Rubens R, Maisey MN, Fogelman I. Detection of bone metastases in breast cancer by 18FDG PET: differing metabolic activity in osteoblastic and osteolytic lesions. J Clin Oncol 1998;16:3375–33799

Schirrmeister H. Detection of bone metastases in breast cancer by positron emission tomography. Radiol Clin North Am 2007;45:669–676, vi

Shie P, Cardarelli R, Brandon D, Erdman W, Abdulrahim N. Meta-analysis: comparison of F-18 fluorodeoxyglucose-positron emission tomography and bone scintigraphy in the detection of bone metastases in patients with breast cancer. Clin Nucl Med 2008;33:97–101

Case 40.3: Brown Fat

Case History

A 40-year-old woman presents with a palpable left breast mass.

Physical Examination

- Palpable mass in the left breast at the 4 o'clock position

Mammogram

Mass (Fig. 40.8)
- Margin: ill defined and obscured
- Shape: oval
- Density: equal

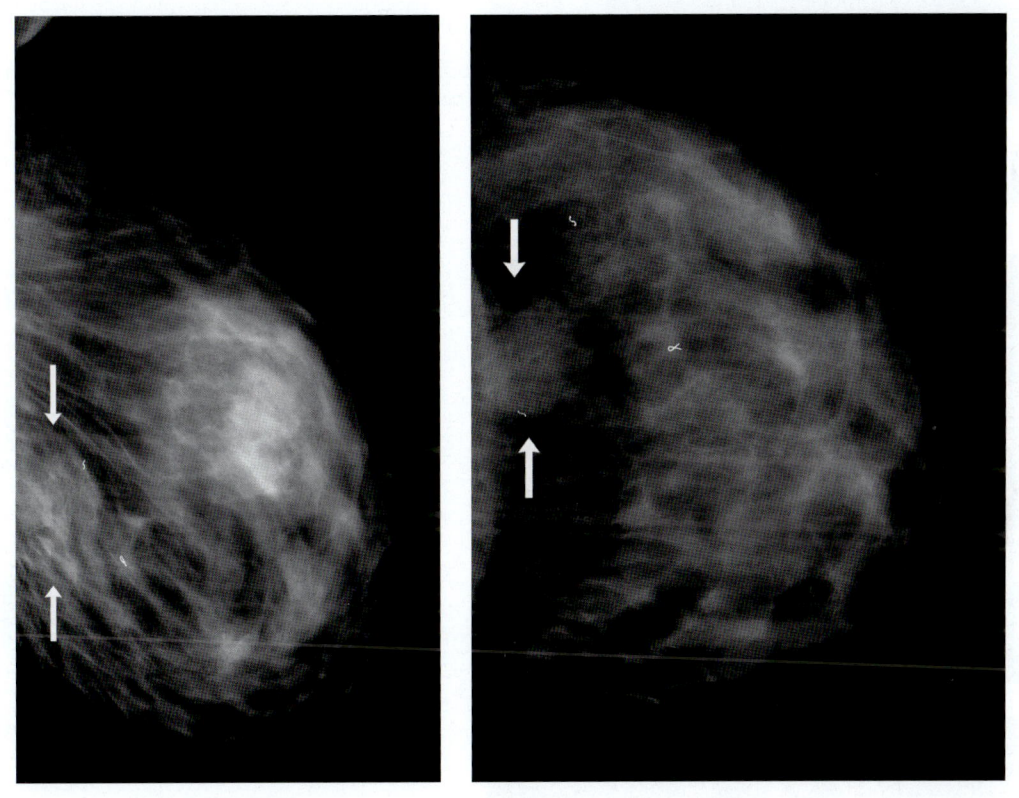

Fig. 40.8 In the inferior central breast, there is an oval, ill-defined mass (*arrows*). (**A**) Left MLO mammogram. (**B**) Left CC mammogram.

Ultrasound (Fig. 40.9)

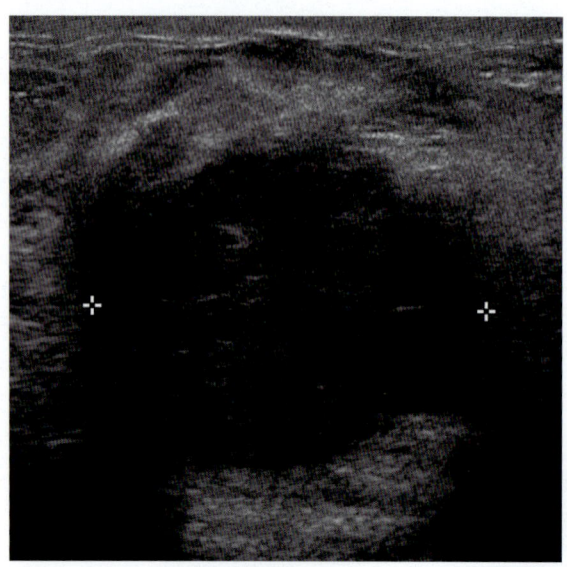

Fig. 40.9 Left breast radial sonogram. The mammographic mass corresponds to a solid hypoechoic mass.

Other Modalities (Fig. 40.10)

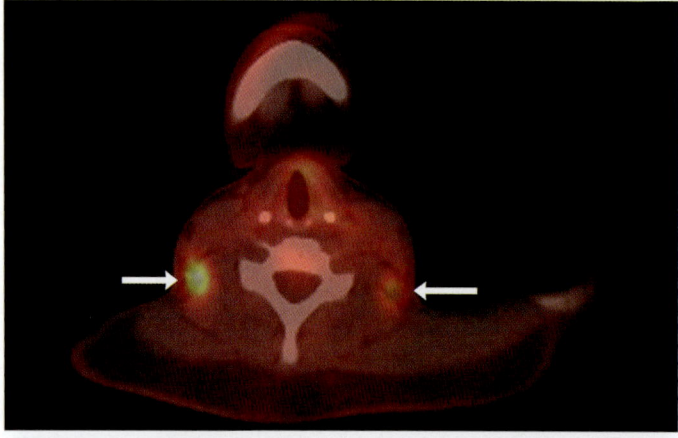

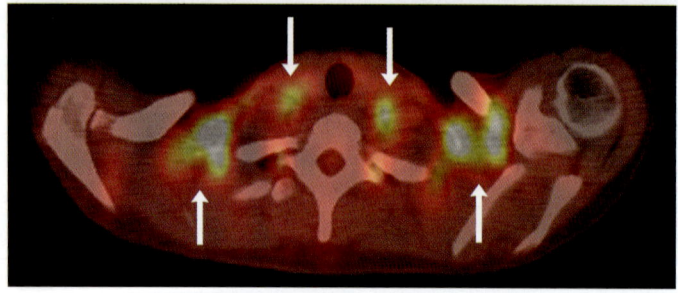

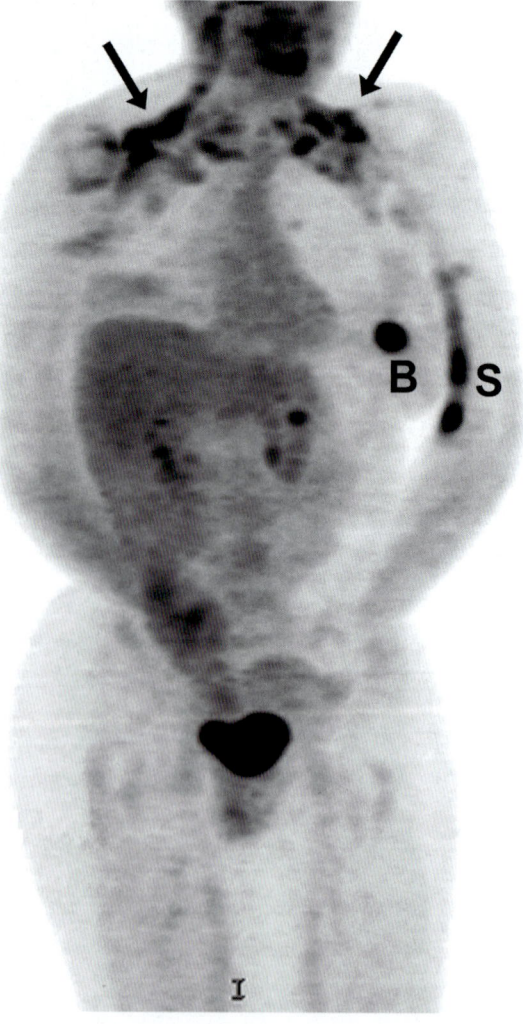

Fig. 40.10 Multiple focal areas of symmetrical uptake (*arrows*) are identified on PET-CT in the neck without lymphadenopathy. These findings are characteristic of hypermetabolic brown fat uptake. Uptake is also present in the left breast cancer (B). The uptake in the left arm (S) is due to extravasation of radiopharmaceutical in the antecubital fossa. (**A**) Axial PET-CT of neck. (**B**) Axial PET-CT at base of neck. (**C**) Maximum intensity projection (MIP) PET image.

Pathology
- Ultrasound-guided biopsy produced high-grade infiltrating ductal carcinoma. After 6 months of chemotherapy, lumpectomy demonstrated no residual malignancy, with zero of two sentinel nodes negative for metastatic disease.

Management
- Left mammographic and sonographic mass: BI-RADS assessment category 5, highly suggestive of malignancy

Pearls and Pitfalls
- There are two types of human fat: white and brown fat. Whereas white fat stores energy, brown fat has a high metabolic rate and generates heat. This case illustrates that hypermetabolic brown fat may simulate metastatic disease on PET by taking up FDG. Brown fat is located in the neck, supraclavicular region, around the mediastinal vessels, axilla, paraspinal areas, and intercostal spaces. Brown fat uptake is sometimes also present around the kidneys, liver, and colon. The main method to differentiate this benign process from malignancy is the lack of lymphadenopathy on CT and the symmetric distribution around the neck.

Suggested Reading
Cohade C, Osman M, Pannu HK, Wahl RL. Uptake in supraclavicular area fat ("USA-Fat"): description on 18F-FDG PET/CT. J Nucl Med 2003;44:170–1761

Hany TF, Gharehpapagh E, Kamel EM, Buck A, Himms-Hagen J, von Schulthess GK. Brown adipose tissue: a factor to consider in symmetrical tracer uptake in the neck and upper chest region. Eur J Nucl Med Mol Imaging 2002;29:1393–1398

Rousseau C, Bourbouloux E, Campion L, et al. Brown fat in breast cancer patients: analysis of serial (18)F-FDG PET/CT scans. Eur J Nucl Med Mol Imaging 2006;33:785–791

Case 40.4: Granulocyte Colony-Stimulating Factor

Case History
A 64-year-old woman presents with a left axillary mass.

Physical Examination
- Palpable mass in the left axilla

Mammogram (Fig. 40.11)
- Normal exam

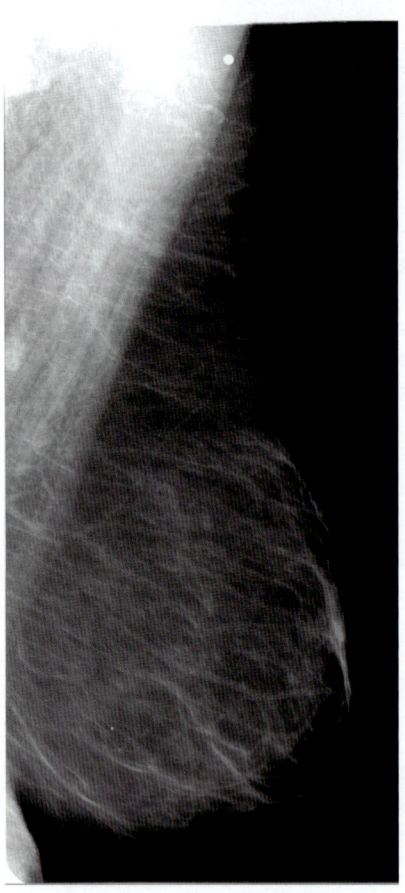
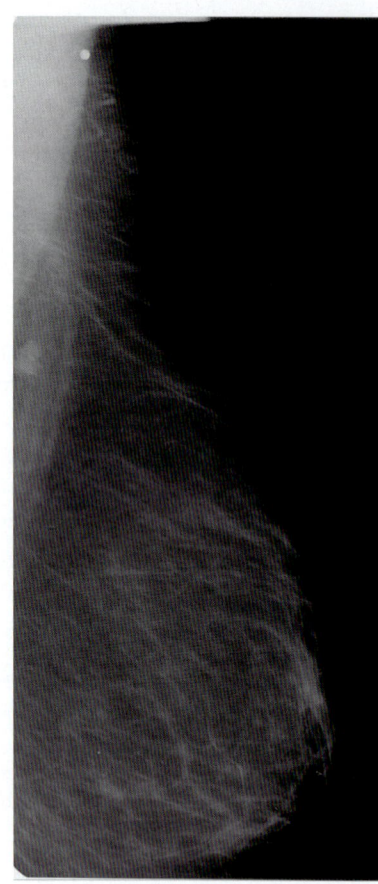

Fig. 40.11 The left breast has predominantly fatty composition. The palpable mass is outside of the field of view even with exaggerated views. (**A**) Left MLO mammogram. (**B**) Left XCC mammogram.

Ultrasound (Fig. 40.12)

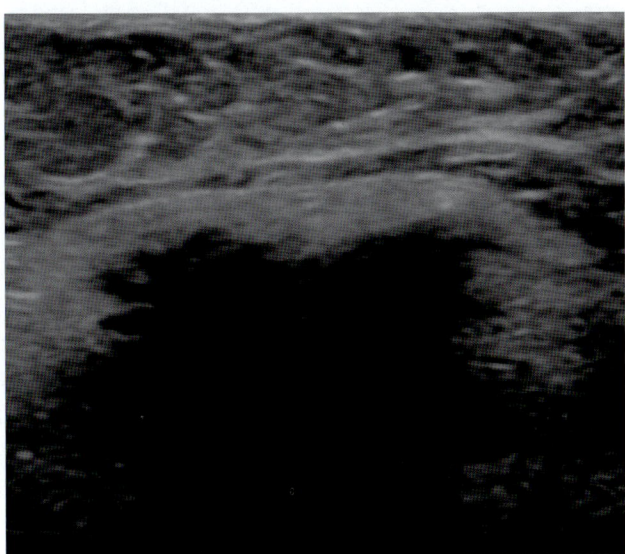

Fig. 40.12 Left longitudinal breast sonogram. The palpable mass corresponds to an irregular, hypoechoic, heavily shadowing mass.

Other Modalities (Figs. 40.13, 40.14, and 40.15)

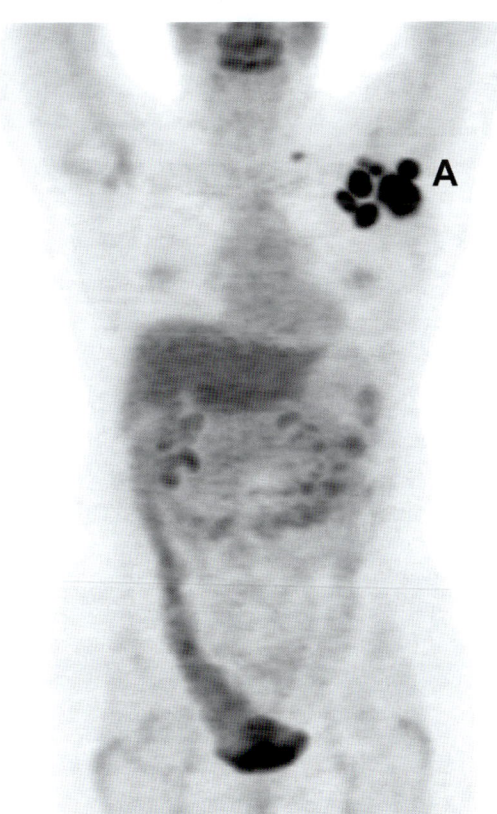

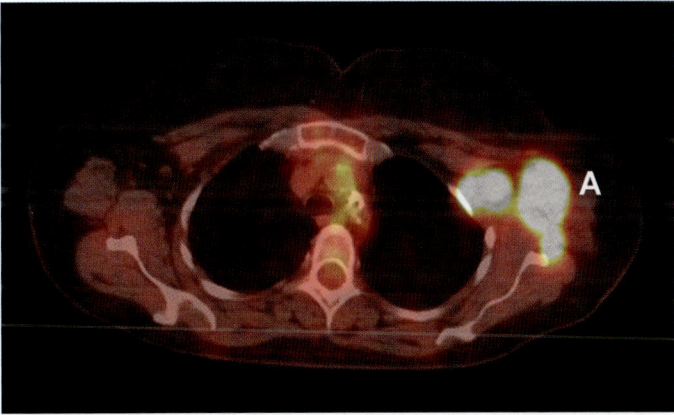

Fig. 40.13 Positron emission tomography (PET) study performed prior to chemotherapy. This image demonstrates FDG uptake in the left breast upper outer quadrant and axilla (**A**). (**A**) Maximum intensity projection (MIP) PET image. (**B**) Axial PET-CT image of the chest.

Applications of PET-CT

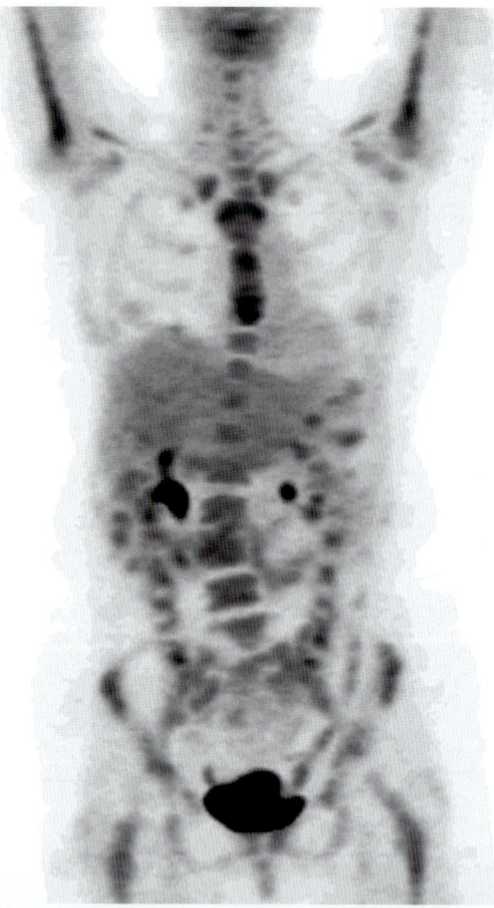

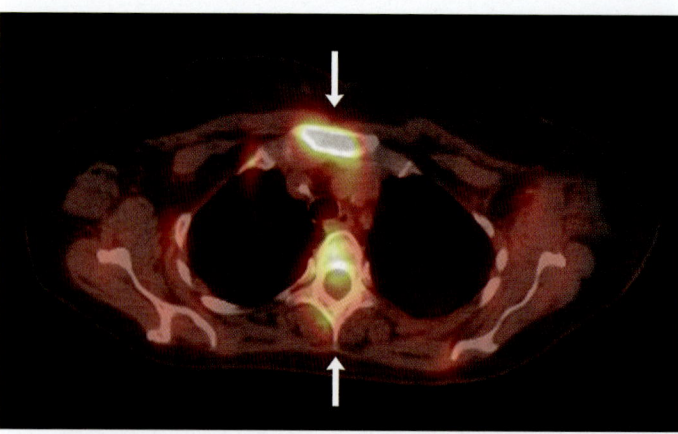

Fig. 40.14 PET study performed in a patient after 6 months of chemotherapy. This examination demonstrates resolution of the abnormal FDG uptake in the left breast and axilla. However, there is new diffuse skeletal uptake. (**A**) PET MIP image. (**B**) Axial PET-CT image of the chest. (*Arrows* point to increased FDG uptake in the sternum and spine.)

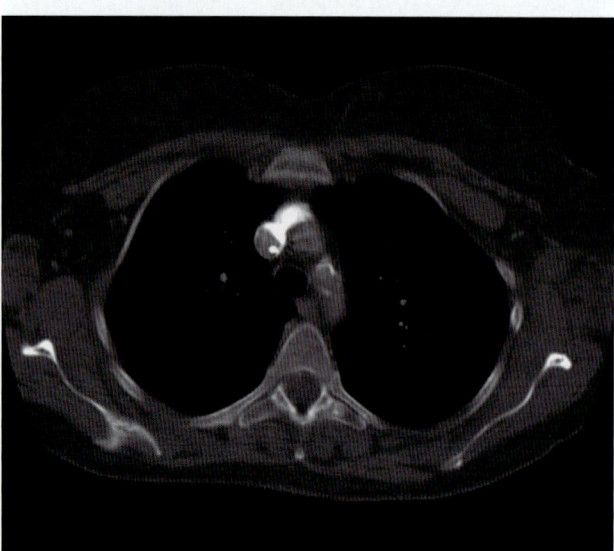

Fig. 40.15 Axial CT of the chest. This study was done at the same time as that in **Fig. 40.14**. There is no evidence of metastatic bone disease. The skeleton appears normal.

Pathology
- High-grade infiltrating ductal carcinoma

Management
- Sonographic left breast mass: BI-RADS assessment category 5, highly suggestive of malignancy

Pearls and Pitfalls

- The increased skeletal FDG activity is due to diffuse bone marrow uptake. During chemotherapy, this patient has received granulocyte colony-stimulating factor (G-CSF) treatment, which stimulates the bone marrow to produce white blood cells and therefore increases the metabolic activity of the bone marrow. This diffuse marrow uptake in the skeletal system simulates diffuse bony metastases. However, CT substantiates the benign etiology of the diffuse FDG uptake because CT exhibits no evidence of metastatic bone disease.
- If G-CSF is administered, most researchers recommend at least a 5-day interval between the final administration and PET examination to allow for reduction of bone marrow stimulation and to reduce the chance of increased skeletal uptake with FDG.

Suggested Reading

Gundlapalli S, Ojha B, Mountz JM. Granulocyte colony-stimulating factor: confounding F-18 FDG uptake in outpatient positron emission tomographic facilities for patients receiving ongoing treatment of lymphoma. Clin Nucl Med 2002;27:140–141

Hollinger EF, Alibazoglu H, Ali A, Green A, Lamonica G. Hematopoietic cytokine-mediated FDG uptake simulates the appearance of diffuse metastatic disease on whole-body PET imaging. Clin Nucl Med 1998;23:93–989

Kazama T, Swanston N, Podoloff DA, Macapinlac HA. Effect of colony-stimulating factor and conventional- or high-dose chemotherapy on FDG uptake in bone marrow. Eur J Nucl Med Mol Imaging 2005;32:1406–1411

Mayer D, Bednarczyk EM. Interaction of colony-stimulating factors and fluorodeoxyglucose f(18) positron emission tomography. Ann Pharmacother 2002;36:1796–1799

Sugawara Y, Fisher SJ, Zasadny KR, Kison PV, Baker LH, Wahl RL. Preclinical and clinical studies of bone marrow uptake of fluorine-1-fluorodeoxyglucose with or without granulocyte colony-stimulating factor during chemotherapy. J Clin Oncol 1998;16:173–180

Index

Page numbers followed by f indicate figures.

A

Abnormality patterns, 1–14
Abscess, 6
  in male breast, 370–371
    mammography, 370f
    pearls and pitfalls, 371
    ultrasound, 371, 371f
  poorly identified on mammogram, 502–503
    mammography, 502f
    pearls and pitfalls, 503
    ultrasound, 503, 503f
Absorption, shadowing and, 25
Adenoid cystic carcinoma, 96–97
  mammography, 96, 96f
  pearls and pitfalls, 97
  ultrasound, 97, 97f
Adenolipomas, 47
Adenoma, lactating, poorly identified on mammogram, 500–501
  pearls and pitfalls, 501
  ultrasound, 500f
Adenomyoepithelioma, 290–292
  mammography, 290, 290f, 291f
  pearls and pitfalls, 292
  ultrasound, 291, 291f
Adenosis, 132–133
  mammography, 132, 132f
  pearls and pitfalls, 133
  sclerosing, 6, 9, 348–350
    mammography, 348f
    pearls and pitfalls, 350
    ultrasound, 349, 349f, 350, 350f
  ultrasound, 133, 133f
ADH. *See* Atypical ductal hyperplasia (ADH)
AMC. *See* Atypical medullary carcinoma (AMC)
Amorphous calcification, 8
Anatomical landmarks, 19, 20
Angiolipoma, benign
  as circumscribed mass, 55–56
    mammography, 55, 55f
    pearls and pitfalls, 56
    ultrasound, 56, 56f
  in male breast, 372
Angiosarcoma
  as circumscribed mass, 98–99

    mammography, 98, 98f
    MRI, 99
    pearls and pitfalls, 99
    ultrasound, 99, 99f
  poorly identified on mammogram, 504–505
    mammography, 504f
    MRI, 505f
    pearls and pitfalls, 505
Apocrine carcinoma, 287–289
  mammography, 287, 287f, 288f
  pearls and pitfalls, 289
  ultrasound, 288, 288f
Architectural distortion
  approach to, 333
  causes of, 9
  central, 9, 10f, 348–367
  cross-correlation and, 26, 27f
  overview of, 8–14
  peripheral, 9, 11f, 334–347
  in reduction mammoplasty patients, 452–456
    mammography, 452f, 453f, 454f, 455f
    pearls and pitfalls, 453, 455, 456
    ultrasound, 456 f
  sonographic, 14
Artifacts, calcifications *vs.*, 8
Assessment categories, 1
Asymmetry(ies)
  diffuse, 6
  focal, 324–331
    cross-correlation and, 26, 27f
    definition of, 6
    masses *vs.*, 1
  global, 306–323
  overview of, 6–8
Atherosclerosis, 190–192
  mammography, 190, 191f
  pearls and pitfalls, 192
Atypical ductal hyperplasia (ADH), 245–249
  biopsy, 249f
  mammography, 248, 248f
  pearls and pitfalls, 247, 249
  ultrasound, 246f, 247f
Atypical medullary carcinoma (AMC), 118

Augmentation mammoplasty
  implant bulge, 410–411
    mammography, 410f
    MRI, 410f
    pearls and pitfalls, 411
  implant calcifications, 413–414
    after renewal, 417–418
      mammography, 417f
      pearls and pitfalls, 418
    chest radiograph, 414f
    mammography, 413f
    pearls and pitfalls, 414
  implant fluid, 412–414
    pearls and pitfalls, 412
    ultrasound, 412, 412f
  infected fluid in subglandular implants, 402–404
    mammography, 402f
    pearls and pitfalls, 404
    ultrasound, 403, 403f
  postsurgical approach to, 401
  residual silicone, 415–416
    mammography, 415f
    pearls and pitfalls, 416
  silicone injections, 408–409
    mammography, 408f
    pearls and pitfalls, 409
  subpectoral implants, 405–406
    advantages of, 406
    mammography, 405f
    MRI, 406f, 407f
    pearls and pitfalls, 406, 407

B

Benign findings, on PET, 35
BI-RADS (Breast Imaging Reporting and Data System), 1, 28, 29t
Bone metastases, 619–620
  bone scan, 619f
  CT, 619f
  pearls and pitfalls, 620
  PET-CT, 619f
Branching calcifications, 8, 290–304
BRCA genes, 545
Breast Imaging Reporting and Data System (BI-RADS), 1, 28, 29t
Breast implant rupture, on MRI, 32

Brown fat, 621–623
  mammography, 621, 621f
  pearls and pitfalls, 623
  PET, 622f
  PET-CT, 622f
  ultrasound, 622f

C

Calcifications
  amorphous, 8, 244–259
  artifacts vs., 8
  branching, 8, 290–304
  dystrophic, 216–223
  eggshell, 207–210
    mammography, 207, 207f, 209, 209f
    pearls and pitfalls, 208, 210
  evaluation of, 189
  fine linear, 8, 290–304
  heterogenous, 8, 9f, 260–289
  implant, 417–418
  indistinct, 244–259
  large round, 201–202
    mammography, 201, 201f
    pearls and pitfalls, 201, 201f
  lobular, 250–251
    biopsy, 250f
    mammography, 250, 250f
    pearls and pitfalls, 251
  lymph node, 256–257
    mammography, 256, 256f
    pearls and pitfalls, 257
  milk of calcium, 197–200
    mammography, 197, 197f, 198, 198f, 199, 199f
    pearls and pitfalls, 198, 200
    ultrasound, 200, 200f
  overview of, 7–8
  pleomorphic, 8, 9f, 260–289
  punctuate, 224–243
  rim, 207–210
    mammography, 207, 207f, 209, 209f
    pearls and pitfalls, 208, 210
  round lucent center, 203–206
    mammography, 203, 203f, 205, 205f
    pearls and pitfalls, 204, 206
    ultrasound, 204, 204f
  secretory, 193–196
    mammography, 193, 193f, 195, 195f
    pearls and pitfalls, 194, 196
  shapes of, 8
  small round, 224–243
    assessment of, 232
  vascular, 190–192
    mammography, 190, 191f
    pearls and pitfalls, 192
Carcinoma
  adenoid cystic, 96–97
    mammography, 96, 96f
    pearls and pitfalls, 97
    ultrasound, 97, 97f
  apocrine, 287–289
    mammography, 287, 287f, 288f
    pearls and pitfalls, 289
    ultrasound, 288, 288f
  ductal
    with lobular, underestimated on mammography, 519–520
      mammography, 519, 519f
      pearls and pitfalls, 520
      ultrasound, 520, 520f
  inflammatory
    as irregular mass, 186–188
      color Doppler, 187f
      mammography, 186, 186f
      pearls and pitfalls, 188
      ultrasound, 187, 187f
    in male breast, 394–395
      bone scan, 395f
      chest radiography, 395f
      mammography, 394, 394f
      pearls and pitfalls, 395
  invasive ductal
    as amorphous calcification, 258–259
      mammography, 258, 258f
      pearls and pitfalls, 259
      ultrasound, 259, 259f
    as architectural distortion, 340–341
      mammography, 340, 340f
      pearls and pitfalls, 341
      ultrasound, 341, 341f
    as central architectural distortion, 355–364
      mammography, 355, 355f, 357f, 359, 359f, 360, 360f, 362, 362f
      pearls and pitfalls, 356, 358, 359, 361, 363
      ultrasound, 356, 356f, 358, 358f, 361, 361f
    as circumscribed mass
      mammography, 100, 100f, 102, 102f, 103f, 107, 107f
      MRI, 104f, 105f
      pearls and pitfalls, 101, 106, 109
      ultrasound, 101, 101f, 104, 104f, 105f, 106f, 108, 108f, 109f
    on fatty mammogram, 516–518
      mammography, 516, 516f
      pearls and pitfalls, 518
      ultrasound, 517, 517f, 518f
    as fine linear calcification
      breast sestamibi scan, 303f
      mammography, 299, 299f, 301, 301f
      pearls and pitfalls, 3030, 304
      ultrasound, 302, 302f
    as global asymmetry, 323–325
      mammography, 323f
      MRI, 325f
      pearls and pitfalls, 325
      ultrasound, 324, 324f
    as heterogenous microcalcification, 277–286
      lymphoscintigraphy, 282f
      mammography, 277, 277f, 280, 280f, 284, 284f
      MRI, 279f, 285f
      pearls and pitfalls, 279, 283, 286
      ultrasound, 278, 278f, 281, 281f, 282f, 284f, 285f
    as irregular mass
      bone scan, 156, 156f
      mammography, 155, 155f, 157, 157f, 159, 159f, 162, 162f, 165, 165f, 168, 168f
      microscopy, 161f
      MRI, 166f, 169f, 170f
      pearls and pitfalls, 156, 158, 161, 164, 167, 171
      ultrasound, 158, 158f, 160, 160f, 163, 163f, 166, 166f, 169, 169f
    with lobular carcinoma, 343–345, 346–347, 365–367
      mammography, 343f, 346f, 365, 365f
      MRI, 347f, 366f
      pearls and pitfalls, 345, 348, 367
      ultrasound, 344, 344f, 347f, 367, 367f
    as mammographically occult lesion
      mammography, 543f, 546, 546f, 550f
      MRI, 544f, 547f, 548f, 551f, 552f
      pearls and pitfalls, 545, 553
      ultrasound, 544f, 547f, 548f, 551f, 552f
    in patients unable to tolerate mammogram, 495–496
    poorly identified on mammogram, 508–509
      mammography, 508f
      pearls and pitfalls, 509
      ultrasound, 509, 509f
    as small round calcification
      mammography, 242, 242f
      pearls and pitfalls, 243
    staging of
      CT, 577f
      mammography, 570, 570f, 574, 574f, 577, 577f, 581f, 587, 586f
      MRI, 571f, 572f, 582f, 583f, 589f, 590f

pearls and pitfalls, 573, 576, 579, 585, 591
PET, 572f, 575f, 576f, 578f, 590f
PET-CT, 578f, 583f, 584f, 590f
ultrasound, 571f, 575f, 582f, 587f, 588f
underestimated on mammogram, 521–523, 524–526
color Doppler, 526f
mammography, 521, 521f, 524, 524f
MRI, 525f
pearls and pitfalls, 523, 526
sestamibi scan, 522f
ultrasound, 522, 522f, 525f
in unusual location, 529–530
mammography, 529, 529f
pearls and pitfalls, 530
ultrasound, 530, 530f
lobular
as circumscribed mass, 112–113
mammography, 112, 112f
pearls and pitfalls, 113
ultrasound, 113, 113f
with ductal, 343–345, 346–347, 365–367
mammography, 343f, 346f, 365, 365f
MRI, 347f, 367f
pearls and pitfalls, 345, 348, 367
ultrasound, 344, 344f, 347f, 367, 367f
with ductal, underestimated on mammogram, 519–520
mammography, 519, 519f
pearls and pitfalls, 520
ultrasound, 520, 520f
as focal asymmetry, 328–331
mammography, 328f
MRI, 330f
pearls and pitfalls, 327, 331
ultrasound, 329, 329f, 330, 330f
as irregular mass, 172–174, 175–177
mammography, 172, 172f, 175, 175f
microscopy, 172f
pearls and pitfalls, 174, 177
ultrasound, 173, 173f, 176, 176f, 177, 177f
as mammographically occult lesion
mammography, 546, 546f
MRI, 547f, 548f
pearls and pitfalls, 545
ultrasound, 547f, 548f
medullary, 117–118
atypical, 118
mammography, 117, 117f
pearls and pitfalls, 118

typical, 118
metaplastic, 119–120
lymphoscintigraphy, 120f
mammography, 119, 119f
pearls and pitfalls, 120
ultrasound, 119, 120f
mucinous, 123–125
mammography, 123, 123f
pearls and pitfalls, 125
ultrasound, 124, 124f
papillary
intracystic, in male breast, 399–400
mammography, 399, 399f
pearls and pitfalls, 400
ultrasound, 400, 400f
invasive, 110–111
mammography, 110, 110f
pearls and pitfalls, 111
ultrasound, 111, 111f
in situ ductal
as amorphous calcification, 254–255
biopsy, 254f
mammography, 254, 254f
microscopy, 255f
pearls and pitfalls, 255
as global asymmetry, 321–322
mammography, 321f
pearls and pitfalls, 322
intraductal, 535–538
ductogram, 538f
mammography, 535f, 537f
pearls and pitfalls, 536, 538
ultrasound, 536, 536f
in male breast, 392–393
mammography, 392f
pearls and pitfalls, 393
mammography, 611f, 612f
MRI, 610f, 617f
pearls and pitfalls, 614, 619
PET-CT, 611f, 617f
poorly identified on mammogram, 506
mammography, 506f
pearls and pitfalls, 507
ultrasound, 507, 507f
as small round calcification
biopsy, 236f, 237f
mammography, 235, 235f, 237, 237f, 240, 240f
pearls and pitfalls, 236, 239, 241
ultrasound, 238, 238f, 239, 239f
thick wall ducts, 539–540
mammography, 539f
pearls and pitfalls, 540
ultrasound, 540f
ultrasound, 612f, 613f
tubular
as irregular mass, 181–185

mammography, 181, 181f, 183, 183f
microscopy, 185f
pearls and pitfalls, 182, 185f
ultrasound, 182, 182f, 184, 184f
as peripheral architectural distortion, 348–349
mammography, 348, 348f
pearls and pitfalls, 349
ultrasound, 349, 349f
Categories, assessment, 1
Central architectural distortion, 9, 10f, 348–367
Chest wall, in breast anatomy, 20, 21f
Circumscribed masses, overview of, 1
Clips, dynamic, 18
Clumped enhancement, 29
Color Doppler, 16–18, 18f
Contrast resolution, 15–16, 17f
Cooper's ligaments
in breast anatomy, 20, 21f
on poor mammogram, 512–513
mammography, 512f
pearls and pitfalls, 513
ultrasound, 512, 512f
Cross-correlation
anatomy in, 20, 21f
architectural distortion and, 26, 27f
of MRI and sonography, 106
rules of, 20–23
shadowing and, 24–26
of sonography and mammography, 19–23, 24f
Curve analysis, kinetic, 28, 549
Cutaneous paraneoplastic syndromes, 495
Cyst, 57–58, 59–60, 61–62. *See also* Fibrocystic change, benign
definition of, 58
as eggshell/rim calcification, 207–208
mammography, 207, 207f
pearls and pitfalls, 208
incidence of, 60
mammography, 57, 57f, 59, 59f, 61, 61f
oil
as circumscribed mass, 51–52, 53–54
mammography, 51, 51f, 53, 53f
pearls and pitfalls, 52, 54
ultrasound, 52, 52f, 54, 54f
as large round calcification, 201–202
mammography, 201, 201f
pearls and pitfalls, 202
as round lucent center calcification, 203–206
mammography, 203, 203f, 205, 205f
pearls and pitfalls, 204, 206

Cyst (*continued*)
    ultrasound, 204, 204f
  pearls and pitfalls, 58, 60
  sebaceous, 84–85
    in male breast, 392–393
      mammography, 392, 392f
      pearls and pitfalls, 393
      ultrasound, 393, 393f
    mammography, 84, 84f
    pearls and pitfalls, 85, 85f
    ultrasound, 85, 85f
  ultrasound, 57–58, 58f, 59–60, 60f, 62, 62f
Cystic carcinoma, adenoid, 96–97
  mammography, 96, 96f
  pearls and pitfalls, 97
  ultrasound, 97, 97f

D
Deodorant
  as amorphous calcification, 244–247
    mammography, 244, 244f
    pearls and pitfalls, 245
Diabetic mastopathy
  as circumscribed mass, 63–65
    mammography, 63, 63f
    pearls and pitfalls, 65
    ultrasound, 64, 64f
  poorly identified on mammography, 496–498
    mammography, 496f
    pearls and pitfalls, 498
    ultrasound, 497, 497f
Diffuse asymmetry, 6
Ductal abnormalities, 531–541
Ductal carcinoma
  invasive
    as amorphous calcification, 258–259
      mammography, 258, 258f
      pearls and pitfalls, 259
      ultrasound, 259, 259f
    as architectural distortion, 340–342
      mammography, 340, 340f
      pearls and pitfalls, 341
      ultrasound, 341, 341f
    as central architectural distortion, 357–364
      mammography, 357, 357f, 358f, 360, 360f, 362, 362f, 363, 363f
      pearls and pitfalls, 357, 359, 364
      ultrasound, 356, 356f, 359, 359f, 363, 363f
    as circumscribed mass, 100–101, 102–106, 107–109
      mammography, 100, 100f, 102, 102f, 103f, 107, 107f
      MRI, 104f, 105f
      pearls and pitfalls, 101, 106, 109
      ultrasound, 101, 101f, 104, 104f, 105f, 106f, 108, 108f, 109f
    on fatty mammogram, 516–518
      mammography, 516, 516f
      pearls and pitfalls, 518
      ultrasound, 517, 517f, 518f
    as fine linear calcification
      breast sestamibi scan, 303f
      mammography, 299, 299f, 301, 301f
      pearls and pitfalls, 300, 304
      ultrasound, 302, 302f
    as global asymmetry, 324–327
      mammography, 324f
      pearls and pitfalls, 327
      ultrasound, 326f
    as heterogenous microcalcification, 280–289
      lymphoscintigraphy, 282, 282f
      mammography, 280, 280f, 284, 284f
      MRI, 285f
      pearls and pitfalls, 283, 286, 289
      ultrasound, 281, 281f, 282, 282f, 284f, 285f, 288f
    as irregular mass, 155–171
      bone scan, 156, 156f
      mammography, 155, 155f, 157, 157f, 159, 159f, 162, 162f, 165, 165f, 168, 168f
      microscopy, 161f
      MRI, 166f, 169f, 169f
      pearls and pitfalls, 156, 158, 161, 164, 167, 171
      ultrasound, 158, 158f, 160, 160f, 163, 163f, 166, 166f, 169, 169f
    with lobular, 341–343, 344–347, 362–364
      mammography, 340f, 344f, 362, 362f
      MRI, 345f, 363f
      pearls and pitfalls, 342, 345, 364
      ultrasound, 341, 341f, 344f, 363, 363f
    as mammographically occult lesion
      mammography, 543f, 546, 546f, 548f
      MRI, 541f, 544f, 547f, 553f, 554f
      pearls and pitfalls, 545, 549
      ultrasound, 544f, 547f, 548f
    in patients unable to tolerate mammogram, 494–495
    poorly identified on mammogram, 508–509
      mammography, 508f
      pearls and pitfalls, 509
      ultrasound, 509, 509f
    as small round calcification
      mammography, 240, 240f
      pearls and pitfalls, 241
    staging of
      CT, 578f
      mammography, 570, 570f, 574, 574f, 577, 577f, 580, 581f, 586, 586f
      MRI, 571f, 572f, 583f, 584f, 590f, 591f
      pearls and pitfalls, 573, 576, 579, 585, 591
      PET, 572f, 575f, 575f, 578f, 590f
      PET-CT, 578f, 583f, 584f, 590f
      ultrasound, 571f, 575f, 582f, 587f, 588f
    underestimated on mammogram, 521–523, 524–526
      color Doppler, 526f
      mammography, 521, 521f, 524, 524f
      MRI, 525f
      pearls and pitfalls, 523, 526
      sestamibi scan, 522f
      ultrasound, 522, 522f, 525f
    in unusual location, 529–530
      mammography, 529, 529f
      pearls and pitfalls, 530
      ultrasound, 530, 530f
    with lobular, underestimated on mammography, 519–520
      mammography, 519, 519f
      pearls and pitfalls, 520
      ultrasound, 520, 520f
  in situ
    as amorphous calcification, 254–255
      biopsy, 255f
      mammography, 254, 254f
      microscopy, 255f
      pearls and pitfalls, 255
    as fine linear calcification, 293–298
      mammography, 293, 293f, 294, 294f, 297, 297f, 298f
      microscopy, 298f
      MRI, 296f
      pearls and pitfalls, 294, 296, 298
      ultrasound, 295f
    as global asymmetry, 321–323
      mammography, 321f
      pearls and pitfalls, 323
    as heterogenous microcalcification
      mammography, 273, 273f, 275, 275f
      MRI, 276, 276f

pearls and pitfalls, 274, 276
ultrasound, 274, 274f
intraductal, 535–538
ductogram, 538f
mammography, 535f, 537f
pearls and pitfalls, 536, 538
ultrasound, 536, 536f
in male breast, 394–395
mammography, 394f
pearls and pitfalls, 395
mammography, 611f, 615, 615f
MRI, 610f, 617f
pearls and pitfalls, 614, 618
PET-CT, 611f, 617f
poorly identified on mammogram, 506–507
mammography, 506f
pearls and pitfalls, 507
ultrasound, 507, 507f
as small round calcification
biopsy, 237f, 238f
mammography, 236, 236f, 238, 238f, 240, 240f
pearls and pitfalls, 236, 239, 241
ultrasound, 238, 238f, 239, 239f
thick wall ducts, 539–540
mammography, 539f
pearls and pitfalls, 540
ultrasound, 540f
ultrasound, 612f, 613f, 616f
Ductal enhancement, 29
Dynamic clips, 18

E
Echoes, in benign cysts, 62
Eggshell calcification, 207–210
mammography, 207, 207f, 209, 209f
pearls and pitfalls, 208, 210
Encephalomyelitis, 495
Endocrine paraneoplastic syndromes, 495
Enhancement
clumped, 29
ductal, 29
kinetics, 549
rim, 28
Equipment, sonography, 15
Estrogen effect, 313–315
mammography, 313f, 314f
pearls and pitfalls, 315
Extent of disease, on MRI, 31
Extremely dense mammogram, 502–513

F
Fascia, in breast anatomy, 20, 21f
Fat
brown, 621–623
mammography, 621, 621f

pearls and pitfalls, 623
PET, 622f
PET-CT, 622f
ultrasound, 622f
on mammography vs. sonography, 20, 22f
types of, 624
white, 624
Fat necrosis, 51–52, 53–54
as amorphous microcalcification, 252–253
mammography, 252, 252f, 253f
pearls and pitfalls, 253
as architectural distortion cause, 9
as benign entity producing irregular mass, 6
as circumscribed mass, 51–52, 53–54
mammography, 51, 51f, 53, 53f
pearls and pitfalls, 52, 54
ultrasound, 52, 52f, 54, 54f
as dystrophic calcification, 216–221
mammography, 216, 216f, 218, 218f, 219f, 220, 220f
pearls and pitfalls, 217, 219, 221
ultrasound, 221, 221f
as eggshell calcification, 209–210
mammography, 209, 209f
pearls and pitfalls, 210
on fatty mammogram, 516–517
mammography, 516f
pearls and pitfalls, 517
ultrasound, 517, 517f
as global asymmetry, 316–318
mammography, 316f, 317f
pearls and pitfalls, 318
ultrasound, 18, 318f
as heterogenous microcalcification, 268–270
mammography, 268, 268f
pearls and pitfalls, 270
ultrasound, 269, 269f
as irregular mass, 134–137
mammography, 134, 134f, 136, 136f
pearls and pitfalls, 135, 137
ultrasound, 135, 135f, 137, 137f
in male breast, 375–376
mammography, 375, 375f
pearls and pitfalls, 376
ultrasound, 376, 376f
in neoplasm procedure patients, 471–475
mammography, 471, 471f, 473, 473f
pearls and pitfalls, 472, 475
ultrasound, 474, 474f
in reduction mammoplasty patients, 458–459
mammography, 458f, 459f

pearls and pitfalls, 459
Fatty mammogram, 514–518
FDG. See 18F-fluorodeoxyglucose (FDG)
Fibroadenolipoma, 47
Fibroadenoma, 6, 66–67
adenoma vs., 501
as focal asymmetry, 324–325
mammography, 324f
pearls and pitfalls, 325
ultrasound, 325, 325f
as heterogenous calcification
mammography, 262, 262f, 263, 263f
pearls and pitfalls, 263, 267
ultrasound, 265f
as irregular mass, 138–139
mammography, 136, 136f, 140, 140f
MRI, 141f
pearls and pitfalls, 140, 143
ultrasound, 137, 139f, 141, 142f
juvenile, poorly identified on mammogram, 496–498
pearls and pitfalls, 598
ultrasound, 497, 497f
mammography, 66, 66f
pearls and pitfalls, 67
ultrasound, 67, 67f
Fibroadenomatoid hyperplasia, 335
mammography, 335f
MRI, 335, 335f
pearls and pitfalls, 335
ultrasound, 335f
Fibroadenomatous hyperplasia
mammography, 264, 264f
pearls and pitfalls, 264
Fibrocystic change
as amorphous microcalcification, 248–251
biopsy, 250f
mammography, 248, 249f, 250, 250f
pearls and pitfalls, 249, 251
as circumscribed mass, 68–69, 70–71 (See also Cyst, benign)
focal solid mass vs., 71
mammography, 68, 68f, 70, 70f
pearls and pitfalls, 69
stages of, 69
ultrasound, 69, 69f, 71, 71f
as heterogenous microcalcification, 262–263
mammography, 262, 262f
pearls and pitfalls, 263
ultrasound, 263, 263f
as small round calcification, 226–228, 229–230, 231–232, 233–234
biopsy, 230, 230f

Fibrocystic change (*continued*)
  mammography, 226, 226f, 229, 229f, 231, 231f, 233, 233f
  pearls and pitfalls, 228, 230, 232, 234
  ultrasound, 227, 227f, 234, 234f
Fibrosis, focal, 6, 9
Fibrous histiocytoma, poorly identified on mammogram, 510–511
  mammography, 510f
  pearls and pitfalls, 511
  ultrasound, 511, 511f
Fine linear calcifications, 8, 290–304
18F-fluorodeoxyglucose (FDG), 34
  in benign findings, 35
Focal asymmetries, 324–331
  cross-correlation and, 26, 27f
  definition of, 6
  masses *vs.*, 1
Focal fibrosis, 6, 9
Focus(foci)
  definition of, 345
  as mammographically occult lesion, 553–555
  single *vs.* multiple, 28
Foreign body, 222–223
  mammography, 222, 222f
  pearls and pitfalls, 223
Frequencies
  shadowing and, 25
  in sonography, 15

G

Galactocele, 42–43
  definition of, 43
  mammography, 42, 42f
  pearls and pitfalls, 43
  ultrasound, 43, 43f
Gastrointestinal paraneoplastic syndromes, 495
Glandular tissue, in breast anatomy, 20, 21f
Global asymmetry, 308–325
Glucose level, PET study and, 35
Granular cell tumor, 129–130
  mammography, 129, 129f
  pearls and pitfalls, 130
  ultrasound, 130, 130f
Granulocyte colony-stimulating factor, 624–627
  mammography, 624f
  MRI, 626f
  pearls and pitfalls, 627
  PET, 625f, 626f
  PET-CT, 625f, 625f
  ultrasound, 625f
Gynecomastia
  causes of, 383
  definition of, 376
  dendritic pattern
    mammography, 379f, 380f
    pearls and pitfalls, 381f
  diffuse glandular pattern
    mammography, 382f
    pearls and pitfalls, 383
  incidence of, 376
  nodular pattern
    mammography, 375f, 377f
    pearls and pitfalls, 376, 378
    ultrasound, 376f, 378, 378f
  patterns of, 378

H

Hamartoma
  as circumscribed mass, 44–45, 46–47
    definition of, 45
    mammography, 44, 44f, 46, 46f
    pearls and pitfalls, 45, 47
    ultrasound, 44–45, 45f, 46–47, 47f
  smooth muscle, 527–528
    pearls and pitfalls, 528
    ultrasound, 527, 527f
Hemangioma, venous, 92–93
  mammography, 92, 92f
  pearls and pitfalls, 93
  ultrasound, 93, 93f
Hematologic paraneoplastic syndromes, 495
Hematoma
  as benign entity producing irregular mass, 6
  as circumscribed mass, 72–73
    mammography, 72, 72f
    pearls and pitfalls, 73
    ultrasound, 73, 73f
  as irregular mass, 144–145
    mammography, 144, 144f
    ultrasound, 145, 145f
  in neoplasm procedure patients, 466–468, 469, 469f, 468f
    mammography, 466, 466f, 467f
    pearls and pitfalls, 468
  pearls and pitfalls, 144
Heterogenous calcifications, 8, 9f
High-frequency ultrasound, 15, 16f
High-risk women, MRI screening of, 31
Histiocytoma, fibrous poorly identified on mammogram, 510–511
  mammography, 510f
  pearls and pitfalls, 511
  ultrasound, 511, 511f

I

Implants
  bulge, 410–411
    mammography, 410f
    MRI, 410f
    pearls and pitfalls, 411
  calcifications, 413–414
    after renewal, 417–418
      mammography, 417f
      pearls and pitfalls, 418
    chest radiograph, 414f
    mammography, 413f
    pearls and pitfalls, 414
  fluid, 412–414
    pearls and pitfalls, 412
    ultrasound, 412, 412f
  neoplasm and, 442–447
    mammography, 442, 442f, 446f
    MRI, 442f
    pearls and pitfalls, 445, 447
    ultrasound, 443, 443f, 447, 447f
  pseudocapsule, 419–421
    mammography, 419f, 420f
    pearls and pitfalls, 421
  residual silicone, 415–416
    mammography, 415f
    pearls and pitfalls, 416
  rupture, 422–441
    extracapsular, 433–438
      mammography, 433f, 436f
      MRI, 434f, 437f
      pearls and pitfalls, 435, 438
      ultrasound, 437f
    false positive, 439–441
      mammography, 439f
      MRI, 441f
      pearls and pitfalls, 441
      ultrasound, 440f
    intracapsular, 429–432
      mammography, 431f
      MRI, 429f, 432f
      pearls and pitfalls, 430, 432
    mammography, 422f, 424f, 427f
    MRI, 32
    pearls and pitfalls, 427, 430, 432
    ultrasound, 423f, 425f, 428f
  subglandular
    infected fluid in, 402–404
      mammography, 402f
      pearls and pitfalls, 404
      ultrasound, 403, 403f
  subpectoral, 405–407
    advantages of, 406
    mammography, 405f
    MRI, 406f, 407f
    pearls and pitfalls, 410, 411
Inclusion cyst, 84–85
  mammography, 84, 84f
  pearls and pitfalls, 85, 85f
  ultrasound, 85, 85f
Inflammatory carcinoma
  definition of, 312
  as global asymmetry, 313–314
    mammography, 313f
    pearls and pitfalls, 314
  as irregular mass, 186–188

color Doppler, 187f
mammography, 186, 186f
pearls and pitfalls, 188
ultrasound, 187, 187f
in male breast, 394–395
bone scan, 395f
chest radiography, 395f
mammography, 394, 394f
pearls and pitfalls, 395
Intracystic papillary carcinoma, in male breast, 399–400
mammography, 399, 399f
pearls and pitfalls, 400
ultrasound, 400, 400f
Intraductal ductal carcinoma in situ, 537–540
ductogram, 540f
mammography, 537f, 539f
pearls and pitfalls, 538, 540
ultrasound, 538, 538f
Intraductal papilloma, 533–536
mammography, 533f, 535f, 536f
pearls and pitfalls, 534, 536
ultrasound, 534, 534f
Invasive ductal carcinoma
as amorphous calcification
mammography, 260, 260f
pearls and pitfalls, 261
ultrasound, 261, 261f
as central architectural distortion, 353–361
mammography, 353, 353f, 355f, 357, 357f, 358, 358f, 360, 360f
pearls and pitfalls, 354, 356, 357, 359, 361
ultrasound, 354, 354f, 358, 358f, 359, 359f
as circumscribed mass, 100–101, 102–106, 107–109
mammography, 100, 100f, 102, 102f, 103f, 107, 107f
MRI, 104f, 105f
pearls and pitfalls, 101, 106, 109
ultrasound, 101, 101f, 104, 104f, 105f, 106f, 108, 108f, 109f
on fatty mammogram, 516–518
mammography, 516, 516f
pearls and pitfalls, 518
ultrasound, 517, 517f, 518f
as fine linear calcification
breast sestamibi scan, 303f
mammography, 299, 299f, 301, 301f
pearls and pitfalls, 300, 304
ultrasound, 302, 302f
as global asymmetry, 321–323
mammography, 321f
MRI, 323f
pearls and pitfalls, 323
ultrasound, 322, 322f
as heterogenous microcalcification, 277–286
lymphoscintigraphy, 282f
mammography, 277, 277f, 280, 280f, 284, 284f
MRI, 278f, 285f
pearls and pitfalls, 279, 283, 286
ultrasound, 278, 278f, 281, 281f, 282f, 284f, 285f
as irregular mass, 155–171
bone scan, 156, 156f
mammography, 155, 155f, 157, 157f, 158, 158f, 161, 161f, 165, 165f, 168, 168f
microscopy, 161f
MRI, 166f, 169f, 170f
pearls and pitfalls, 156, 158, 161, 164, 167, 171
ultrasound, 158, 158f, 160, 160f, 163, 163f, 166, 166f, 169, 169f
with lobular, 343–345, 346–348, 365–367
mammography, 343f, 346f, 365, 365f
MRI, 347f, 366f
pearls and pitfalls, 345, 348, 367
ultrasound, 344, 344f, 347f, 366, 366f
with lobular carcinoma, 343–345, 346–348
mammography, 345f, 346f
MRI, 347f
pearls and pitfalls, 345, 348
ultrasound, 344, 344f, 347f
as mammographically occult lesion
mammography, 543f, 546, 546f, 550f
MRI, 544f, 547f, 548f, 551f, 552f
pearls and pitfalls, 545, 553
ultrasound, 542f, 547f, 548f, 551f, 552f
in patient unable to tolerate mammogram, 494–495
as peripheral architectural distortion, 340–342
mammography, 340, 340f
pearls and pitfalls, 342
ultrasound, 341, 341f
poorly identified on mammogram, 508–509
mammography, 508f
pearls and pitfalls, 509
ultrasound, 509, 509f
as small round calcification
mammography, 242, 242f
pearls and pitfalls, 243
staging of
CT, 577f
mammography, 570, 570f, 574, 574f, 577, 5787f, 581f, 586, 586f
MRI, 571f, 572f, 582f, 583f, 589f, 590f
pearls and pitfalls, 573, 576, 579, 585, 592
PET, 572f, 575f, 576f, 578f, 590f
PET-CT, 578f, 583f, 584f, 590f
ultrasound, 571f, 575f, 582f, 587f, 586f
underestimated on mammogram, 521–523, 524–526
color Doppler, 526f
mammography, 521, 521f, 524, 524f
MRI, 525f
pearls and pitfalls, 523, 526
sestamibi scan, 522f
ultrasound, 522, 522f, 525f
in unusual location, 529–530
mammography, 529, 529f
pearls and pitfalls, 530
ultrasound, 530, 530f
Invasive lobular carcinoma, 172–174, 175–177
mammography, 172, 172f, 174, 174f
microscopy, 173f
pearls and pitfalls, 174, 177
ultrasound, 173, 173f, 176, 176f, 177, 177f
Invasive papillary carcinoma, 110–111
mammography, 110, 110f
pearls and pitfalls, 111
ultrasound, 111, 111f
Inverted nipple, 79–80
in ductal carcinoma, 159
mammography, 79, 79f, 80f
Irregular masses
approach to, 131
benign entities producing, 6
overview of, 6

J
Juvenile fibroadenoma, poorly identified on mammogram, 498–499
pearls and pitfalls, 499
ultrasound, 499, 499f

K
"Keyhole" sign, 429f, 430
Kinetic curve analysis, 28, 549

L
Lactating adenoma, poorly identified on mammogram, 500–501
pearls and pitfalls, 501
ultrasound, 500f
Landmarks, anatomical, 19, 20

Large round calcification, 203–204
   mammography, 203, 203f
   pearls and pitfalls, 204
Leiomyoma, 74–75
   mammography, 74, 74f
   pearls and pitfalls, 75
   ultrasound, 75, 75f
"Linguine" sign, 32, 428
Lipoma, 48–49, 50–51
   in male breast, 384–385
      mammography, 384f
      pearls and pitfalls, 385
      ultrasound, 385, 385f
   mammography, 48, 48f, 50, 50f
   pearls and pitfalls, 49, 51
   ultrasound, 49, 49f
Lobular calcifications, 250–251
   biopsy, 250f
   mammography, 250, 250f
   pearls and pitfalls, 251
Lobular carcinoma
   as circumscribed mass, 112–113
      mammography, 112, 112f
      pearls and pitfalls, 113
      ultrasound, 113, 113f
   with ductal, 343–345, 346–347, 365–367
      mammography, 343f, 346f, 365, 365f
      pearls and pitfalls, 345, 347, 367
      ultrasound, 345f, 347f, 367, 367f
      underestimated on mammogram, 521–523
         mammography, 521, 521f
         pearls and pitfalls, 523
         ultrasound, 522, 522f
   as focal asymmetry, 328–331
      mammography, 328f, 330f
      pearls and pitfalls, 331
      PET-CT, 330
      ultrasound, 329, 329f, 330f, 334f
   as irregular mass, 172–174, 175–177
      mammography, 172, 172f, 175, 175f
      microscopy, 173f
      pearls and pitfalls, 174, 177
      ultrasound, 173, 173f, 176, 176f, 177, 177f
   as mammographically occult lesion
      mammography, 546, 546f, 556f
      MRI, 547f, 548f, 558f, 559f
      pearls and pitfalls, 545, 559
      ultrasound, 547f, 548f, 557f
Location estimation, 19
Low standardized uptake value, 615–618
Lymphedema
   as global asymmetry, 308–309
      mammography, 308, 308f

      pearls and pitfalls, 309
   in neoplasm procedure patients, 479–482
      mammography, 480f
      pearls and pitfalls, 482
      ultrasound, 481, 481f
Lymph node
   benign, 76–78
      mammography, 76, 76f
      ultrasound, 77, 77f, 78f
   in male breast, 386–387
      mammography, 386, 386f
      pearls and pitfalls, 387
   malignant, 114–116
      mammography, 114, 114f
      MRI, 115f
      pearls and pitfalls, 116
      ultrasound, 115, 115f
Lymph node calcifications, 256–257
   mammography, 256, 256f
   pearls and pitfalls, 257
Lymphoma, 178–180
   mammography, 178, 178f
   pearls and pitfalls, 180
   ultrasound, 179, 179f
Lymphoscintigraphy, metaplastic carcinoma on, 120f

M

Magnetic resonance imaging (MRI)
   applications of, 31–32
   contrast administration in, 171
   disease extent definition with, 31
   identifying suspicious lesions on, 28–29
   implant rupture on, 32
   improving identification with, 106
   mammographically occult masses on, 541–568
   recurrent disease on, 31
   residual disease on, 31
   for screening high-risk women, 31
   "second look" sonography and, 29–31
   in staging of lobular cancer, 559
   therapeutic response assessment on, 31
   unknown primary on, 31–32
Male breast
   approach to, 369
   benign, 370–391
   malignant, 392–400
Mammography
   cross-correlation with sonography, 19–23, 24f
   ductal abnormalities poorly identified with, 531–540
   extremely dense, 504–515
   fat on, vs. sonography, 20, 22f
   fatty, 516–520

   inability to tolerate, 494–495
   occult MRI masses, 541–568
   palpable masses poorly defined on, 496–518
   scattered heterogenous, 502–513
   underestimation of tumor size with, 519–526
   unusual locations and, 527–530
Mammoplasty
   augmentation
      implant bulge, 410–411
         mammography, 410f
         MRI, 410f
         pearls and pitfalls, 411
      implant calcifications, 413–414
         after renewal, 417–418
         chest radiograph, 414f
         mammography, 413f
         pearls and pitfalls, 414
      implant calcifications after renewal
         mammography, 417f
         pearls and pitfalls, 418
      implant fluid, 412–414
         pearls and pitfalls, 412
         ultrasound, 412, 412f
      infected fluid in subglandular implants, 402–404
         mammography, 402f
         pearls and pitfalls, 404
         ultrasound, 403, 403f
      postsurgical approach to, 401
      residual silicone, 415–416
         mammography, 415f
         pearls and pitfalls, 416
      silicone injections, 408–409
         mammography, 408f
         pearls and pitfalls, 409
      subpectoral implants, 405–407
         advantages of, 406
         mammography, 405f
         MRI, 406f, 407f
         pearls and pitfalls, 406, 407
   reduction, postsurgical approach to, 449
Margins, well-defined, 2–3, 4f
Masses, 1–6
   circumscribed, overview of, 1
   density analysis of, 1
   in diabetic mastopathy, 65
   focal asymmetries vs., 1
   irregular
      approach to, 131
      benign entities producing, 6
      overview of, 6
   palpable
      poorly identified on mammogram, 496–518
      sonographic approach to, 18–19
   on PET, 35

on sonography vs. mammography, 21
Mastitis
  as global asymmetry, 308–310
    mammography, 308, 308f, 309f
    pearls and pitfalls, 310
    ultrasound, 310, 310f
  plasma cell, as large linear calcification, 190–194
    mammography, 190, 190f, 193, 193f
    pearls and pitfalls, 192, 194
Mastopathy, diabetic
  as circumscribed mass, 63–65
    mammography, 63, 63f
    pearls and pitfalls, 65
    ultrasound, 64, 64f
  poorly identified on mammography, 496–499
    mammography, 496f
    pearls and pitfalls, 498
    ultrasound, 497, 497f
Medullary carcinoma, 117–118
  atypical, 118
  mammography, 117, 117f
  pearls and pitfalls, 118
  typical, 118
Melanoma, metastatic, 121–122
  mammography, 121, 121f
  pearls and pitfalls, 122
  ultrasound, 121, 122f
Menopause, fibrocystic changes and, 69
Mesothelioma
  chest radiograph, 608f
  mammography, 607f
  pearls and pitfalls, 609
  PET-CT, 609f
Metaplastic carcinoma, 119–120
  lymphoscintigraphy, 120f
  mammography, 119, 119f
  pearls and pitfalls, 120
  ultrasound, 119, 120f
Metastases, bone, 619–620
Metastases to male breast, 396–398
  CT, 397f, 398f
  mammography, 496, 496f
  pearls and pitfalls, 498
  ultrasound, 497, 497f
Metastatic melanoma, 121–122
  mammography, 121, 121f
  pearls and pitfalls, 122
  ultrasound, 121, 122f
Microcysts, with milk of calcium, 197–200
  mammography, 197, 197f, 198, 198f, 199, 199f
  pearls and pitfalls, 198, 200
  ultrasound, 200, 200f
Microglandular adenosis, 132–133

mammography, 132, 132f
pearls and pitfalls, 133
ultrasound, 133, 133f
Microlobulations, 6
Milk of calcium, 197–200
  mammography, 197, 197f, 198, 198f, 199, 199f
  pearls and pitfalls, 198, 200
  ultrasound, 200, 200f
Mixed ductal and lobular carcinoma, 343–345, 346–347, 362–364
  mammography, 343f, 346f, 362, 362f
  MRI, 363f
  pearls and pitfalls, 345, 347, 364
  ultrasound, 344, 344f, 347f, 363, 363f
  underestimated on mammogram, 521–522
    mammography, 521, 521f
    pearls and pitfalls, 522
    ultrasound, 522, 522f
Mole, 86–87, 88–89
  mammography, 86, 86f, 88, 88f
  pearls and pitfalls, 87, 89
MRI. See Magnetic resonance imaging (MRI)
Mucinous carcinoma, 123–125
  mammography, 123, 123f
  pearls and pitfalls, 125
  ultrasound, 124, 124f
Multicentricity
  incidence of, 167
  multifocality vs., 164
Multifocality, multicentricity vs., 164
Muscle(s)
  in breast anatomy, 20, 21f
  sternalis, 90–91
    mammography, 90, 90f
    pearls and pitfalls, 91
    ultrasound, 91, 91f
Myofibroblastoma
  as irregular mass, 153–154
    mammography, 153, 153f
    pearls and pitfalls, 154
    ultrasound, 154, 154f
  in male breast, 388–389
    mammography, 388, 388f
    pearls and pitfalls, 389
    ultrasound, 389, 389f

N

Neoplasm procedures, findings after
  fat necrosis, 469–472
    mammography, 469, 469f, 471, 471f, 472f
    pearls and pitfalls, 472, 472
    ultrasound, 470, 470f
  hematoma, 466–468, 469, 469f, 470f
    mammography, 466, 466f, 467f

    pearls and pitfalls, 468
  lymphedema, 475–479
    mammography, 475f
    pearls and pitfalls, 479
    ultrasound, 476, 476f
  pseudoaneurysm, 473–475
    mammography, 473f
    pearls and pitfalls, 475
    ultrasound, 474, 474f
  radiation changes, 477–478
    mammography, 477, 477f, 478f
    pearls and pitfalls, 478
  recurrent neoplasm, 479–491
    mammography, 479, 479f, 480f, 483f, 486, 486f, 488, 488f
    MRI, 485f, 489f
    pearls and pitfalls, 482, 485, 487, 490
    ultrasound, 481, 481f, 484, 484f, 487, 487f, 489, 489f, 490f
  scar, 460–466
    mammography, 460, 460f, 461, 461f, 462f, 464f
    pearls and pitfalls, 461, 463, 466
    ultrasound, 462, 462f, 463f, 465f
Neurologic paraneoplastic syndromes, 495
Nipple out of profile, 79–80
  in ductal carcinoma, 155
  mammography, 79, 79f, 80f
"Noose" sign, 429
Normal structures, poorly identified on mammogram, 512–513
  mammography, 512f
  pearls and pitfalls, 513
  ultrasound, 512, 512f

O

Occult MRI lesions, mammographically, 541–568
  benign, 541–542
    MRI, 541f
  malignant, 543–555
    mammography, 543f, 546, 546f, 550f
    MRI, 544f, 547f, 548f, 551f, 552f
    pearls and pitfalls, 545, 549, 553
    ultrasound, 546f, 549f, 550f, 553f, 554f
Oil cyst
  as circumscribed mass, 51–52, 53–54
    mammography, 51, 51f, 53, 53f
    pearls and pitfalls, 52, 54
    ultrasound, 52, 52f, 54, 54f
  as large round calcification, 201–202
    mammography, 201, 201f
    pearls and pitfalls, 202

Oil cyst (*continued*)
   as round lucent center calcification, 203–206
      mammography, 203, 203f, 205, 205f
      pearls and pitfalls, 204, 206
      ultrasound, 206, 206f
Ointment
   mammography, 260, 260f, 261f
   pearls and pitfalls, 261

P

Paget's disease, 561–568
   mammography, 561f, 565f
   MRI, 562f, 563f, 566f, 567f
   pearls and pitfalls, 564, 567
   ultrasound, 562f, 563f, 566f
Palpable mass
   as normal structure, 514
   poorly identified on mammogram, 496–518
   sonographic approach to, 18–19
Papillary carcinoma
   intracystic, in male breast, 402–403
      mammography, 402, 402f
      pearls and pitfalls, 404
      ultrasound, 403, 403f
   invasive, 110–111
      mammography, 110, 110f
      pearls and pitfalls, 111
      ultrasound, 111, 111f
Papillary lesions, 6, 145–147
   mammography, 145, 145f
   pearls and pitfalls, 147
   ultrasound, 146, 146f, 147, 147f
Papilloma
   as circumscribed mass, 81–83
      mammography, 81, 81f, 145, 145f
      pearls and pitfalls, 83, 147
      ultrasound, 82, 82f, 83f, 147, 147f
   as heterogenous microcalcification, 271–272
      mammography, 271, 271f
      pearls and pitfalls, 272
   intraductal, 533–534
      mammography, 533f
      pearls and pitfalls, 534
   types of, 271
Paraneoplastic syndromes, 495
Patterns of abnormality, 1–14
Perception, of abnormalities, 1
Peripheral architectural distortion, 9, 11f, 336–350
PET. *See* Positron emission tomography (PET)
PET-CT. *See* Positron emission tomography-computed tomography (PET-CT)
Phyllodes tumor, 126–128
   mammography, 126, 126f
   pearls and pitfalls, 128
   ultrasound, 127, 127f
Plasma cell mastitis, 194–196
   mammography, 195, 195f
   pearls and pitfalls, 194, 196
Pleomorphic calcifications, 8, 9f
Positron emission tomography-computed tomography (PET-CT), 34
   for additional malignancies, 607–609
   for recurrent disease identification, 602–606
   for therapeutic response assessment, 592–601
Positron emission tomography (PET)
   benign breast findings on, 35
   blood glucose and, 35
   breast cancer applications of, 35–37
   18F-fluorodeoxyglucose in, 34
   history of, 34
   limitations of, 37–38
   mass identification with, 35
   mechanism of, 34
   patient preparation for, 35
   pitfalls of, 37–38, 615–627
   recurrent disease on, 37
   scanner schematic, 35f
   staging with, 35, 36f, 570–591
   therapeutic response assessment on, 37
Power Doppler, 16–18, 18f
Pregnancy, lactating adenoma in, 500–501
   pearls and pitfalls, 501
   ultrasound, 500f
Premenopause, fibrocystic changes and, 69
Pseudoaneurysm, in neoplasm procedure patients, 473–475
   mammography, 473f
   pearls and pitfalls, 475
   ultrasound, 474, 474f
Pseudoangiomatous stromal hyperplasia, 94–95
   mammography, 94, 94f
   pearls and pitfalls, 95
   ultrasound, 95, 95f
Pseudogynecomastia, 386–387
   mammography, 386, 386f
   pearls and pitfalls, 387
"Pull-away" sign, 430

R

Radial scars
   as architectural distortion cause, 9
   as benign entity producing irregular mass, 6
   as central architectural distortion, 351–352
      mammography, 351f
      pearls and pitfalls, 352
      ultrasound, 352, 352f
   as irregular mass, 148–150
      mammography, 148, 148f
      MRI, 149f
      pearls and pitfalls, 150
      ultrasound, 149, 149f
   as mammographically occult lesion
      MRI, 541f
      pearls and pitfalls, 542
   as peripheral architectural distortion, 340–342
      pearls and pitfalls, 342
      ultrasound, 341, 341f
Radiation changes, in neoplasm procedure patients, 479–482
   mammography, 479, 479f, 480f
   pearls and pitfalls, 482
Recurrent disease
   CT, 604f
   mammography, 602f
   MRI, 31, 603f
   in neoplasm procedure patients, 479–491
      mammography, 479, 479f, 480f, 483f, 486, 486f, 488, 488f
      MRI, 485f, 489f
      pearls and pitfalls, 482, 485, 487, 490
      ultrasound, 481, 481f, 484, 484f, 487, 487f, 489, 489f, 490f
   pearls and pitfalls, 604f, 606
   PET, 605f
   on PET, 37
   PET-CT, 604f
   ultrasound, 603f
Reduction mammoplasty
   architectural distortion after, 453–456
      mammography, 453f, 455f, 456f
      pearls and pitfalls, 453, 454, 456
   fat necrosis after, 455–456
      mammography, 455f, 456f
      pearls and pitfalls, 456
   postsurgical approach to, 449
Reflection, shadowing and, 24–25
Renal paraneoplastic syndromes, 495
Residual disease, on MRI, 31
Resolution, contrast, 15–16, 17f
Rim calcification, 207–210
   mammography, 207, 207f, 209, 209f
   pearls and pitfalls, 208, 210
Rim enhancement, 28
Round lucent center calcification, 203–206
   mammography, 203, 203f, 205, 205f
   pearls and pitfalls, 204, 206
   ultrasound, 204, 204f

Index

S

Scar
- architectural distortion and, 9
- malignancy vs., 6
- mammography, 151, 151f
- in neoplasm procedure patients, 458–466
  - mammography, 458, 458f, 462f, 464, 464f
  - pearls and pitfalls, 461, 463, 466
  - ultrasound, 462, 462f, 463f, 465f
- radial
  - as architectural distortion cause, 9
  - as benign entity producing irregular mass, 6
  - as central architectural distortion, 351–352
    - mammography, 351f
    - pearls and pitfalls, 352
    - ultrasound, 352, 352f
  - as irregular mass, 148–150
    - mammography, 148, 148f
    - MRI, 149f
    - pearls and pitfalls, 150
    - ultrasound, 149, 149f
  - as peripheral architectural distortion, 336–337
    - pearls and pitfalls, 337
    - ultrasound, 337, 337f
- ultrasound, 152, 152f

Scattered heterogenous mammogram, 504–515

Sclerosing adenosis, 6, 9, 348–350
- mammography, 348f
- pearls and pitfalls, 350
- ultrasound, 349, 349f, 350, 350f

Screening, MRI for, 31

Sebaceous cyst, 84–85
- in male breast, 390–391
  - mammography, 390, 390f
  - pearls and pitfalls, 391
  - ultrasound, 391, 391f
- mammography, 84, 84f
- pearls and pitfalls, 85, 85f
- ultrasound, 85, 85f

Seborrheic keratosis, 86–87
- mammography, 86, 86f
- pearls and pitfalls, 87

"Second look" sonography, 29–31

Secretory calcification, 195–198
- mammography, 195, 195f, 197, 197f
- pearls and pitfalls, 196, 198

Shadowing, in sonography, 24–26

Silicone injections, 408–409
- mammography, 408f
- pearls and pitfalls, 409

Single focus, 28

Skin
- in breast anatomy, 20, 21f
- as small round calcification, 224–225
  - mammography, 224, 224f

Skin lesions, 86–87, 88–89
- mammography, 86, 86f, 88, 88f
- pearls and pitfalls, 87, 89

Skin powder
- as amorphous calcification, 244–247
  - mammography, 244, 244f
  - pearls and pitfalls, 245
- as heterogenous calcification
  - mammography, 260, 260f, 261f
  - pearls and pitfalls, 261

Smooth muscle hamartoma, 527–528
- pearls and pitfalls, 528
- ultrasound, 527, 527f

Sonography
- approach to palpable mass in, 18–19
- architectural distortion and, 14
- color, 16–18, 18f
- contrast resolution in, 15–16, 17f
- cross-correlation with mammography, 19–23, 24f
- 3D, 18
- dynamic clips in, 18
- echoes on, in benign cysts, 62
- equipment, 15
- fat on, vs. mammography, 20, 22f
- frequencies in, 15
- high-frequency, 15, 16f
- mammography vs., masses on, 21
- scar vs. mass in, 6
- "second look," 29–31
- shadowing in, 24–26
- special problems in, 24–26, 27f
- techniques, 15–18

Staging
- advanced disease, 574–591
- with PET, 35, 36f, 571–591

Standardized uptake value (SUV), 34–35
- low, 615–618

Sternalis muscle, 90–91
- mammography, 90, 90f
- pearls and pitfalls, 91
- ultrasound, 91, 91f

Subcutaneous fat, in breast anatomy, 20, 21f

Subglandular implants
- infected fluid in, 402–404
  - mammography, 402f
  - pearls and pitfalls, 404
  - ultrasound, 403, 403f

Subpectoral implants, 405–407
- advantages of, 406
- mammography, 405f
- MRI, 406f, 407f
- pearls and pitfalls, 410, 411

Superficial fascia, in breast anatomy, 20, 21f

SUV. See Standardized uptake value (SUV)

T

Tattoos, 244–245
- mammography, 244, 244f
- pearls and pitfalls, 245

Team, composition of, 1

"Teardrop" sign, 430

"Tent sign," 9, 13f

Therapeutic response assessment
- mammography, 592, 592f, 597f
- MRI, 31, 593f, 599f
- pearls and pitfalls, 595, 601
- PET, 37, 594f, 600f
- PET-CT, 594f
- ultrasound, 593f, 598f, 599f

3D sonography, 18

TMC. See Typical medullary carcinoma (TMC)

Transducer position, 19

Tubular carcinoma
- as central architectural distortion, 365–367
  - mammography, 365, 365f, 366f
  - pearls and pitfalls, 367
  - ultrasound, 367, 367f
- as irregular mass, 181–185
  - mammography, 181, 181f, 183, 183f
  - microscopy, 185f
  - pearls and pitfalls, 182, 185f
  - ultrasound, 182, 182f, 184, 184f
- as peripheral architectural distortion, 346–347
  - mammography, 346, 346f
  - pearls and pitfalls, 347
  - ultrasound, 347, 347f

Typical medullary carcinoma (TMC), 118

U

Ultrasound. See Sonography

Underestimation of tumor size, on mammography, 519–526

Unknown primary
- mammography, 610f
- MRI, 31–32, 610f
- pearls and pitfalls, 614
- PET-CT, 611f
- ultrasound, 611f, 612f

V

Vascular calcification, 190–192
- mammography, 190, 191f
- pearls and pitfalls, 192

Vascularity, color Doppler and, 16

Vascular lesions, benign, 92–93, 94–95
- mammography, 92, 92f, 94, 94f
- pearls and pitfalls, 93, 95

Vascular lesions (*continued*)
　ultrasound, 93, 93f, 95, 95f
Venous hemangioma, 92–93
　mammography, 92, 92f
　pearls and pitfalls, 93
　ultrasound, 93, 93f

W
Warts, 86–87
　mammography, 86, 86f
　pearls and pitfalls, 87
Well-defined margins, 2–3, 4f